COUNSELING THE NURSING MOTHER

THE LACTATION CONSULTANT'S REFERENCE

COUNSELING THE NURSING MOTHER

THE LACTATION CONSULTANT'S REFERENCE

THIRD EDITION

Judith Lauwers
Executive Director
Breastfeeding Support Consultants

Debbie Shinskie
Project Director
Breastfeeding Support Consultants

with the assistance of

Sandra Breck
Research Consultant
Breastfeeding Support Consultants

JONES AND BARTLETT PUBLISHERS
Sudbury, Massachusetts
BOSTON   TORONTO   LONDON   SINGAPORE

World Headquarters
Jones and Bartlett Publishers
40 Tall Pine Drive
Sudbury, MA 01776
978-443-5000
info@jbpub.com
www.jbpub.com

Jones and Bartlett Publishers Canada
2100 Bloor Street West
Suite 6-272
Toronto, ON M6S 5A5
CANADA

Jones and Bartlett Publishers International
Barb House, Barb Mews
London W6 7PA
UK

PRODUCTION CREDITS
SENIOR ACQUISITIONS EDITOR   Greg Vis
PRODUCTION EDITOR   Linda S. DeBruyn
MANUFACTURING DIRECTOR   Therese Bräuer
DESIGN   UG / GGS Information Services, Inc.
EDITORIAL PRODUCTION SERVICE   UG / GGS Information Services, Inc.
TYPESETTING   UG / GGS Information Services, Inc.
COVER DESIGN   Stephanie Torta
TEXT PRINTING AND BINDING   Courier Westford
COVER PRINTING   John Pow Company

Cover illustration by Marcia Smith

The Library of Congress has catalogued this edition as follows:
Lauwers, Judith, 1949–
    Counseling the nursing mother : a lactation consultant's guide /
Judith Lauwers, Debbie Shinskie, with the assistance of Sandra
Breck. — 3rd ed.
      p.   cm.
    Includes bibliographical references and index.
    ISBN 0-7637-0975-1 (hc)
    1. Breast feeding.   2. Lactation.   I. Shinskie, Debbie.
II. Breck, Sandra.   III. Title.
RJ216.L354   1999
649'.33—dc21   99-29436
                                      CIP

Printed in the United States of America
03 02 01 00   10 9 8 7 6 5 4 3 2 1

The selection and dosage of drugs presented in this book are in accord with standards accepted at the time of publication. The authors, editor, and publisher have made every effort to provide accurate information. However, research, clinical practice, and government regulations often change the accepted standard in this field. Before administering any drug, the reader is advised to check the manufacturer's product information sheet for the most up-to-date recommendations on dosage, precautions, and contraindications. This is especially important in the case of drugs that are new or seldom used.

CONTENTS

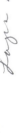

C H A P T E R

5

C H A P T E R

6

C H A P T E R

7

C H A P T E R

8

C H A P T E R

9

PRENATAL CONSIDERATIONS   **161**

C H A P T E R

10

**HOSPITAL PRACTICES THAT SUPPORT
BREASTFEEDING**   **175**

C H A P T E R

11

INFANT ASSESSMENT AND BEHAVIOR   **193**

CHAPTER
12

GETTING BREASTFEEDING STARTED   221

CHAPTER
13

INFANT ATTACHMENT AND SUCKING   233

CHAPTER
14

BREASTFEEDING ISSUES IN THE EARLY WEEKS   247

CHAPTER

15

BREASTFEEDING BEYOND THE FIRST MONTH 273

CHAPTER

16

PROBLEMS WITH MILK PRODUCTION AND TRANSFER 295

CHAPTER

17

CHANGES IN THE FAMILY 307

CHAPTER

18

SPECIAL COUNSELING CIRCUMSTANCES 323

CHAPTER 19

BREASTFEEDING TECHNIQUES AND DEVICES   339

CHAPTER 20

TEMPORARY BREASTFEEDING SITUATIONS   363

CHAPTER 21

HIGH-RISK INFANTS   379

CHAPTER 22

WHEN BREASTFEEDING IS INTERRUPTED   395

CHAPTER 23

MOTHERS AND BABIES WITH LONG-TERM SPECIAL NEEDS   407

CHAPTER 24

PROFESSIONAL CONSIDERATIONS   429

PREFACE

Breastfeeding mothers are helped most effectively by those who demonstrate a belief in breastfeeding as the natural way to nourish an infant. It is not enough to believe in theory that breastfeeding is best. Caregivers must put that theory in practice. Some health workers are reluctant to promote breastfeeding for fear that they will create guilt in mothers who choose not to breastfeed. A caregiver who appears to be ambivalent about breastfeeding sends mixed messages and creates personal doubts for mothers. Those who enthusiastically promote and support breastfeeding serve as a powerful motivator for mothers and staff alike.

The caregiver's approach with breastfeeding women greatly determines the effectiveness of the support and advice they offer. Establishing a partnership with mothers builds confidence and self-esteem—these in turn foster parental independence and growth. Providing an effective learning climate will help you to achieve the goal of actively involving mothers in problem-solving and decision-making. Using humor in your interactions with mothers will help them gain perspective during challenging times and will increase your teaching effectiveness. Finally, understanding the components of communication that affect the messages you send to mothers will help them gain perspective during challenging times and will increase your teaching effectiveness.

Women reach their breastfeeding goals more effectively when they receive consistent encouragement, help and guidance at appropriate times. When a preventive approach is used in the management of breastfeeding, parents have more positive experiences. Caregivers will also find this a time-saving approach that is far more effective than crisis management. Some situations can be handled through telephone contact whereas others require personal visitation. There may be times when a problem is quite advanced by the time contact occurs, which will require more intense problem solving. By entering into problem solving with mothers you will help them recognize problems, their possible causes, and practical actions that can be taken. Using appropriate counseling skills will help you to determine the problem, gain insights into what caused the situation and work toward a solution with the mother.

Lactation consulting is an immensely rewarding arm of the medical profession in which to practice. Being instrumental in promoting a supportive climate for mothers and babies and empowering breastfeeding families reaps benefits for the whole of society. It is our hope that the advice and information in this third edition of *Counseling the Nursing Mother* will guide you in your care of breastfeeding mothers and their children and in your participation in their health care team.

Judith Lauwers
Debbie Shinskie

ACKNOWLEDGMENTS

This third edition of *Counseling the Nursing Mother* would not have been possible without the guidance, support and involvement of scores of people. The entire staff of Breastfeeding Support Consultants' Center for Lactation Education participated in the completion of this edition, whether directly or indirectly. Sandra Breck devoted hundreds of hours to researching journals and other literature so that the clinical information would be current, correct and useful to the reader. In many cases, she helped to write and edit much of this information. Jan Barger, Linda Kutner, and Carole Peterson shared material from their teaching in several topic areas. Entire chapters would not have been possible without their generosity and sincere dedication to sharing their expertise and insights with the entire lactation profession. Other faculty, Michelle Angelini, Sonya Barnett, Genevieve Becker, Karen Krezinski-Bergwall, Cathy Clark, and Mary Alice Tinari have all been instrumental in helping to refine BSC's teaching curriculum over the years. Those refinements are reflected in much of the clinical material throughout the text. The BSC office continued to run smoothly despite weeks of concentrated writing, due to the unflagging professionalism and dedication of Bernadette Zotter, Susan Eggleston and Alexa Jauss. Thank you to all of our staff for each of your individual contributions.

We owe a special heartfelt thanks to Candace Woessner, who was a coauthor on the first two editions of this text. Candace's natural warmth and wisdom continue to weave their magic throughout the text to maintain its original flavor. As one of the "old guard" in the lactation profession, her presence will always be felt in the essence of *Counseling the Nursing Mother*. Candace was instrumental in the growth of the profession in its early years, and we appreciate having this opportunity to thank her for her twenty years of dedication and guidance.

We are appreciative of the tireless reviewing efforts of Marsha Walker and Jan Barger and the insights and improvements their editing provided. Many other colleagues provided artwork, guidance, and review of material throughout the text. We gratefully acknowledge the assistance of:

Kelly, Brian and Brianna Adkins	Miriam Labbok
James Akré	Mary Grace Lanese
Tammy Arbeter	Chele Marmet
Lois Arnold	Debbie Matisse
Helen Armstrong	Carol Mavity
Genevieve Becker	James McKenna
Cheston Berlin	Maureen Minchin
Debi Bocar	Chris Mulford
Pris Bornmann	Jack Newman
Sarah Coulter Danner	Molly Pessl
Deanna Diodato	Ellen Petok
Dianne Flury	Kathy Romberger
Karen Foard	JoAnne Scott
Linda Gort-Walton	Barb Shocker
Thomas Hale	Ruth Solomon
Kay Hoover	Carol and Niki Silcox
Pat Houck	Amy Spangler
Kathleen Huggins	Evalin Trice
Sharon Kelly	Mary Rose Tully
Connie Kishbaugh	Marsha Walker
Kyle Knisely	Barbara Wilson-Clay
La Leche League	Michael Woolridge
of Blacksburg, VA	

We offer a special thanks to Marcia Smith, our superb artist, who captures so exquisitely on canvas the love between a breastfeeding mother and child. She was able to put the essence of our words to form and enhance the learning experience within the text.

We also acknowledge the contributions of numerous volunteers and personnel of the Childbirth Education Association of Greater Philadelphia for their combined efforts in developing the training materials which evolved into the first edition of *Counseling the Nursing Mother* in 1983. Individuals who merit special acknowledgment include Barbara Bernard, Ditta and Frank Hoeber, Louise Stevens, Joanne Hill, M. Elaine Adams, Celeste Marx, Gerry Mckeegan, and Mary Jo Stine.

Our thanks also to Linda DeBruyn, Greg Vis, and John Danielowich of Jones and Bartlett, and Sandra Gormley of UG/GGS Information Services, Inc. for their expert and patient guidance throughout the production process. We are especially indebted to the Internet technology that made it possible to entertain spirited debates, receive input quickly from reviewers, and meet publishing deadlines!

Finally, we express our gratitude and appreciation to our families, David, Michael, Christopher, Don, Christianne, Katelyn, Jon, and Andy, for their patience and understanding throughout the long process of researching, writing, editing such a major production. We thank you for supporting and nurturing us both personally and professionally.

Judith Lauwers
Debbie Shinskie

FOREWORD

The publishing of the third edition of *Counseling the Nursing Mother* by Judith Lauwers and Debbie Shinskie coincides with major changes in the management of breastfeeding mothers and their babies. As we move to close normal newborn nurseries and permit newborns to decide when to take their first feed, allowing them to crawl on their own to the breast, our colleagues in the hospital will look to the lactation consultant for expertise and advice.

A renewed interest in the first minutes, hours, and days of life has been stimulated by several recent provocative behavioral and physiologic observations in both mothers and infants. These assessments and measurements have been made during labor, birth, the immediate postnatal period, and the beginning breastfeedings. They provide a compelling rationale for major changes in care in the perinatal period for both mother and infant. Surprisingly, these findings fit together to form an exciting and novel way to view the mother-infant dyad. This new third edition describes in a lucid fashion the changes in care that are required to make use of this new knowledge.

It is necessary to appreciate that the time period of labor, birth, and for the next several days can probably best be identified in biology as a "sensitive period." During this time, the mother, and possibly the father, are especially open to significantly changing their behavior with their infant dependent on the quality of their care during this sensitive period.

Winnicott also reported a special mental state of the mother in the perinatal period that involves a greatly increased sensitivity to the needs of her baby. He noted this state of "primary maternal preoccupation" starts near the end of pregnancy and continues for a few weeks after the birth. A mother needs nurturing support and a protected environment to develop and maintain this state. Winnicott wrote that "Only if a mother is sensitized in the way I am describing, can she feel herself into her infant's place, and so meet the infant's needs." In the state of "primary maternal preoccupation," the mother is better able to sense and provide what her new infant has signaled. If she senses the needs and responds to them in a sensitive and timely manner, mother and infant will establish a pattern of synchronized and mutually rewarding interactions.

As we make the many changes in care described in *Counseling the Nursing Mother*, it will be especially important to reconstruct the entire environment of the maternity floor, including the attitudes of personnel. They must try to always be thoughtful, warm, caring and able to listen—never judgmental or critical. Since we are all working in a "sensitive period" of the mother when she is open to change in either a positive or negative direction, in part dependent on the approach of the caregiver. In this era of change this new third edition is an especially valuable guide for us all.

Dr. Marshall Klaus
Adjunct Professor of Pediatrics
University of California,
San Francisco

COUNSELING THE NURSING MOTHER

THE LACTATION CONSULTANT'S REFERENCE

BREASTFEEDING PROMOTION IN THE MODERN WORLD

The issue of breastfeeding and its promotion among caregivers and parents is much more complex than it may seem on the surface. The superiority of **human milk** over substitutes is well documented and accepted by the scientific and medical communities and the general population. The fact that many parents still choose artificial milk in spite of that knowledge is not easily explained. Likewise, the fact that some caregivers fail to recommend breastfeeding to their clients or provide questionable advice when complications arise is also complex. To understand these contradictions requires careful examination of all the issues involved. Infant feeding practices have evolved, and will continue to evolve, along with other changes in society. Understanding the dynamics of this evolution, and the political and sociologic factors involved, is essential to effecting tangible and enduring change that will enhance maternal and infant health.

INFANT FEEDING PRACTICES HISTORICALLY

For millions of years, human infants have been nurtured predominantly by human milk—either by the milk of the baby's mother or by the milk of another woman. Throughout history, some women have made a conscious choice *not* to breastfeed. Women of wealth have chosen to employ **wet nurses** or hand feeding in order to stay beautiful, get pregnant again, or merely for the status of being able to afford to hire someone else to feed their baby. Although human milk substitutes have been available for centuries, it is only in recent history that more infants are fed in this way than are breastfed.

During the 17th and 18th centuries, the advent of modern medicine, science, and technology generated great changes in infant feeding. Feeding bottles and rubber nipples made it easier for infants to be fed human milk substitutes. Cow's milk became available in increasing supply, and scientists turned to this form as an acceptable substitute for human milk. When the increase in artificial feeding caused greater numbers of infant deaths, efforts were poured into improving the artificial baby milk rather than working toward increasing breastfeeding rates. Formula feeding continued to increase, with cow's milk products promoted as the *modern and civilized* way to nourish babies. Breastfeeding conveyed low social status, and women who chose to breastfeed were given little support or encouragement. The prevailing cultural belief evolved to one in which bottle feeding is the *norm* and breastfeeding is the *exception*.

Increased Separation of Mothers and Babies

Bottle feeding provided options to women that they had not had previously. Although they still gave birth to babies, they did not have to invest themselves totally in feeding and raising them throughout their infancy. Women were free to take a job or pursue other activities outside the home. Although their female ancestors had been bound by their biology to nurture their young, modern women had a *choice* and the ability to determine their own future. Feeding practices that liberated mothers from continually being with their babies offered an attractive option to some women.

Dramatic changes took place in birth practices, which also affected infant feeding. By the middle of the 19th century, industrialized medicine had removed much of the danger from the birth experience. Traditionally, women had given birth at home with female family members and a midwife in attendance. Birthing women enjoyed a strong and continuous support system throughout labor and delivery. As medical technology advanced, childbirth was moved from the home to a hospital, compromising both the mother's and baby's personal needs. Women now gave birth primarily in a sterile hospital setting surrounded by technology and without the support of female relatives, as was the practice in the past. Birthing practices separated mothers from their babies, regimented infant care, and interfered with the initiation of breastfeeding.

▼ Breastfeeding Revisited

Early in the 20th century, efforts increased within the medical community to question the wisdom of the prevalence of feeding babies artificial baby milk. In 1921, Julius P. Sedgwick advised that more time be given in medical school to observing and studying breastfeeding, and that less time be spent on the study of artificial feeding and formula making (Sedgwick, 1921). The inclusion of breastfeeding instruction in postgraduate medical education was addressed in 1924 by the Brooklyn Pediatric Society. They concluded that breastfeeding was a matter of medical education and lay instruction (McKay, 1924). The scarcity of lactation education in medical and nursing schools continues to be a problem in the 1990s (Freed, 1995, 1996).

Researchers soon demonstrated a correlation between cognitive development and method of infant feeding. A 1929 report stated that breastfed babies walked more than 2 months earlier than artificially fed babies. It also noted that all of the babies studied with IQs over 130 were breastfed (Hoefer, 1929). Recognition of the importance of breastfeeding in the health of infants, books for parents, and professional articles on breastfeeding and infant feeding began to appear in the early 1950s (Fig. 1.1). Mother-to-mother breastfeeding support groups emerged at around the same time. In the mid-1950s, grassroots efforts by La Leche League and other breastfeeding support groups began to promote breastfeeding actively as the preferred method of infant feeding. By the 1960s, a movement had begun among women whose lifestyles advocated healthful living. Breastfeeding was regarded as the natural and culturally appropriate method of infant feeding for these women.

▼ Breastfeeding Rates

Despite a renewed interest in breastfeeding, there was still a general lack of encouragement and advice from the medical community. By the early 1980s, breastfeeding rates reached a peak and then began to decline. In 1984, the U.S. Surgeon General convened a work group to study breastfeeding and human lactation. Yet breastfeeding rates continued to decline. Regrettably, the greatest decline occurred among the most vulnerable high-risk mothers, whose infants would gain the most from being breastfed (American Academy of Pediatrics [AAP], 1991).

Because definitions of **exclusive breastfeeding** vary from one country to another, compiling meaningful statistics presents a challenge. Exclusive breastfeeding means that breastfeeding babies receive no drinks or foods other than their mother's milk. The **World Health Organization** (WHO) established a Global Data Bank on Breastfeeding in 1982. Figures released in 1996, representing 58 percent of the world's total infant population, estimated that 35 percent of the world's infants younger than 4 months of age were exclusively breastfed (Fig. 1.2). Globally, the median length of time infants were breastfed was 18 months (WHO, 1996). One of the goals of WHO is to disseminate identical indicators and definitions worldwide to ensure consistent and comparable results in breastfeeding studies.

Breastfeeding rates vary significantly from one part of the world to another part. In the African region, the median duration of breastfeeding in 1996 was 21 months. However, only 19 percent of infants younger than 4 months were being breastfed exclusively. Nearly half of infants younger than 4 months of age in Southeast Asia

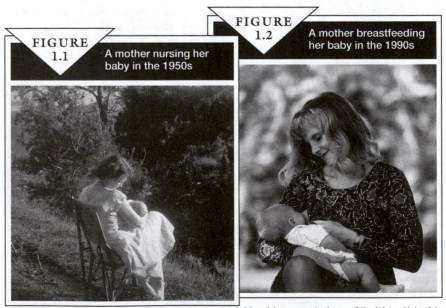

FIGURE 1.1 A mother nursing her baby in the 1950s

FIGURE 1.2 A mother breastfeeding her baby in the 1990s

Used by permission of Debbie Shinskie.

Used by permission of Debbie Shinskie.

were exclusively breastfed in 1996. The median duration of breastfeeding was 25 months. Australia has one of the highest breastfeeding rates in the developed world. In 1996, rates were as high as 90 to 95 percent in many parts of Europe, as low as 35 percent in other parts, and as low as 20 percent in some parts of Central America.

BREASTFEEDING AS AN INFANT HEALTH ISSUE

Studies such as those discussed earlier are conducted because the medical community recognizes the impact breastfeeding has on infant **morbidity** (disease) and **mortality** (death). The medical community acknowledges that breastfeeding is healthiest for infants. Human milk is, in fact, a baby's first immunization. It is uniquely constituted to foster the infant's health and growth, and is easily digested and efficiently used by the body. Human milk can help protect the baby from infectious diseases and reduce the chance of respiratory and digestive infections. Exclusive breastfeeding in the first month delays the onset of wheezing and reduces the severity (Porro, 1993). The multitude of health benefits for the baby, as discussed in Chapter 8, is a clear testimony to the importance of human milk.

Breastfeeding is a physical embodiment of the mother-baby relationship that continues long after birth. The **bonding** that accompanies breastfeeding fosters a special closeness that develops into a deep and lasting attachment between mother and child. In addition to bonding, breastfeeding promotes good oral development in the baby and satisfies his sucking needs. It has also been associated with higher intelligence (Lucas, 1992). Some experts debate whether the correlation between breastfeeding and intelligence results from human milk or from the inclination of breastfeeding mothers to be more nurturing toward their infants. Results of a 1994 British study suggest that "some aspects of intellectual attainment can be demonstrated to be superior among children who were exclusively breastfed for at least three months, compared with their bottle-fed counterparts" (Pollock, 1994). It may be that breastfed children have different early relationships with their mothers.

Immediate gratification of a breastfeeding baby's needs develops in him a sense of security and trust. This may help him accept the demands of socialization later in life. A breastfeeding mother is able to respond quickly to her baby's hunger cries without the delay of preparing and heating a bottle. The early sensory stimulation from skin-to-skin contact that takes place during breastfeeding helps develop the baby's perceptual and response mechanism. It also aids respiration by stimulating blood flow. This may be one reason for the reduced incidence of respiratory ailments in breastfed babies (Ludington-Hoe, 1993).

BREASTFEEDING AS A WOMEN'S HEALTH ISSUE

In many ways, breastfeeding is as much a women's health issue as an infant feeding issue. Traditionally, women's health has received little attention in the U.S. health care agenda. Part of the challenge in promoting breastfeeding in today's climate stems from this failure in the health care system. Breastfeeding needs to be viewed as part of women's health and treated as such in the health care arena. Whatever health care providers can do to help empower the women in their care will benefit women and their families for years to come.

Birth and breastfeeding are empowerment issues for women (VanEsterik, 1994a). The more control women have over their birth and breastfeeding experiences, the greater will be their sense of power, self esteem, and ego (Locklin, 1993). Medical technology often strips a woman of this power by placing external controls on pregnancy, birth, and breastfeeding—three life functions that belong solely to women. Breastfeeding is a part of the entire childbearing cycle. The female body is designed to progress from pregnancy to birth and then on to breastfeeding. Interrupting this cycle by *not* breastfeeding interrupts the normal continuum. Anthropologist Ashley Montagu, author of *Touching: The Human Significance of the Skin*, perceived an 18-month **gestation**, with a baby spending 9 months in utero and 9 months being nurtured at the breast. Breastfeeding, then, is the normal transition from **intrauterine** maternal-based nutrition to **extrauterine** maternal-based nutrition.

In order for breastfeeding to be a real choice for all women, society needs to become more woman-friendly. Breastfeeding and mothering are only two strands in the weaving of women's lives. To ignore the rest of the fabric is to fail to see how connected are all the strands. Lactation consultants and other caregivers who help breastfeeding women need to take care not to ignore the rest of the fabric. Van Esterik states that " . . . breastfeeding is a holistic act and is intimately connected to all domains of life: sexuality, eating, emotion, appearance, sleeping, and parental relationships" (Van Esterik, 1994b). As you study this text and in your daily interactions with women, consider breastfeeding as part of the whole fabric of women, and strive to meet each of their needs on an individual basis.

Physical and Emotional Effects of Breastfeeding on Women

Breastfeeding has a significant impact on women's health. **Oxytocin** that is released while breastfeeding contracts the uterus and helps stop bleeding after delivery. This factor makes it important that breastfeeding begin immediately after birth and that it continues frequently. **Prolactin** and oxytocin both play a role in maternal feelings of well-being, relaxation, and mothering. Oxytocin is known as the "cuddle" hormone, and may be transmitted to the infant (Lawrence, 1999). A positive breastfeeding experience can contribute to a woman feeling good about herself. This can raise her self-esteem and empower her as a woman. She will feel fulfilled in knowing that she is doing something no one else can do for her baby.

Breastfeeding women are energy efficient (Illingworth, 1986). They can produce milk, even with limited caloric intake. The increased caloric demand that accompanies breastfeeding allows the mother to supplement her usual eating pattern—provided that it is nutritionally sound—and still control her weight and return to her prepregnancy size more quickly. As discussed in Chapter 17, exclusive breastfeeding is 98 percent effective in delaying pregnancy naturally without the use of artificial contraceptives.

In a retrospective case-control study, Newcomb found that lactation was associated with a slight reduction in the risk of breast cancer among premenopausal women. With an increasing cumulative duration of lactation, there was a decreasing risk of cancer in that group (Newcomb, 1994). The risk of premenopausal breast cancer is reduced, and the longer a woman breastfeeds, the greater the protection (McTiernan, 1986). The risk of ovarian cancer is also decreased (Schneider, 1987).

Cummings suggests that breastfeeding increases bone density, which decreases the risk of **osteoporosis** (Cummings, 1985). In 1992 and 1993, several researchers studied the effect of breastfeeding on bone mineral density and the occurrence of osteoporosis. Commenting on the previous study that suggested an association between breastfeeding and loss of bone density, Naylor (1993) suggests that research needs to separate women who are still breastfeeding at a particular time from those who are not. Another researcher, Kritz-Silverstein (1992), found no association between history of breastfeeding and lesser bone density.

CULTURAL INFLUENCES ON INFANT FEEDING

Most people will acknowledge that breastfeeding is best for babies. Even the infant formula companies make that declaration in their advertising. However, the messages that permeate the media in the United States do little to support breastfeeding. Despite a renewed interest in breastfeeding, bottle feeding is still recognized as the cultural norm. Adolescent girls and boys are generally uncomfortable at the prospect of observing or even discussing breastfeeding. Young girls, unless they are raised

in a home where the mother breastfeeds, usually "feed" their dolls with a bottle. Infants and toddlers of all ages are seen in public with feeding bottles or pacifiers. Shelves in grocery stores, toy stores, and discount stores abound with bottle feeding devices and infant formula. News media, children's books, parenting magazines, and medical journals carry scores of bottle feeding messages. Several states even have found it necessary to pass legislation safeguarding a woman's right to breastfeed in public or making it illegal to interfere with breastfeeding in public. A large segment of the U.S. population finds the topic of breastfeeding to be uncomfortable to discuss or to view.

In order for breastfeeding promotion to be effective, it must be accompanied by a **paradigm shift**, that is, a change in the way in which society views infant feeding. Promotion efforts for the past several decades have reflected a defensive posture of stating the benefits of breastfeeding and counting off all the reasons why mothers should breastfeed their babies. To promote healthful practices such as breastfeeding more effectively, public awareness needs to shift to the hazards of not breastfeeding and why mothers should not feed their babies artificial baby milk.

Results of a study by Alan Lucas referred to earlier can illustrate this shift in approach. Lucas (1992) found that preterm infants receiving human milk have higher IQ levels than those receiving infant formula. The biologic norm is for infants to be fed human milk. Therefore, it is not that breastfed infants have higher IQs. They have normal IQs! Artificially fed infants have IQs lower than normal because they have been deprived of human milk. Likewise, it is not that breastfed infants have lower rates of otitis media. Rather, formula-fed infants have higher rates. When the general public becomes aware of this subtle shift in attitude, parents will make more informed and healthy choices.

CURRENT BREASTFEEDING RECOMMENDATIONS

WHO recommends that all babies around the world be breastfed with appropriate complementary food for up to 2 years and beyond (WHO/UNICEF, 1990). Their recommendations are based on optimal health of both the baby and the mother, as well as minimal cost to the family, community, and environment. The AAP (1997) recommends that mothers breastfeed exclusively for 6 months and continue breastfeeding with appropriate complementary food through 12 months and beyond. In an effort to improve breastfeeding rates throughout the world, **UNICEF** and WHO have carried out major initiatives to promote good breastfeeding practices and policies worldwide and to remove barriers. Their 1989 joint statement entitled *Protecting, Promoting and Supporting Breastfeeding* established guidelines that breastfeeding proponents know as the *Ten Steps to Successful Breastfeeding* (WHO, 1989). These guidelines form the basis for transformations in maternity practices worldwide in support of breastfeeding. This effort is known as the *Baby Friendly Hospital Initiative*, as described in Chapter 26. UNICEF's late Executive Director, James P. Grant, referred to the *Ten Steps to Successful Breastfeeding* as a road map to get us back on course after a brief detour in infant feeding practices.

The ultimate goal of the global promotion, protection and support of breastfeeding is to empower and enable women to breastfeed exclusively for about the first 4 to 6 months, and to create circumstances that enable mothers to continue to breastfeed for 2 years or longer with complementary foods. Exclusive breastfeeding means that breastfeeding babies receive no drinks or foods other than their mothers' milk, although they may receive vitamin and mineral drops or medicines. For exclusive breastfeeding to go easily, infants should be given no pacifiers or artificial teats (nipples). The mother (or caregiver providing expressed milk) feeds the baby in response to feeding cues, and no limits are placed on frequency or length of breastfeeds. When they are exclusively breastfed, most infants receive at least 8 to 12 breastfeeds in 24 hours, including night feeds.

The Ten Steps to Successful Breastfeeding

A hospital that wishes to achieve the international Baby Friendly Hospital designation must fulfill the following ten steps. They also eliminate free and low-cost supplies of all artificial baby milks, feeding bottles and teats. Artificial feeding supplies needed by any part of a Baby-Friendly Hospital are purchased through the ordinary procurement channels, and are not obtained as free or low-cost supplies. The *Ten Steps to Successful Breastfeeding* state that every facility providing maternity services and care for newborn infants should

1. Have a written breastfeeding policy that is routinely communicated to all health care staff.
2. Train all health care staff in skills necessary to implement this policy.
3. Inform all pregnant women about the benefits and management of breastfeeding.
4. Help mothers initiate breastfeeding within a half hour of birth.
5. Show mothers how to breastfeed and how to maintain lactation even if they should be separated from their infants.
6. Give newborn infants no food or drink other than breastmilk unless *medically* indicated.
7. Practice **rooming in**—allow mothers and infants to remain together—24 hours a day.
8. Encourage breastfeeding in response to feeding cues.
9. Give no artificial teats or pacifiers (also called dummies or soothers) to breastfeeding infants.
10. Foster the establishment of breastfeeding support groups and refer mothers to them on discharge from the hospital or clinic.

SUMMARY

The infant feeding climate today is one in which many parents embrace the idea of breastfeeding. For the most part, health care providers share a conviction that breastfeeding is the optimal method for infant nutrition. Despite this conviction, breastfeeding women need support and advice in a society that is still dominated by bottle feeding messages and attitudes. Caregivers, agencies, and volunteer counselors can provide this support, can educate parents about breastfeeding management, and can empower parents to reach their breastfeeding goals. Breastfeeding is a woman's right, and being breastfed is an infant's choice. The *Baby Friendly Hospital Initiative* and the *Ten Steps to Successful Breastfeeding* will help ensure these rights. They provide a framework within which real progress can be made in breastfeeding promotion.

REFERENCES

American Academy of Pediatrics. Breastfeeding and the use of human milk. *Pediatrics* 100:1035–1039; 1997.

American Academy of Pediatrics Commentary. Breast-feeding trends: A cause for action. *Pediatrics* 88:4; 1991.

Cummings and Nevitt. Epidemiology of osteoporosis and osteoporotic fractures, *Epidemiol Rev* 7:178–208; 1985.

Freed G et al. National assessment of physicians' breast-feeding knowledge, attitudes, training, and experience. *JAMA* 273:472–476; 1995.

Freed G et al. Methods and outcomes of breastfeeding instruction for nursing students. *J Hum Lact* 12:105–110; 1996.

Hoefer C and Hardy MC. Later development of breastfed and artificially fed infants. *JAMA* 92:615; 1929.

Illingworth PJ et al: Diminution in energy expenditure during lactation. *Br Med J* 292:437; 1986.

Kritz-Silverstein D et al. Pregnancy and lactation as determinants of bone mineral density in postmenopausal women. *Am J Epidemiol* 136:1052–1059; 1992.

Lawrence R. Breast-feeding trends: A cause for action. *Pediatrics* 88:(4)867–868; 1991.

Lawrence R. *Breastfeeding: A Guide for the Medical Profession.* St. Louis, MO: Mosby; 1999.

Locklin M and Naber S. Does breastfeeding empower women? Insights from a select group of educated, low-income minority women. *Birth* 20:30–35; 1993.

Lucas A et al. Breast milk and subsequent intelligence quotient in children born preterm. *Lancet* 339:261–264; 1992.

Ludington-Hoe S et al. Skin-to-skin contact beginning in the delivery room for Colombian mothers and their preterm infants. *J Hum Lact* 9:241–242; 1993.

McKay F. Infant mortality in relation to breastfeeding. *New York State Journal of Medicine* 24:433–438; 1924.

McTiernan A and Thomas D. Evidence for a protective effect of lactation on risk of breast cancer in young women: Results from a case-control study. *Am J Epidemiol* 124:353–358; 1986.

Montagu A. *Touching: The Human Significance of the Skin.* Harper & Row, New York; 1972.

Naylor A. Letter. *JAMA* 270:2300; 1993.

Newcomb P et al. Lactation and a reduced risk of pre-menopausal breast cancer. *N Engl J Med* 330:81–87; 1994.

Pollock JI. Long term associations with infant feeding in a clinically advantaged population of babies. *Dev Med Child Neurol* 36:429–440; 1994.

Porro E et al. Early wheezing and breast feeding. *J Asthma* 30:23–28; 1993.

Van Esterik P. Breastfeeding and feminism. *Int J of Gynaecol Obstet* 47:S41–S54; 1994a.

Van Esterik P. Guest editorial. *J Hum Lact* 10(2):71; 1994b.

World Health Organization. *WHO Global Data Bank on Breast-feeding.* Geneva, Switzerland: Nutrition Unit, WHO; 1996.

World Health Organization. *Protecting, promoting, and supporting breastfeeding: A joint WHO/UNICEF statement.* WHO: Geneva, Switzerland; 1989.

▼

BIBLIOGRAPHY

Apple R. The medicalization of infant feeding in the United States and New Zealand: Two countries, one experience. *J Hum Lact* 10:31–37; 1994.

Carter CI and Altemus, M. Integrative functions of lactational hormones in social behavior and stress management. *Ann NY Acad Sci* 807:164–174; 1997.

Cunningham A et al. Breastfeeding and health in the 1980s: A global epidemiologic review. *J Pediatr* 118(5):659–66; 1991.

Cunningham A. *Breastfeeding, Bottlefeeding & Illness: An Annotated Bibliography.* Nursing Mothers Association of Australia and ALMA Publications, Australia: 2 vols.; 1986 and 1990.

Deering C. *A Review of Infant Feeding Related Messages in Lay Parenting Magazines: July 1991–December 1991.* Unpublished research; 1992.

Feldblum P et al. Lactation history and bone mineral density among perimenopausal women. *Epidemiology* 3:527–531; 1992.

Garrett S. *Going It Alone.* Hampshire, England: Gower; 1991.

Hamosh M. *Breastfeeding: Unraveling the Mysteries of Mother's Milk.* Medscape Womens' Health; 1996.

Jackson EB et al. Statistical report on incidence and duration of breast-feeding in relation to personal-social and hospital maternity factors. *Pediatrics* 17:700–715; 1956.

Liebman B. Breast cancer. *Nutrition Action Health Letter* 23:4–7; 1996.

Mepham TB. Science and the politics of breastfeeding: Birthright or birth rite? *Breastfeeding Review* 1(15):5–13; 1989.

Minchin M. *Breastfeeding Matters: What We Need To Know About Infant Feeding.* Victoria, Australia: Alma Publications; 1998.

Newton N. *Maternal Emotions.* New York: Hoeber; 1955.

Rosenblatt K et al. Prolonged lactation and endometrial cancer. *Int J Epidemiol* 24:499–503; 1996.

Schanler R. Pediatricians' practices and attitudes regarding breastfeeding promotion. *Pediatrics* 103(3):E33; 1999.

Schneider AP III. Risk factor for ovarian cancer. *N Engl J Med* 317:508–509; 1987.

Sedgwick JP and Fleischner. Breastfeeding in the reduction of infant mortality. *Am J Public Health* 11:153–157; 1921.

Silva PA and Fergusson DM. Socio-economic status, maternal characteristics, child experience and intelligence in pre-school children. *New Zealand Journal of Educational Studies* 2:180–188; 1976.

Work Group on Cow's Milk Protein and Diabetes Mellitus. *Pediatrics* 94(5):752–754; 1994.

2

THE LACTATION CONSULTING PROFESSION

Contributing Authors: Linda Kutner, Jan Barger, and Carole Peterson

Until breastfeeding becomes the societal norm, with several generations of women comfortable with breastfeeding self-care and management techniques, breastfeeding care will be an integral part of the mother's and infant's health care. The mother and baby form a nursing **dyad**—two individuals who form one unit, each dependent on the other. All members of the health care team must support the nursing dyad in order for mothers to achieve their breastfeeding goals. They can then provide the consistent care that benefits mothers as they are establishing breastfeeding.

Breastfeeding is most enjoyable when the mother and baby function smoothly as a team. Likewise, breastfeeding assistance is most effective when breastfeeding caregivers work collaboratively as a team—both among one another and with parents. The **lactation consultant** emerged in the mid 1980s as the member of the mother's and baby's health care team whose primary focus is breastfeeding. Volunteer **lay counselors** are important members of this team as well. They provide peer support and guidance as a complement to the assistance provided by health professionals.

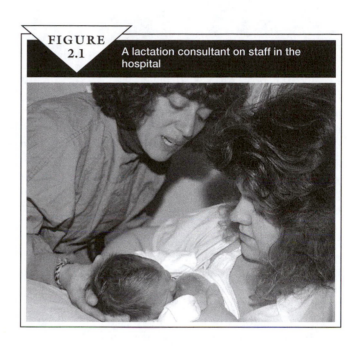

A lactation consultant on staff in the hospital

THE LACTATION CONSULTANT AS PART OF THE HEALTH CARE TEAM

The lactation consultant is the primary member of the mother's health care team who provides support and advice for breastfeeding. During the past two decades, lactation consulting has become a profession in its own right. Many individuals who have been working in maternal/child health are electing to specialize in this new field (Fig. 2.1). Some possess advanced degrees in the medical field and, because of their professional education and experience, are in a unique position to expand their services into lactation consulting. Some lactation consultants began their careers as lay counselors and then acquired the advanced education and skills that enable them to work on a professional level as part of the health care team. Some come into lactation consulting from unrelated fields after having breastfed their own children and wanting to help other mothers do the same.

Professional education for lactation management became available in the early 1980s through various programs. Texts on lactation management were published, some directed to the medical profession and others directed to lay counselors. In 1984, U.S. Surgeon General, C. Everett Koop, convened a "Workshop on Breastfeeding and Human Lactation," identifying professional education as one of six core arenas to be addressed. The **International Board of Lactation Consultant Examiners** (IBLCE) was established in 1985 for the purpose of offering a certification examination to identify the qualified lactation consultant. The **International Lactation Consultant Association** (ILCA) was formed soon after as an association for professional lactation consultants.

As a lactation consultant, you are an advocate first for the nursing dyad and secondly for the infant, with the knowledge, skills, and willingness to work at the baby's pace. As the only member of the health care team whose primary focus is breastfeeding, you may need to suggest alternate plans of care if what is prescribed by other members of the health care team could impact negatively on breastfeeding.

All caregivers—physicians, nurses, midwives, physician assistants, dieticians, physical therapists, occupational therapists, and childbirth educators—need to incorporate breastfeeding teaching and support into their existing practices. Although many mothers benefit from the services of a lactation consultant, in the ideal situation, women would receive appropriate advice about basic breastfeeding management from all their health care providers.

 ## Functioning as a Lactation Consultant

Because the profession is so new, lactation consultants today may find it challenging to establish themselves as integral members of the health care team. Demonstrating the need for a lactation consultant, developing credibility, overcoming medical elitism, and addressing practical employment issues are some of the challenges you may face while trying to establish yourself in the profession. You can keep current by reading relevant research and literature from all disciplines that may impact on lactation and breastfeeding management. Sharing this information as it is appropriate among the different disciplines will help broaden your sphere of influence. Communicating with the nursing dyad's primary care providers will help establish you as part of the health care team.

Your position and function as a lactation consultant may be new to many medical professionals. The services you offer and the manner in which you work with the health care providers will build your reputation and determine the amount of cooperation you will receive from them. It is helpful to realize that those with whom you come in contact—parents, nurses, physicians, educators—all share your goals of ensuring the health of mothers and babies. Exchanging information with medical professionals and working with them to provide parents with the kind of health care they desire can be personally rewarding, as well as a welcome contribution to your community.

Sharing Information with Physicians

Many physicians are in need of, and often will welcome, practical information on the normal management of lactation. When giving any information to patients, a physician must rely on his or her own background and training in a particular field. Unfortunately, little time, if any, is devoted to the practical management of breastfeeding in most medical schools. Emphasis is generally placed on biochemistry or breastfeeding problems of a medical nature. Keeping up with all of the latest information in journal articles can be difficult for busy physicians. Therefore, when it comes to breastfeeding management, many physicians may need to rely on conferences, seminars, breastfeeding experience within their own family, and their patients' experiences. Perhaps their own personal experience with breastfeeding may not have been positive. Patients' breastfeeding experiences may have been unsatisfactory due to lack of information and support. This may bias their opinions either in favor of or against breastfeeding. Many physicians change their practices after they or their spouses have breastfed.

You can inform physicians of your services and help them understand your aims. As a lactation consultant, you will offer an adjunct service that builds on the physician-patient relationship. Provide physicians with evidence-based breastfeeding materials. Much infant feeding literature that physicians receive pertains to the use of artificial formula. Many times, the breastfeeding literature they receive is published by an infant formula company. Physicians have a need for sound breastfeeding information as it relates to infant feeding and growth, received from a non–formula company source.

Encourage mothers to share with their physicians the positive aspects of breastfeeding. Because there is a tendency for mothers to concentrate on problems, physicians often react by prescribing unnecessary practices for what they perceive to be the mother's concern. If a mother mentions that her baby is fussy, her physician may prescribe a formula supplement in an effort to comfort her. The mother may not have considered breastfeeding to be related to the fussiness and may have had general questions about caring for a fussy baby. When mothers also share the positive aspects of their breastfeeding experience, they can help modify or change physician attitudes, opinions, and practices. Remind mothers that physicians are usually very busy and may not readily recall all the details of a situation. A mother needs to be prepared to remind her physician of her desire to breastfeed and of any specific plans that they have previously discussed. She and the physician then can decide how to adapt the plans to her present situation.

Lack of Support From Physicians

If the mother's or infant's physician seems indifferent to breastfeeding or gives questionable advice, the mother will benefit from close contact with you or another breastfeeding support person. Physicians generally are aware of the benefits of human milk as published in current literature. Their practices, however, may not reflect an understanding of the practical aspects of breastfeeding. The best way to change physicians' practices is through the sharing of clinical data and positive comments from mothers. Some physicians are reluctant to advocate breastfeeding too strongly in order to avoid having mothers feel pressured or guilty about their choice to bottle feed. Parents would not expect their infant's physician to be noncommital about the importance of immunizations, dental checkups, or avoidance of cigarette smoking or other **social toxicants**. Adopting a middle-of-the-road stance regarding breastfeeding transmits to parents an attitude that artificial formula is equally healthy for their infant.

You can help physicians recognize that mothers need to be supported and validated in their decisions. They need to be empowered as parents and integrated as an equal member of their baby's and their own health care team. Physicians need to understand the important role they play in protecting the continuation of breastfeeding for mothers and babies in their care. When they encounter a problem that requires specialized care, they can be encouraged to refer mothers to a lactation consultant. They can also facilitate referral to a support group that will provide mother-to-mother support.

THE LACTATION CONSULTANT'S ROLE WITH MOTHERS

It is important that you recognize how your function in the health care system applies to the mothers in your care. Promoting **health consumerism** encourages parents to assume an active role in their family's health care. Parents may need guidance in assuming this new role. You can assist them by providing options and advice, and by suggesting ways in which they can interact with their physicians. Your primary function is to coordinate the mother's breastfeeding care and empower her to breastfeed with minimal intervention or complications. Your role is to serve as a facilitator who educates and gently guides the mother. Acting as a true consultant, you will use your scientific knowledge and practical experience to nurture the relationship between the mother and her infant.

Services to Mothers

Several basic elements are important to developing a comprehensive program of breastfeeding education and support for parents. Ideally, you will provide prenatal and **postpartum** instruction, and be available to advise the mother during her hospital stay. Mothers benefit most from a program that provides the following range of services:

◆ Prenatal and postpartum classes.
◆ Daily rounds to all postpartum breastfeeding mothers.

◆ Assistance with breastfeeding problems before and after discharge.
◆ Routine long-term follow-up.
◆ Telephone **warm line** for counseling new mothers.
◆ Periodic development or review of parent literature.
◆ Referral to a peer support group.

Educating Mothers About Breastfeeding Management

You will share with breastfeeding women practical information on normal breastfeeding management. Pointing out options and offering useful suggestions provides the women in your care with the kind of information they need. Explaining why a certain technique works the way it does and giving the mother the reasons behind your suggestions will help her to understand and relate them to her situation. This will enable her to determine whether or not she can adapt the suggestions for her own use.

In order for you to share information in this manner, you must thoroughly understand the science of lactation regarding **milk production**, typical breastfeeding patterns, and factors that may affect them. If you are incorporating lactation consulting as one aspect of a wider practice—such as a hospital-based nurse—you may focus primarily on basic breastfeeding management. You will then need to be aware of potential complications and unusual circumstances as well as resources for making appropriate referrals. If you are specializing in the lactation field as a board-certified lactation consultant, you will need expertise in the more complicated or unusual breastfeeding circumstances. Whatever your level of involvement, it is important that you keep up to date with new breastfeeding literature and practices. Periodically reviewing the basic information in this text will prepare you for sharing your knowledge with mothers.

Sharing Medical Information

It is especially important that the information and advice you give to mothers is obtained from a reliable source. Anything that is beyond the scope of the lactation consultant must be presented in a manner of educating the mother, not of prescribing treatment. For instance, information on drugs changes based on current research. As a consultant, you must be sure to have the most up-to-date information when you relate it to mothers. Although there may be no studies to show the ill effects of a particular drug, that does not rule out the possibility that such ill effects can exist for either the mother or infant. You can read to her from an authoritative source on medications and lactation (Briggs, 1998; Hale, 1998). When discussing drugs with a mother, always recommend that she consult her baby's physician concerning its advisability. The baby's physician ultimately has the final decision.

Take care to avoid alienating people in your medical community. There have been great strides in family-centered maternity care and breastfeeding in recent years. Unfortunately, breastfeeding advice in some situations may conflict with that of other health care providers. This is not because one side is incorrect but because there are a variety of medical opinions concerning obstetrics and pediatrics. You can present information to the mother and urge her to make her own choices and to work toward suitable solutions with her physicians. Because your advice may contradict that of the physician, it can cause confusion and concern for the mother. Acknowledge this with her and help her to develop a plan.

In essence, you are creating a conflict that the parents must resolve with their other caregivers. In some situations, you may communicate directly with the mother's or baby's physician. In other cases, you may share information with the mother that she will, in turn, discuss with her physician. Demonstrating assertiveness and willingness to work with the physician and the mother to resolve the problem to their mutual satisfaction will strengthen the parents' position. Informing and educating parents places this responsibility on them. At times, however, parents fail to act and do not accept this active role. If this occurs, recognize that you have fulfilled your responsibility of informing parents of their options, whether or not you agree with their decision.

When you share information with mothers, be sure to communicate clearly and simply. Offer the simplest, least complicated explanation in lay terms. Relate the information in a friendly and low-key manner, neither overwhelming a mother nor making her appear uninformed. Relate only information that you are certain is up to date, correct, and evidence-based—not opinion or one person's experience. Whenever your information conflicts with information the mother has obtained from another source, check your sources for accuracy and try to help the mother resolve the conflict. Always check your sources if you are uncertain. If you cannot answer a question, tell the mother you will research it and contact her later.

▼
PRACTICE SETTINGS FOR LACTATION CONSULTANTS

Breastfeeding mothers and babies are cared for by health care professionals in a variety of practice settings. Lactation consultants are employed in hospitals, physician's offices, public health clinics, home health care, and private practice. In some ways, the choice of practice setting will be dictated by other experience you bring to the job. In many cases, hospitals, physician offices, and home health agencies prefer that the lactation consultant possess additional training in health care, such as nursing. Health clinics, especially those in the Special Supplemental Food Program for Women, Infants, and Children (WIC), may employ a lactation consultant who is also a registered dietician. The lactation consultant in private practice should have many years of experience with a great variety of babies and breastfeeding situations. Each of these practice settings are explored in this chapter.

▼
Practicing in a Hospital

One of the most important jobs of a hospital-based lactation consultant is ensuring that every breastfeeding mother in that facility is observed breastfeeding her baby before discharge by someone who is skilled in breastfeeding assessment. That person would preferably be the staff nurse, and the lactation consultant is often responsible for educating staff to provide consistent management guidelines. As the lactation consultant, it is important that you are not the only person who is responsible for helping mothers with breastfeeding problems. Your primary responsibility is to train other maternity staff in basic breastfeeding management and some of the more common challenges encountered in the immediate postpartum period. The lactation consultant is the one contacted for more complex problems.

Making the Decision to Practice in the Hospital

There are a number of factors to consider in choosing to practice in a hospital setting. As a member of the hospital staff, you will be part of a team and will have the support of peer relationships. Being a staff member carries the advantage of a steady income and work, as well as benefits such as vacations, holidays, and sick days. Your work hours will depend on the total number of lactation consultants on staff. Ideally, the hospital should provide 24-hour coverage for breastfeeding mothers and babies. When there are limited lactation consultants on staff, coverage may be provided only during the daily work week. Although you may not be able to see every breastfeeding mother, you will most likely see any who are having problems. Your client base will be steady, and you will not need to seek referrals, as is the case in private practice. Because necessary records and resources will be readily available, you will not need to acquire these on your own. The hospital will process the fees for your services, which frees your time for seeing mothers.

Working as a hospital-based lactation consultant may present some challenges as well. Many lactation consultants work longer hours than other staff positions in an effort to see every breastfeeding mother and baby.

This is especially the case for those who are the sole lactation consultant on staff. When the staff is well trained to help mothers with basic breastfeeding management, you may see only mothers and babies with complicated problems. This can increase the potential for **burnout**. There may be no other lactation consultant with whom to share problems or frustrations. If staff or administrators are unsupportive, this may create obstacles or frustrations for you, especially when there is a conflict in philosophy or priorities. Your role as a breastfeeding advocate may be restricted because of hospital policies and limitations. As a hospital employee, you are accountable to staff and may be expected to see all breastfeeding patients. The work schedule will be less flexible than if you were in private practice. When hospitals experience downsizing, your position may be regarded as less critical than other positions. Consequently, you may be terminated or asked to assume other duties unrelated to breastfeeding.

Despite these potential challenges, most lactation consultants choose to work in a hospital setting. Having a large group of colleagues helps provide a source of reference as well as moral support. You will be viewed as an expert by the rest of the staff. Being on staff will make it convenient for inpatient and staff education. Breastfeeding equipment and other necessary supplies will be provided by the hospital. Many times, hospitals will fund attendance at conferences as well as memberships to professional organizations. The hospital-based lactation consultant also has an opportunity to develop a strong lactation program and be instrumental in designing the care received by breastfeeding mothers and babies.

Services Offered

The hospital setting can permit you to influence large numbers of people. Hospital-based lactation consultants function differently in different settings. You may provide services to both inpatients and outpatients, and serve as a resource for hospital staff in the care of normal breastfeeding couples. This includes assisting with the care of couples who are having difficulty, providing inservice education and training for staff, and advising staff on the standards of care for breastfeeding couples. You will make rounds on some or all breastfeeding mothers and babies, including those who are patients elsewhere in the hospital. On the other hand, you may see only those mothers and babies who are referred by other medical or nursing staff. Administratively, you will assist with developing breastfeeding policies and procedures, develop handouts and reading materials for breastfeeding mothers, and develop appropriate documentation forms for use in the hospital.

Because patient follow-up is an essential element of breastfeeding management, it is important that contact with the mother continue following her discharge from the hospital. Therefore, you may make follow-up phone calls to breastfeeding mothers. When needed, you may provide outpatient visits, either on a fee-for-service basis or as part of your contract with the hospital. You will make referrals to mother support groups and, when necessary, to another lactation consultant or other health professional. You can assist the mother in obtaining breastfeeding devices, when appropriate, and teach her how to use them. Another outpatient service provided by many lactation consultants is conducting prenatal education about infant feeding, incorporating practical information about breastfeeding, and the realities of formula feeding.

Financial Considerations

Some who enter the lactation profession may find it difficult to determine how much to charge for their services. In a hospital, the salary range often is comparable to that of a nurse clinician or a Registered Nurse certified in a specialty. Lactation consultants in the hospital are generally paid an hourly wage, although some may be salaried. You may work full time or part time, or job share—an attractive option if you have small children at home. In order to keep the service viable, it is helpful to work with the billing department to determine the amount patients should be charged for your services. You may, for example, choose to charge only for outpatient services or complex inpatient problems that you see.

▼ Practicing in a WIC Clinic*

The Special Supplemental Food Program for Women, Infants and Children, commonly referred to as WIC, is a special supplemental food and nutrition program. It helps pregnant women choose nutritious foods to have healthier babies. WIC also provides services to breastfeeding mothers, infants, and children up to 5 years of age. It is WIC's philosophy to help participants become healthier and more self-sufficient through education and application of good nutrition principles. WIC provides, at no cost to participants, nutritious foods to supplement the diet, information on healthy eating, and referrals for health care.

As background to a discussion of lactation consultants in WIC, it is helpful to understand the extensive breastfeeding promotion efforts in which WIC is engaged at the local, state, and national levels. The **U.S. Department of Agriculture (USDA)** encourages breastfeeding among WIC participants through regulatory provisions, the development of publications, coop-

*Printed by permission of Breastfeeding Support Consultants.

erative efforts with other federal agencies and private organizations, and funding of breastfeeding grants and studies.

WIC has access to a significant segment of America's low-income, at-risk mothers and infants. Therefore, the USDA has an opportunity to contribute toward achieving the Department of Health and Human Services Healthy People 2010 goals for breastfeeding as well as the program's own nutritional goals. The USDA's national breastfeeding promotion campaign is intended to augment breastfeeding efforts already underway in communities across the country. The campaign promotes breastfeeding awareness and support among women of childbearing age, their families, and others who influence their infant feeding decisions. Promotional and educational publications about breastfeeding and the WIC Program/Population are available from USDA Food and Nutrition Service, Room 607, 3101 Park Center Drive, Alexandria, Virginia 22302.

The breastfeeding rate among WIC participants in 1997 was 50.4 percent initiation rate in the hospital and 16.4 percent at 5 to 6 months postpartum. This compares with the non-WIC population rates of 73.4 percent and 35.5 percent, respectively (Ross, 1998). Many socioeconomic characteristics common among the WIC population are associated with lower rates of breastfeeding and may contribute to this discrepancy. These include race, age (younger than 20 years), family income (185% of poverty), and education (less than high school graduation). It is important to note that breastfeeding rates among WIC participants is increasing, whereas overall population rates remain the same. The WIC program has demonstrated that these programs save tax dollars by encouraging healthy eating, which, in turn, lowers health care costs.

In WIC, a variety of approaches have contributed to increasing the rates of breastfeeding among low-income participants. These include peer support counselors, special incentives, prenatal classes, toll-free telephone lines, and health professional training. The current federal regulations for WIC contain provisions to encourage women to breastfeed and to provide appropriate nutritional support for breastfeeding participants. These regulations, condensed from a USDA document dated July 1993, include

◆ Breastfeeding women are favored in the priority system. When the demand for WIC services exceeds available resources, breastfeeding women are among the first to be considered for benefits.

◆ Breastfeeding participants can continue to participate in the Program for up to 1 year postpartum. Other nonbreastfeeding, postpartum women can continue on WIC only up to 6 months. A breastfeeding woman not at nutritional risk may be certified for WIC based on the eligibility of her at-risk breastfed infant.

◆ Through enhanced food packages, breastfeeding participants receive a greater variety and quantity of food than nonbreastfeeding, postpartum participants.

◆ During WIC nutrition education contacts, all pregnant participants are encouraged to breastfeed unless **contraindicated** for health reasons. Agencies are required to produce a nutrition education plan every 2 years. The plan must include an emphasis on breastfeeding by devising a study group.

◆ Funding incentives are made available to WIC state agencies serving large proportions of **high-risk** persons, which include breastfeeding women and their breastfed infants.

◆ Annually, WIC state agencies are required to spend federal funding specifically designated for breastfeeding promotion and support.

◆ WIC state agencies may use WIC administrative funds to purchase breastfeeding aids such as breast pumps, breast shells, and nursing supplementers that directly support the initiation and continuation of breastfeeding. These purchases are governed by regulations in the individual state.

◆ An enhanced food package is available to breastfeeding women whose infants do not receive formula from the WIC Program. The enhanced package contains additional amounts of juice, cheese, legumes, carrots, and canned tuna. It is intended to support the special nutritional needs of a woman who exclusively or mostly breastfeeds as well as to support her breastfeeding decision.

Qualifications of a Lactation Consultant in WIC

A portion of WIC funding for breastfeeding is targeted for salaries of health care professionals and peer counselors. This funding offers an ideal opportunity for the establishment of a lactation consultant position. Qualifications for funding of a breastfeeding promotion position vary from state to state and from agency to agency. USDA funds are administered on a percentage basis. State and local agencies make independent purchasing and hiring decisions within WIC guidelines. Some states or agencies have breastfeeding promotion positions funded on a percentage basis. For example, a registered dietician's job position may be divided 80 percent for regular WIC job functions and 20 percent for breastfeeding promotion and support.

Most states designate a breastfeeding coordinator for each agency. Funds can be used for the salary of the breastfeeding coordinator. It may be preferred that the lactation consultant be certified through the IBLCE. If a percentage of the position involves nonbreastfeeding WIC functions, an RN or RD degree may be required. An educational credential such as Bachelor of Arts may be required as well, depending on the job responsibilities. In many locations, WIC has become a community resource for breastfeeding. Therefore, other professional or business experience may be required. Marketing and promotional activities to encourage breastfeeding are required in many areas. WIC's promotional activities may involve fund raising in order to sponsor incentive packages and participation in **community outreach**.

As a lactation consultant in WIC, you may encounter many diverse lifestyles. It is important that you be sensitive both culturally and socioeconomically, and that you meet a woman at her own level and her own value system. Lifestyles and priorities among WIC clients may be quite different from your own personal experience. Therefore, you need to remain flexible and adaptable. Many clients have no telephone or move frequently, making home visits a priority. Because a lactation consultant in WIC can be involved in the community in so many ways, you will need to be well trained and have current information in breastfeeding management. You will interface with many levels of health care and other professionals.

Working with Peer Counselors

WIC promotes the use of peer counselors in order to provide ongoing support to their clients. As a lactation consultant in WIC, you may be responsible for training and supervising peer counselors. If a peer counselor program does not already exist, you may be asked to develop the program. WIC believes that peer counselors can reach mothers on their own level. They are able to dispel cultural myths and offer advice on other lifestyle issues because of their own personal experience. For that reason, peer counselors must be representative of the community they serve. (See Chapter 18 for a discussion of cultural issues.) Peer counselors are used for breastfeeding promotion, whereas lactation consultants are used for breastfeeding management and problem solving. Most peer counselors are paid either by the hour or per visit or phone call.

Position Description of the Lactation Consultant in WIC

The variety of tasks and responsibilities for a lactation consultant in WIC may include

◆ Counsel mothers and work with other WIC staff.

◆ Teach breastfeeding classes and facilitate postpartum support groups.

◆ Develop promotion programs and nutrition education programs focused on breastfeeding.

◆ Participate in state breastfeeding workshops, consortiums, and committees.

◆ Establish a system of **networking** for WIC breastfeeding resources.

◆ Provide breastfeeding in-service programs.

◆ Supervise and train WIC peer counselors.

◆ Develop and evaluate breastfeeding materials for WIC clients.

You can make a real difference working in a WIC clinic. Although the WIC population of women represent the lowest breastfeeding rates, they also have the largest increase in breastfeeding rates. WIC serves as a breastfeeding resource within the community and fosters a whole clinic approach to maternal and infant care.

▼ Practicing in a Physician Group

Working with an obstetrician, a pediatrician, or a family practice physician group might possibly be the best of all worlds for a lactation consultant. In this type of practice, you will see healthy normal babies, along with mothers and babies who are experiencing difficulties. Most of the practice is preventive rather than crisis management. Working with only a few physicians will make it easier for you to come to agreement on breastfeeding issues. Therefore, the potential for burnout is less.

There are a few challenges with this arrangement. Your patient load will be dependent on the physician's patient load. When you make rounds in the hospital, you may be there at a time when the baby is not ready for a feed. Early discharge can make it difficult for you to see every breastfeeding mother in a timely manner. You may need to become creative with your schedule in order to visit all mothers and observe a breastfeed. Just as with a hospital-based lactation consultant, downsizing could eliminate your position. Be prepared with documentation that illustrates your importance to the practice.

Developing a Proposal

If you wish to develop a lactation program for a physician or group of physicians, you will want to have a brief proposal ready that outlines the services you could provide for their patients. Be specific about the potential services you can provide to that particular practice. Also see further discussion of developing a job proposal or job description in Chapter 24. Services may include

◆ Teach breastfeeding classes.
   If you are working with a group of obstetricians, nurse midwives, or family practice physicians, you will have a good number of clientele to whom you can offer breastfeeding classes. If you are working with a pediatrician, you may be able to offer prenatal breast-

feeding classes by sending a notice to the offices of the obstetricians who generally refer to that pediatric practice. See the sample class outlines in Chapter 9.

◆ Meet with each pregnant woman at least once during her prenatal course.

The purpose of this visit is to discuss her breastfeeding goals, to evaluate her previous history and the present condition of her breasts and nipples, and to begin appropriate intervention, if necessary. This visit may take place in the office, or in the context of prenatal breastfeeding or childbirth education classes.

◆ Make rounds on breastfeeding mothers in the hospital.

If you are working exclusively with a group of pediatricians, this may be your first contact with these mothers.

◆ Provide a series of follow-up telephone calls.

These calls usually are placed at about 2 to 3 days after discharge, 3 to 4 days after that, and again at around 2 weeks. Initiating such follow-up calls helps the mother to avoid complications. Further follow-up can be provided more frequently as warranted. An office visit or home visit can be scheduled as necessary to evaluate specific problems or concerns.

◆ Provide a warm line for breastfeeding mothers.

You might consider installing a separate phone line in your home to use for a warm line 24 hours a day. An answering machine or voice mail system can be attached to the phone to record calls that you can return later. Depending on your service, you may also wish to carry a pager.

◆ Serve as a resource person to the physicians and their staff.

Update them on new research and recommendations concerning the compatibility of medications with breastfeeding. Provide in-service programs for the nursing staff periodically, especially the nurses in a pediatric or family practice group because they will receive the bulk of the breastfeeding calls. Encourage them to transfer such calls to you so that mothers receive accurate and consistent information.

◆ Maintain a supply of breastfeeding products and literature to make available to parents.

You may find it helpful to write your own breastfeeding handouts. Breast pump rentals and other devices are other possible services to provide, either through the physician's office or directly from you.

◆ Record breastfeeding statistics.

In order to document your effectiveness for the practice, record the numbers of mothers initiating breastfeeding, those who breastfeed for 6 weeks, 3 months, 6 months, and 1 year.

◆ Facilitate a postpartum support group for mothers in the practice.

◆ Make recommendations on specific treatments that impact breastfeeding.

These conditions may include **thrush, failure to thrive**, and **ankyloglossia**.

Benefits to the Physician's Service

Breastfeeding consultations can be time consuming. A lactation consultant can free up the time physicians and office personnel spend with prenatal and postpartum breastfeeding related telephone calls. Preventive education, counseling in the hospital, and telephone follow-up are far more effective than crisis management in dealing with concerns such as low weight gain in infants, sore nipples, and decreased milk production. Being able to turn the management of a slow-gaining infant over to a lactation consultant relieves the physician. This approach identifies the cause of the problem and preserves breastfeeding more effectively. Offering the services of a lactation consultant will attract mothers to the practice. If yours is the first physician practice in the area to have a certified lactation consultant on staff, there is great marketing potential.

Business Issues

You may choose to work specific hours, using the physician's office as your base, or you may decide to work on call out of your own home. In either case, you will contact the hospital in the morning to determine which mothers need to be seen. You will then make follow-up calls and home or office visits as needed. You will need a private room with a comfortable chair, a variety of pillows, charting forms, a breast pump, other breastfeeding devices, literature, diapers, and other items discussed under private practice. You may wish to incorporate breast pump rentals and other breastfeeding devices into the physician's practice or to provide them as a service separate from your arrangement with the physician.

Breastfeeding complications are not limited to specific hours. Just as with a private practice, you will need to be available around the clock. Mothers will need a way to contact you directly. A beeper or voice mail system will allow you to contact clients at your convenience. It will also be important to provide coverage by another lactation consultant or other caregiver for times when you are unavailable.

Financial Issues

You may request to be paid by the physician either on a per-hour or a per-client basis. A third alternative is to be paid directly by the client on a fee-for-service basis. The client would subsequently submit the bill to her insurance company for reimbursement. This may be the least desirable arrangement. Many mothers will not use your services until they are in full-blown crisis to avoid the cost.

The physician can include your services on the bill that is submitted to the insurance company. Individual insurance companies will determine whether or not to reimburse for your services. Billing for your services can be negotiated with the physician at the time of your interview, with a specific contract drawn up specifying your services and salary. You may want to renegotiate at the end of the first year to reflect any changes in your services. ILCA can provide further information on third-party reimbursement.

Wages in a physician's practice will probably be in a range between that of an office staff nurse and a hospital-based lactation consultant. Compensation may be on a per-client basis to cover hospital rounds, follow-up phone calls, establishment of a basic chart, and a warm line. Breastfeeding classes and office or home visits can be billed separately to the client, or may be included in the physician's fee. The physician practice may prefer to compensate for your services with an hourly salary. If the position is not regarded as full time, there may be no employment benefits such as health insurance or vacation time.

▼ **Practicing in Home Health Care**

The home care lactation consultant provides follow-up to mothers and babies after discharge from the hospital. Home health care presents many opportunities to the lactation consultant. Home health services begin with discharge planning and continue through home visits and community referrals. It is essential that the home care nurse be well educated in breastfeeding management in order to give effective care and advice. Ideally, every home care agency that provides maternity services will have a lactation consultant on staff. Hospitals that provide home care services customarily contract with managed care companies that provide this coverage, and only those mothers with coverage are seen by the home care staff.

In the context of short hospital stays, home care services are essential to mothers and babies. If the mother does not stay at least 48 hours after birth, the hospital staff may not be able to observe a breastfeed for every mother and baby. Knowing that a home care lactation consultant will visit the mother shortly after discharge provides a level of comfort that these mothers will be given the breastfeeding advice and care they need.

Breastfeeding advocates experience varying degrees of success from health maintenance organizations for coverage of these services. Some may be more likely to provide coverage for lactation services if the lactation consultant is also a registered nurse. One health management organization (HMO) in the Chicago area canceled an existing home nurse visit program because it was determined that having the mother take her baby to the pediatrician's office was more cost effective. In some places, mothers are seen by home health staff only if they have a health problem.

An Example of a Home Health Lactation Consultant Service

This section provides a description of home health care services provided through a home health agency in central Pennsylvania. Although other programs may vary, this agency serves as a model for a continuum of breastfeeding support. The home health care staff received comprehensive instruction in breastfeeding management and support; the WHO/UNICEF 18-hour course *Breastfeeding Management* and *Promotion in a Baby-Friendly Hospital* was tailored to fit the needs of home care staff.

Discharge Planner

A maternity discharge planner reviews hospital charts each morning to determine which mothers will go home and which ones will stay another day. This is determined primarily by what the mother's particular insurance company will allow. In 1996, many American states reacted to the negative consequences of early discharge by passing legislation that would guarantee that new mothers and babies are kept in the hospital long enough to receive necessary care. Typically, this legislation ensures a 48-hour stay. The legislation covered only about 50 percent of mothers. Therefore, federal legislation is now in place to protect all mothers.

The discharge planner sees every patient who will be leaving that day. She evaluates both the mother and baby, and reviews their charts. She then gives the mother instructions to get her through until her first visit by the home care nurse. If the mother is breastfeeding, she asks how breastfeeding is going and discusses any concerns the mother voices. Breastfeeding mothers receive a home visit by a lactation consultant, who is also a nurse. The discharge planner documents sufficient information to provide to the home care lactation consultant in preparation for this visit.

A packet of information is given to the mother that includes warning signs and symptoms that will help the mother detect potential problems. Mothers who are eligible for home health services also receive information about the home care lactation consultant and are encouraged to make use of her 24-hour access to home care services. After hospital discharge of the mother, the lactation consultant contacts the home care department to arrange for follow-up.

Home Care Lactation Consultant

Agencies differ in their policies for determining which mothers are eligible for home visits as well as the duration of the visits. The average length of a lactation visit in this home health agency is 90 minutes. When the home care lactation consultant is also a nurse, the scope of care includes much more than breastfeeding. If a problem surfaces during the first visit, an interim phone call is made to monitor progress until the next visit. Some agencies require that visits be no longer than 45 minutes. Some also limit visits to mothers who are at risk, have given birth by cesarean, or have preterm babies.

The initial phone call to schedule the patient's first visit also can serve as an opportunity to learn how the mother is doing. In preparation for the visit, the mother can be encouraged to think of herself still as a patient. She is not expected to be dressed or showered and is encouraged to not worry about a clean house or to think of the nurse as a visitor. Helping the mother to lower her expectations of this visit will encourage her to continue getting the rest she needs.

Because a home environment will not be as controlled as a hospital environment, you will need to be flexible in your expectations and the manner in which you provide care. On the first visit, you may be greeted at the door by an excited **sibling** or by a frantic mother who needs reassurance. So, the visit may begin with social amenities and emotional support that is substantially different from what is experienced by hospital staff. Family dynamics may be different as well, with the baby's father, siblings, and grandparents often present. Although these people may be present also during hospital visits, being on one's home turf can provide for a more realistic and comfortable communication style. You are able to assess the mother's support system and capitalize on teaching opportunities with other family members. Often, speaking loudly enough for a family member in another room to hear what the mother is being told may go a long way in enlisting support from a skeptical relative.

A home visit should include breastfeeding assessment and observation of a breastfeed, whether the provider is a lactation consultant or a nurse. The goal is to assess breastfeeding technique and build the mother's self-confidence. You can begin by asking the mother what she knows about breastfeeding. Check the mother's **breastfeeding diary** and discuss how everything is going. Talking with the mother about her labor and delivery will indicate if there are potential problems with breastfeeding, such as the possibility of a sleepy infant. It also gives the mother an opportunity to talk through her birth experience. Helping the mother get past her birth experience and verbalize concerns or dis-

appointments will help her to gain perspective and move onto other parenting issues such as breastfeeding.

The home care lactation consultant who is also a nurse will perform a complete assessment of both mother and infant, assess breastfeeding technique, and teach infant care. The infant assessment may take place on the couch, on the dining room table, or in the nursery—wherever the mother wishes. You may check the baby's bilirubin level according to the home care agency's guidelines. You will provide **anticipatory guidance** to avoid potential complications such as low milk production, nipple soreness, or **engorgement**. It is important to keep in mind that on this first visit, the mother may be stressed and tired, and she may not take in all that is being taught and discussed. If a nurse who is not a lactation consultant is making this first visit and she encounters breastfeeding difficulties, a referral to the agency's lactation consultant or a community-based lactation consultant is warranted.

On the second home visit, the mother may seem more relaxed and reassured than she was on the first visit. She may be more rested and her breasts may feel full, which brings a sense of relief. She is now able to "take in and take hold," as described by Reba Rubin (1961). She may ask about long-term issues such as returning to work and the use of supplemental bottles. This is the vital link the home care nurse provides. Hospital staff assisted the mother in the first 2 days. The home care staff can help the mother after hospital discharge, and prepare her for later by educating her and helping her to access community support.

Another complete assessment on the mother and baby may be done on the second visit, including a breast exam. By this second visit, which occurs around day 5 or 6, the mother should report at least six wet diapers and four stools. Weight loss should be stabilized or less than 7 percent of birth weight.

The home health lactation consultant is in a position to serve as a critical advocate for the mother in terms of further follow-up care. You can call the insurance company with concerns about breastfeeding, and encourage the company to pay for lactation visits or additional nursing visits. You may notify the pediatrician if you feel the baby needs to be seen earlier than the customary well-baby visit. You also may use your contacts with the insurance company representatives as a means to increase their breastfeeding knowledge and work toward better coverage of lactation services as preventive health care.

▼
Working in Private Practice

Many lactation consultants elect to open a private practice in their community. Private practice is a reasonable option for a seasoned lactation consultant who has several years of experience working with a large variety of breastfeeding mothers and infants. Customarily, private practice lactation consultants have some form of medical credential beyond their IBCLC credential (i.e., RN, MD, or RD). These credentials allow the lactation consultant to be viewed as an expert when working on a referral basis. Licensed credentials also make it more likely that insurance companies will provide reimbursement.

Many private practice lactation consultants enjoy the autonomy of being their own boss. You are able to set your own hours and work around family functions. Electing to go into private practice means that you will be dependent on referrals from other lactation consultants, hospitals, physicians, and clients themselves. Establishing a referral base large enough to support you can take years to develop. However, because your referral base is not tied to one single source, you will be in a better position to be an advocate for breastfeeding. It is easier to speak your mind when you are autonomous.

Working in private practice usually permits minimal contact with the staffs at the various hospitals. Because you will be working alone, there will be limited opportunity for peer relationships. Working on community coalitions is an effective way for private practice lactation consultants to network with other professionals. They will learn more about you and your practice, and you will have an opportunity to become acquainted with new colleagues. Some of the tips in Chapter 26 regarding breastfeeding promotion may help guide the manner in which you relate to other professionals. It may be difficult to gain access to medical libraries for needed references. Therefore, avenues for acquiring journal articles and books will need to be developed. These are challenges that can be overcome. Ultimately, the key to your success will be sound business practices, committing time to seeing clients, following through with all necessary paper work, and marketing your services.

Business Issues

Deciding to open a private practice is a serious business decision. Be prepared to work to make it succeed. It may be helpful to take a small business course from your local community college and to read books about how to set up a small business or open a home office (Gower, 1991). Being in private practice means that you will do your own billing and collection of fees. Although there will be no employee benefits, being self-employed does provide you with some tax breaks, which an accountant can help you identify.

You will need to decide whether to work at home or to locate your office elsewhere in the community. Should you decide to base your practice in your home,

you will want to check with your local zoning board to determine whether there are any restrictions on signs, parking, or storage of supplies. If you plan for clients to enter and leave your home, you may need additional coverage on your home owners insurance. Some insurance companies charge higher rates when pregnant women will be coming and going from the home. No matter which location you choose, you will need to arrange for adequate space for seeing clients and for office work, equipment, and supplies.

Home Office

If you choose a home office, make sure you can offer your clients complete privacy for the entire consult. Mothers should not see or hear others in the house. You need privacy to examine and evaluate a mother in a room where family members will not be walking through. Conversation between you and your client is confidential, and you do not want to risk others overhearing anything that is said. Many mothers tell things to a lactation consultant that they have never told anyone before. You and a mother may discuss issues such as abuse, rape, and sexually transmitted diseases. You will want an environment that is conducive to a mother who chooses to confide such issues. Often, such delicate issues may be the hidden motivation for the visit. Keep in mind that you are not qualified to counsel in these situations and will need to refer the mother to qualified professionals. Other things to consider in deciding on a home office are bathroom facilities, safe and easy access into and out of your home, and ease of parking. Also consider whether your home is easy for mothers to locate without long and complicated directions.

Off-Site Location

Deciding to locate your office in a professional or office building is accompanied by greater expenses and additional issues. You might want to consider sharing space with another health professional until you are well established. Some of the things you will need to budget for in addition to your inventory is rent, insurance, utilities, a business sign, and maintenance. A carefully selected location can be your key to a successful practice. Other things to address are good outdoor lighting for evening appointments, security, snow removal, adequate parking, and other tenants in the building. You want to be sure that clients will feel comfortable visiting you at this location.

Office Equipment and Furniture

You will need standard office equipment such as desks, chairs, filing cabinets, and any other furnishings that will provide for efficiency and comfort. A dedicated telephone line and a telephone with an answering machine or voice mail will ensure that calls are not missed and that they are answered professionally. You will want your reference library accessible to you during the consultation and when writing physician reports. A computer and printer will enable you to maintain client records and produce professional reports and correspondence.

Your lactation consulting practice will also require equipment and furniture specific to your profession. Select a comfortable chair with arms for mothers to sit in and nurse, preferably one that can be wiped clean. A footstool placed in front of the chair will help you to teach mothers good body positioning. Pillows of various shapes and sizes will enable mothers to get comfortable for feeds and position their babies at the breast. A baby sling will allow you to hold the baby while the mother is pumping and complete your paperwork at the same time. You will need space where you can lay the baby for examining it and where you can secure the baby while you are assessing and working with the mother. A digital scale is standard equipment in a lactation consultant's offices. If you cannot afford to purchase one, you might consider acquiring one on a rental basis. You will need either paper products or linens for use on your changing table and scale. Many lactation consultants provide toys for toddlers to keep them busy while they work with the mother and baby. If you do so, make sure the toys can be cleaned adequately.

Breastfeeding Supplies and Inventory

You may wish to provide various breastfeeding devices for rental or purchase by parents. Identify a place for these items that will be easily accessible. In the beginning, you may wish to serve as a rental station on consignment with a breast pump company. Later, after you have firmly established a rental station, changing to a flat rate may be better for you financially. In the beginning, you will want to limit your inventory because inventory ties up your money. As your practice grows you can keep track of the products and supplies about which clients question you, and consider carrying those items. Providing replacement parts for breast pumps and breast pump kits is a convenience that mothers appreciate; it is also an excellent marketing tool.

Make sure you have supplies you will be using during consultations, such as nursing supplementers, medicine dropper, small cups, and nipple shields. Some lactation consultants keep small amounts of formula in their office to use when calories are needed and expressed breastmilk is not available. If you use olive oil to improve the vacuum of the breast pump flange, make sure you have small medicine cups to provide individual amounts to mothers. As you develop your practice, keep track of items you did not have that either would have made the consult go more smoothly or would make

breastfeeding more enjoyable for the mother. Weigh the cost of such items with how quickly they would be used or would sell. Order as few of a new item as possible to test the market. If it is an item you use or sell frequently, you might consider purchasing it in quantity and prepaying to save money on shipping and handling.

Marketing Your Private Practice

Your marketing strategy will greatly impact the success of your practice. You can talk with other lactation consultants who work in private practice to find out which marketing strategies have worked best for them. What mistakes did they make that you can avoid? Most lactation consultants will be happy to share their experience in setting up a private practice. Take advantage of the successes and mistakes of others. You do not have to reinvent the wheel!

Your clients will come primarily from medical referrals, referrals from past clients, and your listing in the telephone directory. Your marketing dollars are best spent by placing an ad in the Yellow Pages of your local directory. You can also contact local physicians, hospitals, clinics, birthing centers, and childbirth educators to acquaint them with the services you provide. Letters to such groups and individuals can serve to introduce your service to the community. A follow-up visit to personnel in charge will allow them the opportunity to ask questions and get to know you. Be sure to keep a file of all business cards you receive so that you may contact people at a later date. Note on the back of the card the date you received it and a brief note about the circumstances. Such contacts may prove useful to you at various times in your practice.

There are many aspects of functioning as a private practice lactation consultant that will be helpful to you in marketing your practice. You can meet with physicians and their staff at their offices to confer about clients or to discuss breastfeeding management issues. Offer to present a free in-service session on breastfeeding management to the staff. After you have seen a client, send a report to the physician involved. In some circumstances, you may also want to enclose copies of any relevant research articles. All of this helps reinforce your credibility as a member of the mother's and infant's health care team. This approach increases the likelihood that the physician will refer other mothers to your care. Satisfied clients are the best sources of referrals. Your attention to meeting the needs of mothers in your care will reap marketing benefits as those satisfied clients recommend your services to friends and family.

Consulting with Mothers

In order to create a professional appearance, remove all family items from the area being used for consultations.

If you have a busy practice, your office may become cluttered with paperwork and other items. Clear away any clutter before the client arrives so that you will appear organized. You can store items in a drawer or closet until after the consultation.

You can save time by preparing several client charts ahead of time and giving the client a clipboard containing a consent form and an intake form at the beginning of the consult. While the mother is completing the forms, you can leave the room to wash your hands. You will most likely not have a sink in your office, as is the case in a physician's office. In order to relay the message that you are washing your hands before touching the mother or her baby, you can return to the room drying your hands with a towel. You may also choose to wear a cover gown over your clothes. This is especially important if you have been outdoors or involved in household chores. All of these things show mothers that you are concerned about their health and safety and that of their infants.

Home Visits

If your private practice will involve visits to mothers' homes you will need to equip your car with the necessary supplies and equipment. When making a home visit, you will not be able to run back to your office easily for something you forgot! Recognize that mothers may not have such items as footstools or comfortable pillows. A cellular phone is recommended, in case you become lost or if you anticipate that you may drive to an unsafe neighborhood.

Telephone Calls

As a private practice lactation consultant, you will need to be available to clients at established times. Telephone calls must be able to get through to the office at all times. You will therefore need either an answering machine or voice mail. Be aware that you are legally required to respond if a client leaves a message for you. Maintain a professional demeanor during all telephone contacts with clients—both when answering the telephone and with the message you leave on your answering machine or voice mail. If you are unable to see a client because of a personal commitment, simply say that you are unavailable at that time and suggest the next available time. It is not necessary, nor professional, to offer an explanation of the reason you are not available. Make sure that family members know not to answer the business phone.

At times when you are away from your practice, coverage will need to be provided. Carefully select the person who will cover for you in your absence. Agree ahead of time how she will respond to clients. You will want to know that she approaches breastfeeding with a philosophy that is compatible with yours. Also learn if she has an answering machine and if there are any potential times when the practice may not be covered.

Documentation

It is important that all aspects of a consultation be documented in an organized and consistent manner. You can begin by preparing a consent form for clients to sign at the beginning of every consultation. You may wish to include in the consent form a statement granting permission for any photographs you may use for teaching purposes. As a courtesy, you can ask permission again before taking any pictures. You will also want to develop standard assessment forms that will elicit the information you need from each client. If you make it a practice to use these forms with all clients, you will avoid forgetting to ask an important question.

At the end of the consultation, you will need to complete a report to the client's physician. If you use the same format in this report as you do in the assessment forms, it will help you remember to include all important information. Plan time at the end of the consultation to write the physician's report immediately after the client leaves. Do not consider your consultation completed until this important report has been written and sent. Processing the report by computer will produce a professional appearance and also provide you with a permanent record. Always spell check the document; you may wish to invest in a medical dictionary to aid you in this process. Many caregivers take advantage of the convenience and cost savings of faxing reports rather than mailing them.

Lactation consultants in private practice advise that you retain copies of all records for at least 7 years. This includes appointment books, telephone logs, financial records and receipts, and the like. You can place everything for each calendar year in a separate box and label it clearly. At some time in the future, you may need a duplicate of a client's records, financial records for the Internal Revenue Service, or some other such paperwork. Your diligence in retaining files will assist you in locating the necessary materials. See Chapter 24 for further discussion of documentation as it relates to legal liability.

Financial Issues

It is important that clients know what your charges will be before a consultation. When the nature of a telephone call indicates that a consultation is needed, you can inform the mother of this in such a way as, "I will be happy to see you. I have an opening at the following times. You will need to be here for about 1½ hours and the fee for my services is. . . ." If a mother says she cannot afford your services, it may help to share with her that formula feeding will cost her much more than your services. Help her to see that she is paying the same amount for 1 hour of your time as she does for about 10 minutes of the physician's time. At that rate, your services are quite a bargain! You can help mothers to be comfortable paying for your services if you approach the topic in a self-assured and practical manner. Post your fees on the wall in your office as well, so that clients can see them during the visit. This will help to avoid misunderstandings.

Because many lactation consultants began in the field as volunteers, some may find it difficult to charge a fee for their services. Remember that you are a professional who is providing a professional service. You may find it more comfortable to keep your eyes focused on the bill rather than the client when discussing payment. One way to address payment is to ask, "Will you be paying by cash or check?"

Billing for your services must be done on a regular schedule. Few private practice lactation consultants have the luxury of relegating this task to another person. Plan a regular time slot into your month to update your records and mail bills for any outstanding accounts. If you do not have provider status with the mother's insurance carrier, it is advisable that you collect the fee directly from the client rather than from the insurance company. The client can send your receipt to her insurance company for reimbursement. If you allow a partial payment, you can give the client mailing envelopes printed with your address for the balance of the payment. You may also write the amount due and the date you expect payment on the flap of the envelope.

Financial Record Keeping

You will need to keep a monthly record of all business expenses and income. Investing in an inexpensive accounting software program such as Quickbooks or Quicken will simplify this process for you. Your accounts will be retained easily and be quickly available for reference. Spreadsheets will enable you to note your profits and losses, assisting you in business planning. Some of the items you may wish to include are

Income received
    Consultations and services
    Speaking engagements
    Breast pump rentals
    Breastfeeding classes
    Resale items sold

Expenditures
    Office supplies
    Teaching materials
    Equipment
    Phone
    Fees and memberships
    Journals

    Books
    Resale items purchased
    Conference and meeting expenses
    Insurance
    Advertising
    Donations
    Breast pump rental fees
    State tax

Third-Party Reimbursement

Be sure to provide the client with appropriate forms with which she can seek reimbursement from her insurance company. Contact ILCA for more information on third-party reimbursement. Third-party reimbursement is a legislative and policy issue based within the United States. ILCA can provide information or referral, or both, to the regional representative or delegate within your respective area who might provide you with the names of specific individuals who have successfully achieved reimbursement for services. You can also contact specific managed care providers in your area to negotiate fee payment.

A three-part carbonless superbill has been designed by the UCLA Lactation Alumni Association, specifically for reimbursement of lactation consulting services (see Appendix A). The client submits one copy to her insurance company. This copy must have your name printed on it as the lactation consultant. The client keeps the second copy for her records. It can be submitted with tax records at the end of the year as a child care expense if the client is a working mother. Some insurance companies will require that their own insurance form be completed rather than the superbill. Encourage the client to contact her insurance carrier to learn its requirements. You will want to retain the third copy for your files in case it is needed at a later date.

Attach a Prescription. It may help to attach a physician's prescription requesting your services. The prescription must be dated and made out in the client's name. It is important that the specific services be reflected on the prescription. You may create a form with the information below that tells the physician what needs to be reflected on the prescription. Some codes may apply only if the physician is present for the consultation. The ICD•9 Code is the International Classification of Diseases.

◆ For a consultation: Consult (your name) for evaluation, assessment and treatment of . . . (Diagnosis and ICD•9 Code).

◆ For breast pump rental: Feed baby mother's milk. Obtain the mother's milk by use of a hospital-grade electric breast pump. Classified as durable medical equipment.

◆ Or, for breast pump rental: Electric breast pump for treatment of . . . (Diagnosis and ICD•9 Code).

◆ For infant feeding supplies: "To insure adequate caloric intake use a . . . (name of device)".

Attach a referral letter from the physician. Below is a sample letter that may be helpful in seeking reimbursement for a breast pump rental. It can be attached as a cover letter to the mother's insurer.

(Date)

To insurance carrier for: (client's name)

Name of policyholder:

              Policy number: _____

The following explanation of medical need is provided in order to expedite insurance coverage for the rental of an electric breast pump.

    (Name of mother) delivered the high-risk infant (name of baby) on (date). The child is too immature or ill to nurse directly at the breast. However, it is well established that human milk provides optimal infant nutrition for the first several months of life. Thus, the mother of a **premature** or high-risk newborn is encouraged to pump her breasts in order to supply milk for her hospitalized baby and to maintain lactation until the baby can nurse at the breast.

    The intermittent electric breast pump is by far the most efficient, effective, and physiologic means of stimulating the sucking action of a normal infant. Inexpensive manual, battery-operated, or small electric breast pumps are an adjunct to milk expression for occasional use when a large intermittent suction pump is unavailable. A piston-type electric breast pump is essential for the maintenance of an adequate **milk supply** whenever a child is unable to breastfeed normally. Such pumps cost approximately $1400 and thus are far more economical to rent.

    The electric pump will be necessary until the baby is able to take all required nutrition by feeding at the breast. An electric breast pump is not a convenience for the mother; rather it is a medical necessity in the best interest of the child's health.

Sincerely,

(Pediatrician)

Rental of Breast Pumps

Most private practice lactation consultants provide electric breast pumps for rental by clients. Pumps are available from a variety of breast pump companies. See Appendix A for a listing. Breast pump rental programs may allow clients to lease a pump at a daily, weekly, or monthly rate. There are often special rates for long-term use (i.e., 5 or 6 months). This information will be provided by the individual rental station. There are a number of items you may wish to make available to clients. In addition to large rental electric breast pumps, you can provide smaller electric pumps for purchase, motor adapters, power paks, feeding cups, and bottles. You might also provide clients with instructions that address common questions regarding refunds for early returns, special rental rates, care of the pump, and arranging for its return.

RELATIONSHIP OF THE LACTATION CONSULTANT AND PEER COUNSELOR

Your impact on breastfeeding can be greatly enhanced by a reciprocal and cooperative working relationship with breastfeeding counselors and other support people. As discussed earlier in this chapter, WIC employs peer counselors who receive training and are usually of the same ethnic origin as the other women in the community. Lay counselors are used by La Leche League and Nursing Mothers groups to provide mother-to-mother support. Whether the counselor is working for an agency or as part of a mother-to-mother support group, you can all work together toward accomplishing the breastfeeding goals for women in your community.

Mother-to-Mother Support Groups

The mother-to-mother support group primarily will offer mothers emotional support and the mother-to-mother contact acquired through regular meetings and telephone counseling. Customarily, these counselors will acquire training in counseling and breastfeeding management. You will need to ascertain the degree of education and experience among the counselors with whom you plan to work and to tailor your relationship accordingly.

    The importance of services provided to mothers by a mother-to-mother support group cannot be minimized. Counselors contact mothers before difficulties arise and offer anticipatory guidance and emotional support. Mothers benefit from a variety of resources during their breastfeeding experience. Participating in group activities will increase their satisfaction and self-confidence in their role as mothers. Mutual sharing and seeing other mothers breastfeed greatly enhances their breastfeeding and parenting experiences. The support group also can provide access to a lending library as well as breast pumps and other devices. See Chapter 18 for further discussion of support groups for breastfeeding mothers.

    Lay counselors are capable of dealing with many types of breastfeeding situations without a background of extended lactation education. The **outreach counseling** and emotional support provided by these **paraprofessionals** contributes greatly to mothers' reaching their goals. Mothers are educated about their options, which encourages them to participate actively in decisions concerning their baby's care. If a mother-to-mother support group does not exist in your community, you may wish to consider beginning one from among the population of women in your care. Through your association with a mother-to-mother support group, you can ensure that mothers receive continuing care and consistent information.

The Lactation Consultant's Services to the Group

Services you offer to mother-to-mother support groups generally will be voluntary. Often, the value of good public relations outweighs the benefit of monetary gain. Judge each service according to its impact and scope of commitment when deciding whether a fee will be charged. Following are some suggestions for ways in which you can work with a mother-to-mother support group. These suggestions represent a variety of possibilities for increasing your own effectiveness as well as that of the support group. Working together as a team, you can present a unified program of support to breastfeeding mothers.

◆ Maintain a reciprocal referral system. You will refer mothers to the support group for continuing outreach support. The support group, in return, will refer mothers to you when a special situation exists that requires a higher level of expertise. This system will ensure that a greater number of mothers are reached and given necessary support and information.

◆ Maintain quality counseling and accurate information within the support group by training counselors in counseling skills and breastfeeding information. You can provide such training at periodic intervals or when the need presents itself.

◆ Serve as an advisor to the support group, making yourself available to answer questions from counselors.

◆ Co-sponsor and help organize outreach programs run by the support group. Encourage community programs that address both parents and the medical community.

◆ Offer continuing education for counselors, in the form of study nights, seminars, and workshops.

◆ Offer your services as a speaker at parent or counselor meetings.

◆ Serve as a liaison between the support group and the medical community. Maintain a two-way line of communication concerning mothers who are referred for problems. Keep both physicians and the support group informed.

◆ Review written materials that are distributed by the support group for educating counselors and parents.

Non-Salaried Volunteer in a Breastfeeding Center

Some hospitals use the services of volunteer counselors in place of or in addition to a lactation consultant. To be considered for such a position, the counselor is usually approved by the local breastfeeding support group. She needs a clear understanding of client confidentiality and criteria for referring nonroutine calls to you. The hospital should provide an orientation and tour of the areas where the counselor will work.

The counselor can assist lactation consultants and other staff with routine phone calls, office tasks, and cleaning breast pumps. She can work under the direction of a staff lactation consultant and make routine follow-up phone calls to newly discharged breastfeeding mothers. When mothers call into the hospital with questions or a problem, the counselor can give immediate assistance in your absence. Make sure that the counselor writes or charts all contacts.

SUMMARY

The professional lactation consultant has a variety of employment options to consider. Each particular work setting varies from others in many ways. One constant thread among all settings is the role of the lactation consultant. You serve as part of a strong health care team that provides the consistent care that benefits mothers as they are establishing breastfeeding. Whether you choose to work in a hospital, clinic, physician group, home health care, or private practice, a commitment to breastfeeding mothers and babies is a driving force. Volunteer counselors continue to play a valuable part in the mother's support. You can help coordinate this care by maintaining a reciprocal relationship with community support groups. Mothers who are supported by a strong health care team will be empowered to participate as informed health consumers.

REFERENCES

Briggs et al. *Drugs in Pregnancy and Lactation*; Baltimore: Williams & Wilkins; 1998.

Hale T. *Medications and Mother's Milk.* Amarillo, TX: Pharmasoft Publishing; 1999.

Ross Laboratories Mothers' Survey; 1998.

Rubin R. Puerperal change. *Nurs Outlook* 753; 1961.

BIBLIOGRAPHY

Cadwell K. Using the quality improvement process to affect breastfeeding protocols in United States hospitals. *J Hum Lact* 13:5–9; 1997.

Elder S and Gregory C. The "lactation game": An innovative teaching method for health care professionals. *J Hum Lact* 12: 137–138; 1996.

Hirschman J. Impact of the special supplemental food program on infants. *J Pediatr* S121–S122; 1990.

Howard C et al. Attitudes, practices and recommendations by obstetricians about infant feeding. *Birth* 24:240–257; 1997.

MacGowan R et al. Breast-feeding among women attending Women, Infants, and Children clinics in Georgia, 1987. *Pediatrics* 87 (3):361–366; 1991.

www.usda.gov/fcs/brfdcpgn.htm

3

EMPOWERING WOMEN THROUGH YOUR ATTITUDE AND APPROACH

Breastfeeding mothers are helped most effectively by those who demonstrate a belief in breastfeeding as the natural way to nourish an infant. It is not enough to believe in theory that breastfeeding is best. Caregivers must put that theory into practice. Some health workers are reluctant to promote breastfeeding for fear that they will create guilt in mothers who choose not to breastfeed. A caregiver who appears to be ambivalent about breastfeeding sends mixed messages and creates personal doubts in mothers. Those who promote and support breastfeeding enthusiastically serve as a powerful motivator for mothers and staff alike.

The caregiver's approach with breastfeeding women determines the effectiveness of the support and advice they offer. Establishing a partnership with mothers will build confidence and self-esteem—these characteristics, in turn, will foster parental independence and growth. Providing an effective learning climate will help you to achieve the goal of involving mothers actively in problem-solving and decision-making. Using humor in your interactions with mothers will help them to gain perspective during challenging times and will increase your teaching effectiveness. Finally, understanding the components of communication that affect the messages you send to mothers will enhance your interactions.

EMPOWERMENT THROUGH BREASTFEEDING

It stands to reason that mothers who have a good self-image and who feel confident in their parenting will form more positive attachments with their children. In fact, studies have shown that a mother who lacks confidence has difficulty establishing a relationship with her baby (Zahr, 1991). This underscores the important role you and other health workers play in enhancing the mother's confidence. Locklin reported in 1993 that achieving a positive and rewarding breastfeeding experience produces feelings of power and accomplishment in a woman. Women may view breastfeeding as the one thing they can control in their immediate postpartum situation. It is important that the caregiver take a gentle approach that minimizes interventions and builds on the

mother's confidence and self-direction (Auerbach, 1994).

The experience of giving birth to a child is a major turning point in the lives of many women. Mothers often identify childbirth as their most significant learning experience. The act of creation brings to the woman a new awareness of her own creative capacities. A mother will reassess her capabilities and her capacity to assume a new role of parent. One mother said that as she found that she could hear, understand, and remember the things she was taught about breastfeeding, she began to think of herself as a learner for the first time (Belenky, 1986). You and other caregivers can capitalize on this powerful time in a woman's life by helping her gain skills and knowledge in breastfeeding.

MAKING THE BREASTFEEDING ASSUMPTION

Because Western society has embraced artificial feeding as equal to breastfeeding, some health care workers may be uncomfortable actively promoting breastfeeding as the normal way to nourish an infant. Although research supports the health benefits of breastfeeding to both mothers and babies, many health care practices today continue to convey a belief in artificial feeding as equal.

Caregivers need to adopt language that sends a positive message to parents. The manner in which a question is asked can convey the superiority of breastfeeding. Rather than asking a pregnant woman, "Are you going to breastfeed or bottle feed?" she can be asked, "What questions do you have about breastfeeding?" If you were to ask, "How are you going to feed your baby?" the implication is that there is more than one alternative, one of which may be as good as the other.

You can simply make the assumption that all mothers will breastfeed unless you are told otherwise. A pediatrician would not ask a mother, "Are you going to immunize your baby?" Immunizations are important to an infant's health, and the physician would not want to transmit a message that parents can safely choose not to immunize their baby. Unless you believe that an alternative is equally healthy and an equally good choice, you would not want to phrase a question in a manner that leaves the door open for the less healthy choice. And, indeed, human milk is the baby's first immunization! If the woman plans to bottle feed, she may respond, "I'm not breastfeeding." If she is comfortable with that choice, there is no reason to worry about a negative reaction. On the other hand, should she be uncomfortable with her choice and start to question it, you can help her to discuss her concerns and options.

▼ ## Addressing the Issue of Guilt

Although most health workers will tell you they consider breastfeeding to be superior to artificial feeding, the numbers of those who actively promote breastfeeding are much lower. The fear of guilt presents an obstacle for many caregivers—fear of creating guilt in mothers who choose not to breastfeed, fear of causing guilt in mothers who choose to breastfeed and fail, and fear of pressuring mothers to choose to breastfeed. The common theme in all of these fears is the question of choice—the issue of informed consumerism and informed choice. Informed choice implies rights and responsibilities. Parents have a right to the information necessary in making an informed choice about infant feeding. Caregivers have the *responsibility* to inform parents of their options. This is the basis of health consumerism. In teaching parents about the benefits of breastfeeding and the risks of artificial baby milk feeding, caregivers are not making a choice for parents. They are, in fact, fulfilling their responsibility of making parents aware of the issues involved in both feeding methods.

Believing in Breastfeeding's Superiority

If the medical community truly believes in the superiority of breastfeeding over artificial feeding as the healthiest for babies and mothers, guilt should not be an issue. Why would guilt prevent caregivers from promoting healthy practices? Other health issues carry no guilt. When a health care worker advises parents to use an infant car seat for their baby, there is no worry about offending a parent who elects to place their baby in danger by not using a car seat. A pediatrician does not consider guilt when informing parents of the need for immunizations. There is no guilt associated with advice against cigarette smoking or the use of drugs and alcohol for pregnant women. There is no fear of guilt in recommending diets that are low in cholesterol and fat, or advising good hygiene and dental care.

This issue of guilt can be quite complex and confusing relative to infant feeding choice. Many women feel a sense of personal failure at not breastfeeding that does not accompany the failure to stop smoking, the failure to use car seats, or the failure to meet immunization schedules. A woman assumes a risk in making her baby totally dependent on her ability to breastfeed. For some women, taking that risk can be more painful than the guilt of not breastfeeding. Consequently, while choosing to feed artificial baby milk may cause guilt, the mother stays with that choice anyway.

Caregivers have a responsibility to help women feel confident in their ability to breastfeed. Guilt cannot be allowed to prevent caregivers from promoting breastfeeding. Infant formula feeding is inferior to human milk. Caregivers have a responsibility to inform parents of this without reserve. You can help colleagues understand and appreciate this responsibility.

The driving force behind this issue is the caregiver's own commitment and beliefs. Sending messages that are noncommittal lowers the mother's self-confidence and may cause her to question the wisdom of her decision. A noncommittal attitude by the health worker also carries the danger of unwittingly promoting artificial baby milk. If the important differences between the two feeding methods are not explained, parents will be unable to make the necessary distinctions. An ambivalent approach does not advocate breastfeeding over the feeding of a breastmilk substitute. A positive and assertive approach to breastfeeding promotion will convey the appropriate message to parents.

Guilt about Past Actions

Before we leave the topic of guilt, it is important to dispel another form of guilt—guilt you may feel from your own past actions. Perhaps your past practices included formula supplementation, the use of pacifiers, strict rules about frequency and length of feeds, the use of a nipple shield, or sending mothers home with gifts of formula and bottles. Perhaps, in the past, you have presented breastfeeding as being complicated and reliant on a variety of gadgets and special techniques.

Be kind to yourself and recognize that what you did in the past was based on your level of knowledge and what you considered to be appropriate at the time. As you learn more about breastfeeding management—as you learn about the negative consequences of past practices—you change the way you practice. The lactation field continues to evolve in its recommended practices. As long as you are willing to learn and to change based on what you have learned, you cannot expect more from yourself. There is always room for growth and change.

Guilt in Not Promoting Breastfeeding

Consider for a moment the consequences and guilt at not promoting breastfeeding to the mothers in your care. Family finances will be drained because of the cost of infant formula feeding and accompanying devices. Formula fed babies have a higher incidence of illness, sudden infant death syndrome, and emotional neglect and child abuse. They are at a greater risk for developing allergies and asthma. Learning deficiencies are higher, and IQ levels are lower. Infant health may be compromised by the potential for contamination in artificial baby milk. These are realities that are supported by scientific studies (Minchin, 1987; Walker, 1992, 1993).

Perhaps the greatest potential for feelings of guilt on the part of the caregiver lies in the disappointment of mothers who wanted to breastfeed but were unable due to lack of support and encouragement from a caregiver. Omitting information does not contribute to a trusting relationship with mothers. Consider the guilt a mother may feel later in her child's life after diagnosis of an illness for which breastfeeding affords protection. Perhaps, in order to spare a mother guilt, her caregiver did not educate her about the risks of artificial feeding during her decision-making process. She does not choose to breastfeed, and later, her child develops a condition such as recurrent otitis media, which is known to occur more frequently in infants fed artificial milk.

Through the course of her own research into her child's condition, the mother learns that breastfeeding does decrease the risk. This mother may regard her caregiver unfavorably for not educating her about the risk associated with artificial baby milk. Parents want to feel that they have done all they possibly can for their baby. Learning that their baby is experiencing a condition that was partially avoidable will very likely produce guilt and anger. The parents may question why they were not informed of this relationship between their child's condition and breastfeeding. This can erode their confidence in the caregiver and illustrates an important dimension of the health care worker's role in terms of **informed consent**. Your mandate is to give information and responsible advice to parents, and to trust that they will make appropriate decisions.

Guilt in the Context of Parenting

Guilt or no guilt is not the issue. The issue for me is what is best for babies. If the truth makes mothers feel guilty and they develop some anxiety, perhaps the discomfort will tip the scales in favor of breastfeeding."
FRANK OSKI, MD

Webster defines guilt as "the act or state of having done a wrong or committed an offense." It seems reasonable to suggest that a mother who feels guilty about her choice to not breastfeed believes that she is not doing what is in the best interest of her baby. Oski (1995) suggests that guilt can actually serve a positive purpose to families. If parents feel guilty about their infant feeding

choice, the caregiver can generate a discussion of how they can use this feeling of guilt to make them better parents. Guilt can be viewed as a positive emotion within the realm of personal growth. It can serve as motivation to change a particular behavior or actions by parents on behalf of their children. When you are completely honest with parents regarding the risks of artificial feeding, you will usually find that they appreciate being advised of what to watch for if they later introduce infant formula into their baby's diet. You can help parents make guilt work for them as a means to become the best parents they can be. Make it work for you as well, helping you to provide the best advice and guidance possible.

▼
HEALTH CONSUMERISM

The health care system is a consumer-oriented operation that is concerned with attracting clients and keeping them satisfied and healthy. Those who serve the system, both inpatient and outpatient, must be alert to the needs and wishes of their clients and institute policies that will meet these needs. When a partnership is established between parents and their caregivers regarding decision making, the parents accept responsibility for managing their own lives. Mothers need to be well informed about breastfeeding management so that they can clearly understand their options and develop their own skills. This approach builds confidence and self-esteem. It promotes the mother's growth both as an individual and as a parent. The process of each mother's education can be viewed as a joint venture in which the mother helps determine what she needs to know. It is this philosophy of responsible and knowledgeable self-care that forms the basis of the counseling approach evidenced throughout this text.

▼
Informed Consent

Health consumerism is best explained in terms of informed consent. An informed parent is an advocate of health consumerism, either consciously or unconsciously. In weighing the risks involved in medications, operations, and medical procedures, caregivers may at times interject subjectivity into the decision. Based perhaps on tradition or accepted practice, this subjectivity is the cause, in part, for disagreement concerning the best course of treatment for a given situation.

Informed consent benefits both the caregiver and the health consumer. By gaining as much information as possible about a recommended treatment and by exploring alternatives and possible outcomes, the consumer is able to offer knowledgeable and responsible input.

Mothers then can be actively involved in making decisions and in guiding the course of treatment for themselves and their babies. Providers benefit by having some of this responsibility shifted to the consumer. It reduces the risk of malpractice suits in the event of an unfavorable outcome. It also enables the provider to broaden his or her perspective based on consumer input. See Chapter 24 for further discussion of informed consent in relation to the lactation consultant's practice.

Informed consent means that the consumer is consenting to treatment on the basis of sufficient information and education. Consent given in an emergency situation is most likely not truly informed consent. The consumer has not had sufficient time to explore alternatives and to learn the implications involved in the treatment. To be informed fully requires adequate preparation and education before treatment. Informed consent is possible only when the consumer takes the initiative for self-education and the responsibility for informed decision making. Although caregivers can assist the consumer in obtaining information, it is the consumer who initially must request assistance. The majority of medical situations allow adequate time for the consumer to achieve these goals. Even 20 or 30 minutes can permit time for consultation and research. Below are some suggestions you may share with parents who wish to become informed health care consumers. You might want to incorporate these points into a handout for parents.

Suggestions for the Health Care Consumer

◆ Acquire a medical vocabulary, subscribe to health magazines, acquire a small library of consumer-oriented medical references, or use the public library.

◆ Attend courses for nonprofessionals, such as classes in first aid or home health care. You can check local high schools, colleges, or civic organizations for such programs.

◆ Enlist the services of physicians and hospitals who welcome and encourage actively informed patients.

◆ When choosing **prepared childbirth** classes, select those that will provide information on alternatives, enhance your understanding, and encourage active participation in medical decisions.

◆ Learn to recognize early symptoms of illness, and investigate appropriate methods of treatment before contacting the physician. This will enable you to discuss the situation with the physician in an informed and concrete manner.

◆ If you are unfamiliar with a medical term or do not understand what you are being told, ask to have the point clarified and explained in simpler terms.

◆ Discuss alternatives with your physician, and ask why one course of treatment was chosen over another.

◆ If the situation warrants, seek a second (and even third) opinion. This is your right and your responsibility.

◆ Learn the cost for a recommended treatment, as well as alternative treatments.

◆ If you are uncomfortable or dissatisfied with your physician's advice, you are in most cases not legally committed to comply. You must, however, be aware of the medical risks. You have the right to make your own choices. Even if it seems to the caregiver that you have made a wrong choice, the ultimate consequences and responsibilities are yours.

Informed consent is not a prerequisite for quality health care. It does, however, ensure better chances for the consumer who has accepted the responsibility for becoming knowledgeable and actively involved in his or her own health care. Health care professionals should be chosen wisely and should be used as resources. The ultimate responsibility for informed decisions rests with the consumer.

◆ A Parent's Role in the Health Care System

An active health consumer is an informed person who is a responsible decision maker concerning health care. It is a person who becomes actively involved in the health care of all family members. Until recently, many parents have had few choices about their experiences, with hospital and physician policies dictating the course of their health care. Real change happens when an awareness and attitude shift occurs among caregivers and administrators. A health care delivery system that increases the incidence and duration of breastfeeding will create cost savings over the life span of both the mother and child. If breastfeeding is not actively supported, there will be a financial loss to the system.

If the health care system does not meet the needs of the parents, a change of care providers may or may not be an option. In the years before managed care, satisfaction could be expressed through simply changing providers or hospitals. In managed care, often the option to change providers is limited to once-a-year enrollment through the client's employer. Consequently, consumer action is more concentrated in written expression of both positive and negative experiences while continuing to receive care within the system. You can encourage positive change by urging parents to express their concerns. Those aspects of care that are positive may also be reinforced through positive, written comments.

Parents who have not been accustomed to being actively involved in health care may need guidance from you in assuming a more active role. They will need to know what their rights are and the accompanying responsibilities. Also, they will need to know how to communicate their desires to physicians and hospital staff to ensure effective and positive interaction and a healthy working relationship between physician and patient.

Consumer Rights and Responsibilities

Consumers and providers share a two-way relationship. Rights and responsibilities go hand in hand. Occasionally, parents may need information in order to grow as consumers. You can provide them with the facts they need concerning their rights and responsibilities. A signed consent form is the consumer's best friend. Parents have used this as a means of obtaining their wishes, such as ensuring that no procedure may be done on their hospitalized child without the parents being present. If a mother finds that the hospital is doing something she does not want, such as giving supplemental feeds to her baby, she can ask for the consent form and amend it. Urge mothers to check the patient's bill of rights in their hospital. Below are rights that should be provided to every breastfeeding mother.

The mother has the right

- To understand what she is giving consent to.
- To receive information concerning a drug or treatment prior to its administration.
- To know alternative methods.
- To accept or refuse treatment or advice without pressure.
- To know if a procedure is medically indicated or elective.
- To have access to her complete medical records.
- To seek another medical opinion.
- To be kept informed of the most up-to-date information.
- To be treated as an equal partner in her health care.
- To have her questions answered completely and courteously.
- To be treated with respect.
- To be provided with the best care possible, with a focus on prevention.
- To make decisions regarding her own treatment and that of her infant.
- To care for herself and her infant to the maximum extent she is able.

The mother has the responsibility

- To find out what is available and make an informed choice.
- To find caregivers who can help her reach her goals.
- To listen to her caregivers with an open mind.
- To let her preferences be known in a courteous manner.
- To carry through on an agreed plan or cure.
- To find out the approximate cost of a procedure in advance.
- To state why she changes caregivers, if applicable.

The Lactation Consultant's Role in Health Consumerism

In defining your role as a consultant to consumers in the health care system, it is important to keep in mind that one of your goals is to encourage parents to take responsibility for their own actions. This applies to areas of health care as well as parenting. In your role as an advocate for health consumerism, you may wonder how to educate parents about options that you know they cannot have with their present provider. You might question if you should simply prepare them to deal with the health care available within the framework of their current medical relationships. In your caregiving role, you do not want to suggest to parents that they change providers. It is the parents' responsibility to select and work with their medical services.

A lactation consultant, as a member of the health care team, will be viewed by the mother as a knowledgeable professional. You need to be tactful in counseling mothers regarding their relationships with physicians. You can, however, help parents with choices after their medical relationships have been established. Recognize, too, that parents may at times choose a course of action with which you disagree either personally or professionally. You will need to examine your own position and decide to what extent it is appropriate for you to become involved.

Helping Parents Become Better Health Consumers

Parents are responsible for the health of their children as well as themselves, and so they have compound consumer roles and interests. Your primary means of helping parents become good consumers is by educating the mother about breastfeeding through reading, conversations, classes, and meetings. It is through breastfeeding mothers that we can heighten awareness within the health care system. Encourage a mother to tell her physician how increasing feeding frequency helped increase her milk production. Suggest that she convey to her health care team how the importance of breastfeeding goes far beyond the milk her baby receives. Guide parents to the many consumer-oriented books that are available.

When you answer parents' questions, first determine whether or not they are informed consumers. They may be unaccustomed to questioning statements made by physicians. Often, the first time a mother will realize that she may disagree with a physician is when she is told to supplement her milk with artificial baby milk or to introduce solid foods into her baby's diet. You can help a mother gain confidence in herself and her maternal instincts regarding her baby's needs. Emphasize to her that she is the one who knows her baby best. Help her become attuned to her baby's behavior and to understand her baby's needs. A newborn feeding every 2 hours may appear to her to be a problem unless she understands why. When she understands, she will be less likely to ask her baby's physician, "Do I have enough milk?" By helping mothers progress from where they are to the next step, and then another step, you can develop their awareness of their rights and responsibilities as health care consumers.

You can also help a mother understand the difference between parenting issues and medical advice. For several reasons, parents often turn to medical professionals for answers to parenting concerns. If a mother asks a physician what to do about her baby waking at night and her physician suggests letting the baby cry or giving solid foods at 10 P.M., this is parenting advice, not medical advice. Most issues in the breastfeeding arena are, in fact, parenting concerns that do not require medical advice. What the concerns do require are informed parents who have faith in their abilities to determine what is best for their baby.

A good approach is to present facts to help parents find the options that best suit their needs and goals. This pertains to all aspects of childbirth, breastfeeding, and parenting. You can teach parents the benefits of family-centered maternity care, prepared childbirth, rooming-in, exclusive breastfeeding for 4 to 6 months, and so forth. You are not establishing goals for parents. Rather, you are educating them about alternatives that will help them go about establishing and achieving their own goals—even if you do not always agree. Your role is to stimulate parents in assuming more responsibility for their health care. Many times, all they will need are suggestions for questions they can ask their physicians.

RELINQUISHING CONTROL

Fostering informed consumerism and decision making among parents requires that the caregiver relinquish much of the control that has traditionally been associated with patient care. It is rare to find an adult who has not experienced a hospitalization at some time in his or her life. The majority of hospitalized patients are ill or injured. This, however, is not the case with a woman who enters the hospital to deliver her baby. Despite this, she loses a certain amount of control the moment she passes through the door. Her privacy is invaded, and she

is placed in a dependent role. Often, hospital and physician policies impose unnecessary controls over a mother and her newborn. Decisions are made about her care and that of her baby, decisions that are too often outside the mother's control. The medical community needs to regard a new mother differently than it does an ill or injured patient. New mothers need to be given greater control and options regarding their care and that of their infants.

The caregiver's goal should be one of empowering the breastfeeding mother to be independent and self-reliant. When she feels controlled, she may not recognize ways to help herself. She needs to use her own resources in order to become self-sufficient. If she becomes dependent on others, she may lose sight of her own resources. She will expect others to solve her problems and find solutions; and she may blame those same people when they do not come through for her.

Medical intervention should never be initiated without a clear and specific purpose. Breastfeeding advice often imposes too many rules—advice to always hold the breast during a feed, to wear a bra that gives good support, to avoid certain foods, to watch the clock, to always use both breasts at a feed, and the like. These and other arbitrary rules about separating mothers and babies or giving bottles to breastfeeding babies are not well founded and cause harm to the establishment of breastfeeding. A cavalier attitude about such practices is counterproductive to the goal of empowering the mother. Chloe Fisher (1996), a midwife in London, tells us there is only one rule in breastfeeding. The rule is: There are no rules!

Control is important to a new mother. She may need to re-establish control following birth and may lack control for a new venture such as breastfeeding. Even if this is not her first child, it may be the first child she is breastfeeding. She needs you and other caregivers to help her gain control or retain the amount of control she has already established.

Take care not to allow control issues to compromise the care that is given to mothers and babies. Policies of the medical staff should model self-reliance and parental decision making from the very beginning. This requires a negotiation of control between the caregiver and patient. The vast majority of breastfeeding issues fall within the realm of parenting rather than medical decision making. Caregivers need to become comfortable with relinquishing unnecessary control and placing control with babies and mothers where it belongs.

Trusting in Mothers and Babies

Relinquishing control requires that caregivers trust that mothers and babies are capable of assuming the control. As you proceed through this text, it will become clear that newborns have amazing capabilities from the very moment of birth. If caregivers refrain from interfering with the process, and if mothers are taught how to read infant language, the baby can exert tremendous control in having his needs met. Further, when mothers are allowed to exercise legitimate control, they feel more independent, self-reliant, and confident. They learn to trust themselves and their babies. Consequently, they find it easier to adjust to the maternal role, and become responsible for their own learning. They develop problem-solving skills, accept the consequences of their own decisions and actions, and control their own outcomes. Use words and actions that show that you believe in the mother's abilities. Trust your instincts to put the mother and baby in control, not the staff.

USING AN ADULT LEARNING APPROACH

A mother's control over her care will be enhanced when the caregiver uses an adult learning approach during consultations and discussions. The adult learning approach is one of learning rather than being taught. With this concept, you serve as a facilitator rather than a teacher. Simply telling a mother what to do and prescribing a course of care are not as effective as including the mother in the learning process. In other words, the sage on the stage needs to be replaced by the guide on the side. As a facilitator of the mother's learning, you explore options with the mother and guide her as she

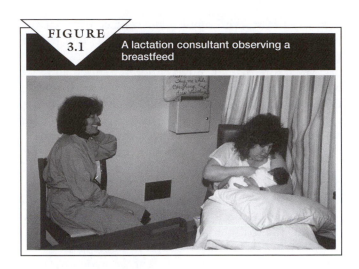

FIGURE 3.1 A lactation consultant observing a breastfeed

plans her course of care with you. This requires that she be an active participant in the learning. Your role is to provide choices and encourage the mother to select those that will work for her.

Your goal is to develop a partnership with the mother and baby, to form a problem-solving team. One of your most important functions is to observe at least one breastfeed with every mother and baby in your care, watching how they learn to respond to one another (Fig. 3.1). Observe how the first breastfeed goes, and realize that the baby may want only to nuzzle at the breast in the early hours. There is no need to rush the first feed. Remember that you are moving at the baby's pace, not yours and not the mother's. Holding the baby

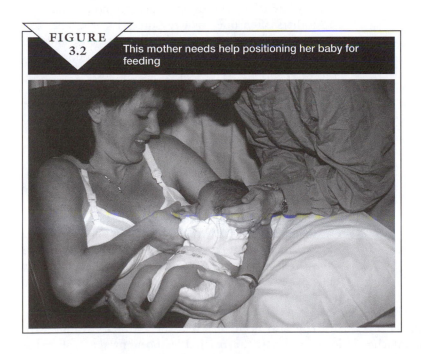

FIGURE 3.2 This mother needs help positioning her baby for feeding

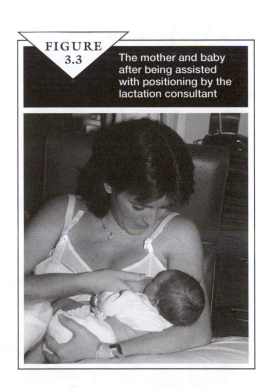

FIGURE 3.3 The mother and baby after being assisted with positioning by the lactation consultant

near the breast, with ample skin contact between the baby and mother, will help them bond and initiate breastfeeding when the baby is interested.

Make sure that any intervention is focused and that you have a good reason for becoming actively involved. Confine your interactions to guiding more than directing unless intervention is needed. Recognize times when you need to become more actively involved with a mother and times when you should keep your hands in your pockets. For instance, if the baby is not positioned well enough to get a good latch, you can gently instruct the mother how to adjust her hold (Figs. 3.2 and 3.3). This does not require that you take charge and put the baby to the mother's breast yourself. Rather, you can talk her through it, perhaps modeling it yourself with a teaching doll. This approach puts the mother in control and actively involves her in the learning process.

Making Positive Impressions on Adult Learners

Adult learners respond to a learning experience in much the same way as adolescent learners. However, their expectations may be greater in some areas more than in others. The manner in which adults interact and their assessment of the facilitator's credibility make the dynamics quite different from interactions with adolescents. Some guidelines follow that will help you make positive impressions on adults.

◆ A display of self-confidence.
◆ A desire to share knowledge.
◆ An ability to relate to people.
◆ A willingness to be flexible and adapt.
◆ A sense of humor.
◆ A strong knowledge base.
◆ Enthusiasm.
◆ A comfortable tone of informality.
◆ Respect for the learner.
◆ Frequent eye contact.
◆ Positive **body language.**
◆ Neat, clean, and stylish attire.
◆ A strong voice with carefully pronounced words.

Creating an Effective Learning Climate

You will want to create an effective atmosphere for interactions with mothers. An effective learning environment is one that encourages the learner to be an active participant. Malcolm Knowles says that "People attach more meaning to learnings they gain from experience than those they acquire passively" (Knowles, 1980). Through your body language and the effective use of communication and counseling skills, you can create a climate that is relaxed, trusting, mutually respectful, informal, warm, collaborative, and supportive.

Within this climate, planning is accomplished mutually by you and the mother. A partnership is formed as you and the mother explore issues together. This approach encourages self-direction and risk taking among mothers. The mother develops problem-solving skills and becomes more self-reliant. When the mother takes an active part in setting her goals, she has ownership for the plan and is responsible for the outcome. As partners, you mutually evaluate the mother's needs and set objectives. You can present choices and ask, "What will work for you?" Such learning actively involves the mother, as she practices techniques you have shown to her. Similarly, urge the mother to evaluate her own learning, because she knows best what has been learned. You may ask, for instance, "How will you change your breastfeeding pattern when you get home?" With this approach, the mother develops increased competence and confidence, which fosters greater self-esteem and independence.

Individualizing Your Approach

Recognize that every mother and baby are unique and that your approach will vary with each contact. Every mother you see will have her own array of experiences and resources that will make her needs different from others. Learning will be more effective and personalized when you respect the mother's background and tap into it. Mothers often offer rich resources for learning. You may find at times that the mother is the teacher and you are the learner! Remaining open to such opportunities will help you grow as a lactation consultant.

Be sure to assess each mother's learning needs before you enter into problem solving. Is this her first baby, or does she have previous parenting experience? What exposure has she had to breastfeeding—does she have relatives or friends who breastfed, has she breastfed before, what has she read or heard about breastfeeding? Inquire about her support system and resources. Does she have someone to help her with caring for her baby or with breastfeeding? Help the mother accommodate breastfeeding to her lifestyle. Will she be separated from her baby because of employment? Is she a teen mother? Does she live with her extended family? Does she have an active social life? All of these areas will help you determine your approach with this particular mother and baby.

You also need to assess the mother's readiness to learn. When is the **teachable moment** that will maximize her ability to learn and process information? How is her health and that of her baby? Is she in any physical discomfort? What is her confidence level—her emotional state? If she is anxious about her baby's health or discouraged because of difficulty with breastfeeding, you must first address her emotional needs before addressing breastfeeding issues. Until these issues are addressed, she may be unable to focus on learning or problem solving.

Using this approach will help you individualize your objectives and your problem-solving techniques with each dyad. You want to avoid using an established agenda and be ready to adjust your objectives based on input from the mother and baby. Remember, too, that you do not need to teach everything to every mother. Assessing her needs and her readiness to learn will help you recognize what to teach each mother. Keep pace with the mother and slow down if you sense that she is not taking in what you are saying. Using her language style and imagery will help you relate to one another. Matching her intensity and her sense of humor will help you adopt an appropriate approach. Watch for responses, and tailor your actions accordingly. Mothers respond well to this personalized approach.

Each mother brings with her a rich background of experience and capabilities. Some appear confident and knowledgeable. Others have a greater need for increasing their self-esteem and confidence. You will want to capitalize on each mother's strengths and build on her present capabilities. When she has learned a technique or overcome an obstacle, praise her for her accomplishment. Find something to praise about her baby as well, for example, "See how your baby looks at you." When you relate to mothers on a personal level, your helping relationship will be strengthened. Make it a point to use the mother's and baby's names, and to focus on the whole person, rather than the mother's breasts or particular condition. Regarding every mother and baby as a unique dyad and broadening your scope beyond the immediate situation will enhance your effectiveness as their caregiver.

The Learning Process

Involving the mother as an active participant in her learning will improve her outcome. Learning takes place at three levels. The most effective learning is achieved when the learner is actively involved. The lowest level of learning takes place when information is shared verbally. Learning increases when something visual is added to the verbal instruction. However, the level at which learning is most effective is one in which the learner participates actively in the learning process. This demonstrates the importance of the mother taking an active part in her learning. One way to characterize this learning curve is "I hear and I forget, I see and I remember, I do and I

understand." Stated in a similar fashion, the three levels are "Tell me and I may remember, show me and I may understand, involve me and I may master." Some examples of breastfeeding teaching at these levels follow:

- *Tell me and I may remember:* There will be times in your interactions with mothers when verbal instructions are sufficient and appropriate. A discussion of **contraception,** nutrition, or medications, for instance, can be approached in this way. You are sharing information that does not require visual or interactive reinforcement.

- *Show me and I may understand:* Much of the teaching you do with mothers will be enhanced by demonstrations of some sort. When you teach a mother how to position her baby at the breast, for example, you can demonstrate this process with a doll. A chart showing the anatomy of the breast will also be helpful. In teaching **manual expression,** a cloth breast can be used to show the location of the lactiferous sinuses and the expression technique. Use of a breast pump requires demonstration as well. Discussions such as engorgement, mastitis, nipple soreness, and thrush may also benefit by the use of a cloth breast and photographs (Fig. 3.4).

- *Involve me and I may master:* Although demonstrations are helpful, the mother's learning will be enhanced even more when she practices the various procedures with you. While you are positioning the doll for feeding, at the same time the mother can position her own baby at the breast. While you are demonstrating manual expression or the use of a breast pump, the mother can attempt to do so with her own breast. This learning method provides you with visual reinforcement to show that the mother

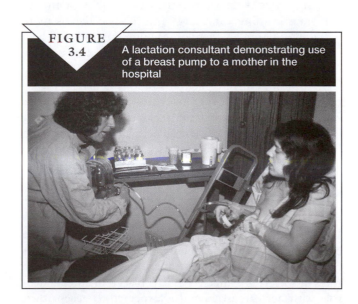

FIGURE 3.4 A lactation consultant demonstrating use of a breast pump to a mother in the hospital

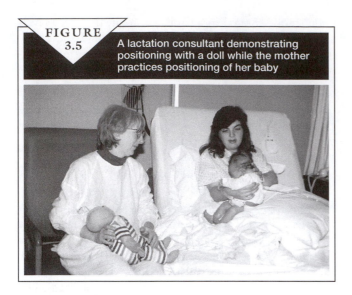

FIGURE
3.5
A lactation consultant demonstrating positioning with a doll while the mother practices positioning of her baby

has mastered the technique being taught. Such return demonstrations are essential to the mother's learning and growth (Fig. 3.5).

Learning Styles

Your approach also needs to correspond to the mother's own learning style. People tend to favor one side of the brain over another in their learning styles. Generally, those with dominance in the left brain learn better from verbal instruction. They respond well to analytic and logical information. Right brain learners respond more readily to images, symbols, intuition, and emotion. Although you may not be able to determine the learning style of every mother in your care, there are things you can do regardless of learning style to make the learning more effective.

You can adopt an approach that helps merge both learning styles. Characteristics of both right brain and left brain learning can merge into a style that is more integrated. Using a variety of teaching methods will help you achieve this integration. Written instructions, verbal instructions, visual aids, videotapes, and interactive learning in the form of demonstrations and verbal feedback are techniques you may use. Also, humor helps open both sides of the brain, making it more likely that integrative learning will take place. Therefore, infusing humor into your interactions with mothers will enhance their learning. It also makes your job more enjoyable!

▼ Using Humor as a Communication Tool

Humor serves as an indirect form of communication between caregivers and clients. When a woman enters the hospital or physician's office, many of the typical rules of society are affected. She is placed in a dependent role with her caregivers and is expected to accept their

concern and competency almost on faith. Humor can help the caregiver establish trust with the mother. With so little time to build a relationship in the health care setting, you will want to use any tools that are available to you to facilitate this process. The relaxed atmosphere created by the use of humor will help you develop relationships in which mothers will heed your advice and follow through with their plan of care.

Your goal is to make learning fun for breastfeeding mothers. This sounds so simple. Yet mothers who lack self-confidence, who are anxious about their ability to breastfeed, or who have little support from family or friends may find it difficult to access their sense of humor and find enjoyment. You can help by approaching mothers in a friendly manner that shows your humanness. When they are first initiating breastfeeding or when they confront challenges, help them see humor in their situation so that they can learn to not take it too seriously. Incorporating laughter into learning helps ensure that the lesson is learned well. Humanizing your interactions will help you achieve your ultimate goal of a happy mother and baby.

Using humor as a tool may not be as easy as it sounds. We adults, and especially those who work in the medical profession, tend to take ourselves too seriously! As lactation consultants, we are often so intent on becoming better in our profession that we do not take the time to enjoy ourselves in the process. We need to become comfortable with having fun and incorporating humor in our work. Humor is something we choose, just as we choose to be in a foul mood or we choose to see the negative side of things. As members of the health profession, we need to be able to laugh at ourselves and learn to take ourselves more lightly. Learning to laugh at life and at the challenges we face will help us keep perspective and find solutions. Humor, therefore, can help our clients as well. It can help them to deal with their own stresses, tensions, and frustrations (Fig. 3.6).

The Role of Humor in the Health System

In order to tap into our own sense of humor, we need to first understand the nature of humor. Humor is more than an occasional witticism—it is a way of life, an attitude. Humor has a direct effect on both mental and physical health, and as such, it is important in all aspects of one's life. Two books that serve as wonderful resources are *Humor and the Health Professions: The Therapeutic Use of Humor in Health Care,* by Vera Robinson (1991) and *Anatomy of an Illness,* by Norman Cousins (1979).

A sense of humor helps you give the best of yourself to others. Humor in the health system is essentially humanism. Approaching clients in a humanistic manner shows each mother that you accept her as a person. It

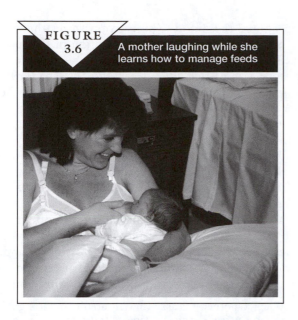

FIGURE 3.6 A mother laughing while she learns how to manage feeds

shows that you respect and care for her, and that you genuinely want to help her. You are, in essence, accepting the mother's own humanness. Humor evolves naturally in a relaxed climate of warmth and caring. Such an atmosphere enhances a mother's self-concept and helps her be more tolerant and more understanding of herself and her baby. The warmth and caring that you transmit to the mother will help her use humor to relieve the stresses of learning how to be a mother and how to breastfeed her new baby. She is better able to laugh at herself and shake off missteps as she and her baby learn to respond to one another.

It is not always the big stresses that get to us. Life is full of daily events and obstacles that pile up. We can choose to let those things make us miserable, or we can choose to use our humor and a positive outlook to help us put it all into perspective. In the world of health care, the stresses may seem even more monumental, primarily because the stress is accompanied by a loss of privacy and a loss of control. Traditionally, health care professionals are socialized not to interject humor into interactions with patients. However, humor has many faces. It may come through in the form of a warm and friendly approach, a smile, or a light touch. Such pleasantries are a valuable use of humor in your work as a lactation consultant.

The Health Benefits of Humor

In *Anatomy of an Illness*, Cousins wrote about events in his own life that were reported in 1976 in the New England Journal of Medicine. He used humor therapy to recover from a life-threatening disease that produced intense pain and paralysis. His health improved by eliminating all medications, taking heavy doses of vitamin C, and scheduling laughter sessions—videos of Candid Camera and the Marx Brothers, along with humor books. Cousins found that 10 minutes of genuine laughter had an anesthetic effect that gave him at least 2 hours of pain-free sleep. Gradually, he was able to regain movement and recover.

Humor actually causes a biochemical change in the body that is enormously healing and therapeutic. Eliciting laughter from a mother can produce positive effects in most of her body's major physiologic systems. Laughter speeds up heart rate, raises blood pressure, accelerates breathing, and increases oxygen consumption. It can stimulate muscles and relax muscle tension, thereby reducing pain and anxiety. Laughter stimulates the cardiovascular system, the sympathetic nervous system, and the production of catecholamines and endorphins, thus boosting the immune system. Laughter increases adrenaline in the brain, which stimulates alertness and memory and enhances learning and creativity. Following this arousal state, respiration, heart rate, and muscle tension actually return to below normal levels (Robinson, 1991). Perhaps it is for this reason that there are Laughter Clubs in India, whose members meet in the town square for a short period of laughter before beginning the work day!

Physiologic benefits of laughter demonstrate that humor and a positive outlook can help in the healing process and disease prevention. Clearly, negative emotions can create organic changes within the body such as headaches and ulcers. It stands to reason, therefore, that positive emotions can produce positive biochemical changes in the body. When mothers have a positive outlook, they will be more likely to meet new challenges with enthusiasm and optimism.

Humor Enhances Learning

It was stated earlier that humor enhances learning and productivity. Humor and laughter reduce tension and anxiety and contribute to learning enjoyment, interest, motivation, and creativity. A humorous approach with mothers helps stimulate divergent thinking. It opens the way to the mother accepting new ways of looking at a situation. It frees the flow of ideas so that mothers can consider new alternatives and solutions. Humor stimulates both the right and left hemispheres of the brain at the same time, to create a level of consciousness and of brain processing that enables the brain to work at its fullest capacity. When the right and left brain are integrated and functioning simultaneously, the capacity for learning is at its highest level. Humor helps achieve this goal.

As part of the mother's health care team, you can lighten the mood to facilitate a mother's learning and make learning fun. Shared laughter will energize both of you, enabling you to get back to helping the mother. Humor also increases a mother's ability to take risks.

She will be more comfortable and will feel more welcome to ask questions and offer input. She will also be more receptive to your advice. Humor gets people to listen. Humor is graphic. It creates images in the learner's mind and helps the learner to remember better and longer. When you can get a humorous reaction, you relax enough so that you can give the best of yourself to the mother.

The appropriate use of humor can help mothers gain perspective and see that a situation is not so serious. When humor is blended in the right atmosphere, with the right timing, and the right style and is offered to a receptive mother, it will enhance your interactions. You can learn to determine the need for humor and your purpose in using humor with breastfeeding clients. Humor is as much a form of preventive medicine as breastfeeding. It will help mothers to relax, which facilitates oxytocin release. It increases a mother's self-confidence and improves her frame of mind and perspective. Humor helps the mother enjoy her baby. Your use of humor with the mother will teach her to see and use humor herself.

Using Humor to Relieve Stress

The value of humor was recognized in the emergency room of St. Christopher's Hospital for Children in Philadelphia. The June 1992 issue of *Pediatrics* reported on a retrospective review of their most interesting chief complaints over a 20-year period. "Some complaints that were charted and recorded in a notebook included "Needs circumcision because his tonsils and adenoids are so big"; "Can't find the baby's birthmark"; "Drank the dog's milk—from the dog's nipple"; "Lump down in his tentacle"; and "Swollen asteroids." Among the interesting telephone inquiries were "Hello, I would like to schedule an emergency" and "My little girl just kissed a dead chicken. Should I bring her in?" The staff recognized that these statements would help to buoy the spirits of an Emergency Department staff stressed by long hours and a hectic work environment" (Nelson, 1992).

Lactation consultants might develop a similar notebook with humorous lactation situations. Using amusing terminology or a play on words may help you teach techniques to a mother. One lactation consultant makes it a point to use humor frequently with mothers. Linda Kutner (1996) refers to the **cross-cradle hold** as the chicken hold. "I show the mother how her elbow is pointed out like the wing of a chicken. I wave it up and down and go 'cluck, cluck.' This gets the mother laughing and relaxes her." That mother is also more likely to remember the technique she was being taught. People tend to remember stories more than any other form of teaching.

If a mother develops sore nipples, she may be very discouraged about the prospect of breastfeeding. To help lighten the mood, Kutner sympathizes that there are two things necessary for propagation of the species that should be pleasurable and not hurt—and the second one is breastfeeding. If a mother has had a long labor and her baby will not nurse, she is probably very concerned that something is wrong, that her baby will starve, and that breastfeeding will not work for her. Kutner points out to this mother that her baby was standing on his head for 16 hours knocking at the door, and he probably has a headache! A humorous image can help the mother relax, chuckle, and realize that things will be okay.

You can also share an amusing anecdote that may have happened to another mother in similar circumstances. Keeping a humor diary will help you to capture such moments. The humor is out there just waiting for you to capitalize on it in your interactions with mothers.

> When a mother was asked, "Why aren't you going to breastfeed?" she answered, "It doesn't run in my family."
> A mother at a dinner party had her baby pull off just as her milk let down. Her dinner partner, mystified by the sudden droplets on his sleeve, brushed them off and gazed at the ceiling to find the leak.
> A mother and father were in the recovery room following a cesarean delivery. The father turned to the nurse and asked, "Did they pierce her nipples yet to let the milk out?"

The use of humor in communication, when used appropriately, will enhance your effectiveness and enrich the lives of your clients and colleagues. We all need to stay in touch with the child inside us. In the words of a favorite song sung by the Brownies,

> I have something in my pocket that belongs across my face.
> I keep it very close at hand in the most convenient place.
> I'm sure you couldn't guess it if you guessed a long long while,
> So I'll take it out and put it on as a great big Brownie smile!

▼

COMPONENTS OF COMMUNICATION

The process of communication requires two basic elements: the delivery and the reception of a message. When transmitting a message from one person to another, the way in which the message is received depends on a combination of three factors—body language, tone of voice, and the spoken message (Fast, 1970). As you will discover below, a far greater impression is made by nonverbal language than by the words that are spoken. A person may be highly knowledgeable about every aspect of breastfeeding management and lactation. However, that knowledge will be lost if it is not shared in an effective manner.

The Importance of the Spoken Word

The actual words you speak have a relatively low bearing on the message the mother receives. The message that is conveyed is determined only 7 percent by the spoken word. On the face of it, this statement seems quite startling. You will study a variety of books, attend classes and conferences, and network with colleagues in an effort to learn all that is necessary about breastfeeding management in order to help mothers. Yet, the verbal communication of that information alone has relatively little impact on the mother. There are, however, certain words and phrases that may impact negatively and therefore need to be avoided.

Negative Terminology

The words and phrases you use can influence the mother's emotional reaction to what is said. Negative messages can be conveyed with poorly chosen words. Therefore, you want to avoid terminology that will impact negatively on the mother's impression or suggest that she is doing something incorrectly. There are two specific words you can eliminate from your vocabulary in order to be an effective communicator with breastfeeding mothers.

The first word to avoid is the word "but". When you join two thoughts with but, you may not achieve your intended outcome. It actually negates the first half of the thought. You may say to a mother, "You are holding your baby in a good position, but if you turn him slightly toward you he can get a better latch." Without intending to, you have told the mother that she was not holding her baby correctly. The mother might think, "I'm not holding my baby right. I feel so dumb!" As soon as the mother hears the word "but," a negative impression is created and the first part of the statement is forgotten. Your intention was to teach the mother how to hold her baby during breastfeeding. However, with your phraseology, you have undermined her self-confidence as a new mother.

If you wish to connect two thoughts and at the same time correct the mother, you can simply replace the word "but" with "and." With the same statement, you could rephrase it like this: "You are holding your baby in a good position, and if you turn him slightly you will find that he can get an even better latch." Another way to phrase it is: "That's a good start. Now, you can turn him slightly toward you so that he can get a better latch." You have succeeded in helping the mother improve the manner in which she holds her baby and at the same time you have avoided any suggestion that the mother is doing something incorrectly. You have preserved her self-confidence and helped her to grow as a mother.

The other word to eliminate from your vocabulary is the word "should". Consider these statements by a consultant who is attempting to teach the concept of **need feeding** and the avoidance of artificial nipples. She advises: "You should feed your baby whenever he wants." "You shouldn't give your baby a pacifier." With such phrasing, you risk sounding judgmental to the mother. The implication is that the mother should breastfeed in the way which you consider to be correct and appropriate. To state that a mother should do something implies that she was doing something she should not have done, or that she is doing something incorrectly.

Advice can be offered in a more effective manner without diluting the message. How, then, can you teach the concept of need feeding and the avoidance of artificial nipples? You may reword the above-mentioned statements in this way: "When you feed your baby whenever he wants, you will be meeting his needs." and, "Because a baby sucks so differently on an artificial nipple and the breast, if a breastfed baby receives a pacifier it can confuse him when he tries to suckle at the breast." Notice that incorrect or inappropriate practices are being corrected and at the same time you are educating the mother about the reasons for the advice. You are avoiding sending a judgmental message or undermining the mother's confidence.

Negative Imagery

You also need to avoid words that create negative images. It seems that such words abound in women's health—an *incompetent* cervix, *failure* to progress, *inadequate* milk supply, a baby who is *not* satisfied. Even words that are intended to be positive can suggest the possibility of something negative. If you refer to a mother as being *successful* with her breastfeeding, you raise the possibility that she may be unsuccessful. If you talk to a mother about establishing an *adequate* milk supply, you may be suggesting that her milk supply might be inadequate. You can rephrase both of these messages by referring to the mother as reaching her breastfeeding goals and producing enough milk to meet her baby's needs.

Mixed Messages

Take care not to use phrases that will create doubt in a mother's mind, send mixed messages, or compromise her self-confidence. Consider the message you may be sending to a mother with the following statements:

> Statement: You need your rest. I'll take your baby to the nursery for you.
> Message: You cannot get enough rest if you keep your baby with you. It does not really matter if you skip a feeding. We can give the baby a bottle of formula. Formula is just as good as your milk.

Statement: Are you going to try to breastfeed?
> Message: You might not be able to breastfeed. A lot of mothers try and fail. You can go ahead and try but do not be surprised if it does not work.

Statement: Do you have any milk yet?
> Message: You might not have enough milk for your baby. We might need to give your baby a bottle. You should have more milk by now. Some women never establish a good enough supply of milk.

These certainly are not the messages you intended to send. Be certain that the words you use create the effect you want. You can tactfully help other caregivers recognize the effects of such phrases as well. Knowing that much of your spoken message will be eclipsed by other elements of communication, you can supplement your verbal messages with demonstrations, visual aids, written instructions, and careful attention to your voice tone and body language.

▼ The Effect of Voice Tone

You can undoubtedly recall a time when you talked with another person on the telephone and could tell by the sound of his or her voice that this was a person you hoped you would never have to deal with again! You can probably also recall a time when the sound of another person's voice was so pleasant that it enhanced your exchange. You sensed this was a person with whom you would enjoy interacting. Your tone of voice has a dramatic effect on the manner in which mothers respond to you. In fact, your voice tone is responsible for 38 percent of the message received by the mother.

Make sure that your voice tone matches the message you want to send, both to mothers and to colleagues. You can create a warm, friendly, even humorous atmosphere through your manner of speech. The warmth of a smile even comes through in your voice. Take a moment to evaluate your speech. How is the volume—is your voice too loud or too low? Consider your rate of speech. Do you talk too fast or too slow? Do you remember to breathe, or do you seem rushed because you run out of breath? And how about pitch—does your voice get higher when you are angry or excited? All of these aspects of your speech can have an effect on the message you convey. Moderating the rate and pitch of your voice and talking slowly enough to pause and breathe will help you achieve an effective voice tone.

▼ The Effect of Body Language

Of the three components in communication, body language has the greatest effect on the manner in which a message is received—55 percent. Body language is based on the behavioral patterns of nonverbal communication and is a study of the mixture of all body movements. These include smiling, eye contact, posture, space, and touching. Body language ranges from the very deliberate gesture to the unconscious. It may apply in only one culture or span across cultural barriers. In addition to sending and receiving messages, body language can also serve to break through defenses. The manner in which you capitalize on your nonverbal messages will determine your effectiveness in the care you give to mothers.

Smile

A pleasant facial expression adds to a warm and inviting atmosphere. A calm, relaxed smile says that you enjoy your work and enjoy meeting people. That kind of smile will put mothers at ease. When you smile, you elicit a smile from the mother as well. She cannot help it—it is human nature! It is almost impossible not to return a smile.

Eye Contact

The eyes are the most important of all the body parts in transmitting information. When you are involved in an interchange with another person, try to maintain eye contact at least 85 percent of the time. Eye contact has a powerful impact on your message. Establishing eye contact with a mother conveys your desire to communicate with her. It establishes a warm, caring, and inviting climate. Eye contact can also be a powerful tool for influencing others. The next time you are competing for a parking place or trying to merge into traffic, if you are able to establish eye contact with the driver in the other car, the driver will probably bend to your wishes. If you are standing in line for a movie and another person tries to cut into the line, look the other person straight in the eye. Chances are the other person will turn away and go to the back of the line.

Be aware of the power your eye contact has on the messages you send. Failing to establish eye contact sends a message as well. We all use this tactic to avoid talking with someone or being seen by them. Consider, therefore, the message you send if you talk to a mother with your back turned or your eyes focused on what you are writing (Fig. 3.7). You have a powerful communication tool, two of them! Consciously engaging in eye contact with mothers in your care will enhance your interactions and your effectiveness.

Posture

Posture is another aspect of body language that sends a strong message. To create a warm and inviting climate, you want your body to be relaxed and comfortable. Try to avoid crossing your arms or legs, because this can

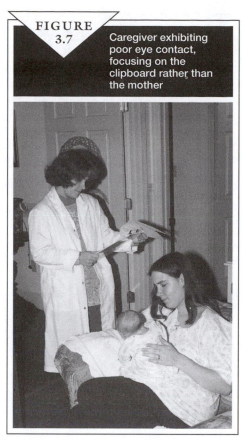

> **FIGURE 3.7**
> Caregiver exhibiting poor eye contact, focusing on the clipboard rather than the mother

Used by permission of Debbie Shinskie.

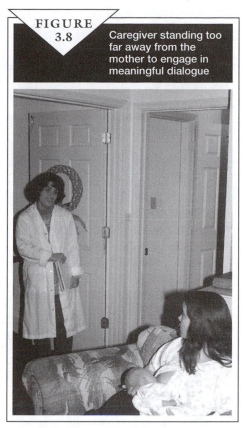

> **FIGURE 3.8**
> Caregiver standing too far away from the mother to engage in meaningful dialogue

Used by permission of Debbie Shinskie.

convey an attitude of disinterest and emotional distance. Instead, you can sit or stand squarely with both feet flat on the floor. Rest your arms at your side or, when sitting, on your knees. This open body posture shows an openness to communicate on a meaningful level. Leaning forward further conveys your interest in interacting with the mother.

Body Position

Everyone has a certain amount of space surrounding them that creates their comfort zone. People vary in the amount of space they require in order to be comfortable. How we guard our zones and how we react when others invade our zone is an integral part of how we relate to other people. Be careful not to invade a mother's comfort zone and cause her to feel uneasy or awkward. At the same time, if you position yourself too far away, you may convey a message that you are too busy or uninterested in engaging her in any meaningful way. Poking your head in the door and asking a mother how breastfeeding is going does not suggest a willingness to help or an interest to interact (Fig. 3.8). Neither does standing on the other side of the room. Establish a position that is comfortable for both of you—not too far away and not too close.

Another aspect of body position is altitude. When two people interact, the height each person assumes in relation to one another will determine who is perceived as having the greatest importance or control. When the mother's caregiver stands over her, it can be intimidating to the mother and does not empower her to be the one in charge (Fig. 3.9). Placing the mother at an equal or greater height establishes that the mother is the person of greatest importance. It will lead to greater self-reliance, which is one of the goals of your consultation with the mother. You can position a chair near to the mother or even kneel on the floor next to her. In the hospital, you might sit on the bed next to her. Realize that sitting on the bed will invade the mother's space. So be sure to ask her permission and use her comfort as a guide.

Touch

Any posture that involves body contact must be used judiciously. Some people are comfortable touching others, and some are not. Some will be receptive to being touched, and some will not. The touch of a hand, or an arm placed around someone's shoulder, can convey warmth, caring, and encouragement. However, such a touch must come at the right moment and within the right context. On your first contact with a mother, she

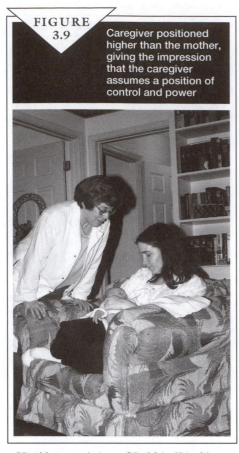

FIGURE 3.9 Caregiver positioned higher than the mother, giving the impression that the caregiver assumes a position of control and power

Used by permission of Debbie Shinskie.

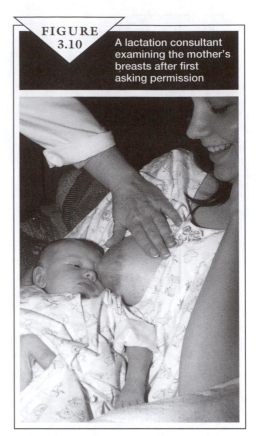

FIGURE 3.10 A lactation consultant examining the mother's breasts after first asking permission

Used by permission of Debbie Shinskie.

may respond favorably to your arm around her shoulder as you observe her baby at the breast. However, if you were to immediately touch her breast, she may react in an embarrassed or negative manner. When you need to examine a woman's breasts, be sure to ask her permission first—"May I examine your breasts?"—and explain the purpose (Fig. 3.10). These same rules apply to touching her baby. If you would like to examine the baby's mouth or help comfort him, explain this to the mother and ask her permission before invading her space and taking her baby from her.

Cultural Differences

To make it even more complicated, a particular form of body language may send different messages from one culture to another. In Western culture, for instance, a person shakes his head up and down to indicate yes and from side to side to indicate no. However, there are some societies in which just the opposite is true. Side to side means yes and up and down means no! Smiling, eye contact, space, touching, and posture may vary greatly from one culture to another. Learn the special nuances of the cultures that

influence your clients so that you send the messages you intend (Fig. 3.11).

Reading the Body Language of Others

In addition to gaining an awareness of the body messages you send, you need to be alert for nonverbal messages the mother sends to you as well. Observe and respond to her body language (Fig. 3.12). Does she appear to be comfortable, or is she in pain? Does she welcome eye contact or does she avert her eyes? How is her tone of voice? Does she sound stressed or anxious? Is her facial expression animated or listless? Is she comfortable being touched? Does her body sag, or does she sit or stand with an erect posture? Does she have an air of self assurance, or does she seem passive and unsure of herself? Does she shift her body and fidget? What is her posture while she is breastfeeding her baby? Are her shoulders hunched and tense? If so, perhaps she needs some pillows to help her get comfortable. Does she curl her toes when her baby is feeding? This may indicate that she is in pain and needs to reposition her baby. It is important that you pay careful attention to all of these nuances of the mother's body language as you gather impressions about her.

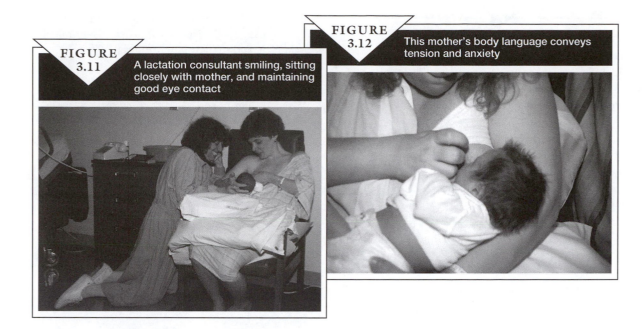

FIGURE 3.11 A lactation consultant smiling, sitting closely with mother, and maintaining good eye contact

FIGURE 3.12 This mother's body language conveys tension and anxiety

SUMMARY

The caregiver's commitment, beliefs, attitude, and approach are clearly a driving force behind a mother's ability to reach her breastfeeding goals. The caregiver who presents breastfeeding as the natural way to feed babies, and who demonstrates a belief in the superiority of breastfeeding over artificial feeding will increase the mother's self-image and confidence. When you serve as a facilitator, exploring options and developing a partnership with the mother in problem solving, mothers will grow as active health consumers who are informed and responsible concerning their health care and that of their infants. Relinquishing medical control, limiting interventions, and trusting in the abilities of mothers and babies will further this growth. A personalized approach with every mother, one that assesses her needs, capitalizes on her strengths, and praises her accomplishments will lead to the mother's long-term satisfaction. Keeping a sense of humor and using effective communication skills will help you establish an optimal learning climate and a meaningful rapport with mothers.

REFERENCES

Auerbach K. Maternal mastery and the assisting "hand" of the lactation consultant. *J Hum Lact* 10:223–224; 1994.

Belenky M et al. *Women's Ways of Knowing.* New York: Basic Books, Inc.; 1986.

Cousins N. *Anatomy of an Illness.* New York: Norton; 1979.

Fast J. *Body Language.* New York: Pocket Books; 1970.

Fisher C. Breastfeeding Basics, Annual Conference, *Breastfeeding: The Cross Cultural Connection*, Kansas City, MO; July, 1996.

Knowles M. *The Modern Practice of Adult Education/From Pedagogy to Androgogy.* Chicago: Follett Publishing; 1980.

Kutner L. Lactation Management Course, Breastfeeding Support Consultants Center for Lactation Education; 1996.

Locklin M and Naber S. Does breastfeeding empower women? Insights from a select group of educated, low-income minority women. *Birth* 20:30–35; 1993.

Minchin M. Smoking and breastfeeding: An overview *J Hum Lact* 7: 183-188; 1991.

Nelson DS. Humor in the pediatric emergency department: A 2—year retrospective, *Pediatrics* 89:6, 1089–1090; 1992.

Oski F. In defense of guilt. *Contemporary Pediatrics* 12:9; 1995.

Robinson VM. *Humor and the Health Professions: The Therapeutic Use of Humor in Health Care.* Thorofare, NJ: Slack, Inc.; 1991.

Walker M. *Summary of the hazards of infant formula*, International Lactation Consultants Association; 1992.

Zahr L. The relationship between maternal confidence and mother-infant behaviors in premature infants. *Res Nurs Health* 14:279–286; 1991.

Ziv A. The influence of humorous atmosphere on divergent thinking. *Contemporary Educational Psychology* 9:413–421; 1983.

Ziv A. Humor and creativity. *The Creative Child and Adult Quarterly* 5(3):159–170; 1980.

▼

BIBLIOGRAPHY

Fine GA. Sociological approaches to the study of humor. In McGhee PE, Goldstein JH, (eds). *Handbook of Humor Research*, Vol 1. New York: Springer-Verlag; pp. 159–181; 1983.

Foster S. Does your style block your message? *MCN* 13:207; 1988.

Fry WF Jr. *Mirthful Laughter and Blood Pressure*. Paper presented at the Third International Conference on Humor, Washington, D.C.; 1982.

Fry WF Jr. Humor and the human cardiovascular system. In Mindess H, Turek J. (eds). *The Study of Humor*. Los Angeles: Antioch University; 1979.

Jackson M. The comedy of management. In: Simms, Price, Ervin (eds). *The Professional Practice of Nursing Administration*. New York: Wiley; pp. 339–351; 1985.

McGhee (ed). *Humor and Aging*. New York: Academic Press: pp. 81–98; 1986.

Meichenbaum D and Turk D. *Facilitating Treatment Adherence*. New York: Plenum Press; 1987.

Mozingo J. Empowering women to breastfeed. *Advance Feb* 43–44, 46, 65; 1996.

Northouse PG. *Health Communication. A Handbook for Health Professionals*. Englewood Cliffs NJ: Prentice-Hall; 1985.

4

COUNSELING: LEARNING TO HELP MOTHERS

Whether you are a health care professional, lactation consultant, or a lay counselor, your primary role with breastfeeding mothers is that of a counselor. Counseling is the most basic part of the helping process. In order to carry out the process of helping parents, you need to become acquainted with general breastfeeding information and be able to convey it to parents. And you need to acquire the skills that will lead to effective communication. The focus of this chapter is the demonstration of counseling skills which enhance the helping relationship between you and the mother. Suggestions to simplify the practical aspects of counseling are presented to aid you in day-to-day contacts with mothers.

UNDERSTANDING THE COUNSELING PROCESS

Basic counseling techniques provide the means for giving mothers the support they need to develop confidence in their mothering and breastfeeding abilities. Counseling skills involve ways of encouraging the mother to express herself, educating the mother, and providing problem-solving techniques. The skills will aid you in helping the mother toward self-sufficiency and satisfaction. These skills are the essence of breastfeeding counseling. With effective counseling techniques, you can better use breastfeeding knowledge to work toward a positive experience for the mother.

The ultimate goal of each individual counseling contact is increased satisfaction for the mother. When emotional stress and physical discomfort are relieved, her satisfaction increases. When you and the mother have talked through a situation and the mother feels good about her participation in the outcome, her self-confidence increases. Increased self-awareness and understanding will lead to the mother's personal growth. This enables her to take responsibility for her situation and to be self-sufficient. Table 4.1 lists the general skills that will assist you in helping the mother reach her goals. The mother's satisfaction comes about through your perception of her needs, your use of coun-

seling skills, and your own personality traits. All of these factors are explored in the following sections.

Counselor Traits

Your own personality will have a direct effect on your rapport with the mother. Mothers respond best to a person who has a warm and caring attitude that shows deep and genuine concern and empathy to help the mother feel understood. Your openness in disclosing feelings and thoughts will encourage trust and openness in the mother. Positive regard and respect, which acknowledge the mother's individuality and worth without judgment, will give the mother freedom to be herself. It is important that you accept mothers without judging their decisions based on your own expectations. Show the mother that you approve of her and that you value what she has to say. Clear, accurate communication will reduce confusion and frustration. Flexibility will help you to move along freely, using a full range of skills, so that you can respond appropriately to the mother at different stages in the counseling process.

Expanding briefly on the concept of openness may clarify when it is appropriate for you to share personal experiences. As a professional member of the mother's health care team, it is recommended that you not share opinions or personal experiences with mothers within the counseling context. If you are operating in the capacity of a peer counselor, it may be appropriate for you to relate with the mother in a less formal manner. As such, the sharing of personal experiences may prove helpful to the mother. As a general rule, however, you are trying to guide mothers to their own solutions.

By relating your own opinions or experiences, you set yourself up as a standard, implying that the mother should follow your example. This tends to limit the mother's resourcefulness in arriving at alternative solutions. It may discourage her from being honest with you if she does not like your solution. Such personal responses tend to focus the conversation on you rather than the mother. This could minimize the mother's

	TABLE 4.1		
	Ideal Counseling Model		
Mother's Needs +	**Counseling Skills +**	**Counselor's Traits =**	**Satisfaction for Mother**
emotional support	listening	empathy and warmth	reduced stress
	influencing	concern	increased self-confidence
immediate physical comfort	facilitating	openness	personal growth
understanding	informing	positive regard and respect	acceptance of responsibility
positive action	problem solving	clear, accurate communication	
		flexibility	

concern and cause her to feel unimportant or left out. When you begin your response with "You . . ." you will immediately focus the conversation on the mother and away from you. For example, you might say, "You're wondering when (or how) you should . . ." Mothers generally are not interested in what other mothers did. They want to know what will help *them* in their breast-feeding. Focusing the discussion back on the mother will help to achieve this goal.

▼ ### The Mother's Needs

The counseling process helps the mother fulfill her needs for emotional support, physical comfort, under-standing, and action. With each contact, make sure that you have covered these four areas, when the need is indicated, so that the mother is satisfied by the contact. As shown in Table 4.1, each of the mother's needs may be met by using the counseling skills described later in this chapter. Some needs are met most easily through the use of specific skills. For example, listening and influencing are effective in giving emotional support, and problem solving leads to the development of some type of action. The variety of skills you can use to meet each need are discussed in the following sections.

Emotional Support

Providing emotional support to a mother validates her feelings, emotions, and concerns. It helps the mother arrive at a state at which she can take in information and join in problem solving. Visualize your grandmother preparing a stew in her pressure cooker. She knows that when the stew is cooled, she must slowly vent the steam to relieve the pressure before she can remove the top of the cooker. If she opens it too soon, the stew will end up on the ceiling instead of on the plate! This same prin-ciple can help you to appreciate all the pressure and anx-iety that is felt by mothers in your care. A flurry of

emotions may be boiling and ready to explode. What will happen if you jump in to try to resolve a mother's engorgement or sore nipples before you have addressed these emotions?

You can use counseling skills to help the mother lower pressure and stress. Help her verbalize her feelings and validate her concerns. Show acceptance and praise her actions or attempts. Listen to hear what she is saying as well as what she is not saying. Learn to read between the lines at her underlying message. When she is in a receptive state and is able to process the information, you can then enter into problem solving and begin to deal with information and education.

Factors that cause emotional distress can build up. Your emotional support will provide a sense of security and a climate that encourages the mother to express her feelings and anxieties. Remember this important princi-ple used in an advertising campaign for a realty firm: *People won't care how much you know until they know how much you care.* In providing emotional support, you are sending the message that you genuinely care about the mother's well-being and concerns. It shows that you are interested in helping the mother to achieve her goals. We all give support to those we love, unconsciously at times, simply as an outpouring of our concern for them. Likewise, support is an essential element in the care you give to a mother. It helps her feel secure and at ease, reduces her anxiety, and gives her someone with whom to share her concerns.

Emotional support can be given most effectively by careful use of listening skills and influencing skills—**attending, active listening, empathetic listening, reassuring, praising**, and **building hope**. When you understand and become experienced in the use of these skills, you will find yourself giving support almost auto-matically. New mothers often feel inadequate at fulfilling all that is required of them as mother, wife, professional, and homemaker. Praise a new mother at frequent inter-vals for how well she is doing with all her responsibilities. You may be the only person telling this mother she is doing a good job at this time in her life. Your interest in her and in her concerns, your frequent contacts with her, your enthusiasm for the things she is happy about, and your acceptance of her, her situation, and her decisions are all ways of showing support.

Immediate Physical Comfort

Often a mother needs to take some immediate action in order to reduce physical stress. Perhaps she is tired, her nipples are uncomfortable at the beginning of feeds, or her baby has slept through the night and her breasts are engorged. Before she can address ways to resolve her situation, she will first need immediate physical relief from her discomfort. When such a condition exists, you can first offer emotional support and then suggestions to help her feel better physically. This approach temporarily deviates from the usual problem-solving process, in which you would carefully work toward defining the problem before suggesting any action. After the mother is more comfortable, you can work with her to develop a better understanding of the problem. Intermediate actions that will relieve the mother's discomfort will enable her to work with you later to find the cause of the difficulty and eliminate it. Figure 4.1 shows how immediate physical comfort fits into the counseling process as a temporary measure. Giving physical comfort is not always necessary. If a problem exists and it is not urgent, or the mother seems calm and relaxed, then you can follow the usual counseling process.

Understanding

Understanding on the part of the mother is basic to the success of the counseling process. In order to develop satisfaction from a contact with you, the mother needs to understand herself and her feelings about the problem or concern. She needs to define and understand the problem clearly, the events or actions that led to it, and what actions will help resolve it. She also needs to understand her options in resolving the problem in order to make informed choices and assume responsibility for her actions. Such understanding comes from use of the counseling skills of listening, influencing, facilitating, informing, and problem solving.

Positive Action

As stated earlier, the goal of the counseling process is the mother's satisfaction and self-sufficiency. After having received the appropriate support and having gained an understanding of her problem, it is hoped that the mother will be able to take positive action in dealing with her concern. Even if the problem is not immediately solved, she will gain satisfaction in knowing that she is actively working on it and she can modify her action appropriately. You can initiate positive action through the use of problem-solving and decision-making processes and skills. By developing a plan together, both you and the mother can mutually agree upon the action to be taken.

◢ Methods of Counseling

In order to meet the mother's needs for emotional support, physical comfort, understanding, and action, a systematic counseling process is used. In the context of breastfeeding support, counseling encompasses more than the typical definition of counseling as a "process of advising." The three distinct aspects which characterize this process are the methods of guiding, leading and follow-up.

The Guiding Method

The guiding method will help you really listen to the mother and to empathize with her through understanding her feelings, goals, and other factors that influence her actions. The skills used in this method serve two purposes. They keep the conversation going and help you gather the information you need in order to determine the situation. Guiding skills encourage the mother to express her ideas and concerns openly. She is able to listen to herself so that she, as well as you, understands the situation better. They help you to hear what the mother is not saying, that is, the hidden messages that

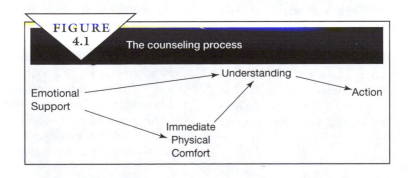

FIGURE 4.1 The counseling process

are not verbalized. Guiding skills help transmit a message of acceptance of the mother's viewpoint and positive regard for her well-being. They help you say, "I care."

The Leading Method

The leading method requires you to take a more active role in directing the conversation. This method is useful when the mother has identified a problem or concern that she is unable to solve with her available resources. The skills used in this method help both you and the mother see her situation more accurately and define options open to her so that she can work with you to develop a plan of action. It is through the use of these skills that you and the mother form a partnership in finding solutions.

The Follow-up Method

In order to be fully aware of the mother's progress, you need to analyze the effectiveness of every contact. You can then determine how and when to plan the next contact and what preparation is needed. Following up each counseling session with a subsequent contact will help you determine whether you have achieved your goal of increasing the mother's satisfaction and self-sufficiency. It will help you learn if your suggestions have been useful and if the mother needs further emotional support. The follow-up method lets the mother know how actively concerned you are in helping her. It encourages you to review the situation and to research other sources of information.

▼ USING COUNSELING METHODS AND SKILLS

The individual skills within each method of the counseling process are tools that need to be developed in order to create the climate of acceptance that makes counseling possible. To use these tools effectively, you need to understand thoroughly what they encompass, in what circumstances each skill is most helpful, and how each is used in a counseling situation. Numerous examples are given as an aid to the practical application of skills. It is hoped that these examples will help you relate the skills to actual counseling concerns. The most effective way to develop counseling skills and become proficient in their use is to practice them as frequently as possible. If you take the opportunity to practice counseling skills in conversations with your friends, colleagues, and family, you can soon develop an appreciation of their effectiveness and make them an important part of your own manner of relating to others.

Table 4.2 presents an outline of the various skills used in each of the three counseling methods. It gives an overview of the counseling process and can serve as a reference for you as you read through the individual discussions of the methods and skills.

▼ The Guiding Method

The guiding method is one in which the mother is helped through emotional support and limited direction by the counselor. In order to carry out this method successfully, you need to be aware of the mother's feelings, values, goals, and physical and emotional environment. This will enable you to better understand her needs. The major responsibility for the direction of the discussion rests with the mother during this guiding process. She, therefore, does most of the talking. This allows you to concentrate on listening carefully to her message. To help you achieve this it may help to remember that you have two ears and only one mouth. During the guiding phase of your counseling contact, you should spend twice as much time listening as you do talking!

The aim of all counseling is self-help and self-sufficiency. By encouraging the mother to talk, reflecting her ideas and clarifying her concerns, you help her see a clear picture of her situation. This ideally results in the mother taking responsibility for what is happening and deciding on her own plan of action. Throughout the contact, continually evaluate the mother's capacity for independence and self-support. If she fails to take responsibility upon herself, you may need to change your approach in order to encourage her to take the initiative while continuing to support her.

In guiding the mother, you will use listening skills that reinforce what she says. These skills will clarify her statements, show acceptance of her situation, and encourage her to arrive at her own solutions. Effective listening lets the mother know that you care about her enough to give her your total attention. While giving the mother the opportunity to hear herself and to sort out her feelings and concerns, listening also enables you to gather information.

At times, you will need to be more actively involved in gathering information by directing the conversation so that the mother will focus on specific points. Facilitating the conversation in this way helps both you and the mother recognize and clearly define her situation. In facilitating, you act as a sounding board for the mother. While gathering information, if you feel the mother needs to increase her self-confidence or gain a new perspective, you can use influencing skills to encourage her and to give her emotional support. Influencing the mother's attitude in a positive way can help her view her

	TABLE 4.2	
	Counseling Methods and Skills	
Method	**Technique**	**Skills**
Guiding	◆ Listening	◆ Attending
		◆ Active listening
		◆ Empathetic listening
	◆ Facilitating	◆ Clarifying
		◆ Interpreting
		◆ Asking open-ended questions
		◆ Focusing
		◆ Summarizing
	◆ Influencing	◆ Reassuring
		◆ Building hope
		◆ Identifying strengths
Leading	◆ Informing	◆ Presenting
		◆ Timing
		◆ Educating
	◆ Problem solving	◆ Listening to your first hunch
		◆ Looking for hidden factors
		◆ Testing your hunch
		◆ Exploring alternative hunches
		◆ Developing a plan
Follow-up	◆ Evaluating the session	◆ Analyzing
	◆ Arranging the next contact	◆ Use skills listed above as needed
	◆ Researching outside sources	
	◆ Renewing the counseling process	

circumstances more optimistically. This reduces stress so that she is able to think more clearly and work toward a solution.

Listening

Everyday listening usually takes place at one of four levels. The lowest level of listening is ignoring. No doubt, anyone who is a parent has probably experienced this level of listening with their child! The next level is pretending. This is done when the listener is trying to be polite and is really not giving any attention to the speaker. It is the noncommittal response you might receive if you interrupted someone who was deeply engrossed in reading a book or newspaper. The third level is selective listening, in which the listener hears only certain parts of what is said. The fourth level of customary listening is attentive listening, in which the listener actively focuses on words.

Listening is a technique that you can develop beyond these everyday listening skills. It is a consciously active process of responding to total messages, perceiving with the ears, eyes, and imagination. It means that you must be silent much of the time and allow the mother to talk. We are all guilty of sometimes listening with half an ear to the speaker while busily figuring out what to say next or how to change the subject to something we would rather discuss. In order to help the mother, you need to listen carefully to what she is saying and avoid the temptation to intervene with your own comments. This requires that you put your own thoughts and interests aside for the moment so that you can give yourself more fully to the job of listening.

Listening requires time and patience, and often means waiting until the mother develops an understanding of her feelings and concerns. Time is a valuable commodity for all of us, and few people take the opportunity to sit down with another individual and really listen to that person. Failure to help the mother is often a result of snap judgments and not taking enough time to hear the whole story. You need to give the mother enough time to collect her thoughts. If a new mother is asked how everything is going, she may quickly reply, "Fine." Ten minutes later, after you have talked about increases in the frequency of feeds at particular stages in her baby's growth, she may say, "No wonder my baby is nursing constantly!" She may then tell you she has been under great stress and had begun to wonder if she has enough milk to satisfy her baby. Many times the mother is not sure about how she feels and needs more time to talk and to feel at ease before you both communicate on the same level. In a situation in which the mother has mixed feelings or several concerns, you will need time and ample conversation before you can be sure of how the mother really feels. Three listening skills that can give you this time are attending, active listening, and empathetic listening.

Attending

Attending is a passive listening skill that involves responses to assure the mother that you are listening without asking questions, taking the topic in new directions, or adding to the mother's meaning. Some phrases used in this manner are "Yes," "I see," "I can appreciate that," "Oh," "Mmmmm," and "Really." The goal of attending behavior is to encourage the mother to continue talking freely. It has a strong reinforcing effect that helps the mother explore her own way and be responsible for the course of the discussion. Attending minimizes your tendency to intervene unnecessarily. Silence is another effective attending technique. At times, pausing in the conversation and waiting for the mother to fill the silence may encourage her to take a more active role.

Other aspects of attending are visual observation and the use of eye contact, posture, gestures, and listening in a noninterfering manner. The absence of any type of attending behavior, whether verbal or nonverbal, may discourage the mother from pursuing a topic and cause her to feel that you are not interested in what she has to say. Your use of eye contact and other nonverbal behavior will send positive messages to the mother. If you avoid eye contact with a mother, cross your arms or legs, and seem unapproachable, you may send a message that you are disinterested. Such a message cannot be altered by any verbal attempt to show interest. You can transmit a positive nonverbal message and show that you are genuinely interested through the use of direct eye contact, leaning toward the mother with a natural relaxed posture, calm gestures, and your facial expression.

Active Listening

Active listening, also called reflective listening, is a very useful technique for gathering information from the mother. Active listening serves three distinct functions: it clarifies, shows acceptance of the mother's viewpoint, and encourages a response. To use active listening, you will paraphrase what the mother has said and reflect her message back to her. This type of exchange encourages the mother to respond and to feel free to explain her situation in detail. It provides an opportunity for the mother to recognize and solve her own problem and creates an atmosphere in which she can grow and be accepting of information.

Active listening clarifies a message and lets the mother know you received her message completely and correctly. It helps the mother hear what she is saying and think about it. Your response may involve some interpretation of her message. Her subsequent response lets you know that you understood correctly. This focuses the conversation and provides better mutual understanding. Active listening is particularly useful when talking to a mother who has only some vague or as-yet unspoken thoughts on a situation herself. It is also useful with a mother who is emotionally upset and is not sure what her concern is or how she feels about it. You cannot begin to offer suggestions until the mother is ready to accept them. She will be ready only after her situation and her feelings are clear. Listening and encouraging the mother to continue talking are crucial in defining her concerns.

Active listening shows acceptance of the mother's viewpoint and goes beyond a more passive type of attending response such as "I see" or "Really." In active listening, you send back what you believe the mother's message meant. This encourages her to continue discussing the issue further. You are letting the mother know that you understand how she feels, that you are interested in what she is saying, and that you validate what she is feeling.

Using the mother's and baby's names helps personalize the exchange and enhances the helping relationship between you and the mother. You will want to make a conscious effort to use both of their names frequently. It is especially important that you use the baby's name with a mother who continually refers to her infant as "the baby" and does not refer to her infant by name. This could indicate that the mother is having difficulty bonding with her baby. Your use of the baby's name will help model it for the mother.

An example that illustrates clarification:

Mother: My nipples hurt.

Counselor: Your nipples are sore when you feed Michael. (Some interpretation that the soreness occurs during a feed; and using the baby's name.)

Mother: Not just when I nurse, but after I wash them, too. (This is a correction, a clarifying message. Note that you have gathered some more information in her response that may help you in problem solving, i.e., the fact that she washes her nipples after a feed.)

An example that shows acceptance:

Mother: I'm not sure I can breastfeed much longer. My nipples are so sore that breastfeeding is really unpleasant!

Counselor: It's no fun to feed Jill when it hurts. We talked about how enjoyable breastfeeding is, and this isn't fun at all.

An example that encourages the mother to respond:

Mother: Adam is 4 months old now and is always looking around the room instead of nursing. I guess he's ready to **wean**.

Counselor: You're wondering if Adam is ready to wean.

With an active listening response, you are first accepting what the mother feels, which usually encourages her to relax and respond openly. It is a warm, sincere, and considerate way of talking that most people cannot resist. Instead of informing the mother right away that most 4-month-old children do not wean themselves and are just distracted, you first accept the mother's feelings, making no judgment. Later, after further discussion, you can begin to offer the mother information about weaning and help her learn and grow.

The following is an example using active listening to encourage a response from a mother who is emotionally upset. This conversation takes place after 20 minutes of interchange. The counselor has been explaining about supply and demand and increases in feeding frequency to the mother of 2-week-old Andrew.

Mother: I don't know if I can make it through a **growth spurt**. Every time I pick up my baby, I start crying.

Counselor: Picking up Andrew makes you start to cry.

Mother: Everything makes me cry. Last night my husband and I were cuddled on the sofa with Andrew and it was terrific. It was everything that I've waited for. It was just as I've imagined it, but all I could do was cry. My husband is more upset than I am, because I'm crying all the time.

The mother did not feel comfortable sharing her personal feelings with the counselor until they had talked for quite a while and trust had developed between them. Using active listening often requires a great deal of time, patience, and interaction. The counselor's use of Andrew's name influenced the mother to use his name as well in her next response. Active listening serves as an important means of developing trust and encouraging the mother to respond.

Empathetic Listening

Listening as part of the counseling process goes beyond merely reflecting words. The highest and most effective level of listening is empathetic listening. Simple reflective or active listening conveys an intent to reply or to manipulate the conversation. Empathetic listening goes even further. The empathetic listener listens with the intent to understand emotionally and intellectually. You listen with your ears, eyes, and heart, tuning in to the feeling, meaning, and behavior that is being conveyed. You use your right brain as well as your left brain to sense and feel what is being said. When you reflect the message back to the mother, you rephrase both the content and the feeling of what has been said. This will help you and the mother work through both her thoughts and her feelings. When you reflect back what the mother seems to be saying, in your own words, you reveal to her the emotions she has expressed.

Example of an empathetic listening response:

Mother: I don't know whether I should nurse my next baby. It might make my 2-year-old child more jealous.

Counselor: You're afraid Christopher will be more jealous if you breastfeed your new baby.

You may not be certain that this is the message the mother is sending. Hearing you say it back to her with your interpretation will help the mother to decide if this is what she meant. She may say, "Yes, that's exactly what I meant." or, "No, that's not what I meant. I mean that . . ."

Empathetic listening helps reveal the mother's meaning. Listening helps you gain information that will clarify the mother's situation. This makes it less likely that you will misinterpret her meaning. To illustrate the need to understand what the mother is saying before offering suggestions, refer to Figure 4.2, which contains a list of possible meanings for several statements. If you misinterpret the mother's initial statement, your explanation or suggestions will be inappropriate and unhelpful. The wide range of possible meanings reinforces the importance of coming to a common understanding with the mother.

When using empathetic listening, at times it may be difficult to think of words to express feelings. To help you, a list of "feeling words" is presented in Figure 4.3. You can add to it other words that assist you in reflecting the feelings of the mother you are counseling. Be specific in your responses and avoid use of the general word "upset," which may communicate that you do not really understand the emotion the mother has expressed. When a mother sends you a "feeling" message, think to yourself, "What is she feel-

> ### FIGURE 4.2
> **Possible meanings from a mother's statements**
>
> *A mother may say:* I think I'll have to give my baby a bottle in the evening so that my husband can do something for the baby."
>
> *Possible meanings:*
>
> ◆ Mother wants to start a bottle.
>
> ◆ Husband wants to start a bottle.
>
> ◆ Husband feels left out.
>
> ◆ Mother wants father to take a more active role in childcare.
>
> ◆ Baby is fussy in the evening.
>
> ◆ Mother wants baby to sleep through the night.
>
> ◆ Mother has other things to do in the evening and wants husband to care for baby.
>
> ◆ Husband doesn't think baby is getting enough nourishment.
>
> ◆ Mother is thinking of weaning her baby.
>
> ◆ Baby is fussy in the evening—mother thinks she doesn't have enough milk.
>
> ◆ Husband wants to help as much as possible.
>
> *A mother may say:* "My mother-in-law is here helping me these first 2 weeks, but she bottle fed."
> *Possible meanings:*
>
> ◆ Mother-in-law is not supportive of breastfeeding.
>
> ◆ Mother-in-law thinks baby isn't getting enough nourishment.
>
> ◆ Mother-in-law is helpful around the house but not with breastfeeding.
>
> ◆ Everything is fine, and mother is just stating a fact.
>
> ◆ Mother may be embarrassed breastfeeding in front of her mother-in-law.
>
> ◆ Mother-in-law envies her for being able to breastfeed.
>
> ◆ Mother-in-law is great. She wants to learn about breastfeeding and thinks it's wonderful.
>
> ◆ Mother-in-law is not familiar with differences between bottle feeding and breastfeeding, and mother needs information to pass on to her.
>
> ◆ Mother needs support and mother-in-law may not know how to provide it.
>
> *A mother may say:* "I have to wean to go to a wedding."
> *Possible meanings:*
>
> ◆ Mother wants to wean, and the wedding is a convenient excuse.
>
> ◆ Mother does not want to breastfeed baby at wedding.
>
> ◆ Husband wants mother to wean.
>
> ◆ Mother doesn't realize she can miss a feed.
>
> ◆ Mother doesn't know how to collect and freeze milk.
>
> ◆ Mother is not comfortable breastfeeding in public.
>
> ◆ Mother wants more freedom.
>
> ◆ Mother cannot wear her favorite dress, due to increased breast size.
>
> ◆ Mother's favorite dress will not accommodate breastfeeding in public.
>
> *A mother may say:* "I don't know how long I'll be able to breastfeed. My sister had to wean at 10 days because her milk dried up."
> *Possible meanings:*
>
> ◆ Mother is worried that her milk may dry up.
>
> ◆ Sister may be unsupportive of breastfeeding.
>
> ◆ Mother may not know about growth spurts.
>
> ◆ Mother is worried about her baby getting enough milk.
>
> ◆ Mother is not getting enough encouragement to breastfeed.
>
> ◆ Mother fears that if she breastfeeds, it may make sister look like a failure.
>
> ◆ Mother has a ready excuse if anything goes wrong.
>
> ◆ Mother is not sure how long she wants to breastfeed.

ing?" Think of a word to describe the emotion being expressed and then put that word into a sentence. If you concentrate on asking yourself this question, you will find that your empathetic listening responses come more easily. Be cautious when using empathetic listening and keep your feedback statements tentative. You cannot be sure you know exactly what a mother is feeling. Watch your tone of voice and avoid sounding like a mind reader.

Facilitating

The term facilitating incorporates skills that actively encourage the mother to give more information and define her situation better, as well as to focus on specific concerns. Facilitating requires you to direct the conversation in order to help the mother pinpoint issues and feelings on which she would like to concentrate or which you believe may be the cause of problems. Five skills that are effective in facilitating a conversation are clarifying, asking open-ended questions, interpreting, focusing, and summarizing.

Clarifying

Clarifying simply means to make a point clear. To do this in counseling, you need to gather enough information from the mother in order to clearly understand her message. One way you can clarify a point is by admitting confusion about the mother's meaning and restating what you heard. You may also clarify what the mother has said by using other guiding method skills such as active listening, asking open-ended questions, and interpreting.

Example of clarifying responses:

◆ "I'm not sure what you mean. Was it . . . ?"

◆ "Let me see if I understand what you said.

◆ "You want to . . . Do I have that right?"

◆ "I'm confused, is this what you are saying?"

◆ "Can you tell me more about . . . ?"

FIGURE 4.3   Words that reflect feelings

Words that reflect "upset"	Words that reflect "happy"
angry	accepted
anxious	appreciated
defeated	better
difficult	capable
disappointed	comfortable
discouraged	competent
disrespected	confident
doubtful	empowered
embarrassed	encouraged
feel like giving up	enjoy
frightened	excited
guilty	glad
hate, hated	good
hopeless	grateful
hurt	great
inadequate	happy
left out	love, loved
miserable	pleased
put down	proud
rejected	reassured
sad	relieved
stupid	respected
unhappy	satisfied
unloved	validated
worried	wonderful
worthless	

Asking Open-Ended Questions

Asking open-ended questions is a useful skill for gathering information. It is the most direct way of finding out what you want to know. In counseling, you need to use questioning in such a way that the mother does not feel she is being interrogated. At the same time, you need to find out important and specific information. An open-ended question is one which cannot be answered by a simple "yes" or "no." Questions requiring only a yes or a no response are those that begin with words such as, "are," "is," "do," or "does." These are closed questions that give you only minimal information and tend to close off the conversation. Open-ended questions require more informative answers. They are the same questions a good newspaper reporter asks: "who," "what," "when," "where," "why," "how," "how much," and "how often."

This technique is probably best explained through examples. If you ask, "Are you eating well?" the mother will probably answer, "Yes," and you gain no helpful information. This question can be changed to an open-ended question, such as, "What did you eat today?" or "What do you usually eat for breakfast?" The mother's answers to these questions will tell you more about her diet and eating patterns.

In another example, you may suspect the baby is feeding infrequently and ask, "Does Rachel nurse often enough?" The mother can reply, "Yes" or "No" and you will not have learned much. Instead, you could ask, "How many times does Rachel nurse in 24 hours?" In this way you will gain more specific information about Rachel's breastfeeding pattern to clarify the situation. Think about what you want to learn, then word the question in your mind before asking it, so that you get more information than a simple "yes" or "no." As with many counseling skills, asking open-ended questions becomes easier and more natural with practice.

When using open-ended questions, take care not to pose too many questions in sequence or in an interrogating manner, which may cause the mother to feel threatened. Continually asking questions can also establish a poor model for the relationship. The mother may learn to expect that when she describes symptoms and complaints you will provide a solution from your wealth of information. You can discourage this pattern from the very beginning of a conversation by setting up a friendly atmosphere that encourages the mother to talk on a conversational level rather than answer a series of questions. Your goal is to encourage the mother to talk freely and to develop her own solutions whenever possible. Balancing open-ended questions with other guiding skills promotes the mother's self-sufficiency, builds her self-confidence, and discourages her dependence on you.

Interpreting

Like active listening, the skill of interpreting will clarify, show acceptance, and encourage a mother to respond. However, it goes one step further. Interpreting is more of an analysis of what the mother is saying. It contains more of your own thoughts and feelings than the simple rephrasing of what the mother said, "So you're saying that . . ." or "It sounds like you are saying . . ." or "That must mean . . ." Drawing together several of the mother's statements and adding your own tentative conclusions is a way to interpret what was said. You will want to make interpretations in such a way that you leave the door open for the mother to process what you have said and correct you if she believes you have misinterpreted her message. The goal of interpreting is to reflect the meaning of the conversation so that the mother can see her situation in new ways and learn to interpret events in her life. It is a skill that is used when you listen and respond empathetically.

In the example in Figure 4.4, the counselor interprets each statement the mother makes. In an actual counseling session, you would not interpret one statement after another. This is simply an illustration of the technique. In the final response, the counselor misinterprets what the mother said and the mother corrects her.

FIGURE 4.4 Interpreting a mother's statements

Mother: I'm 7 months pregnant, and I'd really like to breastfeed my baby. Everybody in my family thinks I'm crazy.

Counselor: It sounds like the idea of breastfeeding is new and unfamiliar to your family.

Mother: My mother can't understand why I'd even want to. It's kind of hard for me to explain it myself. It's just kind of a feeling I have.

Counselor: So you're saying you would like to breastfeed this baby.

Mother: Yes, I do really want to. But my husband kind of thinks of breasts, well, as something that belong in the centerfold of *Playboy.*

Counselor: Your husband doesn't want you to use your breasts to feed the baby.

Mother: No, it's not that exactly. I'm just not sure he understands what breastfeeding is all about.

FIGURE 4.5 Distinguishing between interpreting and active listening

Mother of a 4-week-old infant: "I can't get anything done during the day because I'm nursing all the time." (Frustrated)
◆ You feel your housework is getting away from you. (*Interpreting*)
◆ You're surprised a newborn needs so much time. (*Active Listening*)
◆ You wish you had more time to do other things. (*Interpreting*)
◆ You seem to be nursing all day. (*Active Listening*)

Mother of a 2-month-old infant: "Johnny is still waking up two times during the night, and I feel like a zombie most days." (Yawning)
◆ You're wondering if you'll ever get a good night's sleep. (*Interpreting*)
◆ You feel tired because your sleep is interrupted. (*Active Listening*)
◆ It seems as if this will go on forever. (*Interpreting*)
◆ You're wishing Johnny would sleep longer at night. (*Active Listening*)

Mother of a 2-month-old infant: "My physician said Jimmy was doing very well, but then he said it was time to start cereal twice a day." (Confused)
◆ You're wondering if Jimmy needs solid foods at this time. (*Active Listening*)
◆ You don't feel Jimmy needs solid foods yet. (*Interpreting*)
◆ You're wondering why he suggested cereal at this time. (*Active Listening*)

Mother of a 1-year-old child: "Tommy and I enjoyed breastfeeding so much, and now all of a sudden he would rather do other things than breastfeed." (Disappointed)
◆ You seem to miss the daytime feeds. (*Interpreting*)
◆ Nursing times were such happy and warm times for you and the baby. (*Active Listening*)
◆ Tommy seems to prefer his toys and other activities. (*Active Listening*)

Pregnant woman: "I want to breastfeed but I'm not interested in classes. Natural childbirth is horrible (Fearful)
◆ You don't want to go through that. (*Active Listening*)
◆ You think natural childbirth is painful. (*Interpreting*)
◆ It sounds as though you've heard about some unpleasant experiences. (*Interpreting*)
◆ Natural childbirth is not what you want. (*Active Listening*)

Figure 4.5 presents further examples that distinguish between interpreting and active listening. These examples illustrate the similarity between the two skills. Essentially, interpreting is a form of empathetic listening, which we learned earlier is the highest level of active listening. Although interpreting can be used to analyze a conversation and to help a mother gain perspective, this skill should be used with discretion. Take care not to cause the mother to feel annoyed or offended by your interpretations. Use this technique when you have a clear impression of what she is saying and when the mother seems to need help in sorting out her own feelings.

Focusing

Focusing emphasizes a topic that you think would be helpful to explore. It can be used when the mother seems to be rambling or changing the focus to a topic that is unrelated to breastfeeding. Often a mother will bring up many topics during a conversation. When you believe the mother has raised her main concerns, you can focus the conversation by pursuing one aspect that you feel could be useful to her. The goal of focusing is to pursue a more meaningful dialogue that increases understanding for both of you.

To focus the conversation, you could select one particular point to repeat or condense a number of points into a selective summary in order to concentrate on such things as how the mother feels and how the baby has been acting. Focusing is especially helpful with a very talkative mother. It is a way to bring her back to the important points that may really help her. You might say things like, "Tell me more about . . ." or "Can we talk about . . . again?" Focusing will require that you sort through the various issues to identify any topics that need to be explored. Be aware of hints from the mother that indicate her concerns. Consider the following conversation:

Mother: Hi Sue. I really liked the book you recommended on *Breastfeeding and the Family.* I just wish my husband would have been willing to read it. I gave it to my neighbor. She's going to have a baby next month. . . .

Counselor: You say your husband needs to learn more about breastfeeding?

Mother: He sure could. He's really kind of uptight about what our two kids are going to think when they see me breastfeeding. They're getting older now. My son Bobby is going out for

Little League, and he's really a pretty good pitcher for a kid his age. And my daughter who's in nursery school only knows about bottles.

Counselor: Let's get back to your husband. He's afraid of how your kids will react when they see you breastfeeding the new baby?

The mother had referred to her husband's attitude twice. It was also the first personal topic she mentioned. Often, the mother's first statement will give a clue as to her concerns, as will the number of times she brings up a topic. You can use your own feelings of confusion and sense of direction as a guide in deciding when and how to focus the conversation. This skill becomes almost second nature with practice. After you have focused the conversation, you can be alert to feedback from the mother to make sure that she believes the topic is worth pursuing.

Summarizing

Summarizing entails making a summary of the important points of a conversation. This is especially helpful when you and the mother have talked for a long time. It helps both of you go over the highlights of the conversation and reinforce important aspects. The mother may need to hear the plan of action again, clearly and briefly, so that she is certain of what to try. Summarizing reassures the mother that you have been tuned into her message all along. It also helps you know that you have understood the mother. When possible, urge the mother to do the summarizing. This will indicate her understanding, as well as help her assume responsibility. You may say, for example, "Let's see. In order to change your baby's schedule from daytime to nighttime sleeping, you are going to try which things?"

Example of summarizing responses:

Counselor: You want to learn more about breastfeeding so you can decide how to feed your baby. Would you like me to recommend some parenting books you may want to read?

Counselor: "You're not sure when you want to wean your baby, and you would like to learn more about long-term breastfeeding. Reading one of the books we discussed may be helpful. If you still have questions after reading it, please call me and we'll talk about it some more. How does that sound?"

Influencing

Influencing the mother in a positive way can encourage her to continue to seek help and work toward a solution. Many times, a new mother may be unsure of herself. She may find that the reality of caring for her baby does not match her expectations. This may cause her to become discouraged or to be swayed by poor advice. Heartening words from you can often counteract these negative factors. By using the influencing skills of reassuring, building hope, and identifying strengths you can instill a positive outlook in the mother.

Reassuring

Reassuring is an influencing skill that gives the mother perspective and lets her know that many babies act like her baby—they have fussy periods, do not sleep through the night, do not nap when you want them to, nurse frequently, and so on. Reassuring can help a mother see that her situation is normal. Be careful, however, not to give the impression that you are minimizing the importance of her feelings or concerns. You can gently let her know that it is okay to feel the way she does and assure her that her situation will improve.

Reassuring does have some limitations. Because it is easy to use, there may be a tendency to overuse it. Reassurance efforts sometimes come across as insincere sympathy and as a means of avoiding discussing the mother's concern. Keep in mind that your goal is to build the mother's confidence. This will help you decide when reassuring is appropriate.

Example of reassuring responses:

Counselor: "Even though breastfeeding in front of relatives can be difficult, it gets easier the more you do it."

Counselor: "You are really going through a rough period. The first 10 days of breastfeeding are the most challenging. It will get easier as you and your baby become more experienced."

Building Hope

Hope is the mother's main antidote to discouragement, as well as a source of relief from tension and unmet expectations. It gives the mother the feeling that the future may bring relief. You can begin building hope by encouraging the mother to talk about her feelings. Help her see how her feelings relate to her present situation and how appropriate action can change that situation. Encouraging active participation helps the mother feel better and gets her functioning at an effective level. Mothers with such long-term conditions as persistent sore nipples, a fussy baby, unsupportive family, or returning to work can usually benefit from your use of this technique.

Example of responses that build hope:

Counselor: "Being a parent isn't easy. It does get easier as the baby grows older and you become more experienced."

Counselor: "Your baby's constant fussing seems to be getting on your nerves. We can talk about some ideas that will help you cope."

Counselor: "Your aunt really discourages you by offering your baby a bottle, doesn't she. Would it help to give her some information on the importance of exclusive breastfeeding?"

Counselor: "Since you have returned to work, you seem to feel like you are not giving your baby enough attention. Would it help to set aside the first hour when you get home for just nursing and being together?"

Identifying Strengths

Identifying the mother's strengths is a form of praise that helps her focus on her positive qualities. It counteracts negative factors such as fatigue, a crying infant, or failure to meet preconceived expectations. Reminding the mother how well she handled a situation or what a knack she has for doing something can encourage her to continue to work out an answer to her present concern. Reviewing past experiences from which the mother learned and grew can help her realize that she is capable of handling her present situation. It encourages her to develop and rely on her own resources and is a step in the direction of self-sufficiency. Discussing past problems and how they were resolved is the essence of this technique. Other growth experiences such as childbirth offer fruitful discussions. Be careful to select experiences that you know had positive outcomes so that the discussion is uplifting.

Recalling peak moments can be another way of identifying strengths for the mother. Happy, exciting times such as her baby's first smile, a sibling's helpfulness, and a fun evening with other new parents are enjoyable memories for the mother to recall. These can help a new mother perceive her mothering experience as positive. She will see that she, her baby, and her family are special and that more memorable times are likely to come. Recalling peak experiences is a type of praise that gives the mother a positive outlook and also lets her know that you have taken an interest in her by the fact that you can recall important events in her life.

Example of responses that identify strengths:

Counselor: "You handled that well."

Counselor: "You seem really tuned into your baby's needs."

Counselor: "You certainly manage to get a lot done!"

Counselor: "You're the only one who can do that for your baby."

Counseling Example Using Guiding Method Skills

There are a number of listening, facilitating and influencing skills that may be used in a given situation. The example in Table 4.3 illustrates the use of each of these skills. Table 4.4 presents less helpful responses to the same statement.

TABLE 4.3
Example of the Effective Use of Guiding Method Skills

A pregnant woman says, "I'm afraid that breastfeeding might make my child too dependent."

Listening responses	◆ Attending	*Hmmm, you do . . .*
	◆ Active listening	*You're worried that breastfeeding will make your child too dependent on you.*
	◆ Empathetic listening	*You want your baby to grow into an independent child and you're not sure that breastfeeding will make that possible.*
Facilitating responses	◆ Clarifying	*I'm not sure what you mean. Could you explain what you mean by 'too dependent'?*
	◆ Interpreting	*You believe the close breastfeeding relationship will keep your child from exploring his world.*
	◆ Asking open-ended questions	*In what ways do you think breastfeeding will make your child too dependent?*
	◆ Focusing	*Let's get back to your concerns about. . . . (This would be used later if it becomes necessary to focus on the mother's primary concern— dependence, or feelings of inadequacy as a prospective parent, or other concern.)*
	◆ Summarizing	*We talked about. . . . (This would be used later to go over the main points of this topic.)*
Influencing responses	◆ Reassuring	*Being a parent can be confusing. Many bottle-feeding mothers also wonder how the attention they give their infant relates to later independence.*
	◆ Building hope	*You know, research has actually shown otherwise. Babies given more attention and physical contact in the early years grow up to be more independent.*
	◆ Identifying strengths	*It's great that you are concerned about your baby's independence. How do you feel you can encourage your baby to become independent?*

TABLE 4.4

Example of Less Helpful Responses to a Mother's Concern

A pregnant woman says, "I'm afraid that breastfeeding might make my child too dependent."

Less helpful responses	◆ Disagreeing	No, it makes him more independent.
	◆ Criticizing	That's because you don't know how babies learn to be independent.
	◆ Ordering	You need to read a book on parenting.
	◆ Sharing experiences	I used to think that way too. I remember when . . .
	◆ Changing topic	I really wanted to talk to you about . . .
	◆ Moralizing	You really don't want your child to be so independent . . .

Practicing the Use of Guiding Skills

Below are some statements that you can use to practice your use of guiding skills. You can first consider the types of responses that would be least helpful or encouraging to the mother. These may even be comments you have heard others make to mothers. Then you can practice with responses based on the skills discussed earlier.

My labor wasn't what I expected.

I'm not sure what to do when the nurse brings my baby to me.

I wish the doctor would spend more time with me.

I have to go back to work in 6 weeks.

My doctor says I have to give my baby a bottle.

My baby cries all the time.

▶ The Leading Method

The leading method in counseling is distinguished from that of guiding by the presence of a problem or concern that the mother is unable to solve with her existing resources. By using informing and problem-solving skills, you provide her with additional resources to lead her toward a solution. The use of leading responses changes the nature of the relationship between you and the mother from what it was during the guiding phase. In guiding, you encourage the mother to do most of the talking. The leading method places more responsibility for the direction of the discussion on you rather than the mother. The goal of leading is for both you and the mother to understand her problem and to develop a plan of action. During the guiding phase, you will have gathered sufficient information and impressions from the mother so that you now are able to enter into effective problem solving.

You can help the mother toward understanding by educating her and offering her two or three possible solutions. The mother then will decide which suggestions she will try according to her perception of the situation. Dur-

ing the leading phase, it is important that the decision of specific action rests with the mother in order to develop her self-sufficiency. The mother may need this kind of reinforcement especially at a time when she is doubtful of her parenting abilities in other areas. "When do I pick up my baby?" "How do I know how warmly to dress him?" "How do I care for him so that he will grow up to reach his potential?" The mother needs to be encouraged to make her own decisions on these issues.

The leading method is used when the mother clearly needs additional information or direction. When you have gathered enough information through listening and facilitating so that your leads are not premature or incorrect, your evaluation of the situation will be more accurate and you will be able to determine when leading is appropriate. You first need to take sufficient time to gain the mother's trust and clarify the situation so that you will know when leading will be helpful. Then you can intervene and educate the mother, working with her to overcome obstacles and find solutions.

Informing

Informing, or educating, is a skill used to explain how something functions and the reasons behind it. It can range from stating a simple fact about nutrition to educating parents on the manner in which human milk is produced. By providing parents with the proper information at the appropriate time, you help them grow as parents. Parents learn about breastfeeding at childbirth preparation and breastfeeding classes, at support group meetings, and from caregivers, friends, and relatives. You can educate them by suggesting appropriate reading material, whether it be a page of literature, a pamphlet, or an entire book. Following up with discussions of parents' questions and ideas enhances reading material and inspires parents to educate themselves further.

Explaining why things happen the way they do often makes basic facts more meaningful and more acceptable. For example, stating to a mother, "The more frequently you breastfeed, the more milk you will produce," may not convince her to feed her baby more frequently. Explaining briefly how nipple stimulation increases hormone production, which, in turn, increases milk production, will help her understand the process. When the mother develops understanding, she is more likely to institute changes that make her actions compatible with her new knowledge.

Before giving any information to a mother, allow her enough time to explore her concerns and to determine what she needs to know. Ask yourself, "Does this mother need information?" If so, "How much information does she need?" And then, "Is this the best time to educate her?" Determining the appropriate time—the teachable moment—for educating the mother can be critical to her accepting and processing the information. After you have determined what facts the mother needs, you can give her new information to take in. You will want to limit the amount of information so that it does not confuse or overwhelm her.

Example of responses that inform:

Counselor: "Maybe it would help to understand what happens when a baby has a growth spurt. As your baby grows. . . ."

Counselor: "One way to tell if you are having letdown is by the leaking you're noticing from the other breast. When your baby suckles. . . ."

Correcting a Misconception or Mismanagement

There will be times when you need to correct a mother's perception of something or the way she is managing her breastfeeding. If a mother is convinced, for instance, that she will need to wean her baby when he gets teeth, you might first start with an active listening response such as, "It seems like it will hurt when your baby has teeth." Then continue with something like, "You will find that your baby's tongue covers his bottom teeth when he breastfeeds." You have cleared up the mother's misconception and at the same time you are giving support by accepting her statement. And note that you corrected her perception without saying "but!" With a warm and friendly tone of voice you can supply her with information without making the mother feel foolish or uninformed. Remember that you want to avoid telling a mother she "should" do something. Rather than saying, "You should . . ." or "I think . . .", you can say "You may want to . . ." or. "You will find that when you. . . ." These types of responses will educate her and preserve her self-confidence.

Example of a response to tactfully clear up a misconception:

Mother: Isn't it great the way you don't get your period while you're breastfeeding?

Counselor: That's true for some women. It doesn't always happen that way. There's a lot of variation among individuals. When you are lactating, . . . (You can then go on to explain about the effect of lactation on menstruation and ovulation. The mother had the general idea and just needed some clarification.)

Problem Solving

An important element in your role as a consultant to the mother is helping her when problems arise with her breastfeeding. By using guiding skills to gather information, you can sort through the facts and help the mother clarify her situation. While guiding the mother, you may become aware that she has a problem. However, this is not always the case. You want to avoid jumping in with problem-solving advice when it is not needed. To begin the problem-solving process, you will form your first hunch about what the mother's problem may be. Based on that hunch, you will look for additional factors to confirm that your hunch is correct. You can then test your hunch by suggesting to the mother what you consider her problem to be. If you both agree that this is a correct interpretation of the situation, you can go on to develop a plan of action together. If the mother provides additional information that reveals your hunch to be incorrect, you will need to explore alternative hunches, reverting back to guiding skills to gain more insight and information. After you and the mother have identified the problem, you are ready to develop a plan. Each of the steps in the problem-solving process are discussed in more detail in Chapter 5.

▼ Combining the Guiding and Leading Methods

The most effective approach to counseling places an emphasis on the use of guiding skills. These skills clarify the mother's message best. You want to begin each contact with those listening techniques that help "feel the mother out" and provide her with emotional support. Guiding skills will help you encourage the mother to determine the direction of the conversation. They will produce the information and impressions you will need before going on to problem solving.

When the conversation reaches the point that you realize the mother either has no problem or is adequately handling her own problem, you can end the conversation with a summary of what was said and any plan of action to be taken. If you realize that the mother needs further assistance, you can use your leading skills to educate or problem solve as you see the need. By avoiding active participation early in the contact, you allow the mother the maximum opportunity to resolve her situation and thus encourage her emotional growth and increased self-confidence. The conversation may swing back and forth from guiding to leading as different topics are introduced. It is not our intent to develop a strict model for the counseling process. Rather, we wish to emphasize the importance of balancing leading skills with guiding skills that will help provide a clear picture of the situation and build the mother's confidence.

The counseling conversation in Table 4.5 concerns a mother and her 3½-month-old infant. It shows how

TABLE 4.5

Use of Guiding and Leading Skills in a Counseling Example

Mother	Counselor Response	Comments
(Sounding weary and discouraged) I'm so tired. My baby has been getting up three times a night for the last three nights.	You really sound discouraged, Linda.	Counselor uses *active listening* to provide emotional support. Also uses the mother's name to personalize the exchange.
Yeah. I thought we were really getting somewhere when Michael slept through the night last week. And now he acts starved at night. He eats and eats.	It seems to you like Michael is backsliding.	Counselor continues to give emotional support through *active listening*. Uses the baby's name to personalize the exchange.
I'll say. And just when my sister and her three kids have come for a week's visit.	Mmmm. That's a lot of company.	Counselor uses an *attending* response and *forms a hunch* that the mother is too active and her milk production has decreased. The mother did not say anything about her activities with her sister, whether she's doing too much, and so on. So the counselor can't assume immediately that the mother is too tired and the baby isn't getting enough milk. She needs to wait for the mother's response to know if this hunch is correct.
It *is* a lot of people, but my sister is very helpful. She's doing most of the cooking, and she keeps my house in better shape than I do!	That's great for you, Linda. So she's really more help than work for you.	Counselor finds that her first hunch was incorrect. She uses *active listening* to encourage the mother to talk so that she can gather more information.
Definitely.	Let's get back to Michael. What's he like during the day?	Counselor *focuses* the mother back on the baby and uses the baby's name to personalize the exchange. She uses an *open-ended question* to seek additional information. She is *looking for hidden factors* that will help identify the problem.
Well, he eats around 8:00 when he wakes up, then again around 10:30 before his nap. He sleeps until 1:00, then eats again. He eats again around 3:00, then takes another nap until about 6:00. Then he fusses and eats a couple of times during the evening and goes to bed about 10:00. At least that's what he's done the last couple of days.	Let's see, Linda, that's about six feeds during the day, that's nine in 24 hours. How does each feed go?	Counselor uses the mother's name again to personalize the exchange. She *summarizes* what the mother has told her and asks an *open-ended question* to gain more information.

(continued)

TABLE 4.5 (CONTINUED)

Use of Guiding and Leading Skills in a Counseling Example

Mother	Counselor Response	Comments
Well, he fools around a lot, eating, looking around, watching my sister's kids.	You know, Linda, this is the age when babies are easily distracted by people and motion and noise.	Counselor uses the mother's name and then responds with *interpreting* to test whether these distractions are the cause of the problem.
Michael is definitely distracted. Every time someone comes near he lets go and looks at them.	It's hard for Michael to pay attention to eating with so many people around.	Counselor uses baby's name in an *active listening* response to voice an *alternative hunch*.
That's right.	So you're saying that Michael is distracted a lot during the day and seems really hungry at night.	Counselor uses baby's name in an *interpreting* response to *test the hunch*.
Do you think he might be making up for not getting enough milk during the day? (This interpretation makes sense and she is pondering it.)	That seems to be a possibility.	Counselor uses an *attending* response to encourage the mother to add information that might shed more light on the situation.
That makes sense. When Michael and I were alone for a feeding yesterday, he ate for a long time and took an exceptionally long nap.	He seemed to sleep better when he ate with no distractions.	Counselor received confirmation that the *hunch* was correct and uses an *interpreting* response.
Yeah. He did.	Linda, perhaps it might help if you breastfed Michael in a quieter place during the day.	Counselor uses mother's and baby's names and *suggests an alternative action*.
I could go into the living room. The kids pretty much stay in the family room, and my sister and I could talk quietly.	Good idea. You might also try waking Michael sooner from his long afternoon nap and giving him an extra feed in the afternoon.	Counselor uses baby's name and *suggests an alternative action*. The mother has accepted the first suggestion and is trying to adapt it to her own situation. The counselor will want to document this. It is the beginning of a *plan of action*.
Well, I could, but that would interfere with my making supper. I really like that quiet time to make supper, and I hate to work on supper in the morning.	It wouldn't work for you. Okay, so you're going to try to breastfeed Michael in a quieter place, to see if you can satisfy him during the day so he'll sleep better at night.	Counselor realizes the mother does not like the second suggestion and uses *active listening* as a graceful way to withdraw the rejected suggestion. By not pushing it, the counselor shows that she supports the mother and recognizes her right to make her own decisions on how to handle her situation. She uses the baby's name while *summarizing* what they have discussed and arriving at a *plan of action*. Although this example limits the plan to one option, there undoubtedly would be more suggestions in a real life situation.
Yes.	Great Linda. Please give me a call next week to let me know how this has worked. Feel free to call me before then if you need to.	Counselor uses mother's name and *arranges follow-up*.

counseling skills are used to define a problem and work through the problem-solving process. Notice how guiding and leading skills are intermingled. The counselor takes the lead only when the mother's conversation wanders from the main concern or when she needs options pointed out to her. This nonassertive role of the counselor encourages the mother to become an active participant in the problem-solving process. This helps her understand the problem and become eager to work out a solution that will suit her circumstance.

◤ **The Follow-up Method**

Follow-up is an ongoing process. It takes place during and after each counseling contact. By objectively analyzing the contact, you can determine what you and the mother accomplished and how to plan subsequent contact that will be most beneficial to her. You can also research outside sources—such as literature and resource people—to obtain information to meet the mother's special needs. You will then renew the counseling process with new information and a new perspective. Generally, follow-up is needed after each individual contact. The mother's level of need and the urgency of the situation will determine how soon and how frequent the follow-up should be. The elements of follow-up—evaluating the session, planning, and arranging for the next contact, researching outside sources, and renewing the counseling process—are discussed in the following section.

Evaluating the Session

In evaluating a contact, examine it from the point of view of the mother's need for support, comfort, understanding, and action. You will also want to evaluate your use of skills and your own satisfaction from the contact. This approach enables you to determine the areas that need to be explored further. The questions in the following list will help you evaluate your contacts.

Questions for Evaluating a Counseling Contact

1. What support did I give? In what other ways could I have supported the mother?
2. Did the mother require immediate physical comfort? If so, what suggestions did I offer?
3. Did I gather enough information so that the mother and I both understood the problem? If not, what further information do I need?
4. Did I give appropriate information? Did the mother understand it? If not, what information do I need to give to the mother during the next contact?
5. Did the mother seem relaxed and talkative? If not, what skills can I use in a new approach for the next contact in order to encourage her to talk freely?

6. What plan did the mother and I make? Is it workable? If not, what alternative actions could I suggest?
7. Did the mother seem satisfied with the contact? If not, what areas should I explore in future contacts?
8. What follow-up did the mother and I arrange? Is it adequate, or should I contact the mother sooner?
9. Did I take usable notes during or after the contact? How were notes from previous contacts with this mother helpful? How can I improve my method of documentation?
10. Did I form a partnership with this mother and empower her to be self-sufficient in her problem solving?
11. Am I satisfied in my helping role with this mother? If not, what can I do to bring about greater satisfaction?

Evaluating can be very encouraging for you. It shows you how you have been helpful through the use of counseling techniques such as supporting, clarifying, and educating. You will know that you have done a good job of counseling a mother if you can say some of these things to yourself:

- "The mother freely talked about her concerns."
- "The mother figured out what to do about her problem."
- "The mother understood why the baby acted that way and knows what to do the next time."
- "The mother seemed willing and eager to carry out the plan we developed."

It is sometimes more spontaneous to evaluate yourself after you feel you have failed to help a particular mother. The best thing you can do is learn from such failures. You might find it helpful to discuss it with a colleague. You can plan how you will improve future contacts and recognize that as you gain more experience, you will increase your effectiveness and success. Be good to yourself! It is through our failures and mistakes that we learn and grow.

Arranging the Next Contact

As the final step in your evaluation, you will want to plan for your next contact with the mother. From your analysis of the mother's satisfaction and needs, you will be able to determine when the next contact needs to occur if any. This may be through a follow-up telephone call or suggesting that she schedule a visit with you. You can also decide who will initiate the contact and what additional information or assistance you will need to provide.

You can judge how soon to get back to a mother by the urgency of her situation. Is she having difficulty at every feed? If so, daily or even more frequent support and information from you would probably be helpful. Whenever the mother needs emotional support, frequent contact is important. Less critical or short-term problems usually require less frequent contact. For example, a mother who is becoming discouraged trying to use an electric breast pump to get milk for her premature infant in the hospital might benefit from your contacting her every day for a while. A mother whose problem is an interfering family member might want to talk with you periodically but not as frequently. You will want to contact the mother any time you gain important new information, need to correct information you have given a mother, or realize that you need to gather more information to resolve a problem. The mother will appreciate such concern about her welfare.

Always make sure the mother understands that she may call you before the prearranged time. "Remember, you can call me any time if you have a question or want to talk." If you have asked a mother to call you and she does not, you may want to contact her. If you work in a busy practice and are unable to initiate frequent contact with mothers, you will need a referral relationship with a support group in your community. You may then refer the names of mothers in your care to the support group or give mothers the name of a contact person.

Researching Outside Sources

At times, you may need to gain further input and a fresh outlook on a problem. This is especially true if a situation is outside the realm of your usual counseling. It is important that you recognize your own need for assistance. There may be issues you have overlooked. You are not expected to have every piece of information about breastfeeding immediately available. You do, however, need to know where to find the information, and you need to know when to use your resources. You can review the topic in this text and other breastfeeding literature. Contacting another lactation consultant to discuss the issue may provide you with a new perspective. Your colleague may lead you to additional information you need to obtain from the mother, such as how the infant is acting between feeds or what the infant's physician says about the weight gain. You can also gain valuable support from a colleague. It is important that you ask for help whenever you are involved in a situation that you are not able to resolve with your own resources.

Renewing the Counseling Process

Regardless of who initiates the contact, when you begin a follow-up contact, the counseling process starts all over again. You will begin with your guiding skills and progress to leading skills just as in the original contact. You might start with an opening question such as, "Hi Marsha. This is Amy. How have things been going since we last talked?"

Next, listen carefully to what the mother says. Perhaps everything you suggested worked and the problem is resolved. More likely, there is still some problem or concern that you can continue to help the mother work out.

▼

COUNSELING EXAMPLES

Three examples of counseling scenarios are provided in the next section to illustrate further the use of counseling skills in a consultation. Pay particular attention to the lactation consultant's listening skills and use of emotional support for the mother. Guiding skills are interspersed throughout the contact. Note the plan of action and follow-up arrangements between the mother and lactation consultant. Counseling skills are identified by the abbreviations below. As a general rule, the elements will progress roughly in the order in which they appear in the list.

▼

Counseling Example with Pregnant Woman

Let us examine the techniques used by the lactation consultant in the counseling example in Figure 4.6. Jan started with open-ended questions to learn more about Kelly's situation. Then she used active listening to clarify Kelly's feelings. She focused on Kelly's main concern by asking why she felt that some women have difficulty breastfeeding. When it became clear that a lack of information contributed to Kelly's hesitation to commit herself to breastfeeding, Dana began to educate her and offer her suggestions on how to learn more about breastfeeding. Notice that Dana did not overwhelm Kelly with information about the importance of human milk or reasons why she should breastfeed. (Although that is all important information, and may be addressed at another time.) Together, Dana and Kelly formed a plan of reading and attending the breastfeeding class. Dana summarized the plan and arranged for follow-up.

▼

Comparison of Two Lactation Consultants

Perhaps it would be helpful to illustrate the differences between effective and ineffective counseling scenarios for the same mother. Figure 4.7 presents ineffective communication techniques. Figure 4.8 portrays the same scenario with the lactation consultant using the techniques that have been presented in this chapter. In each of the scenarios, try to recognize what you have learned in this discussion.

In Figure 4.7, Pam fails to provide emotional support, and does not listen and respond to the mother's concerns about the emergency cesarean birth and failed

FIGURE 4.6   Counseling example with a pregnant woman

Kelly, a pregnant woman, arrives for an appointment with Jan, the lactation consultant.

Jan: Hi Kelly! I'm glad you came to see me. When is your baby due? (OEQ)

Kelly: Oh, the baby's due in about 6 weeks. We are really getting excited!

Jan: It is exciting having a baby! (AL) Is this your first child?

Kelly: Yes it is, and I wanted to talk to you about breastfeeding. I can't decide if breastfeeding is the right thing for me.

Jan: You're not positive you want to breastfeed. (AL)

Kelly: Well, at first I kind of wanted to breastfeed, but my sister recently had a baby and she had so many problems that I just don't know. . . .

Jan: So, you would like to breastfeed, and you want to make sure you don't have any problems. (I)

Kelly: Yes, it seems like I have talked with so many people who had problems that I don't think I want to even begin.

Jan: That's understandable. Why do you think some women have difficulty breastfeeding? (F) (LC acting on hunch that Kelly doesn't know much about breastfeeding.)

Kelly: I'm not sure. Maybe they don't know enough or just haven't got what it takes.

Jan: It's true that many women have problems because they don't have the correct information about breastfeeding. (E) What kind of problems did your sister have? (OEQ)

Kelly: Oh, I can't exactly remember. It seems to me she had sore nipples, the baby was crying all the time, and she just didn't have enough milk. She just decided it wasn't worth it and then she quit. And then I have a friend who started breastfeeding and quit because her baby wanted to nurse all the time and she never could go anywhere. I really don't want to be tied down.

Jan: It's too bad your friend felt so hassled because it is possible for a mother to do a number of things to make breastfeeding less demanding. As we learn more about breastfeeding, we find ways that make it easier for women to blend it into their life. Problems like your sister had can be prevented now through better understanding of the baby's needs and how the breast makes milk. (E) Would you consider postponing your decision about breastfeeding until you learn a little more about it?

Kelly: Well, I've got time to make a decision, and I would like to try breastfeeding if I could be sure that it wouldn't be an ordeal like my sister had.

Jan: Although there is no way to guarantee breastfeeding will be completely trouble free, through educating yourself you can avoid most problems. You could start by reading some of our pamphlets on breastfeeding. Here's one on common questions mothers have and another one on how the breast makes milk. It would also help for you to attend a breastfeeding class. There is one coming up next week on Thursday night that you could attend with your husband. I can also give you the number of a support group near you. (PS) Where would you like to start? (OEQ)

Kelly: Well, these pamphlets look interesting. Do they cover how to keep from having problems?

Jan: Some problems are covered. See, sore nipples and low milk supply are in here. If you read this first, then we can talk about other obstacles and I can suggest more reading if you like. What about the breastfeeding class? (OEQ/F)

Kelly: Yeah, that would probably be okay. I'll have to check with my husband and make sure he's free. Next Thursday night did you say?

Jan: Yes. The class meets right here in our office from 7:30 to 9:30, and because I'm teaching, we'll have an opportunity to talk again. There are a number of couples signed up for the class, so that will give your husband a chance to talk to some prospective breastfeeding dads, too. So, you are going to read the pamphlets, and then come to the class on Thursday night. (S) I will plan to see you then. If you have any questions before Thursday and you want to talk, don't hesitate to call me. (FU)

Kelly: Great. I'll see you next week. Thanks a lot!

Abbreviations for Skills

ES	emotional support
AL	active listening
I	interpreting
OEQ	open-ended question
IS	identifying strengths
F	focusing
E	educating
PS	practical suggestion
S	summarizing
FU	follow up

birth plan. She does not pick up on Steph's feelings of inadequacy—that the nurses did such a good job and Steph feels as though she cannot do anything right. Steph needs to know that her feelings are normal and that a sleepy infant is normal. Pam may inadvertently contribute to underlying feelings of guilt by saying that the sleepiness was caused by Steph's pain medication. Steph needs help in learning to respond to her baby's feeding cues and wakeful times. She needs to see that she is capable of caring for and breastfeeding her baby. This could have been accomplished by Pam offering some specific suggestions on infant care and breastfeeding. Most of all, in this example, Pam is very impersonal and dismissive, failing to respond to Steph as an individual.

FIGURE 4.7   Ineffective counseling technique

Steph is in her hospital room with her 2-day-old infant Michael. Pam, the lactation consultant, comes to visit.

Pam: Hi Steph! How are you doing today?

Steph: Oh, not very good.

Pam: Why? What's the matter?

Steph: I don't know. You know, I planned to have a natural childbirth with Bob in the delivery room, but I had to have an emergency c-section, and well, things just aren't going well.

Pam: Well, these things happen. You know the important thing is that you have a healthy baby, and my gosh, c/sections nowadays are almost as common as vaginal deliveries. It really isn't such a big deal any more.

Steph: I suppose. And I should just be grateful that he's healthy. But the other problem is that he isn't breastfeeding very well.

Pam: Really? Well, he sure looks content. Most c-section babies don't nurse very well the first couple of days anyway. He'll pick up.

Steph: All Michael wants to do is sleep all the time, and the nurses take real good care of him because I'm not moving around very well yet. His head is so floppy, and the nurses handle him so well. I'm afraid I might hurt him.

Pam: Isn't it great the nurses are so good with him! That saves you from having to do much, and you can get your rest. You'll have plenty of opportunity later on to take care of him!

Steph: Yeah, but I never get a chance to even hold him, and he's always too sleepy to nurse.

Pam: It's probably all the pain medication you are taking and the anesthesia you had during the c-section. Don't worry about it. He'll wake up and start breastfeeding better when you get home. You just take care of yourself and get plenty of rest while you have people around who can wait on you.

Steph: I guess you're right. I hope he'll do better. I'm really worried about him. I'm afraid he's starving.

Pam: Oh goodness, I'm sure they are giving him some formula in the nursery. Don't you worry. They won't let him starve. Well listen, I've got to scoot. Nice seeing you. You look great! Give me a call if you need anything else.

In Figure 4.8, as with many breastfeeding problems, the mother's state of mind and self-esteem are the factors that most influence her outcome. Pam listens to Steph and focuses on her concerns—disappointment over her birth experience and overall feelings of inadequacy. By building on the mother's ability to handle her infant and letting her know that awkwardness is common at first, Pam encourages Steph and helps her feel competent. By teaching Steph how to watch for Michael's cues and encouraging Steph to put Michael to breast on her own, she shows that she believes Steph can resolve her problem herself.

FIGURE 4.8   Effective counseling technique

Steph is in her hospital room with her 2-day-old infant Michael. Pam, the lactation consultant, comes to visit.

Pam: Hi Steph! How are you doing today?

Steph: Oh, not very good.

Pam: Oh Steph, that's too bad. (ES) What seems to be the problem? (OEQ)

Steph: I don't know. You know, I planned to have a natural childbirth with Bob in the delivery room, but I had to have an emergency c-section, and well, things just aren't going well.

Pam: What a disappointment! (ES) It is really hard when your birth experience doesn't go the way you planned. (AL).

Steph: I *am* disappointed. And, I feel guilty for feeling disappointed, because Michael is beautiful and healthy, and that is all I should be concerned about. But I can't help wishing Bob could have been there to see him being born, and I feel as though both of us missed out somehow. To top it off, he isn't even breastfeeding well. He's too sleepy.

Pam: Steph, there is nothing wrong with feeling disappointed or even really angry. You need to have time to grieve your lost birth experience. Your feelings are part of the grieving process, and you need time to work it through. Being upset does not make you a bad person or ungrateful for your beautiful little boy. Expressing your feelings is healing. And this is important. (E/S) You feel as though you can't do anything right because first of all you had to have a c-section, and now he won't even breastfeed! (I/AL)

Steph: That's right. Talk about being inadequate. And I feel so awkward with the baby. The nurses all know just what to do. They make it look so simple to hold up his floppy head, and change his diaper. And they wrap him perfectly in that blanket, just like a cute little mummy! When I do it, the blanket just falls apart.

Pam: You feel that because you are Michael's mom, you should be able to care for him better than anyone else. (I)

Steph: Yeah.

(continued)

FIGURE 4.8 Effective counseling technique (continued)

Pam: Learning all the best ways of caring for Michael takes time. Most first-time mothers feel inadequate at first. You and Michael just need time to adjust to each other, time to learn to communicate with one another. You can trust your intuition about how to care for him and respond to his needs. (IS/E) For example. You seem upset about his sleepiness. Have you been wondering if you should wake Michael up to feed him?

Steph: Umhm. I wondered if I should, if it would be all right. I wanted to try feeding him again, but then I wasn't sure how or when to go about it.

Pam: One of the best things to do is what you are doing right now, and that is keeping Michael with you as much as possible. That way, you can watch for his feeding cues, things like bringing his hands to his mouth or around his head, making little sucking motions, rapid eye movement, or rooting toward the breast when you hold him. Sometimes unwrapping him completely will rouse him out of a light sleep and remind him that it might be time to nurse. (IS/E)

Steph: But won't he get cold if I do that?

Pam: Your breasts are the warmest part of your body, and when Michael is snuggled up to you with skin-to-skin contact, he will stay warm and cozy. You can put his blanket over the two of you after he starts breastfeeding. (E)

Steph: Well, he's beginning to stir and looks as though he wants to suck on his hands. Should I try feeding him?

Pam: Super. Using a position like this (demonstrates) that holds your baby to the side is especially good so you can avoid putting pressure on your incision. Hold your breast so your fingers don't touch the dark part of your nipple. Now, gently touch his lower lip with your nipple. Look, there, he's opening his mouth really wide. Pull him quickly to your breast nice and tight. He's got it! By George, I think he's got it! See, you know just what to do! Notice those long, drawing sucks? He's having a lovely lunch. (E/PS/IS)

Steph: It really helped having you here to get us started. How long should I let him nurse?

Pam: As long as he continues to breastfeed with those long **nutritive** sucks. After he's feeling pretty content, his hands will probably relax, and he'll drift off to sleep or come off your breast spontaneously. In either case, you can then put him to breast on the other side. If he wakes up and breastfeeds some more, that's fine. If he continues to sleep, that's okay, too. (E)

Steph: He's really nursing well now. I think we'll be okay. Thanks so much for your help.

Pam: I think you'll both be fine. Just trust your judgement, and if you can't figure out what to do, don't hesitate to ask for help. I'll stop in again tomorrow to see how you're getting along. (FU)

SUMMARY

With the use of basic counseling techniques, you can provide mothers with the support and teaching that will help them develop confidence in their mothering and breastfeeding. Approaching mothers with a warm, caring attitude will show deep, genuine concern and empathy that help the mother feel understood and take positive action in dealing with her concern. Guiding skills help keep the conversation going while you gather information and provide emotional support. With leading skills you will take a more active role in directing the conversation and help the mother work toward developing a plan of action. The final stage of a contact is arranging appropriate follow-up and analyzing the effectiveness of your assistance and support. Developing and continuing to improve your use of these counseling skills will enhance your effectiveness in communicating with parents.

BIBLIOGRAPHY

Brammer LM. *The Helping Relationship*. New Jersey: Prentice Hall; 1973.

DeVito JA. *The Interpersonal Communication* Book, 5th ed. New York: Harper & Rowe; 1989.

5

CLIENT CONSULTATIONS

Contributing Author: Linda Kutner

Women will reach their breastfeeding goals more effectively when they receive consistent encouragement, help, and guidance at appropriate times. When a preventive approach is used in the management of breastfeeding, parents will have more positive experiences. Caregivers will also find this to be a time-saving approach that is far more effective than crisis management. Some situations can be handled through telephone contact, whereas others require a personal visit. There may be times when a problem is quite advanced by the time contact occurs, which will require more intense problem solving. By entering into problem solving with mothers, you will help them recognize problems, their possible causes, and practical actions that can be taken. Using the counseling skills that were presented in Chapter 4 will help you determine the problem, gain insights into what caused the situation, and work toward a solution with the mother. This chapter describes a step-by-step process for consultations, as well as several methods of documentation.

REACHING OUT THROUGH ANTICIPATORY GUIDANCE

Breastfeeding rates are higher when mothers receive consistent encouragement, help, and guidance prenatally, during their hospital stay, and throughout lactation. Preventive counseling will help mothers avoid or minimize breastfeeding problems. A mother's breastfeeding education needs to be viewed in the context of a preventive approach to health management, much in the same way that dental checkups help prevent cavities.

By receiving continuing support and information prenatally and throughout lactation, the mother becomes prepared and knowledgeable. She is then better able to meet the challenges of mothering with confidence. Through frequent contacts at key times, problems can be diminished or avoided entirely. These contacts help establish a foundation of knowledge, as well as good management practices. This investment of time and energy pays off in fewer problems and more enjoyment for the nursing couple. A positive experience

for parents, coupled with less time spent in problem solving, makes this both a parent-friendly and time-saving approach.

A challenge facing today's practicing lactation consultant is the lack of time to do anticipatory guidance outreach in addition to the many other responsibilities in a busy hospital, clinic, or group practice. If outreach is not part of your practice, you might refer mothers to a local support group for such contact. Peer counselors are also a wonderful resource for the mother to receive continued support and guidance.

The Timing of Anticipatory Guidance

Anticipatory guidance is as much a part of routine health supervision as the history and physical examination. It is an integral part of preventive health care for the breastfeeding mother. This guidance needs to occur at an appropriate time—when retention of information will be high and at a moment when decision making takes place. Such an appropriate time is referred to as a *teachable moment.*

Experts generally agree that the decision to breastfeed is made long before a mother delivers her baby (Beske, 1982). In fact, this decision may occur even prior to pregnancy. Therefore, earlier exposure is even more effective (Sarett, 1983). Several studies indicate that adolescents are interested in learning about breastfeeding during their high school years (Neifert, 1988) a time when many misconceptions could be corrected early enough to help adolescents form their perceptions of sexuality and parenthood (Yeo, 1994). Anticipatory guidance and education at this critical stage in an adolescent's development promotes positive attitudes and establishes a sound knowledge base. These early concepts can then be reinforced later as the adolescent approaches adulthood.

Contact with women during pregnancy will help build rapport and establish trust. The new mother then will accept advice more readily from the support person during breastfeeding. Specific needs can be addressed more effectively after a comfortable relationship has been established. A climate of acceptance, flexibility, and cooperation will set the stage for a positive breastfeeding experience.

When initial learning about breastfeeding has taken place before delivery, the postpartum period can then be a time of reinforcement. A typical postpartum hospital stay does not allow sufficient time for presenting all of the information necessary for teaching breastfeeding. Studies support the importance of prenatal education regarding infant feeding in promoting a positive breastfeeding outcome (Axelson, 1985; Grossman, 1990; Sable, 1998; Valdes, 1993; Wiles, 1984). After a program of comprehensive prenatal breastfeeding education, you can spend your valuable time with postpartum mothers and babies reinforcing and reviewing issues presented earlier.

▼ Comparing Anticipatory Guidance and Crisis Intervention

An outreach approach of anticipatory guidance in the care of breastfeeding mothers is not a new concept. It forms the basis of breastfeeding counseling in support groups and breastfeeding programs throughout the world. All areas of the medical community engage in preventive medicine. It is most easily recognized in the form of well-baby checkups, dental exams, routine breast exams and Pap smears, routine eye exams, and so on. Modern medicine clearly recognizes the benefits of early detection.

The breastfeeding mother is no exception when it comes to a need for preparedness. She often lacks role models, an experienced support person, practical and timely information, and the self-confidence to anticipate her own needs. Her only source of breastfeeding information may be skimpy literature or a brief discussion at a childbirth or postpartum class. At a time when her energies and concentration are centered on her infant's birth and her changing role, retention of breastfeeding information may be minimal at best. Half-remembered instructions may join with incorrect information from well-meaning friends and relatives to place her breastfeeding at risk. A knowledgeable caregiver, therefore, becomes a key to the mother meeting her breastfeeding goals.

Anticipatory guidance may save both the mother and infant from potential difficulties by guiding the mother one step at a time through her breastfeeding. When done on a timely basis, you can teach and inform a mother well in advance of critical periods. Her preparedness and self-confidence are often enough to prevent problems. Any problems, if they do occur, will be of shorter duration and the chances of recurrence decreased.

Crisis intervention, on the other hand, is engaged in by the caregiver after a problem has already been encountered. It may seem to some that crisis intervention is less time consuming than educating the mother before the delivery and supporting her throughout her breastfeeding experience. However, time spent later in problem solving negates any time saved. Even more important, the results for the mother are less positive. The mother's immediate problem may have been alleviated. However, the crisis might never have presented itself at all had she been educated adequately beforehand. Additionally, her sense of well-being and self-assurance are compromised. Breastfeeding needs to be viewed as a normal part of childbearing and family life. A problem-oriented approach must be replaced with one of prevention and preservation of the healthy normal phenomenon—the breastfeeding dyad of mother and baby.

Counseling Examples of the Differences in Approach

Perhaps an example of a counseling situation will help to illustrate the benefits of prevention counseling. We will follow two women who attended a breastfeeding class you offered for pregnant women. In Figure 5.1, Lynn is referred to a mother-to-mother support counselor who begins contacting her regularly 1 month before her due date. In Figure 5.2, Denise is given the phone number of a lactation consultant and told to call if she has questions or problems. The log of each lactation consultant's contacts illustrates how the degree of contact can affect the results.

Over about a 3-week period, we see the differences in breastfeeding experiences for these two women. Lynn, who is equipped with information and support, is enjoying breastfeeding. She experiences a bit of nipple tenderness on the second day. Because her lactation consultant visited her the previous day, she feels comfortable calling her to ask for help with the nipple soreness. The soreness clears up after she is reminded about correct positioning and attachment and makes the necessary adjustments. Anticipatory guidance about growth spurts and what to expect at the baby's first checkup helps Lynn anticipate these events. During her baby's growth spurt, the lactation consultant refers Lynn to the additional support of her breastfeeding counselor. Lynn is well on the road to long-term breastfeeding.

Denise has no contact with a lactation consultant until her problems are advanced to a point that is irreversible. She lacks the knowledge and self-confidence to see her through the normal occurrence of a growth spurt, and begins supplementing her baby with formula. She endures the discomfort of engorgement, sore nipples, and

FIGURE 5.1

Example of anticipatory guidance

8/15   Saw Lynn at 9 A.M. in hospital. Baby was born at 1 P.M. yesterday. 3-hour labor. Apgars 9 and 9. Baby was put to breast within 1 hour. Feedings are on demand and going well. Baby has had 6 feeds. Lynn indicated a support counselor had called her several weeks ago. They discussed putting baby to breast as soon as possible after delivery. Suggested she read *Breastfeeding Today* and attend breastfeeding class, which she did. Counselor had given her my name as the LC who would see her in the hospital. Will return when baby is ready for the next feed.

8/15   Visited Lynn at 10:30 A.M. Baby had good feed, needed some help with positioning. Reviewed basics of breastfeeding management while baby nursed.

8/16   Lynn called from home. Her nipples are tender. We discussed positioning and latch on again. Asked her to call tomorrow if no improvement.

8/18   Lynn called. Nipples are not as tender. She notices a difference with the way she positions baby. Realizes he wasn't getting a good latch before. Feels she finally has the hang of it. Breasts seem fuller. Reminded her to rest, and follow baby's feeding cues. Also discussed typical growth spurt at about 10 days.

8/25   Lynn called. Is having rough day. Baby nurses constantly. She's ready to give a bottle. Reminded her about growth spurts and gave encouragement. Lynn says she will hold off one more day. Suggested she contact her breastfeeding counselor to find out when the next support group meeting will be held.

8/27   Called Lynn. Baby is nursing less frequently now. Nipples no longer tender. She spoke with counselor and plans to attend a support group meeting in 2 weeks. Discussed what to expect at baby's first checkup. Asked her to call after checkup.

9/1   Lynn called. Weight gain is good and breastfeeding going great. Lynn in high spirits and enjoying breastfeeding.

12/6   Saw Lynn at the grocery store. Breastfeeding is going very well. She plans to become a counselor with her support group. Said, "I couldn't have done it without you!"

FIGURE 5.2

Example crisis intervention

8/12   Contacted by mother, Denise. Denise delivered her baby on 7/29 and began breastfeeding within 6 hours. Baby was fussy at feeds for the first 2 days, and popped on and off the breast. Denise figured this was because she didn't have any milk yet. On day 3 Denise's nipples became very tender. She applied breast cream that was given to her by the hospital. Two days later, Denise's nipples were cracked and bleeding. Her breasts were full and uncomfortable. She remembered that she was given my phone number but could not find it. After another 5 days, baby wanted to nurse all the time. Denise began giving a bottle of formula two times a day. She believed that she did not have enough milk for her baby. Nursing was still painful at this time. After another 3 days, baby began to prefer the bottle and was still fussy when Denise tried to nurse. Denise contacted the hospital to get my phone number. Denise was in tears. Her baby is taking four bottles of formula a day. She wants to return to exclusive breastfeeding. Scheduled her for 3:00 appointment today.

8/12   Saw Denise and baby at office. Observed a feed. Denise needed much help with positioning and attachment. Baby fussy, popped on and off frequently. Her nipples are red and tender. Evidence of thrush in baby's mouth. Advised her to contact her physician for appropriate treatment of nipples and baby's mouth. Gave her information sheet on treatment of thrush.

8/15   Called Denise. She cannot detect any increase in milk supply. Baby refuses the breast at most feeds. She is using medication for thrush on her nipples and in baby's mouth. Nipples are still tender but getting a little better. Denise is tired and frustrated at balancing bottle and breast. Discussed using nursing supplementer, to increase milk production, but Denise did not wish to use it. Reviewed positioning and treatment of her sore nipples.

8/18   Called Denise. She has decided not to continue trying to breastfeed. She is disappointed but resigned to bottle feeding.

undiagnosed thrush. By the time she contacts a lactation consultant, she is discouraged and her baby prefers bottle feeding over breastfeeding. Despite appropriate assistance, the lactation consultant is unable to help Denise return to exclusive breastfeeding, which is what Denise had wished to do. In fact, within 3 weeks after her baby is born, Denise is no longer breastfeeding at all.

Early contact with Denise could have helped her feel comfortable calling her lactation consultant when she delivered. Learning correct positioning and attachment would have increased her confidence and avoided prolonged nipple soreness. When she developed thrush,

early treatment would have cleared the infection sooner. Not having made personal contact with the consultant before now, she put off placing a call until she was desperate. This type of scenario is all too common and could be avoided with appropriate anticipatory guidance by a lactation consultant or breastfeeding counselor.

▼ Providing Anticipatory Guidance

Providing anticipatory guidance through outreach, or prevention counseling, does require more time in the early stages of breastfeeding. You can see from our ex-

TABLE 5.1

Anticipatory Guidance Through a Breastfeeding Counselor

Initiating contact with mothers: Care providers and other support people need to make a concerted effort to contact women during pregnancy. Encourage the expectant woman to educate herself about breastfeeding through reading, attending meetings, observing other mothers breastfeeding, and having her questions and concerns addressed by a knowledgeable breastfeeding helper. The combination of this early contact and education are most likely to result in a satisfying experience for the mother.

If you contact a mother near her due date and receive no answer, you might try calling the hospital and asking if she is a patient. If she has delivered, be aware that she will have other demands on her and keep your call brief. When you talk to a mother for the first time after delivery, make your initial question general, "How is everything?" "How was your birth experience?" The outcome of the birth may not have met the mother's expectations and you will want to focus on the mother until you learn more.

In preparing to make your first contact with a mother, it is helpful to have all the items you will need organized and easily accessible. These items may include this manual and other references on breastfeeding, paper, pencil, and forms you will use for documentation. In this first contact, you will want to find out the mother's goals for breastfeeding and whether she has already begun. Through the use of listening skills, you can learn how she feels about breastfeeding, the extent of her breastfeeding knowledge, and her need for support. Be sure to give her an opportunity to ask questions.

In closing the initial contact, make certain that the mother does not have any unanswered questions or concerns. Be sure that she has your name, telephone number, and the best times to reach you. Encourage her to call you any time, even if she believes her question is unimportant. Remember, however, that most mothers will be more comfortable receiving calls than initiating them. You will want to contact the mother frequently, showing your interest and concern instead of relying on calls from her. You and the mother can establish the most convenient times for subsequent contacts, taking into consideration family responsibilities and needs, and you need to make specific plans for your next contact.

Continuing regular contact: In the early weeks of breastfeeding, a mother will benefit from frequent contact. As she learns more about her baby and breastfeeding, the frequency of contacts can gradually diminish, unless she is experiencing problems. Initiating contact around times when the potential for problems typically occurs will give mothers the support and advice they need. Detailed records and thorough evaluations of each contact will help you determine when a mother needs to be contacted.

During your conversations, check that every mother understands the basic information about breastfeeding management and the prevention of problems. Help her learn how to know if her baby is positioned at the breast for optimal milk transfer and how to respond to feeding cues. Discuss ways to ensure ample milk production, responding to periods of increased hunger (growth spurts), and typical nursing patterns for babies of different ages. Help her learn to trust her baby and herself. Encourage her to look at him, to listen to him, and to watch his reactions. Following are some general guidelines for deciding how often to contact a mother and what to talk about at the different stages.

TIME PERIOD	ANTICIPATORY GUIDANCE
◆ During pregnancy	Contact the pregnant woman once or twice during her pregnancy. You can recommend books and videos, and urge her to begin acquainting herself with breastfeeding management issues. Invite her to attend a support group meeting. This is an opportune time to begin building a rapport with the mother, perhaps discussing her expectations and preparation for childbirth.
◆ When the baby is born	Hopefully you will be in close enough contact to know when the mother delivers. You can ask her to call and let you know when she has the baby. Ask if she would like you to visit her so that you can help her get started with breastfeeding and answer any questions she may have. If you are unable to visit her in person, a telephone call will be a second best option. Encourage her to talk about her labor and delivery. You may be the only person who shows an interest in helping her verbalize any disappointments or concerns regarding the birth. Find out how she feels and how her baby is doing. Ask her baby's name and start referring to her baby by name. Be sure that she knows when you will contact her again. Because most mothers spend a short time in the hospital, it may be a challenge for you to schedule a contact during her stay. This makes close prenatal contact with her even more critical, because she will be more likely to let you know when she delivers.
◆ Just home from hospital	Contact the mother within 2 to 3 days after she returns home, and more frequently for specific problems. You can first ask, "How do you feel?" and then inquire about the number of feeds, voids, and stools in 24 hours. Discuss, as necessary, common concerns such as fatigue, positioning the baby during feeds, how to know the baby is getting enough milk, and how to avoid problems such as sore nipples and engorgement. Try not to overwhelm her with too much information all at once.

TABLE 5.1 (CONTINUED)
Anticipatory Guidance Through a Breastfeeding Counselor

◆ Baby 1 week old	Call to remind the mother that babies typically seem more hungry and increase feeding frequency at approximately 10 days old. Also remind her that her breasts will reduce in size around this time as she responds to her baby's increased feeds. Make sure she understands how milk production depends on supply and demand, and encourage her to continue to respond to her baby's feeding cues. Discuss typical breastfeeding patterns for this age, and assure her that you welcome calls from her.
◆ Before baby's 2-week checkup	You can help the mother understand what her baby's physician will be looking for at this checkup. Discuss normal weight patterns and normal feeding patterns, and help her form questions to ask the physician. Call the mother again after the checkup, and ask about weight gain and any recommendations the physician has made. Help her integrate the physician's suggestions into her breastfeeding management and clarify any possible misunderstandings.
◆ Baby six weeks old	At about 6 weeks, the mother will be returning for her postpartum checkup. Discuss with her the possible effects of oral contraceptives on her breastfeeding experience. She may be interested in resuming her prepregnant activity level. Caution her about overdoing, and explain how fatigue can reduce milk production. Remind her that her baby may go through another hunger spurt at this time. This may be prolonged if she has been very active and has been missing some feeds.
◆ After the first month	Continue to keep in touch with the mother as the need arises. If you feel confident that the mother will call you whenever she has a question or problem, you could discontinue initiating calls. Some mothers will benefit from routine calls all the way through weaning.

ample, that Lynn received assistance and support twice as often as Denise. This frequency of contact subsides, however, after the first several weeks, by which time the mother and baby have developed together into a harmonious pair. Guiding the mother through her early stages, educating her in advance and building her self-confidence, produce positive results for you, the mother and her infant.

Prevention counseling may not always be an option for caregivers. In many settings, a hot line or warm line may be the most practical method of ensuring contact between the caregiver and mother. A lactation consultant's practice may be so large and busy that little time is available for outreach counseling. In cases in which the caregiver is unable to initiate regular contact with mothers, referral to a community support group is essential. Lay counselors will continue to remain an important partner in the mother's breastfeeding support team.

A study by Alice K. Ladas in 1970 showed that women who received information and support had significantly longer breastfeeding experiences with fewer problems. Her findings revealed that although prenatal support was more effective than support given only after delivery, support both before and after delivery produced the best results. The survey also showed that lack of information was significantly related to all of the reasons why mothers stop breastfeeding before they actually desire to do so.

Occasionally a mother may not desire contact as frequently as anticipatory guidance suggests. Being sensitive to the mother's cues will establish a graceful opportunity for the mother to make her wishes known. Some mothers are more comfortable handling the day-to-day stresses of motherhood in a more private manner. The most effective approach may be simply to explain your availability to the mother and allow her to initiate any contacts.

Breastfeeding Support Counselor

When this text was first written in 1983, breastfeeding support was provided primarily by volunteer lay counselors who would develop a long-term relationship with mothers through a series of contacts. Contacts took place for the most part through telephone counseling. A counselor would contact the mother several weeks or months before delivery and continue to contact her through weaning. Some mothers would attend monthly support group meetings as well. While the climate has changed with the emergence of the lactation consulting profession, the method used by lay counselors serves as a noteworthy model for anticipatory guidance and support. If you do not incorporate this kind of contact into your practice, referral to a support group could provide this guidance. Table 5.1 provides a guide for support by a lay counselor.

▼

USING A PROBLEM-SOLVING APPROACH

Problem solving involves more than simply offering a suggestion for the mother to act on. It requires gathering information and comparing it to the circumstances that fit known patterns of problem development. This is referred to as trouble shooting. As discussed in Chapter 4, problem solving may involve the use of your intuition to develop hunches. You can use these hunches to focus your thinking in order to select those suggestions which will be most helpful to the mother.

An overlying theme of this text is the development of breastfeeding management that will enable the mother and infant to breastfeed with few problems. You may not always be in a position to help a mother prevent problems. Even when sound breastfeeding techniques are practiced, problems may still occur. You can help the mother recognize problems, as well as their possible causes and practical actions the mother can take in order to alleviate them.

Throughout this text a variety of suggestions are presented for the mother. There is no one universal solution to any breastfeeding problem. A number of suggestions may, in fact, be contradictory to one another. They are provided because they have worked for some mothers. It is up to you to decide which action to offer first to a particular mother, according to your perception of her situation and her ability to cope. If your first suggestion does not lead to the solution of her problem, you will need to suggest other actions until she finds the one that works for her. Never offer so many suggestions that the mother is overwhelmed. First suggest two or three things that she can try. If these suggestions do not resolve the situation, be sure that the mother knows other methods may be tried.

▼

Using Counseling Skills to Determine the Problem

Often, breastfeeding problems are complex issues with more than one cause and no specific "right" solution. The many factors that may affect breastfeeding—the infant's physical and medical status, as well as his temperament and ability to **suckle**, the frequency and length of feeds, the condition of the mother's breasts, as well as nutritional and emotional influences, to name a few—make it inappropriate to offer information to the woman without first clearly defining her problem.

You can use the counseling skills presented in Chapter 4 to learn more about the circumstances surrounding the issue and to gather information about symptoms. By patiently listening and encouraging the woman to communicate openly, you show her that you value her perception of the problem and care enough about her to conscientiously work with her toward a solution. In doing this, you may gain additional insight into what caused her situation and more easily determine her needs. Providing her with emotional support can reduce her anxiety and allow her to be more patient and objective in working toward a solution.

Remember that sometimes a mother needs to take immediate action in order to reduce physical discomfort before you can investigate the causes of her problem with her. You can first give her suggestions for physical relief and then continue with the problem-solving process when she is more comfortable. Immediate comfort measures need to be discussed early in the contact. Otherwise, she may be unable to hear or accept the information you share with her.

In order to develop the most satisfaction from her contact with you and to decrease the likelihood of recurrences, the mother needs to understand her problem, the events and actions that led up to it, and the steps that will help her resolve it. Her understanding comes more readily when she is made an equal partner in the problem-solving process. By working with her to define her problem and explore possible actions, you can help the mother understand her situation better and develop her confidence and skills that will enable her to reach her goals for breastfeeding.

▼

Working Toward a Solution

When the nature of a problem begins to take shape through investigation with the mother, problem-solving skills can be used to clarify and suggest some action on the mother's part. The problem-solving method should contain the elements that are essential to meeting the mother's needs. The consultation begins with the gathering of information and impressions before any intervention or active involvement by the helper. The mother is asked to identify the purpose for the visit, and she remains an active participant in establishing a plan of action.

After gathering sufficient information and impressions, taking a maternal-infant history, and doing a maternal-infant assessment, you can form a first hunch and begin to define the problem. While continuing to look for hidden factors, you eliminate related causes and test your hunch. In comparing your ideas with the mother's, you explore alternative hunches and look for other possible causes.

After you have defined the problem, you can develop a plan with the mother. Together, you and the mother will examine the options, selecting one and putting it into action. Try to not give the mother more than three suggestions at a time for fear of overwhelming her with information. Ask the mother to indicate whether your suggestions suit her needs and just how to adapt them to her situation. Involving the mother in the development of a plan will increase the likelihood that she will follow it. These steps are explored in the following section.

Step 1. Form Your First Hunch

When a breastfeeding problem arises, you will first want to check with the mother to determine how she views the situation. What does she think is the cause, and what actions has she taken already? From this, you can form your own hunch about the cause and possible solution to the problem. This is more an unconscious reflex rather than a carefully reasoned analysis. Concentrating on this preliminary hunch is an essential first step to working toward a solution. It helps focus observations and reduces aimless thinking. Your first hunch is only the beginning of the problem-solving process. You can think of it as a point of departure rather than a final destination. While forming your first hunch, you continue to use guiding skills to provide emotional support, and to gather information and impressions to further clarify and define the problem.

Step 2. Look for Hidden Factors

Often, there are hidden factors that contribute to a problem. A mother who has sore nipples may be using soap and water to cleanse her nipples. An infant who nurses all night may be sleeping for long periods during the day. A mother who thinks her milk is not rich enough may have expressed milk from her breasts and noticed the normal, thin watery appearance of human milk. It is important to determine such hidden factors as early as possible in the process. This can be done by getting on the mother's wavelength, encouraging the mother to talk, and actively listening. Guiding skills are essential to this process.

Step 3. Test Your Hunch

While gathering more information, you can continually evaluate your hunch to determine whether the situation is exactly as you expected. Perhaps new information is leading you to the formation of a new hunch. Hidden factors and the mother's lack of breastfeeding information may obscure the problem unless you explore all possibilities diligently. A mother who first complained that it hurt whenever she nursed may have led you to believe she had sore nipples. By exploring further leads from her, you might learn that she is experiencing pain when her milk lets down. You then would need to change your hypothesis accordingly. To test your hunch, you can use interpreting, focusing, and summarizing. "So what you have told me is that . . ." "Let me see if I understand . . ." "You seem to be. . . ." Based on what you know about the topic involved, you can continue to explore your hunch with the mother. If your hunch proves to be correct and the problem becomes clearly identified, you may be ready to develop a plan of action with the mother.

Step 4. Explore Alternative Hunches

Based on additional input from the mother, your initial hunch may prove to be wrong. You then will need to pursue other hunches to resolve the problem. Perhaps when you tested your hunch, the mother corrected you, and so led you in another direction. Exploring alternative hunches may clarify the problem. Sometimes, a problem will remain ill defined throughout several contacts with the mother, perhaps over several weeks. At such times, you and the mother might develop a trial plan that addresses the most obvious symptoms or concerns. Through this tentative plan, the cause of the problem may be revealed by the mother when she observes which actions are most effective. You can also network with other lactation consultants about a situation that puzzles you.

Step 5. Develop a Plan

Throughout the problem-solving process, you and the mother function as a team. Together, you will come up with workable alternatives. Workable means that it fits the mother's situation and is specific to her problem. When you tell her why something is true, the mother is better able to work out her own plan of how to do something. The way in which your facts and hints are received will give you important clues as to whether or not the mother feels they will help her. If the mother likes your suggestions and adapts them to her own situation, you can be fairly certain that she is likely to try them. You can then note them for your summary of the plan of action.

If the mother seems noncommittal or replies with, "Yes, but . . ." she may be telling you that she does not feel that your suggestions will fit her problem. You may need to gather more information in order to define the problem clearly. Occasionally, the mother simply wants to talk about a problem and does not need or want suggestions for changing things. Perhaps she already knows what to do and needs support from you in the form of a listening ear.

After you and the mother have discussed the possible actions to take, you can develop a plan together. In order to eliminate confusion and to learn whether a particular action was helpful, it is best to develop a plan with only two or three actions for the mother. Asking the mother to summarize the plan will help you determine that she understands what has been discussed. Be sure to follow up with her to learn if your plan worked. If it did not work, you can consider further suggestions.

Part of developing a plan is setting a time limit on the actions to be taken by the mother, as well as arranging for follow-up. Be sure to work this out with the mother. "So, you will try . . . for 2 days and will call me on Thursday afternoon to let me know how it worked. In the meantime, please call me if it gets worse or if something else develops." Always leave the door open for the mother to call you whenever she has a concern.

Be sure to document any plan that you and the mother decide on. When you talk to the mother again, you can say, "Let's see, we talked about . . ." or, "You were going to try. . . ." This will show the mother that you are actively concerned about helping her. It also will help you to keep the situation clear in your own mind.

▼ **A Similar Approach to Problem Solving**

A similar problem-solving process was used in a study at the Vancouver Breastfeeding Centre in British Columbia (Ellis, 1993). The Vancouver model progresses through the process of assessment, analysis, diagnosis, care, and counsel. During assessment, the mother's reason for the visit is recorded, as well as any additional problems that are revealed during the visit. A maternal and infant history are taken, and physical assessments of both the mother and infant are performed. The mother is asked to initiate breastfeeding, with no intervention by the staff at the Centre, in order to obtain baseline data. Impressions gained through observing the breastfeed, along with the physical assessment and information obtained from the mother, enable the staff to analyze the situation and factors that contributed to the difficulty. A diagnosis is then made, which provides direction for the appropriate care and counsel for this particular mother. The mother participates in developing the plan of care. Then she returns for a follow-up visit to evaluate the effectiveness of the care and advice that were provided. Any necessary adjustments are then made in her plan of care.

▼ **Telephone Counseling**

Much breastfeeding counseling occurs over the telephone. Certainly, a good deal of follow-up that occurs after hospital discharge or subsequent to a clinic or office visit can be accomplished in a telephone contact. It is important to recognize those situations that require an in-person contact for assessment and appropriate advice. Many breastfeeding contacts concern parenting issues that do not require a clinical assessment. A mother may be concerned that her baby is fussy or fails to sleep through the night. You can review her breastfeeding management to determine if she is feeding frequently enough. If she describes engorgement, you can discuss adjustments in her breastfeeding routine. She may have questions about expressing her milk or returning to work. These are issues that generally do not require your seeing the mother and baby in person in order to provide appropriate assistance.

Be aware of your telephone manner any time you rely on a telephone contact to assist a mother. Remember that body language is a great determinant of the manner in which your message will be received by the mother. In the absence of any visual cues such as body language, you must rely on your tone of voice and your spoken word to relay a message that will be most effective and helpful for the mother. Body language can still enhance the exchange, however, as you can convey warmth and sincerity if you smile when you are speaking.

▼ **Deciding When a Consultation Is Required**

Circumstances sometimes require that the mother or infant, or both, be seen. If the situation is after discharge, you may need to see the mother in her home or in your office. Hospital staff have limited time to prepare mothers to care for their babies at home. Mothers will benefit from at least one home visit following discharge to ensure that breastfeeding is getting off to a good start. Also, counseling is easier, more personal, and much more pleasant when you and the mother can see each other face-to-face. The need to see a mother in person may be indicated for a variety of reasons.

◆ If a mother reports sore nipples, or difficulties that imply latch-on problems or incorrect positioning, you will need to assess her breasts and observe a breastfeed in order to gain sufficient insight into the situation.

◆ Any time there is poor weight gain, you will need to examine the infant and observe a feed. It is advisable, for legal protection, that a lactation consultant insist on a consultation for any poor or slow weight gain.

◆ A mother who is using an electric breast pump will need to be shown how to operate the pump and receive some help using it for the first time. If the need for the pump stems from a problem with the infant or with getting breastfeeding established, the mother may need help dealing with the situation. It is for this reason that mothers should, when possible, acquire their breast pumps from a person experienced in caring for breastfeeding mothers rather than from a pharmacy or other business that does not provide assistance and support.

◆ If the mother seems to be shy or untalkative, or if you sense she has difficulty relating her concerns to you in a telephone conversation, a face-to-face interaction with a breastfeeding counselor may be helpful.

◆ Severe engorgement will require a visit in order to gain further insight into the cause.

These are only a few examples. Any time you feel uneasy about a situation or unable to obtain sufficient information during a telephone contact, advise the mother to see you. Make sure she understands that further consultation will be on a fee-for-service basis, or whatever payment policy you or your institution have established.

▼ Last Resort Help

You may not always be in contact with a mother at an early stage of her problem. She may have received advice from various caregivers that was unhelpful, inappropriate, or contradictory. Consequently, a mother may have lost hope when you see her for the first time (Auerbach, 1993). Although these conditions are less than ideal, the reality is that you will need to be prepared to enter into problem solving at various levels. You also will need to be sensitive to the frustrations and anxiety the mother brings with her to the consultation. There may be times when a problem is so advanced that your only recourse is to assist the mother in weaning and offer emotional support to her. When this happens, help the mother to recall with pleasure the positive aspects of her breastfeeding. She may need reassurance that breastfeeding can follow a more rewarding course for a subsequent baby.

▼ ELEMENTS IN A CONSULTATION

The problem-solving process is integrated into the logical flow of a consultation. Regardless of the reason for the consultation, in order for the mother's needs to be met, guiding skills should be used for the first part of the conversation as described in Chapter 4. After the mother provides her consent to the consult, you can then gather information and assess the mother and baby. Your role then becomes more active after the situation has been determined and you and the mother are ready to discuss a plan of action that includes appropriate follow-up. At the end of the discussion of these steps, Table 5.2 shows how the steps are followed in a counseling scenario.

TABLE 5.2

Example of the Main Parts of a Consultation

Situation: Nancy, the mother of a 2-week-old infant says to you, "My son Justin just had his 2-week checkup. His doctor is concerned because his weight is still just under his birth weight. He thinks I may need to give formula and I am so upset. I wanted to breastfeed totally and now I don't know what to do."

◆ Statement that shows emotional support	"You're upset because your pediatrician recommended that you supplement with formula."
◆ Consent	Have the mother sign and date a consent form before proceeding with gathering information and doing an assessment.
◆ Gather information through a maternal-infant history and assessment	How often is Justin breastfeeding in 24 hours? Does he feed during the day and night? What are his feeding cues to which Nancy responds? Does he swallow audibly during the feeds? Who ends the feeds? How does Justin react during and after feeds? How many voids and stools does he have in 24 hours? What does Nancy already know about breastfeeding? Did Justin's physician prescribe supplements now or is that a future possibility if more immediate breastfeeding measures do not help Justin's weight gain? How is Justin's general appearance and hydration status? What is his present weight, birth weight, and hospital discharge weight? How are Nancy's breasts and nipples? What does she notice about her milk supply? How are latch, position, and milk transfer? *Your hunch: Nancy is unfamiliar with normal feeding cues, and therefore, Justin is not breastfeeding frequently enough for adequate milk intake and weight gain.*
◆ Develop a workable plan with the mother	Be sure Justin is nursing 10 or more times in 24 hours around the clock. Teach Nancy feeding cues and baby-led feeding. Instruct her to watch for audible swallows at feeds. Teach her how to do breast compression to enhance milk transfer. Help Nancy identify sources of support and household help through this time.
◆ Follow-up	Call the next day to evaluate how the changes in Nancy's breastfeeding management are going. See Nancy and Justin for a weight check in 2 days.
◆ Physician's report	If Nancy is unsure about the physician's exact request regarding supplements, a call to the physician's office may be warranted to clarify that issue. A report outlining the plan of care should be sent within 24 hours.

Consent

You can begin the consultation by establishing a receptive climate through the usual social amenities ("It's nice to see you, how may I help you?"). At this time, it is also imperative to have the mother sign a consent form before initiating the consultation. A signed consent form may not be required for a lactation consultant who works in a hospital, pediatric office, or clinic. You may need to determine whether consent is required in your work setting.

Your explanation of why you need consent should convey a caring attitude about the well-being of the mother and the baby. This consent should state that the mother gives permission for you to work with the mother and infant at this and all subsequent visits. In the consent, the mother gives permission for you to touch her breasts or nipples for the purpose of assessment, to perform an examination of the infant including a digital oral examination, to observe a feed, and to demonstrate or use equipment and techniques that may be necessary to ensure an adequate caloric intake for the infant and to improve the breastfeeding experience.

The mother must also give permission for you to release information to the insurance company, to send reports to the mother's and infant's primary physicians, and to consult with them regarding their care. Should you plan on using any information obtained from the consult for educational purposes or if you plan to take pictures, this permission must also be obtained in writing.

If the mother is responsible for any or all payments and charges, it is wise to include this statement on the consent form. Some lactation consultants include a section on their consent forms for the rental of breast pumps and other equipment. If you plan to do so, you must be sure to include all necessary statements in the consent in the event of future collection or legal problems. The consent should be signed and dated by both you and the mother.

It is wise even after the consent is signed to say to the mother, "May I examine your breasts now?" or "May I take your baby and examine him?" Continuing to ask the mother's permission during the consult helps give her some control over what occurs. If a mother refuses to sign the consent form or crosses out significant parts, such as allowing you to communicate with her or her infant's primary physician, it is recommended that you not continue with the consultation. A signed consent form provides the lactation consultant protection. Consulting without one is not recommended. Note that if you are practicing within a hospital or a medical group where a consent form for all care provided within that setting has been signed, you may be covered by that general consent and therefore do not need to have the mother sign a separate form. It is wise to discuss this factor with your employer in such a work setting. See Chapter 24 for further discussion regarding informed consent.

History

You can get in the habit of providing emotional support early in the consultation by feeding back to the woman your best guess as to what she is feeling. Simply diving into a checklist and questioning from your history form will do little to put the mother at ease. Active listening is a tool that helps you accept and validate her feelings. Remember that you are listening to both what she says and how she says it. Continue to provide feedback and give emotional support to the mother throughout the contact. As the discussion progresses, you will pick up on any problem the mother is experiencing. For the lactation consultant in private practice, the problem may be readily apparent. If the mother has initiated contact, she is often forthright about her situation. The lactation consultant working in an environment such as a hospital or clinic may see all the breastfeeding mothers present on a given day, and problems may not be so obvious. You can gather information and impressions through the use of guiding skills and through using your history and assessment forms as a guide.

In order to focus on the nature of the mother's concern, a history of both the mother and baby should be taken. Many lactation consultants use a standard history form or develop their own. Using such forms will help you remember to ask all essential questions. Remember that the history needs to include all information regarding the health of the mother and infant, both past and present. Begin with the mother's perception of her present problem and when it began. Document exactly what the mother says, obtaining an appropriate history relevant to the situation. If you are seeing a 6-month-old infant who is biting, a detailed history of the pregnancy and birth is probably not going to be helpful. But in dealing with a 2-week-old infant with slow weight gain, it is important to obtain such information.

Any history of previous lactation and breastfeeding should be recorded, as well as details about the present breastfeeding situation. Note any medications taken by the mother and baby, both past and present. Many mothers do not consider birth control pills, herbs, or food supplements as medications, so you may want to ask about these individually. Some mothers have been taking insulin or thyroid medication for most of their lives and again may not think of these as medications. It is also important to ask about the mother's diet, including the amount of fluids consumed each day.

Next, explore issues regarding the present situation, using open-ended questions and other guiding skills to gather more information. Be careful to word questions appropriately, for example, "How many times does your baby nurse in 24 hours?" rather than, "How frequently does your baby nurse?" Find out what the mother has tried in attempting to alleviate her problem. What were the results of her efforts? What worked, and what did not work? Include the infant's feeding and growth patterns, as well as a review of his sleeping, crying, and ability to socialize. Record the infant's pattern of stooling and voiding and obtain an estimate of the amounts in the last 24-hour period. Ask the mother if there has been any change in this pattern and, if so, when that change occurred. If you choose to not ask something on your history form, make sure to write "NA" (not applicable) in the space, indicating that you chose not to ask that question. To leave a question blank could imply that you forgot to address that particular issue.

For the lactation consultant practicing within a hospital or medical group, the history taking may not need to be so detailed, because the mother's and baby's charts will include much of the information. In such a setting, you can familiarize yourself with the mother's and baby's histories by reading their charts before the consult. Any information relevant to lactation that is not already included on the charts will then be a part of your consult with the mother. This can be noted on the mother's and baby's charts after the consult.

▼ Assessment

If you are practicing in a setting such as a hospital where the baby has already been assessed before your consult, be sure to familiarize yourself with that information, particularly the baby's daily weight status, intake, and output. In a private practice setting, you may need to do a more detailed assessment of the baby that includes his weight because you will not have access to nursery records. In either setting, you will want to look for signs of the baby's hydration and caloric status and general health, as well as numbers of wet diapers and stools. You can then move onto assessing the mother's breasts and nipples. See Chapter 11 for further discussion of infant assessment.

Moving at the baby's pace, you can then proceed to the feeding assessment. Depending on the situation, you may decide that a full feeding assessment is needed including prefeeding and postfeeding weights to measure milk transfer accurately. To do this, you will need an electronic digital scale that you can either purchase or rent. No matter how involved the feeding assessment will be, first help the mother into a comfortable position and ask her to nurse her baby. Ask her to show you what the infant does while at the breast. Do not tell her you

are going to be watching what she does so that she senses that you are focused on the baby and not on her. This approach is much less threatening and intimidating to the mother. You do not want her to feel that she is on trial and that you are the judge and jury! Allow the feeding to proceed without any suggestions or interventions on your part until you have a clear picture of what is going on. If you perceive a problem, it is then appropriate to suggest to the mother some alternative methods or interventions.

The following factors are important to consider when doing your assessment. They can have both a positive and negative impact on your plan of care and eventual outcome of the situation. Factors include:

◆ Interactions between the mother and infant

◆ The dynamics of the feeding process

◆ The infant's oral and facial structure

◆ The infant's and mother's temperaments, behavior, and emotional status

◆ The appearance and condition of the mother's breasts and nipples

◆ Evidence of milk transfer from the mother to the infant

◆ The mother's economic and employment status

◆ The mother's support network and cultural beliefs and practices

◆ The mother's breastfeeding goals

With the completion of the physical and feeding assessments, you will probably have developed a clear idea of whether a problem exists and, if so, the nature of the problem. You can then begin to think about the overall goals for this mother and baby. If the mother has very sore nipples and the baby is not getting sufficient calories because the mother cannot nurse comfortably, your overall goals will be to decrease the mother's pain while providing sufficient calories to the baby. From these general goals, you can develop a specific plan of care detailing all the steps necessary to achieving the final goal of having the mother nursing without pain and the baby nursing effectively and adequately from the breast.

Develop a Plan with the Mother

After you have determined the nature of the mother's problem, you will be prepared to take a more directive role in the consultation. Based on the identified problem, you next want to determine what the mother needs to know. You cannot enter into a consultation with a prescribed agenda. What this particular mother needs relative to the problem may be different from another mother with the same problem. In developing a plan of care, initially it is wise to limit your plan to the essentials, such as feed the baby, pain relief, and maintaining or increasing milk production. Help the mother understand what produced her situation and how she can avoid its recurrence. Brainstorm with her some of the options available to her. Be mindful of the mother's reactions to your suggestions. Although you know what would be most effective for this breastfeeding dyad, the mother must be able and willing to follow your suggestions. For example, you are aware that cup feeding will provide enough calories to the baby while allowing the mother's nipples to heal. But if this mother does not believe that cup feeding is something she can handle, then you will need to offer an alternate solution that she will find more acceptable. Your role is to provide choices and encourage the mother to decide what will work for her.

After you and the mother have decided on a plan of care, you can ask her to repeat the suggestions that she accepted. You can review them with her, if necessary. It is important that you give her this responsibility of determining her own plan. After she has stated the plan of action, you can summarize it with her to avoid any confusion. If the father is present for the consultation, be sure to include him in developing the plan of care. Remember that your goal is to empower the mother and to increase her self-confidence and self-reliance. Ask yourself if you have accomplished this at the end of every consultation.

Arrange for Follow-Up

Before you end the consultation, learn what support may be available from the mother's family and friends. Refer her to a community support group, especially if you sense that she needs the peer support it offers. Provide the mother with a written plan of care and, when appropriate, other written materials, videos, or breastfeeding products. Mothers tend to not remember much of the discussion from these consultations and they will need something in writing to take home.

As discussed in Chapter 4, follow-up is important to the mother's outcome. Depending on the situation, the follow-up may be another visit in the next day or so, or perhaps in a week or later. If it is a self-limiting situation, follow-up by telephone may be sufficient. The mother who comes in for a consultation regarding her return to work, for example, may not require a set time for follow-up but could be advised to call for any concerns or questions. If you have arranged for the mother to call you and let you know how she is doing and she does not call, you can try to call her several times. Document each call and whether or not you left a message on an answering machine or with a family member. If the situation was one of great concern, such as an infant who is failing to thrive, for example, it would be wise to notify the pediatrician that the mother has not followed up as requested.

▼ Writing Physician Reports

As a part of the mother's health care team, you will need to communicate regularly with other members of the team, specifically, the physician. This is especially important if you are working as an independent, community-based lactation consultant and do not have daily contact with other members of the mother's and baby's health care team. It is good practice to send reports to physicians for both the mother and baby. However, if the purpose of the consultation is primarily pediatric (e.g., slow weight gain), a letter only to the infant's physician is acceptable. By the same token, if the problem is maternal (e.g., a plugged duct or engorgement), a letter to the mother's physician is sufficient. Any time you have immediate concerns on seeing a mother and infant, you may want to contact the physician immediately to discuss your concerns. Be sure to document on your charting forms that you notified the physician.

Send a physician report to all appropriate primary care or referring physicians within 24 hours of seeing the client. You may also want to send a brief report if you rent a breast pump, sell breast shells, or help someone over the telephone, after first having obtained permission to release the information. Take advantage of all opportunities to let any and all members of the health care team know what you do. By educating them through such reports, they will, in turn, be more likely to refer patients to you.

Establish a routine of following up with documentation after every consultation. If you are working in the hospital, you can make notations on the patient chart. If you are working for a physician, you will probably have your own chart form that is copied and placed on the chart. In private practice, you will need to document your findings on a chart, and follow with a report to the physician. The follow-up report should be written on professional letterhead containing contact information such as your name, credentials, address, telephone number, fax number and e-mail address. See Figure 5.3 for elements that need to be included in a physician report.

▼ Evaluation

Any plan of care the mother and you establish needs to be re-evaluated frequently. As the situation changes, the plan of care may also need to change. If you do not see resolution of a problem with your plan of care, there are several areas you can address. Is there more to the problem than you first thought? Do you need to do another complete assessment? Is the mother compliant with the plan of care that she and you developed? Did you overwhelm her or suggest things that she is simply unable to

> **FIGURE 5.3**
>
> **Elements of a physician report**
>
> 1. Date the patient was seen.
> 2. Mother's physician's and baby's physician's names and addresses.
> 3. Regarding: Mother's and baby's names and baby's date of birth.
> 4. Dear Dr............,
> 5. Patient was seen at your request, was self-referred, was referred by (include name if possible)
> 6. If you also called the physician's office to give a verbal report or faxed in a short report, you can mention this in your letter.
> 7. Because of .... (reason for referral)
> 8. Brief description of the mother's history (general health, conception, pregnancy, and birth).
> 9. Assessment of the mother's breasts and nipples.
> 10. Brief description of the baby's history (birth, Apgar scores, in-hospital feeding, current feeds, output, weights, behavior, etc.).
> 11. Assessment and present status of the baby (muscle tone, activity, skin **turgor,** oral cavity, behavior, weight, and so on.).
> 12. Assessment of the feed (include feeding weights, if possible).
> 13. Your assessment of the situation.
> 14. Suggestions you made to the mother and the action plan that was developed.
> 15. Arrangements for follow-up with the mother.
> 16. If the patient was referred to you, thank the physician for allowing you to participate in the care of her/his patient. If the patient self-referred, you may comment about working with the physician with this couple ("It was a pleasure . . .").
> 17. Sincerely yours,........... (use all your credentials behind your name).

do? Are there family members who are interfering? And lastly, are you too rigid? Are you holding a mother to a plan of care that is not working because of your own personal expectations? Remaining flexible, attending breastfeeding conferences, networking with colleagues, and reading current literature will help you offer the mother a variety of options.

Evaluating Your Counseling Skills

Following up with the mother will provide insights into the effectiveness of your consultation. There are other aspects that warrant evaluation as well. Such scrutiny will help you grow in your consulting skills. This evaluation is critical to meeting the needs of the mothers in your care. Figure 5.4 contains a series of questions asked of dietetics practitioners. It serves as a model for develop-

ing an evaluation tool for your use as well (Isselman, 1993). You are encouraged to adapt the questions to your own work setting. Responses to the statements, posed as a means of evaluating the quality of their consultations, were rated on a scale ranging from *strongly agree* to *strongly disagree*.

A series of questions that evaluate your use of counseling skills is another form of evaluation you may wish to use. It is presented in Figure 5.5. These questions are used as a self-evaluation tool for students in a lactation management class to assess the use of counseling skills during a role play of a consultation with a mother (BSC, 1998). Responses are rated on a scale ranging from needs improvement to excellent. This evaluation combines the use of counseling skills with elements of a consultation. It will help you assess your own effectiveness with your clients.

> **FIGURE 5.4**
>
> **Questions to measure the quality of a consultation**
>
> 1. My confidence in my counseling skills has increased over the past 6 months.
> 2. I have identified the counseling style in which I am most comfortable and effective.
> 3. I am able to adapt my counseling style to meet the needs of the patient.
> 4. I am now using more attending and listening skills in my counseling sessions.
> 5. I am now able to recognize when a patient is not attending or listening during the counseling process.
> 6. I am better able to acknowledge my feelings that arise during the counseling process.
> 7. I am better able to acknowledge the feelings of my patients during the counseling process.
> 8. I have altered the way I conduct the counseling session based on the recognition of my own or my patient's feelings.
> 9. I evaluate the counseling environment before beginning the counseling session.
> 10. I take steps to correct the environment before beginning the counseling session.
> 11. I have requested that management make changes in my work site counseling environment that will enhance the counseling process.
> 12. I need further instruction, encouragement, or evaluation to enhance my counseling skills.

FIGURE 5.5

Questions to evaluate counseling skills in a consultation

1. Understanding of the problem: LC understood the mother and helped her.
2. Breastfeeding information: Information was correct and appropriate. Not too much or too little.
3. Clarity of instructions: The mother understood the information and advice.
4. Good counseling skills: LC put mom at ease, encouraged her to share feelings.
5. Partnership with mother: Mother was drawn into the problem-solving process.
6. Encouraged mother's self-reliance: LC fostered greater self-assurance in mother.
7. Balance: LC achieved balance between listening, educating, and problem solving—no lecturing.
8. Arrangements for follow-up: LC made it clear when any further contact will take place and who will initiate it.
9. Overall impressions of mother's satisfaction with consultation.

HOSPITAL DOCUMENTATION

Documentation does not need to be a time-consuming task. If you expect staff to provide complete and useful information about every mother and infant, you want to use a method that is user friendly and one that will not seem daunting to the staff. You can also teach the mother to chart much of her own breastfeeding information. Giving her this responsibility is a step to her becoming self-sufficient and self-assured in her breastfeeding.

There are a variety of methods for charting hospital contacts with breastfeeding mothers and babies. The method you use needs to include essential information about the mother, the baby, and breastfeeding. Charting in the hospital needs to be done at least one time per shift. Avoid using terms such as "good, fair, or poor" to evaluate the feed. These terms, used by themselves, give very little information that would indicate the mother's and baby's progress to anyone else who reviews the chart. Likewise, simply recording the duration of a feed gives no indication of the quality of the feed. Several methods for documenting breastfeeding are presented in the following sections. You are encouraged to find one that works best for you in your own practice setting.

BREASTfeed Observation Form

A form printed by UNICEF and WHO in their manual used for training maternity staff around the world uses the acronym B-R-E-A-S-T to help health workers memorize how they can evaluate a breastfeed (UNICEF), 1993; (Fig. 5.6). The main categories that are evaluated are body position, responses, emotional bonding, anatomy, suckling, and time spent suckling. After having observed a complete breastfeed, the clinician checks off in the left column the signs that breastfeeding is going well. The right column identifies signs of possible difficulty. Hospitals may find this method convenient for

helping staff to recognize good breastfeeding management and to know signs suggesting that a mother and baby may need help. The original intent was not for this form to be used as a checklist for every mother and placed into her hospital records. The purpose is for the elements of the checklist to become ingrained in the clinician's memory so that the essential points are noted when observing breastfeeds.

Charting with Breastfeeding Descriptors

Another useful method uses abbreviations that reflect the level of achievement by the mother and baby (BSC, 1998); Table 5.3). When this method is used, it is important that all staff understand the definitions for each of the abbreviations. You will notice that each rating gives very specific information about the breastfeed and is much more helpful than "good feed" with no definition for what a "good feed" is.

The LATCH Method

Another method of documentation is the LATCH charting system (Jensen, 1994). See Figure 5.7. Each letter of the acronym LATCH represents the scored item: *l*atch, *a*udible swallowing, *t*ype of nipple, *c*omfort (breast and nipple), and *h*old (positioning). Latch assesses the infant's ability to latch onto the breast. Audible swallow is evaluated as a determinant of milk intake. Type of nipple indicates the shape, size, and texture of the nipple as an important factor in the infant's ability to latch on. Comfort of the breasts and nipples is an indicator of the possible need for adjustments in positioning or another aspect of breastfeeding management. Hold, the final component of the LATCH assessment, considers the breastfeeding position used by the mother and her ability to assume a comfortable position that enables her to achieve and maintain a good latch.

FIGURE
5.6

UNICEF BREASTfeed observation form

B-R-E-A-S-T FEED OBSERVATION

Mother's name_____   Date_____

Infant's age_____   [Bracketed items refer only to the newborn infant, not to the older infant who sits up.]

Signs that breastfeeding is going well: **Signs of possible difficulty:**

BODY POSITION
___ Mother relaxed and comfortable   ___ Shoulders tense, leans over baby
___ Infant's body close to mother   ___ Infant's body away from mother's
___ Infant's head and body straight   ___ Infant must twist neck
___ Infant's chin touching breast   ___ Infant's chin does not touch breast
___ [Infant's bottom supported]   ___ [Only shoulder or head supported]

RESPONSES
___ Infant reaches for breast if hungry   ___ No response to breast
___ [Infant roots for breast]   ___ [No rooting observed]
___ Infant explores breast with tongue   ___ Infant not interested in breast
___ Infant calm and alert at breast   ___ Infant restless or fussy
___ Infant stays attached to breast   ___ Infant slips off breast
___ Signs of milk ejection: [leaking, after pains]   ___ No sign of milk ejection

EMOTIONAL BONDING
___ Secure, confident hold   ___ Nervous, shaking or limp hold
___ Face-to-face attention from mother   ___ No mother/infant eye contact
___ Much touching by mother   ___ Little touching between mother and infant

ANATOMY
___ Breasts soft and full   ___ Breasts engorged and hard
___ Nipples stick out, protractile   ___ Nipples flat or inverted
___ Skin appears healthy   ___ Fissures or redness of skin
___ Breast looks round during feed   ___ Breast looks stretched or pulled

SUCKLING
___ Mouth wide open   ___ Mouth closed, points forward
___ Lower lip turned outward   ___ Lower lip turned in
___ Tongue cupped around breast   ___ Cannot see infant's tongue
___ Cheeks round   ___ Cheeks tense or pulled in
___ Slow deep sucks, bursts with pauses   ___ Rapid sucks
___ Can see or hear swallowing   ___ Can hear smacking or clicking

TIME SPENT SUCKLING
___ Infant releases breast   ___ Mother takes infant off breast
  Infant suckled for_____minutes

Notes:

From *Breastfeeding Management and Promotion in a Baby Friendly Hospital: An 18 Hour Course for Maternity Staff,* UNICEF/WHO, 1993.

TABLE 5.3

Breastfeeding Descriptors for Documentation of Feeds

You may chart two types of feeds in one session. For example, a mother and baby may need considerable assistance with attachment. After the latch is achieved, the baby demonstrates nutritive sucking with audible swallows. This would be charted as *FBF → GBF*. Another example: You observe a baby that has some difficulty latching and the mom is poorly positioned. After offering assistance, the mother and baby overcome the obstacles and have an excellent feed with lots of swallows. This would be charted as "*Initial PBF → after assistance EBF*. Any rating below Excellent Breastfeed or Good Breastfeed will require further documentation that describes the problem and any help that is given.

Descriptor	Meaning	Elements observed
EBF	◆ Excellent breastfeed Note: It would be unusual to see an excellent breastfeed in the first 24 to 48 hours of life.	◆ Baby can latch on without difficulty ◆ Sucks are nice and deep with a nice steady rhythm ◆ Pauses are brief, and baby quickly resumes sucking again ◆ Can hear baby swallowing frequently, sometimes with each suck ◆ Mother does not need assistance positioning the baby or latching him on ◆ No nipple discomfort
GBF	◆ Good breastfeed	◆ Baby can latch on without any difficulty ◆ Sucks are nice and deep with a nice steady rhythm ◆ Pauses are brief, and baby resumes sucking again without being moved or prodded ◆ Some swallowing is heard ◆ Mother requires a little help with positioning or latch-on ◆ No nipple discomfort
FBF	◆ Fair breastfeed	◆ Baby is able to latch on to the breast and once on is able to stay on ◆ Sucks are short and quick; only occasionally may there be a nice deep suck; no steady rhythm ◆ Mother has to stroke or prod infant to resume sucking ◆ An occasional swallow may be heard, but usually no swallowing is heard ◆ Mother requires a lot of assistance with positioning and latch-on ◆ Mother could be experiencing nipple discomfort
PBF	◆ Poor breastfeed	◆ Roots for the breast, licks the nipple ◆ Latches on, but has difficulty doing it ◆ Once latched-on he does not stay on the breast or if he does he does not suck ◆ No swallowing is heard ◆ Mother requires a lot of assistance with positioning and latch-on ◆ Mother could have nipple discomfort or pain
ABF	◆ Attempted breastfeed	◆ Roots and licks at the nipple ◆ Unable to latch on to the nipple ◆ Mother requires a great deal of assistance
0BF	◆ No breastfeed	◆ No effort at the breast (too sleepy, lethargic, no interest) ◆ Pushes away from the breast, fights or cries, or both ◆ Despite lots of assistance, unable to accomplish a feed

Printed by permission of Breastfeeding Support Consultants (Barger, Kutner, 1996).

FIGURE
5.7

LATCH method

	0	1	2
L Latch	Too sleepy or reluctant No sustained latch or suck achieved	Repeated attempts for sustained latch or suck Hold nipple in mouth Stimulate to suck	Grasps breast Tongue down Lips flanged Rhythmical sucking
A Audible swallowing	None	A few with stimulation	Spontaneous and intermittent <24 hours old Spontaneous and frequent >24 hours old
T Type of nipple	Inverted	Flat	Everted (after stimulation)
C Comfort (breast/nipple)	Engorged Cracked, bleeding, large blisters, or bruises Severe discomfort	Filling Reddened/small blisters or bruises Mild/moderate discomfort	Soft Nontender
H Hold (positioning)	Full assist (staff holds infant at breast)	Minimal assist (i.e., elevate head of bed; place pillows for support) Teach one side; mother does other Staff holds and then mother takes over	No assist from staff Mother able to position and hold infant

Source: Jenson, D, Wallace, S, Kelsay, P (1994). LATCH: A breastfeeding charting system and documentation tool. *JOGNN,* 23(1):29. Reprinted with permission of Lippincott-Raven Publishers and authors.

FIGURE
5.8

Mother-Baby assessment (MBA) method

	M	B	HELP
Signaling	x	x	
Positioning	x	x	
Fixing	x		
Milk Transfer			
Ending			

Total Score   5 (With Help)

This is an assessment method for rating the progress of a mother and baby who are learning to breastfeed.

For every step, each person—both mother and baby—should receive an *x* before either one can be scored on the following step. If the observer does not observe any of the designated indicators, score 0 for that person on that step. If help is needed at any step for either the mother or the baby, check *Help* for that step. This notation will not change the total score for mother and baby.

(*continued*)

Source: Mulford, C (1992). The mother-baby assessment (MBA): An "Apgar score" for breastfeeding. *J Hum Lact,* 8: 79–82. Reprinted with permission.

FIGURE 5.8   Mother-Baby assessment (MBA) method (continued)

1. SIGNALING

- Mother watches and listens for baby's cues. She may hold, stroke, rock, talk to baby. She stimulates baby if he is sleepy, calms baby if he is fussy.
- Baby gives readiness cues: stirring, alertness, rooting, sucking, hand-to-mouth, vocal cues, cry.

2. POSITIONING

- Mother holds baby in good alignment within latch-on range of nipple. Baby's body is slightly flexed, entire ventral surface facing mother's body. Baby's head and shoulders are supported.
- Baby roots well at breast, opens mouth wide, tongue cupped and covering lower gum.

3. FIXING

- Mother holds her breast to assist baby as needed, brings baby in close when his mouth is wide open. She may express drops of milk.
- Baby latches-on, takes all of nipple and about 2 cm (1 inch) of areola into mouth, then sucks, demonstrating recurrent burst-pause pattern.

4. MILK TRANSFER

- Mother reports feeling any of the following: thirst, uterine cramps, increased lochia, breast ache or tingling, relaxation, sleepiness. Milk leaks from opposite breast.
- Baby swallows audibly; milk is observed in baby's mouth; baby may spit up milk when burping. Rapid "call up sucking" rate (two sucks/second) changes to "nutritive sucking" rate of about 1 suck/second.

5. ENDING

- Mother's breasts are comfortable; she lets baby suck until he is finished. After nursing, her breasts feel softer; she has no lumps, engorgement, or nipple soreness.
- Baby releases breast spontaneously, appears satiated. Baby does not root when stimulated. Baby's face, arms, and hands are relaxed; baby may fall asleep.

Source: Mulford, C (1992). The mother-baby assessment (MBA): An "Apgar score" for breastfeeding. *J Hum Lact*, 8:79–82. Reprinted with permission of Human Sciences Press, Inc., and the author.

The Mother-Baby Assessment Method

Another tool, modeled after the Apgar system, is the Mother-Baby Assessment (Mulford, 1992); Figure 5.8. This tool, developed by a lactation consultant, evaluates the progress of a mother and baby as they are learning to breastfeed. Five steps are assessed: signaling, positioning, fixing, milk transfer, and ending. Signaling is the step in which the mother and baby reach agreement that a feeding will take place. Positioning refers to the placement of the mother's and baby's bodies in relation to one another. Fixing is the point at which the infant attaches to the breast and begins to suckle. Milk transfer

occurs when milk is released and consumed by the baby. The final step, ending, refers to the outcome of the feeding session. The mother and infant are both evaluated on every step, with a total of 10 possible points. Any assistance that was provided is also documented.

The Infant Breastfeeding Assessment Tool

The Infant Breastfeeding Assessment Tool (IBFAT) is another option for documenting information about breastfeeding (Matthews, 1988). This tool assesses the infant's behavior during a breastfeed. (Fig. 5.9) It evaluates overall feeding behavior of the infant, the level of

FIGURE 5.9 Infant breastfeeding assessment tool (IBFAT) method

Check the answer which best describes the baby's feeding behaviors at this feed.

1. When you picked baby up to feed was he/she

(a) deeply asleep (eyes closed, no observable movement except breathing)	(b) drowsy	(c) quiet and alert	(d) crying
_____	_____	_____	_____

2. In order to get the baby to begin this feed, did you or the nurse have to

(a) just place the baby on the breast as no effort was needed	(b) use mild stimulation such as unbundling, patting, or burping	(c) unbundle baby; sit baby back and forward; rub baby's body or limbs vigorously at the beginning and during the feeding	(d) baby could not be aroused
3	2	1	0

3. Rooting (definition: at touch of nipple to cheek, baby's head turns toward the nipple, the mouth opens, and baby attempts to fix mouth on the nipple). When the baby was placed beside the breast, he/she

(a) rooted effectively at once	(b) needed some coaxing, prompting, or encouragement to root	(c) rooted poorly even with coaxing	(d) did not try to root
3	2	1	0

4. How long from placing baby at the breast does it take for the baby to latch-on and start to suck?

a) starts to feed at once (0–3 min)	(b) 3 to 10 minutes	(c) over 10 minutes	(d) did not feed
3	2	1	0

5. Which of the following phrases best describes the baby's feeding pattern at this feed?

(a) baby did not suck	(b) sucked poorly; weak sucking; some sucking efforts for short periods	(c) sucked fairly well; sucked off and on, but needed encouragement	(d) sucked well throughout on one or both breasts
0	1	2	3

6. How do you feel about the way the baby fed at this feeding?

(a) very pleased	(b) pleased	(c) fairly pleased	(d) not pleased
_____	_____	_____	_____

(continued)

Source: Matthews, MK (1988). Developing an instrument to assess infant breastfeeding behavior in the early neonatal period. *Midwifery*, 4(4), 154–165. Reprinted with permission of Churchill Livingstone and the author.

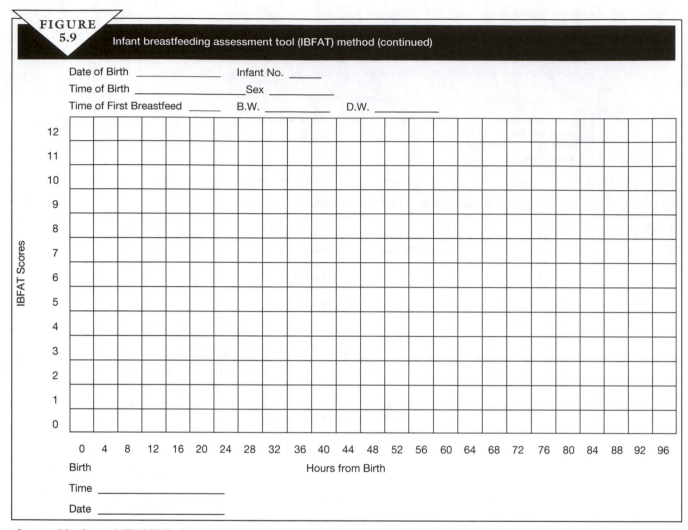

Source: Matthews, MK (1993). Assessments and suggested interventions to assist newborn breastfeeding behavior. *I Hum Lact,* 9:243–48. Reprinted with permission of Human Sciences Press, Inc., and author.

stimulation required to coax the infant to breast, the infant's rooting response, time lapsed from initiating the process until the infant latches, the infant's sucking pattern, and the mother's feelings about the feeding. A score of 0, 1, 2, or 3 is assigned to the first five factors (not including the mother's evaluation of the feed). The total score for a feed ranges from 0 to 12. The IBFAT tool does not assess the mother's physical aspect of the feed, nor does it specifically evaluate the baby's position and latch.

Developing a Plan of Care for Hospital Discharge

A final step in hospital documentation should include instructions that will help facilitate breastfeeding at home. For the mother and baby who are breastfeeding well on discharge, a diary to record the baby's feedings, voids, and stools with instructions regarding what is normal and where to get help will suffice. (See Chapter 11 for an example of such a diary.) When documenting a problem-oriented consultation as opposed to a routine check of breastfeeding management, you will want to give the mother a written plan of care based on an assessment of her needs and her infant. There are a variety of care plans and other forms available. You do not need to develop your own unless you wish to. See Figure 5.10 for an example of a care plan for engorgement. Using a form such as this, you would check off the items that apply to a particular mother. Having a standard form will help you avoid forgetting to include essential information. See Appendix A for sources of care plans.

FIGURE 5.10 Care plan for engorgement

Care Plan for Treating Engorgement

As your milk supply increases, your breasts should feel heavier and full. This normal fullness should not prevent your baby from being able to latch on easily. Your breasts should also be pain free. Breasts that become engorged are very hard, and the nipples can be flattened out because of the swelling inside of the breasts. The breasts may be tender or quite painful. The skin may appear shiny. Engorgement, if left untreated, can cause loss of some or all of the milk supply. It is important to treat engorgement quickly. The goal is to decrease swelling and enable the baby to latch on effectively. Heat (hot moist compresses) will increase swelling. Icy cold compresses and cabbage will reduce swelling.

Suggestions:

❑ 1. Try to breastfeed 10 to 12 times each 24 hours around the clock.

❑ 2. Try to breastfeed at least 15 minutes on the first breast before offering the other breast.

❑ 3. Feed your baby with just a diaper on in order to keep him awake and stimulated.

❑ 4. Hand express some milk from the breast to soften the areola before putting your baby to breast.

❑ 5. Wear breast shells for about 20 minutes before feeds.

❑ 6. Wear a good-fitting, supportive bra.

❑ 7. Lie flat on your back with a bra on between feeds to elevate your breasts.

❑ 8. Apply icy cold compresses to your breasts and under your arms. (Compresses can be made from pouring water onto disposable diapers and placing them in the freezer for 15 to 20 minutes. Or use a bag of frozen vegetables. Do not apply the compress directly on your breast; place a towel over your breast first.) Apply compresses for _____ minutes every _____ hours.

❑ 9. Express your milk after nursing to remove the milk that comes out quickly and easily, or for _____ minutes.

❑ 10. Express between feeds for comfort if necessary, but only as long as the milk comes out quickly and easily.

❑ 11. Apply olive oil to your nipple and areola before pumping to help prevent pulling and soreness.

❑ 12. Take a warm shower and hand-express milk in shower. Have the water flow against your back rather than onto your breasts.

If the areola is swollen and hard, the nipple is flattened, and the baby will not or cannot latch on, follow the instructions below:

❑ 13. Do not breastfeed until the breast has softened enough to let the baby latch on comfortably.

❑ 14. Apply green cabbage leaves to your breasts:
    a. Discard the outer leaves from the cabbage.
    b. Remove the inner leaves. Rinse and dry them. They can be kept in the refrigerator.
    c. Crush the leaves slightly with your hands.
    d. Cover the breasts entirely with the leaves (and under your arms if needed). Put your bra on over the leaves to hold them in place.
    e. Change the leaves every 2 hours or more frequently if they become wilted.
    f. Check your breasts often. As soon as you feel the milk begin to drip, or if your breasts begin to feel "different," remove the leaves and try to express your milk.
    g. Express enough to soften the breast and areola then put your baby to breast.
    h. Reapply cabbage as needed. You can use the icy compresses over the cabbage.
    i. Use only the green leaves. The white inner leaves do not work.
    j. As soon as your breasts are soft enough to nurse comfortably, you may stop using cabbage leaves.

❑ 15. Call _____ if you are not getting any relief or if you have any questions.

_____   Date _____
Mother's signature

_____   Date _____
Lactation Consultant's signature

Printed by permission of Breastfeeding Support Consultants.

SUMMARY

Using a preventive approach of anticipatory guidance will help parents have positive experiences and actually be less time consuming for the health care staff. The most effective method is one in which the helper initiates contact early and continues regular contact at such times that problems can be prevented or minimized. The nature of the situation will determine whether it can be handled through telephone contact or will require a consultation. In a consultation, you want to immediately begin by providing emotional support to the mother in order to establish a climate of receptiveness and solve her problem. Once you have established a supportive environment and obtained the mother's consent, you will gather information through taking the mother's and baby's histories and completing a physical assessment of both. You may then move on to sharing information and offering suggestions, working with the mother to develop a workable plan for her situation. Part of that plan will include a method of follow-up in order to evaluate the mother's and baby's progress. The consultation is completed after necessary documentation is recorded and a written report is sent to the physician.

REFERENCES

Axelson M et al. Primiparas' beliefs about breast feeding. *J Am Diet Assoc* 85:77–79; 1985.

Beske J and Garvis M. Important factors in breastfeeding success. *MCN* 7:174–177; 1982.

Breastfeeding Support Consultants (BSC). Lactation Management Course. Chalfont PA; 1998.

Ellis D et al. Assisting the breastfeeding mother: A problem-solving process. *J Hum Lact* 9:89–93; 1993.

Grossman L et al. The effect of postpartum lactation counseling on the duration of breastfeeding in low-income women. *Am J Dis Child* 144:471–474; 1990.

Isselman M et al. A nutrition counseling workshop: Integrating counseling psychology into nutrition practice. *J Am Diet Assoc* 93:324–326; 1993.

Jensen D et al. LATCH: A breastfeeding charting system and documentation tool. *JOGNN* 23:27–32; 1994.

Matthews M. Developing an instrument to assess infant breastfeeding behavior in the early neonatal period. *Midwifery* 4:154–165; 1988.

Neifert M et al. Factors influencing breastfeeding among adolescents. *J Adolesc Health Care* 9:470–473; 1988.

Sable M and Patton C. Prenatal lactation advice and intention to breastfeed: Selected maternal characteristics. *J Hum Lact* 14:35–40; 1998.

UNICEF/WHO. Breastfeeding Management and Promotion in a Baby-Friendly Hospital: An 18-hour course for maternity staff; 1993.

Valdes V et al. The impact of a hospital and clinic-based breastfeeding promotion programme in a middle class urban environment. *J Trop Pediatr* 39:142–151; 1993.

Wiles L. The effect of prenatal breastfeeding education on breastfeeding success and maternal perception of the infant. *JOGNN* 13:253–257; 1984.

Yeo S et al. Cultural views of breastfeeding among high school female students in Japan and the United States: A survey. *J Hum Lact* 10:25–30; 1994.

BIBLIOGRAPHY

Auerbach K. Last resort help-seeking and breastfeeding behavior. *J Hum Lact* 9:73–74; 1993.

Matthews M. Assessments and suggested interventions to assist newborn breastfeeding behavior. *J Hum Lact* 9:243–248; 1993.

Mulford C. The mother-baby assessment (MBA): An Apgar score for breastfeeding. *J Hum Lact* 8:79–82; 1992.

THE SCIENCE OF LACTATION

The breast is a marvelously complex mechanism. For millions of years, it has promoted the survival of the human race and continues today to feed and nurture our babies. It is only in the past several decades that a study of the anatomy and physiology of the breast have become an issue in lactation. For centuries, mothers instinctively have nurtured their young, confident in their natural abilities to produce and release milk. Today, health professionals study every detail of the breast externally and internally. The growth of functioning breast tissue, **milk synthesis** (production), the **letdown reflex**, and types of nipples all receive intense scrutiny. The information presented in this chapter will help you gain an understanding of these elements.

ANATOMY OF THE BREAST

The breast is a part of the whole intricate system of reproduction. Each breast is an individual exocrine gland that functions and develops independently to extract materials from the blood and convert them into milk. Thus, the breast is called a **mammary gland**. Individuality in size and shape is especially evident during lactation, when a woman's breasts enlarge to accommodate milk synthesis. Uniqueness throughout the breast is also revealed during lactation by the rate of flow and quantity of milk produced. A knowledge of the components of the breast—skin, supportive tissue, and milk-producing and milk-transporting tissue—will enable you to help mothers understand the changes in their breasts during pregnancy and in the early weeks of lactation.

Skin

Most contact with our environment is through our skin, which has many functions. Skin helps hold us together and acts as a defensive covering for deeper tissue. It is flexible and elastic to allow for changes in tissue size. Skin acts as a screen against the damaging effects of light, and performs respiratory and excretory functions—it breathes and perspires. Skin contains hair and **sebaceous** and sweat glands, and is composed of cells with many layers, one upon the other. Dead cells lie on the surface, while living cells are found underneath. Two distinct layers are the **dermis** and the **epidermis**. Located within the surface layer of the breast are the nipple, **areola**, and **Montgomery glands**.

Skin Layers

The **dermis**, composed of connective tissue, is the inner layer of the skin. It contains nerve endings, **capillaries** (small blood vessels), hair follicles; **lymph** channels, and other cells. Muscle cells are generally located under this layer, except in the area of the areola and nipple, where the two intermingle.

The **epidermis**, made up of **epithelial** cells, is the outer skin layer. It covers and protects deeper skin layers from drying out and from invasion by bacteria. The epidermis has three sublayers. Cells progress through the epidermis from initial growth in the germinating layer, to loss of fluid in the transitional layer, and on to the surface layer of dead skin, also called **keratin** (Fig. 6.1).

The skin is unique in that its dead cells serve a vital function. New cell growth in the germinating layer pushes dead cells outward toward the surface of the skin. As the cells move outward through the transitional layer, they undergo changes that cement them firmly together. This creates a tough, hard, waterproof barrier against bacterial invasion. The outer layer of the skin, the epidermis, protects the inner layer, the dermis, from abrasion and water evaporation.

Nipple

The **nipple** is the protruding part of the breast that extends and becomes firmer when stimulated. This provides a means for the baby to latch onto the breast for feeds. The nipple is flexible and able to be molded so that it will conform to the baby's mouth during a feed. Nerve endings in the nipple trigger the production and release of milk. The majority of the nipple is composed

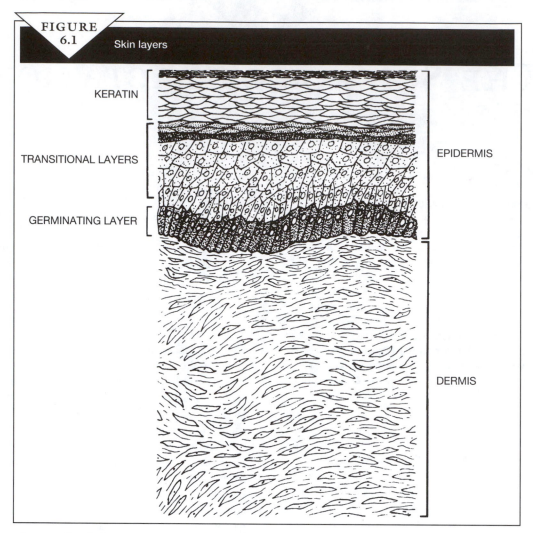

FIGURE 6.1 Skin layers

KERATIN

TRANSITIONAL LAYERS

GERMINATING LAYER

EPIDERMIS

DERMIS

Source: *Gray's Anatomy,* p. 1137, 1977. Reprinted with permission from Lea & Febiger.

of **smooth muscle** fibers that function as a closing mechanism for the **lactiferous sinuses**. Although each nipple contains 15 to 25 **ductule** openings, only six or seven function during a particular feed, and these alternate from one feed to the next. The ductule openings, commonly called **nipple pores**, are located at the end of the nipple and enable the baby to receive the milk (see Fig. 6.2).

Areola

The areola is the dark circular area surrounding the nipple. The size of the areola varies greatly from woman to woman. During puberty, menstruation, and pregnancy, it enlarges and becomes darker in color. The greater contrast in color of the areola and nipple is thought by some to be a visual sign to aid the newborn in locating and latching onto the nipple portion of the breast. Because the areola partially covers the lactiferous sinuses,

the baby's mouth needs to enclose a sizable portion of the areola. This enables his tongue to compress a large amount of breast tissue against his **palate** to squeeze milk out of the lactiferous sinuses.

Montgomery Glands

The **Montgomery glands**, which have a pimply appearance, are located around the areola. They secrete an oily substance that serves as a lubricant and a protective agent for the nipple. With natural lubrication by Montgomery gland secretions throughout lactation, the nipple and areola require no additional creams or lotions to remain soft and flexible. Only when these secretions are removed by washing with anything except water might they need to be replaced temporarily by substitute lubricants.

The Montgomery gland secretions allow the skin to breathe and remain pliable. There is also some speculation that these secretions provide a taste and smell that enables the baby to find the nipple (Widstrom, 1993). Washing the nipples with any substance other than plain water may remove this natural lubrication, dry out the breast skin, and reduce the scent. Lubricating the nipples with creams unnecessarily will coat the skin and thereby reduce the amount of air reaching the tissue, making the skin less healthy. Creams may also introduce a scent or taste that the baby dislikes or does not recognize.

▼ Supportive and Sustaining Tissue

Under the skin and between parts of the milk-producing and milk-transporting tissues lie other tissues that are vital to the function of the breast. Connective tissues support the breast, whereas subcutaneous fatty tissues give it shape. Nerves provide a triggering mechanism for milk synthesis and release. The blood and lymph systems bring nourishment to breast tissues, supply the nutrients for human milk, and filter out bacteria and cast-off dead cell parts.

Nerves

The breast contains sensory nerves that trigger breast function for lactation. From the fourth, fifth, and sixth **intercostal** nerves, these sensory fibers **innervate** the smooth muscle in the nipples and blood vessels. Intercostal nerves are located in the space between two ribs (see Fig. 6.2). Innervation is the distribution of nerve fibers or nerve impulses. There is extensive innervation of the nipple and areola composed of both **autonomic nerves** and sensory nerves. Autonomic nerves have the ability to function independently without outside influence. The epidermis of the nipple and areola are supplied with few nerves, whereas the deeper part, the dermis, is amply supplied. Although these deeper nerves are insensitive to light touch, they are highly responsive to suckling stimulation. A baby who grasps the breast well and suckles vigorously will stimulate the deeper nerves. This stimulation, in turn, starts the milk production and release mechanisms, and activates Montgomery glands and milk duct openings. A baby who is weak or tired, or one who is sucking on the nipple alone, will not provide adequate stimulation to the deeper nerves. Ultimately, this factor may result in lower milk production and less effective letdowns. This explains why a mother whose baby cannot nurse and who must express milk from her breasts will often notice a gradual decline in milk production.

Fatty Tissue

The fatty tissue within the breast cushions the organ and makes it comfortable as well as graceful. Fat cells are found throughout most of the breast, between lobuli, ducts, and lactiferous sinuses, and under the skin. There is no fat deposited immediately beneath the areola and nipple. That area is dominated by muscular tissue and the lactiferous sinuses. The amount of fatty tissue in the breast primarily determines breast size. Fatty tissue does not contribute to milk synthesis or transport. Therefore, the amount of fat or size of the breast is no indication of the quality or quantity of milk that will be produced. Women with large or small breasts may breastfeed equally well.

Connective Tissue

The breast contains fibrous connective tissue that supports and contains the fatty tissue, milk-producing and milk-transporting tissues, and all the other parts of the organ. Some fibrous bands attach the breast to the overlying skin and the underlying fibrous tissue enclosing the muscles. These bands, known as **Cooper's ligaments**, keep the breasts from sagging. Other fibers hold the segments of the breast together and support the ducts as they fill with milk. All of the fibers elongate and increase in number as the breast grows during pregnancy. They expand further with lactation. The fibrous tissue acts in much the same way as does the muscle of the uterine wall. Both grow during pregnancy and follow a pattern of cyclic growth and deterioration throughout the menstrual cycle. The uterine wall retracts when pregnancy ends. Fibrous breast tissue retracts after lactation has ceased.

There are no conclusive studies available to show whether or not fibrous tissue returns to its prepregnancy condition. Some women notice that their breasts sag and their abdomens protrude after pregnancy and lactation. More than likely, these changes are due to the pregnancy rather than lactation. The same effects can be observed in women who do not breastfeed their infants. Many caregivers believe that breast sagging can be lessened by the wearing of a good support bra during pregnancy and lactation, especially during times when the breasts are enlarged and full. However, this belief is not supported by research. Mothers can wear a bra for comfort only if they wish. Caution them against support bras with underwires and other stiff parts which may press on milk ducts.

Blood and Lymph Systems

Everything the breast cells need for nourishment—proteins, fats, carbohydrates, and other substances—is brought to them by the bloodstream. Fluids containing these nutrients pass through the capillaries to the tissue spaces, where they are absorbed by the cells. Capillaries are tiny blood vessels that link the arteries and the veins. The body has a miraculous control over the amount of blood that flows into tissue. Circulation is maintained by the body at a level that meets the needs of each tissue. When the needs of the breast are increased during menstruation and pregnancy, blood flow increases to support tissue building. Later, when frequent suckling signals a need to increase milk production, more blood becomes available to provide the nutrients needed to make milk.

The **lymphatic system** acts like the bloodstream in reverse. The lymphatic system is a complex network of capillaries, thin vessels, valves, ducts, nodes, and organs. Lymph is a thin, clear, slightly yellow fluid. It is about 95 percent water with a few red blood cells and variable numbers of white blood cells. The lymphatic system absorbs the excess blood fluids from the tissue spaces and eventually returns them to the heart. **Lymph nodes** (small rounded masses) function as filters in the lymph vessels to trap bacteria and cast-off cell parts. Each node is a potential dam to arrest the spread of infection. At times, lymph nodes may swell and be painful when functioning in this way. Most of the lymph produced within the breast flows into the nodes in the armpit. There, they will trap bacteria that travels up the ducts from the nipple or from the bloodstream. The swelling of a lymph node in the armpit could suggest that an infection is present in the breast, as well as in the arm or hand.

During breast **engorgement** (swelling or congestion of body tissues), increased pressure from milk in the ducts halts the flow of blood and lymph. This condition causes tissues to become waterlogged, which is referred to as **edema** (abnormal pooling of fluid in tissue) (Hill, 1994). With the lymphatic system at a standstill, the risk of local infection increases. Bacteria and cell particles are not adequately removed from the breast, leading to poor drainage of the duct and the connected alveolus. Generally, bacteria multiply more easily in stagnant fluids than in moving ones. This predisposes a poorly drained breast to **mastitis** (breast inflammation characterized by pain, swelling, redness, and fever). In order to reduce pressure within the breast, the milk needs to be removed as quickly and efficiently as possible. This can be accomplished by the infant feeding frequently for short periods of time or by expressing milk from the breast.

Glandular Tissue

The breast is a highly efficient gland that takes raw materials from blood and creates new and essential nutrients for the baby. It is a gland composed of many smaller individual glands, or lobuli (plural of **lobule**). These lobuli, in turn, are made up of many milk-producing **alveoli** (described later). The lobuli are connected to a system of ducts that provide a passageway for the milk to flow out of the breast and to the infant. This functional portion of the breast that produces and transports milk is called the glandular tissue. Understanding

the structure of the functioning tissue in greater detail will help you assist mothers in preventing and solving breastfeeding problems.

Milk-Producing Tissue

The production of milk takes place in the breast in tiny individual glands called alveoli. The singular form is alveolus, also called **acinus**. The alveoli consist of epithelial cells encased in a smooth muscle layer, known as the **myoepithelial cells**. Numerous capillaries surround the alveoli and bring nutrient-rich blood from which the alveoli select the ingredients to make milk. Through this same system, the alveoli receive oxytocin and prolactin, which signal them to release and produce more milk.

The alveoli are clustered together in groups of 10 to 100 to form lobuli, as shown in Figures 6.2 and 6.3. These lobes are arranged around the nipple as in a pie. About 15 to 20 smaller lobuli make up one lobe. During pregnancy, the alveoli enlarge and the cells undergo rapid multiplication. When lactation begins, the cells in the center of the lobule undergo fatty degeneration. They are then eliminated in the first milk as **colostrum** corpuscles. The outer alveoli remain to produce milk, which is ejected into the cavity in the center of the lobule.

Lobuli are spread throughout the breast. The majority are concentrated in the lower half and toward the **axilla** (underarm) against the chest wall. Breast tissue that extends into the axilla is known as the **tail of Spence**. Only a minimal amount of lobuli extend across the top half of the breast. It is for this reason that women who express milk are advised to concentrate **breast massage** in the bottom portion and toward the underarm.

The myoepithelial cells, or smooth muscle layers, enclose the alveoli and ductules in overlapping bands to form a dense basket-like meshwork (see Fig. 6.3). These cells multiply and greatly increase in size during pregnancy and lactation. They later decrease in size and number when breastfeeding ends. Like other smooth muscle cells in the body, such as those in the uterine wall and the nipple, myoepithelial cells contract when they are exposed to the hormone oxytocin that is released during suckling. The contraction of these cells results in a squeezing effect on the lobule, forcing milk down the ducts.

Milk-Transporting Tissue

The tissue through which the milk flows is a system of **lactiferous** (mammary) **ductules,** secondary ducts, ducts, lactiferous sinuses, and nipple pores, as shown in Figure 6.2. In the young girl, the **duct system** begins with a few small basic ducts in childhood. They sprout

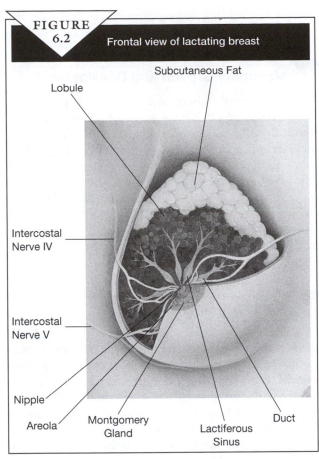

FIGURE 6.2 Frontal view of lactating breast

Lobule
Subcutaneous Fat
Intercostal Nerve IV
Intercostal Nerve V
Nipple
Areola
Montgomery Gland
Lactiferous Sinus
Duct

Illustration by Ka Botzis.

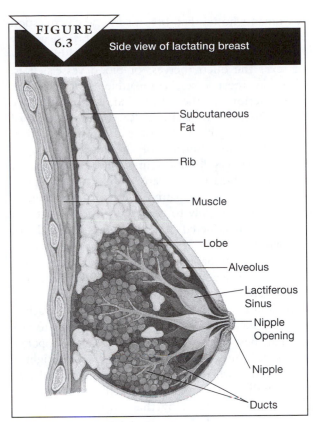

FIGURE 6.3 Side view of lactating breast

Subcutaneous Fat
Rib
Muscle
Lobe
Alveolus
Lactiferous Sinus
Nipple Opening
Nipple
Ducts

Illustration by Ka Botzis.

and branch during puberty, forming tissue buds for the future development of alveoli and lobuli. With each ovulation, the ducts grow lengthwise as alveoli and lobuli develop. During the first 4 to 5 months of pregnancy, sprouting and growth of ducts and alveolar development intensify. In the second half of pregnancy, the duct and alveolar tissues become more specialized in preparation for their milk-related functions.

The mature lactating breast contains 15 to 25 duct systems. These ducts bring the milk out of the breast through an equal number of nipple pores. Each duct widens in the area beneath the areola to form a lactiferous sinus. The lactiferous sinuses—you can help mothers visualize them as small pockets of milk—narrow considerably in the nipple. Feeding each duct are 20 to 40 smaller ducts, or secondary ducts, with a lobule on each one. The lobuli, in turn, are supplied with milk through ductules by 10 to 100 alveoli. The total number of alveoli varies from 3,000 to 100,000 during lactation. This may account for the fact that some mothers have such

an abundant supply of milk, whereas others have just enough to meet their babies' needs.

The Question of Insufficient Mammary Tissue

In rare cases, a woman lacks the functional breast tissue to produce sufficient milk for her infant's total nourishment. Signs of possible duct work insufficiency are (Neifert, 1990)

- No noticeable change in breast size during pregnancy or lactation.
- One breast appreciably smaller than the other.
- Previous or family history of lactation failure.
- Inadequate milk production despite appropriate feeding management.
- Ductal **atresia** (absence of a normal body opening), where the milk duct opening is absent, thereby preventing milk from being ejected from that particular duct.

A woman who has had breast surgery may question her ability to breastfeed. **Breast augmentation** usually does not involve the destruction of functional breast tissue or sever the ducts, nerves, or blood vessels. It is, therefore, in most cases, compatible with lactation. **Breast reduction**, on the other hand, is more intrusive and can interfere with lactation. **Resection** (removal of tissue by surgery) of the breast with **transplantation** (removal and reattachment) of the nipple severs all ducts. This renders lactation impossible. Removal of portions of the breast with transposition of the nipple, areola, and ducts is compatible with breastfeeding, as long as the nerve supply to the breast is left intact. An Austrian study conducted in 1993 indicates that 14 of 16 women who had aesthetic mammary operations breastfed, with no patient reporting severe complications with breastfeeding (Deutinger, 1993). Another source indicates that breastfeeding is possible after modern reduction techniques because less tissue is detached from the nipple (Marshall, 1994). It is important to recognize that these mothers may not be able to support a full milk supply after the baby reaches a certain weight.

Any woman who has had breast surgery is advised to check with her surgeon to learn if any functional breast tissue was affected by the surgery. This would apply to chest or cardiac surgery as well. A recently developed technique measures blood flow and innervation to the nipple following surgery as a means of predicting a woman's ability to breastfeed (Hallock, 1992). This study confirms the occurrence of low milk production following some surgeries. However, it is probably not a practical answer for the mother who asks the question, "Will I be able to breastfeed my baby?" A far simpler answer is for her to breastfeed and, with her physician, to monitor her infant's weight gain carefully.

Women who have had surgery to remove cysts, cancer, or other growths are advised to contact their physicians before attempting to breastfeed. Some health professionals believe that the hormones of lactation increase the probability that such conditions will recur. There is sufficient data, however, to encourage lactation after surgery for early-stage breast cancer. Higgins and Haffty (1994) report that "successful breastfeeding from the untreated, as well as the treated breast, is possible after conservative surgery and radiation." There is also an anecdotal report of a mother who underwent breast surgery, received radiation therapy, and was able to nurse after a 3-month waiting period (Baird, 1989).

Whenever a mother has great difficulty producing enough milk and breastfeeding management issues have been ruled out, consider the possibility of insufficient ductwork. If the mother has tried all means of increasing production and is unable to keep up with her infant's requirements, supplements may be needed. Both the mother and infant can still derive the benefits of breast-feeding while nursing and supplementing. It is to everyone's benefit to encourage this positive outlook.

Mammary Growth and Development

With the onset of puberty and throughout pregnancy, the mammary gland is in a stage of **mammogenesis**, when it develops to a functioning state. During the last **trimester** of pregnancy, it enters into **lactogenesis**, when milk synthesis and secretion are established. With the establishment of **mature milk** and throughout lactation, the breast is in a state of **galactopoiesis. Involution** occurs at the end of lactation, with the breast slowly returning to its prepregnant state. See Figures 6.4 and 6.5 for a comparison of the breast before and during pregnancy.

Mammary Growth during the Fetal Stage

The beginnings of breast development become noticeable in the fetus at 5 weeks of life. At this time, two ridges of tissue called **milk lines** are detectable. They extend from the armpits to the inner thighs. The lower parts of the milk lines disappear after a few weeks. By 20 to 32 weeks, the upper parts develop and form milk ducts. Sometimes, the lower ends of the milk lines fail to regress and the child is born with one or more **supernumerary nipples** along this line. Toward the end of gestation, the ducts form openings in the nipples that are depressed below the surface of the skin. Just before birth, the nipples push outward and become level with the skin. In some females, this step fails, resulting in a nipple that is partially or completely inverted.

When some babies (both male and female) are born, their breasts become congested and secrete a colostrum-like fluid, sometimes referred to as **witch's milk**. This fluid consists primarily of shed epithelial cells. It is thought to be caused by an influx of hormones through the mother's **placenta** at birth. Babies who are born before term do not have this secretion. Left alone, witch's milk disappears in about 20 days.

Mammary Growth between Puberty and Pregnancy

The majority of functional breast tissue development occurs during puberty and pregnancy—two periods of increased hormonal activity. Although the structural growth of the breast is very apparent during puberty, only a small amount of alveolar development takes place. During ovulatory cycles, the development of functional breast tissue is slight. With the advent of pregnancy,

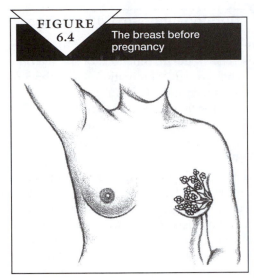

Illustration by Marcia Smith.

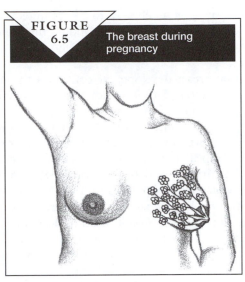

Illustration by Marcia Smith.

hormonal changes cause a spectacular phase of growth and proliferation within the breast.

Because the breast is attached over the bony rib cage, it grows outward. The skin that covers and contains the breast expands and grows to accommodate it. The result is a gland that is evenly rounded with a protruding nipple. With the onset of menstruation, the body's hormonal balance is altered by an increased production of **estrogen**. This produces the growth of ducts and the connective tissue between them. At this time, a thick layer of fat is deposited under the skin and forms the firm and enlarged adolescent breast. The areola and the nipple grow and take on a deeper color during puberty and again in pregnancy.

During puberty, the major changes in functional breast tissue are typically complete approximately 12 to 18 months after the first menstrual period. The formation of fibrous connective tissue and the laying down of fat continue to increase breast size during each adolescent menstrual period. Between the events of puberty and pregnancy, the mammary gland is relatively inactive. Twelve to sixteen days before the onset of menses, the ovaries release an egg and estrogen is released. The reproduction of ductule tissue in the breast and the formation of alveolar cells occur in preparation for pregnancy. However, this proliferation is not significant in terms of breast size. The breast fullness experienced by women just before menstruation is due to an increased blood supply and excessive fluid retained in the tissues. After the menstrual cycle is complete, tissue growth regresses and glandular cells degenerate. Loss of fluid from the tissues causes the breast to return to its previous size. Because regression of tissue growth is incomplete, the

ovulatory cycle slightly enhances mammary growth for younger women (before approximately 30 to 35 years of age). However, in terms of overall breast development and preparation for lactation, breast tissue enhancement during pregnancy is far more significant than any total gain made during menstrual cycles.

Mammary Growth during Pregnancy

With the onset of pregnancy, the mammary gland enters the stage of mammogenesis, when it develops to a functioning state. During the first trimester of pregnancy (0 to 3 months), estrogen and **progesterone** levels cause the duct system to multiply. The skin begins to respond to internal enlargement. The nipple and areola area, in particular, increase in circumference. The darkening or increased pigmentation in this area may make this growth seem more apparent. Montgomery glands, often unnoticed before pregnancy, now enlarge or elongate. They give the area a rough pimply appearance (most noticeable if the breast is cool). The Montgomery glands begin to secrete an oily substance that protects the nipple and areolar skin. This protective lubricant continues to be produced throughout pregnancy and lactation. The Montgomery glands often become noticeable by the first missed menstrual period, giving the experienced mother an early sign of pregnancy.

In the second trimester (4 to 6 months), the duct system continues to develop and the alveoli begin to appear as a result of placental prolactin (see Fig. 6.5). By the end of the trimester, the blood supply and body fluids (lymph) that support alveolar growth and the multiplying number of alveoli have increased the weight of the breast by as much as 1 to 1½ pounds. Production of colostrum is established, and at this point if a woman were to deliver prematurely, she would be able to lactate.

General breast development continues throughout the third trimester (7 to 9 months). Stretch marks may appear, as evidence of the stress on the skin. The nipple and areola darken and enlarge. Their color will lighten somewhat at birth and toward the end of lactation. This process is repeated with each succeeding pregnancy. The change in size and color is more pronounced in younger women, perhaps because their breasts are not fully mature when pregnancy occurs. During pregnancy, from the time that the alveoli begin to develop, alveolar cells wear out and are constantly being replaced. This proliferation of ductwork during pregnancy explains why adolescent mothers are able to lactate despite their recent pubescent changes. The cycle continues throughout lactation, indicating the ongoing process of breast development.

▼ Lactogenesis

Lactogenesis is the phase during which milk synthesis and secretion are established. Lactogenesis occurs in three stages. **Stage I lactogenesis** starts at the beginning of the third trimester of pregnancy. At this time, increases occur in **lactose,** total proteins, and **immunoglobulin**, with a decrease in sodium and chloride. The gland begins to gather the substances needed for milk synthesis. **Stage II lactogenesis** occurs at around the second or third day postpartum. It is referred to as the time when the colostral phase ends and **transitional milk** is produced. Blood flow within the breast increases, and copious milk secretion begins. After about 10 days, **Stage III lactogenesis**, also called **galactopoiesis,** marks the establishment and maintenance of mature milk. Lactogenesis is followed by a period of **involution** (normal process marked by decreasing size of an organ), with the breast slowly returning to its prepregnant state. This process takes about 3 months when accompanied by slow and gradual weaning. Abrupt weaning will cause marked involution in a matter of days or weeks.

Understanding the physical process of lactation will help you advise mothers on the daily management of breastfeeding. An awareness of the factors that influence milk synthesis enables you to explain to mothers the way in which frequent suckling increases milk production. In order to identify problems with milk letdown and to help mothers work out solutions, you need to recognize factors that initiate letdown, the function of hormones in the letdown process, and their effects on breast tissue.

▼ Hormonal Impact on Lactation

Hormones are chemical products of the **endocrine** glands. They regulate functions of specific organs or tissues. The growth, maturation, and function of the breast are the result of stimulation by four major hormones—estrogen, progesterone, prolactin, and oxytocin—described in the following sections.

Estrogen

Estrogen is produced in the ovaries and placenta. It stimulates growth of the uterus, vagina, and other reproductive organs. Estrogen is responsible for the development of female secondary sex characteristics, such as the distinctive female skeleton, skin, body contour, and mammary glands. In the breast, estrogen causes the growth of duct work and of the connective tissue between the ducts.

Progesterone

Progesterone is produced in the ovaries and placenta. The name means, in Latin, for gestation. Progesterone works along with estrogen to maintain the reproductive tract and menstrual cycle. It is essential for the maintenance of pregnancy and aids in the development of the milk-secreting cells in the breast. Progesterone inhibits prolactin's effects during pregnancy. A retained placenta following delivery, and its accompanying progesterone, could impair milk synthesis.

Prolactin

Prolactin is produced in the placenta and in the anterior **pituitary**. It means, in Latin, *for lactation*. Anterior pituitary prolactin stimulates alveolar growth in the breast during pregnancy. Prolactin level in the mother's blood increases soon after initiation of the sucking stimulus. Prolactin tells the breast to speed up milk synthesis. It serves as a natural tranquilizer and stimulates feelings in the mother of restlessness and yearning for her baby. It is for this reason that prolactin is referred to as the "milk-making hormone." The tension created by this yearning is relieved by the relaxing effect of oxytocin, released when the baby is put to breast. The repetition of this cycle provides a physiologically conditioned response in the mother to interact positively with her baby. Thus, prolactin is often credited with inducing maternal behavior.

A mother can do several things to keep prolactin levels high. She can make sure her baby is attached effectively at the breast and is not given any artificial nipples or pacifiers that would cause **nipple preference**. She can give her baby unlimited access to the breast, breastfeeding as frequently as he wants, usually every 1 to 3 hours, and as long as he wants at a feed. Also, she can breastfeed during the night, when prolactin release in response to suckling is greatest.

Oxytocin

Oxytocin is produced in the **hypothalamus** and transported via nerve fibers to the posterior pituitary, where it is stored. The infant's suckling stimulates nerve endings in the nipple. Impulses are carried through the hypothalamic region to the posterior pituitary. Oxytocin is released there and taken by the blood to the breasts. It causes smooth muscle cells to contract, thus producing the uterine contractions of childbirth, **afterpains**, and orgasm. Oxytocin causes the muscle layer around each milk-producing cell to contract during letdown. This is called the **milk ejection reflex**. In response, the high-fat **hindmilk** is pushed down the ducts and out through the nipple pores. Initially, the mother may need several minutes of stimulus to have a high enough level to be effective. She will notice when the milk ejects because the rhythm of the infant's suckling will change from rapid to regular deep, slow sucks (about one per second). **Pitocin** is a synthetic form of oxytocin that sometimes is used for induction or augmentation of labor.

Hormonal Imbalances That Affect Lactation

The lactation process is regulated by hormones in the woman's body. Therefore, a disturbance in her hormone levels has the potential to affect milk synthesis and release. Pituitary, thyroid, and adrenal imbalances can alter a mother's hormone levels, as can certain medications. This imbalance may cause her to produce too little or too much milk, to release milk at inappropriate times, or to fail to release milk at all. Women who have difficulty conceiving or who have become pregnant by any of the new reproductive technologies are at a higher risk for hormone imbalance and milk insufficiency.

If a mother has breastfeeding problems and has had a vague feeling of physical discomfort or a history of previous thyroid problems or menstrual irregularities, she may have a hormone imbalance. Placental retention can inhibit the process of lactation by causing hormones to remain at pregnancy levels. The absence of breast fullness and changes in breast secretions are signs that placental fragments may have been retained. The incidence of hormone imbalances causing breastfeeding problems is extremely low. However, if all other measures have proved ineffective in regulating a mother's milk production or letdown, refer the mother to her physician for a general examination to rule out hormone imbalance as a cause.

Sheehan's Syndrome

Sheehan's syndrome can result from severe postpartum hemorrhage and **hypotension**. In this condition, the mother's blood pressure drops so low that blood fails to circulate to the pituitary gland. This causes some or all of the cells in the gland to stop working permanently. The mother may have produced some colostrum in her breasts before going into shock. However, as a result of the malfunctioning pituitary gland, her breasts will remain soft after delivery and she may not be able to produce any milk. This is an irreversible condition and may rule out the prospect of breastfeeding any future babies as well.

Prolactinoma

A **prolactinoma** is a pituitary tumor that secretes prolactin. Although it can cause secondary amenorrhea or **galactorrhea**, a prolactinoma is not a reason for a mother to not breastfeed. Breastfeeding does not seem to affect the size nor the activity of the tumor (Ikegami, 1987). In some cases, there is an abnormal or lack of breast tissue response to normal hormone levels.

Hypothyroidism

Hypothyroidism is a condition caused by a deficiency of thyroid secretion. This disorder results in sluggishness, low blood pressure, dry skin, possible obesity, and sensitivity to cold. Replacement therapy with natural or synthetic hormone preparations can totally eliminate these symptoms. A mother who is properly managed while receiving a thyroid supplementation can breastfeed without compromising her baby's health. The supplementation she receives merely brings the mother's own thyroid to a normal level. Therefore, the amount of thyroid secretion the infant receives through her milk is equal to that of any other breastfeeding mother.

There is one word of caution, however, for the mother who is severely hypothyroid and receiving unusually high dosages of thyroid supplement. The additional thyroid that passes to her baby through her milk may mask latent hypothyroidism while he is being breastfed. When weaning begins and the level of thyroid intake decreases, the infant with latent hypothyroidism could suffer brain damage. Many hospitals routinely screen for hypothyroidism in newborns in conjunction with screening for phenylketonuria. It is also worthwhile to note that many severely hypothyroid women are unable to become pregnant, so the likelihood of your encountering such a mother is rare.

▼ Colostrum Production

Colostrum is a unique substance that appears as a semi-transparent, thick, and sticky liquid ranging in color from pale to deep yellow. It contains water, minerals, fat droplets, **lymphocytes**, and similar cells. It also contains cast-off alveolar cells, which form a unique combination of nutrients designed to meet the nutritional and **immunologic** needs of the newborn. Colostrum acts as a natural lubricant, and because of its **lysozyme** content, it is **bactericidal** (a substance that destroys bacteria).

Alveoli begin producing colostrum in the fourth month of pregnancy. Only small amounts are released into the center of the lobuli. As pregnancy advances, colostrum continues to be produced and to fill the alveoli. Estrogen and progesterone act directly on the alveolar **epithelium** to suppress the secretion of colostrum. Some colostrum may leak out of the alveoli through the cell pores. Protruding portions of the alveoli may break away into the center of the lobule. Thus, some women find that their breasts leak colostrum during the later months of pregnancy.

▼ Milk Synthesis

When the placenta is delivered, estrogen and progesterone levels in the body drop sharply and prolactin production in the anterior pituitary rises. The high level of prolactin, combined with decreased levels of estrogen and progesterone, signals the alveoli to start producing and secreting milk. If the infant is allowed free access to the breast, colostrum will be replaced with transitional milk and will result in increased milk production and breast fullness between the second and fifth day postpartum. This is sometimes accompanied by a low-grade fever, which is normal and not a cause for concern. With initial milk production, many women experience a **normal fullness** in their breasts. This can be mistaken for engorgement by those who do not understand this normal physiologic response.

Prolactin is the hormone that promotes milk synthesis. It is present in small amounts in all humans, both male and female. Prolactin levels increase gradually during pregnancy. Levels reach a peak of 20 times the normal value near term. The estrogen and progesterone of pregnancy act locally on the alveoli to inhibit milk production and secretion. After delivery, when estrogen and progesterone levels have dropped, prolactin levels are high to stimulate initial milk production. Levels increase again tenfold in response to suckling. After 3 months postpartum, prolactin levels range three to five times above the level of a menstruating female. Further stimulation results in doubling of the level above the baseline through the second year of lactation (Lawrence, 1999).

Recent research suggests that milk synthesis is not based entirely on endocrine control. Milk production becomes dependent on the frequency of drainage and the degree of drainage of each breast. This factor may be due to a constituent present in the milk that suppresses milk synthesis by negative feedback when it remains in the alveoli. Researchers have identified the apparent human whey protein **feedback inhibitor of lactation (FIL)** that enables autocrine inhibition of milk synthesis (Wilde, 1995a). **Autocrine control** is defined as local control within the gland. In the case of the breast, the control agent is a **secretory** product from one type of cell that influences the activity of this same type of cell. This suggests that milk that is left in the breast acts to inhibit the production of more milk. Thus the mother produces only what her baby needs and protects her energy expenditure during lactation (DeCoopman, 1993). This theory helps explain why women are able to nurse with just one breast exclusively through the course of lactation and not develop chronic engorgement or mastitis in the other breast (Ing, 1977).

During times when the baby is not nursing, prolactin is prevented from being released by a substance **prolactin inhibitory factor (PIF)**. Suckling inhibits PIF, thereby allowing the release of prolactin. The level of prolactin released is affected significantly by frequency of feeding and stimulation of the nipple. It is important, therefore, to encourage frequent feeds, good positioning of the baby at the breast, and avoidance of nipple shields. In the absence of effective and frequent suckling to remove milk from the breast, prolactin production decreases and autocrine inhibition begins. This decrease delays Stage II lactogenesis and lowers the mother's milk production. Help mothers understand that milk production changes from endocrine control to autocrine control. Frequent feeds are necessary in the beginning to ensure an increase in the number and sensitivity of prolactin receptors for when prolactin levels fall to normal. This concept and that of frequent feeds are necessary for long-term milk production.

▼ Milk Ejection Reflex (Letdown)

Milk ejection, also referred to as **letdown,** is a reflex that can be triggered by various stimuli. When the baby suckles, contact between his tongue and the mother's nipple stimulates nerve endings to send a message to the hypothalamus. The message is then relayed to the anterior pituitary. This, in turn, lowers the prolactin inhibitory factor and enables prolactin to be released. As suckling continues, the posterior pituitary gland secretes oxytocin. This causes the smooth muscles around the alveoli and the uterus to contract. Milk is forced down through the duct system to the lactiferous sinuses underneath the areola (Fig. 6.6.). The milk is then available to the baby, who, through a combination of suction, rhythmic compression of the gums, and undulating movement of the tongue, can nurse the milk out through the nipple pores.

Milk ejection is **bilateral,** occurring at the same time in both breasts. Milk is prevented from flowing freely from the nonsuckled breast by **sphincters** at the end of the ducts. A sphincter is a circular band of muscle fibers that narrows a passage or closes a natural opening in the body. Letdown brings the milk into the ducts, thus making it accessible to the baby through the activity of suckling. Initially, letdown causes active expulsion

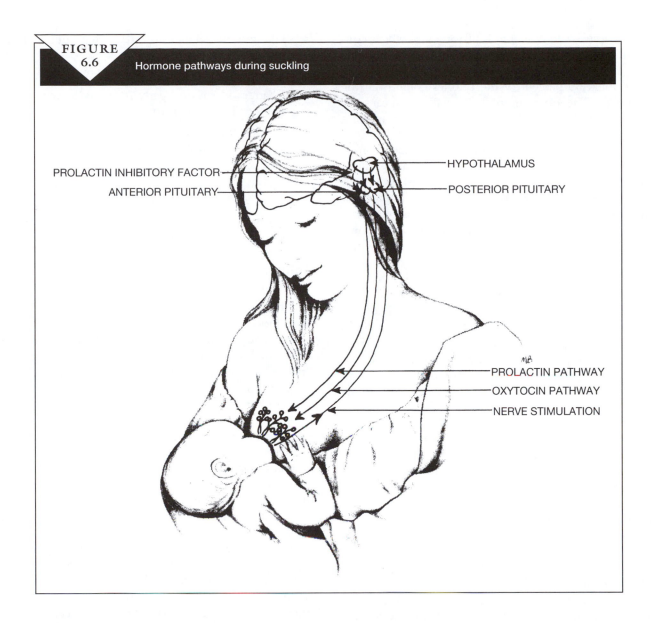

FIGURE 6.6   Hormone pathways during suckling

PROLACTIN INHIBITORY FACTOR
ANTERIOR PITUITARY

HYPOTHALAMUS
POSTERIOR PITUITARY

PROLACTIN PATHWAY
OXYTOCIN PATHWAY
NERVE STIMULATION

of milk through pressure within the lactiferous sinuses and ducts. This lasts for a relatively short time, and then the flow subsides. Positive pressure is maintained within the breast, and milk flow will continue with further suckling. Letdown provides for free flow of milk, which is essential to move fat globules down through the ducts. When milk does not flow freely, engorgement can develop, which could lead to a plugged duct or mastitis.

A woman may become aware that her milk is letting down when her baby's swallowing pattern changes. He may begin gulping or be unable to control the flow of milk and pull away from her breast. Some women notice that milk drips from one breast while the baby is nursing on the other breast. Since letdown is bilateral, this **leaking** is a sign that milk has let down in both breasts. Letdown may cause a tingling or tightening sensation. This feeling is the result of thousands of alveoli contracting and of the pressure of milk being forced through the duct system. The mother may also experience increased

thirst or sleepiness. In the first days postpartum, letdown often is accompanied by uterine contractions due to oxytocin's action on the involuting uterus. Mothers will experience several letdowns in a single feed. The initial letdown is usually the only one that is noticed owing to the large quantity of milk moved at this time.

A functioning letdown reflex is crucial to nourishing an infant. In the absence of letdown, the infant receives only a third of the milk. Letdown enables him to receive the majority of the fat content of the milk that tends to stick to the duct lining. This is the "cream," or hindmilk. As letdown occurs, it forces the hindmilk down into the lactiferous sinuses, where it mixes with the high-protein **foremilk** that collected there since the previous feed. The infant then receives more fatty milk after letdown as the feed progresses. It is important that the infant nurse long enough on each breast to receive sufficient calories. Limiting nursing time on one breast in order to switch to the other breast could cause the infant to receive a large volume of foremilk, which contains fewer calories. This practice may cause gastric upset, as well as low weight gain (Woolridge, 1988). In human milk, 50 percent of the calories come from the fat content. Therefore, an inhibited letdown means the infant is underfed even if a fair amount of fluid is being ingested.

The letdown reflex may not be recognized consistently in the first days and weeks of breastfeeding. This is especially the case for women who are breastfeeding for the first time. Encourage mothers to relax both physically and mentally during the early weeks. The less tension a woman experiences, the more likely she is to let down her milk consistently during a feed. You can also suggest that she choose a quiet location and a comfortable position, as well as set up a routine to begin each feed. This will help ensure that letdown becomes a firmly established part of each feeding session and will condition the mother psychologically for letdown. These techniques are especially helpful to a woman who is separated from her baby and is providing milk through hand expression or pumping. When she becomes conditioned to letdown, the mother may notice that her milk lets down when she picks up her baby, when she hears a baby cry, or whenever she thinks about her baby.

Some mothers experience no physical sensations to indicate that their milk is letting down. They can be encouraged to look for signs in the infant that their letdown reflex is functioning. After letdown has occurred, the infant may begin gulping or even gagging from the sudden rush of milk. Swallowing will also be more pronounced than at the beginning of the feed. She can monitor the number of wet diapers and stools her baby has during a 24-hour period. Six or more wet diapers and four or more stools a day from the end of the first week of life through the first month indicate that her milk is letting down and that her baby is well nourished. Signs that the letdown reflex is functioning are summarized in the next section. The mother's awareness of letdown may diminish as she and her baby become more experienced in breastfeeding and begin to focus on other aspects of their relationship.

Signs of a Functioning Letdown Reflex

◆ Tingling sensation or feeling of fullness or tightening in the breasts.

◆ Leaking from the other breast while nursing.

◆ Leaking when thinking about the baby or hearing a baby cry.

◆ Uterine contractions (afterpains); especially noticeable in **multipara** women.

◆ A feeling of relaxation or well-being.

◆ Increased thirst.

◆ Filling of the lactiferous sinuses that can be felt with the fingers.

◆ Areola is drawn in toward the baby's lips.

◆ Changes in sucking pattern during a feed; sucking slows or baby begins to gulp.

◆ Swallowing is heard.

◆ The baby is satisfied and gaining weight.

◆ The baby has at least 6 wet diapers and 4 stools per day after day 5 with no water or formula supplements.

◆ Change in the baby's stools from dark **meconium** to yellow, soft, and seedy by day 5 postpartum.

Inhibited Letdown

The letdown reflex can be inhibited by such emotional or physical states as fatigue, anxiety, fear, and pain. A new mother may be anxious about her breastfeeding and parenting. She may feel tense and pressured by work and family commitments or unsupportive family and friends. Perhaps she is overtired due to lack of rest or overexertion. She may be experiencing pain from childbirth or resulting surgery. Any of these circumstances could inhibit her letdown. During times of stress or fatigue, the secretion of oxytocin may be inhibited. Adrenaline is released, which is believed to negate the effects of oxytocin on the myoepithelial cell. Letdown also can fail to occur when nipple stimulation is weak, which may happen if the baby is not attached effectively.

A functioning letdown reflex depends on the mother's having a positive attitude about breastfeeding and developing confidence in her ability to do so. Be cautious in discussing any concerns you may have about a mother's letdown reflex. You do not want to plant seeds of doubt that could aggravate poor letdown further. If you become reasonably certain that a woman's letdown reflex is not functioning well, you may need to see her in order to teach her relaxation techniques such as those presented later. You can also build her confidence in her ability to nourish her baby by explaining that her body is able to sustain her baby now, just as it did during pregnancy. A consultation will allow you to discuss pressure from family members and suggest ways of overcoming any opposition to breastfeeding.

When letdown does not occur, it usually becomes evident in the way the baby reacts. He may become frustrated with feeds and pull away from the breast. He may fail to gain enough weight and continually act hungry. A nonfunctioning letdown reflex can also lead to breast engorgement and its related difficulties. The signs of poor letdown and their causes are summarized in Table 6.1, with suggestions for the mother to overcome each problem. Relaxation techniques are presented in Figure 6.7.

TABLE 6.1
Signs, Causes and Treatment of an Inhibited Letdown

SIGNS OF AN INHIBITED LETDOWN

◆ Baby is frustrated after a short time at the breast.

◆ Baby pulls away from the breast repeatedly.

◆ Baby is not gaining weight.

◆ Baby has fewer than 6 wet diapers a day, or has dark concentrated urine.

◆ Baby has fewer than 4 stools a day, or meconium is still present on the fifth day of life or beyond.

◆ Mother has engorged breasts.

◆ Mother has sore nipples.

ACTIONS FOR THE MOTHER

◆ Allow the baby ample time at the breast until he unlatches himself or falls asleep. For a baby who falls asleep and remains latched, try breast compression to encourage further suckling to allow for letdown and good milk flow.

◆ Nurse in a quiet spot away from distractions.

◆ Avoid embarrassing or stressful situations for feeds.

◆ Ask someone to massage her upper back, especially along the sides of the backbone.

◆ Massage her breasts before feeds. (See chapter 19 for a description of breast massage.)

◆ Use warm compresses before feeds.

◆ Express a little milk, and gently stimulate the nipple.

◆ Drink juice, water, or noncaffeine tea before and during feeds.

◆ Condition letdown by setting up a routine for beginning a feed.

◆ Use relaxation and breathing techniques.

◆ Use breast compression while the baby is nursing.

◆ Stimulate the nipples manually before nursing.

◆ Concentrate thoughts on the baby and on milk flow. Turn on a water faucet so that the sound of running water can help to stimulate letdown.

◆ Nap or rest when the baby rests.

◆ Lie down to nurse.

◆ Nurse the baby in bed at night.

◆ Increase skin-to-skin contact with the baby at feeds. Remove her bra and shirt, and have the baby in a diaper only.

◆ Simplify daily chores and establish priorities.

◆ Get help with household, car pooling, and other responsibilities.

◆ Discuss causes of tension, and eliminate or minimize them.

◆ Take a break from the daily routine with an evening out, shopping, a walk, lunch with friends, and so on.

◆ Develop confidence in mothering skills (a personal consultation may help).

CAUSES OF AN INHIBITED LETDOWN

◆ Letdown is not well established.

◆ Mother is overtired or overextended.

◆ Mother is tense or pressured.

◆ Mother is caught in a cycle of little milk, worry, less milk.

◆ Baby is not latched onto the breast effectively.

FIGURE 6.7	Relaxation Techniques for the Mother

◆ Spend a few minutes before going to sleep to analyze your own relaxation techniques, e.g., movements, positions, room darkness. Repeat these techniques at other times for relaxation.
◆ Remove distractions, e.g., find a quiet spot, and take the phone off the hook.
◆ Get comfortable, e.g., empty your bladder; find a cozy chair or bed; get pillows for support; remove eyeglasses, shoes, or tight clothing; adjust room temperature.
◆ Listen to relaxing music.
◆ Take a deep breath and let it out slowly. Repeat this several times.
◆ Breathe steadily and rhythmically, noting the faint movement of your body and breathing slowly to relax further.
◆ Tense your entire body and relax slowly. Concentrate on one muscle at a time, starting from your toes and progressing up to the facial muscles, until your limbs, eyelids and all body parts feel heavy.
◆ Use massage or warm compresses on tense parts of your body.
◆ Take a warm shower or bath.
◆ Close your eyes and move them back and forth or up and down. Then rest your eyes and feel the release of tension. Relax your eyes by thinking about a ship sailing away from you and disappearing over the horizon.
◆ Allow your mind to drift into a sleepy state and think pleasant thoughts, e.g., enjoyable moments, pleasures, dreams.
◆ Think about your baby, of milk flowing, or of water rushing.
◆ Think about, write down or talk with someone about your fears, stresses, tensions, and what you feel causes them. Then let your mind drift or think of pleasant thoughts and feel the release of tension.
◆ Visualize some strenuous or precarious activity, such as walking across thin ice, and then pretend it has ended and you are at ease.
◆ Pray.
◆ Meditate on a passage of a text from a favorite author.

VARIATIONS IN BREAST STRUCTURE AND FUNCTION

Breastfeeding requires something essential from both mother and baby. The mother needs both a desire to breastfeed and breasts that produce and release milk. The infant needs the ability to remove milk from the breast with effective suckling. The manner in which the infant is attached at the breast will determine how much of the mother's nourishing milk is received. The size and shape of a mother's breasts are not indicators of how much milk they are able to produce, nor of how well her baby will thrive on her milk.

The ability to produce and release milk does depend in part on the physical condition of the mother's breast. A wide variety of breast sizes and nipple shapes will accommodate breastfeeding. There are only a few variations in structure that may hinder or contraindicate breastfeeding. Some differences in structure, such as nipple inversion, can be corrected. Other deviations, such as previous breast surgery that has severed milk ducts, may make it necessary to supplement breastfeeding with other foods or to rely totally on an alternative feeding method.

Examining the Mother's Breasts

Caregivers do not need to examine every woman's breasts and nipples. However, if a difficulty arises that you suspect may be due to the mother's nipples or breasts, a careful examination may help. Most women associate breast examination with illness or cancer prevention. Make sure that the mother knows that you are examining her breasts in preparation for breastfeeding. Ensure privacy to help the mother feel comfortable. Before touching the mother's breasts, ask her permission and explain your purpose. Be aware of any customs of modesty that may make this procedure uncomfortable for the mother. Reassure the mother that small and large breasts alike will produce milk.

You can begin by asking the mother if both breasts became larger and the areola became darker during pregnancy. If the answer is yes, this may indicate that there is sufficient functioning tissue in both breasts. Examining both breasts at the same time will enable you to observe the symmetry between them. You can note the skin's elasticity as well as any engorgement, lumps, swelling, or redness. Look for evidence of past breast surgery, which may have severed some ducts. Note the size and shape of the nipples and the size of the areola. Learn how the mother's nipples respond to stimulation, in response to either cold or touching.

Discussing the shape of a woman's nipples needs to be done sensitively and respectfully. If the message the woman hears seems negative, she may be unable to overcome that feeling in order to breastfeed. This type of phenomenon may explain why Alexander and associates (1992) found that just recommending breast shells decreased breastfeeding duration. The researchers did not really measure whether women actually used the shells and, if they did, for how many hours per day, nor

TABLE 6.2

Five Basic Types of Nipples

Type of Nipple	Before Stimulation	After Stimulation
Common nipple The majority of mothers have what is referred to as a **common nipple**. It protrudes slightly when at rest and becomes erect and more graspable when stimulated. A baby has no trouble finding and grasping this nipple in order to pull in a large amount of breast tissue and stretch it to the roof of his mouth.		
Flat nipple The **flat nipple** has a very short shank that makes it less easy for the baby to find and grasp. In response to stimulation, this nipple remains essentially unchanged. Slight movement inward or outward may be present, but not enough to aid the baby in finding and initially grasping the breast on center. This nipple may benefit from the use of a syringe to increase **protractility**.		
Inverted-appearing nipple An **inverted-appearing nipple** may appear inverted but becomes erect after stimulation. This nipple needs no correction and presents no problems with **graspability**.		
Retracted nipple The **retracted nipple** is the most common type of inverted nipple. Initially, this nipple appears to be graspable. However, on stimulation, it retracts, making attachment difficult. This nipple responds well to techniques to increase nipple protrusion.		
Inverted nipple The truly **inverted nipple** is retracted both at rest and when stimulated. Such a nipple is very uncommon and more difficult for the baby to grasp. All techniques used to enhance protractility of breast tissue can be used to improve attachment. Even if the nipple remains retracted, the baby should be able to latch on if the mother helps form her breast into his mouth.		

for how many weeks before giving birth. They measured the recommendation to use shells and found that it was associated with a shortened duration of breastfeeding.

Differences in Nipples

Efficient milk transfer depends on an infant's ability to latch on to the breast, to form it into a conical shape, and to stretch it forward and then upward against the **hard palate** (roof of the mouth). A nipple that protrudes on stimulation aids the infant in finding and centering on the breast. It also provides tissue for the infant to grasp in order to draw the breast into his mouth. Each woman's nipples are unique in shape, size, and the degree to which they protrude. Nipple inversion, in which the nipple retracts inward, is found in 28 to 35 percent of all women in early pregnancy. The skin gains elasticity by the third trimester of pregnancy, and only a small percentage of these women still have some inversion (Blaikeley, 1953; Hytten, 1958; Waller, 1946). The degree of inversion also decreases with each subsequent pregnancy. There seems to be little relationship between the degree of protrusion of the nipple and the ability of the infant to nurse well (Inch, 1989). With a good latch, the infant takes a large portion of the breast into his mouth and forms it into a cone-shaped teat. Milk transfer, therefore, depends more on the pliability of the entire breast than on the configuration of the nipple itself.

There are many variations in types of nipples. For the convenience of discussion, Table 6.2 shows nipples classified into five types. Stimulation—such as touch, cold, or gentle compression—can reveal whether or not inversion is present. Figure 6.8 shows a nipple that appears normal and, on stimulation, becomes inverted (Fig. 6.9). The nipple in Figure 6.10 appears inverted, and yet when it is stimulated, it everts (Fig. 6.11). A **pinch test**, as described in Chapter 19, *Breastfeeding Techniques and Devices,* will help you test the protractility of the mother's nipples.

Working with Nipple Inversion

In order for the baby to receive milk, he needs enough breast tissue in his mouth to reach back to the hard palate. When the breast will not stretch to accommodate this pattern, the baby has difficulty maintaining suction. Only in the very small percentage of women who have a truly inverted nipple will the problem be pronounced to the degree that the baby will have difficulty latching on. Fortunately, in most cases, inversion does not interfere with breastfeeding.

Inverted nipples begin to respond to correction techniques during the last trimester of pregnancy. This is also the time when increased nipple stimulation can induce premature labor in some women. It is for this reason that a woman should be advised to check with her physician before beginning any techniques that involve nipple stimulation.

In the past, the **Hoffman technique** was recommended for correcting nipple inversion. This was a method in which the forefingers would pull outward away from the nipple, in a pattern like rays of the sun, in order to break the **adhesions**. A study by the MAIN Trial Collaborative Group showed that neither the use of breast shells nor the Hoffman technique by randomly assigned women caused nipple elongation (MAIN, 1994).

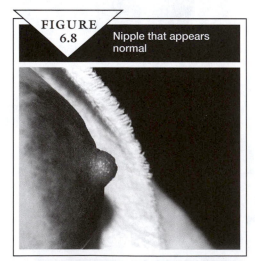

FIGURE 6.8 Nipple that appears normal

Source: Courtesy of Kay Hoover, MEd, IBCLC.

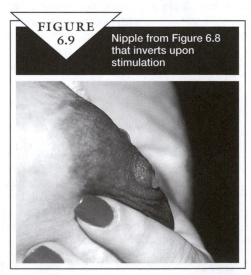

FIGURE 6.9 Nipple from Figure 6.8 that inverts upon stimulation

Source: Courtesy of Kay Hoover, MEd, IBCLC.

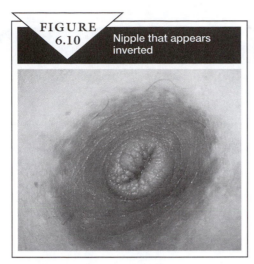

FIGURE 6.10 Nipple that appears inverted

Source: Courtesy of Kay Hoover, MEd, IBCLC.

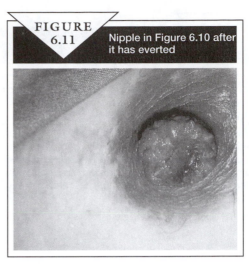

FIGURE 6.11 Nipple in Figure 6.10 after it has everted

Source: Courtesy of Kay Hoover, MEd, IBCLC.

Methods to Decrease Nipple Inversion

There are some techniques that will help **evert** nipples that are difficult for the baby to grasp. A mother may be able to form the nipple by hand or with the aid of ice just before a feed. There is much anecdotal information to recommend wearing breast shells prenatally in order to improve nipple protrusion. It is widely believed that wearing breast shells between feeds improves nipple protractility by gently placing pressure on the skin, stretching and pushing the nipple forward. A study from India indicates that an **inverted syringe** can be used to help elongate the nipple as a preparation for breastfeeding (Kesaree, 1993). Another possibility to encourage protrusion of the nipple is the careful use of suction from a breast pump. Recommended times and frequency of use are similar to those for the inverted syringe. See Chapter 19 for detailed instructions on how to improve the graspability of the nipple with these three methods. In using any of the techniques, mothers need to take care not to increase the suction to painful levels and to limit frequency of use to reasonable levels.

CAUTION

Some hospitals may use a nipple shield as a solution to inversion. However, a nipple shield presents many hazards. Often, the infant may come to prefer the rubber or silicone nipple. Also, the underlying construction of the nipple shield may damage breast tissue. More important, however, the shield interferes with the suckling stimulation that normally induces letdown and subsequent milk production. This is especially the case when the shield is kept in place incorrectly during the entire feed. Use of a nipple shield should be reserved as the method of last resort.

Lumps in the Breast

The general population most frequently associates lumps in the breast with breast cancer. However, there are many breast lumps associated with lactation that are not a health risk. In fact, the normal state of the lactating breast is lumpy due to the enlarged milk-filled alveoli that are distributed throughout the tissues. Other lumps may occur due to a **plugged duct** or **breast infection** (see Chapter 14). These two conditions are usually temporary, and after the cause has been alleviated, the associated lumps disappear.

Regular Breast Self-Examination

Encourage women to check their breasts for lumps regularly and to notify the physician as soon as possible whenever unfamiliar lumps are noticed. The best time for a lactating woman to perform a breast self-examination is immediately after a feed, when her breasts are the least full. If she is menstruating, a good time would be on the seventh to tenth day after menses has ended. The important factor is to do it at the same time each cycle to increase familiarity with the breast in relation to hormonal influences. With regular self-examinations, breastfeeding women will develop a knowledge of their breasts and will notice any changes more readily (Fig. 6.12).

Other Lumps in the Breast

The breasts typically become lumpy during lactation, especially as the lactiferous sinuses fill with milk. Encourage mothers to examine their breasts monthly or even more frequently to develop a knowledge of the way their breasts feel during the various stages of lactation. In this way, a mother will become familiar with her breasts and will quickly recognize a lump if one should

> ## FIGURE 6.12
>
> ### Breast self exam
>
> Pick a regular time of the month to examine your breasts. When you are not pregnant, the best time is right after your menstrual period. Your breasts will feel lumpy and irregular during pregnancy and lactation. The idea is to get to know the particular contours of your breasts. After examining them, ask your physician to do a breast exam during your next visit, so he can confirm that what you felt is normal.
>
> Examine your breasts during a bath or shower. Your fingers will glide easily over wet skin. Keeping your fingers flat, press gently in a circular motion over the entire breast area following the arrows. Use your right hand to examine the left breast; your left hand for the right breast. Check for any lump, hard knot, or thickening.
>
>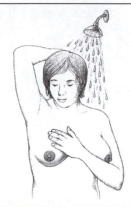
>
>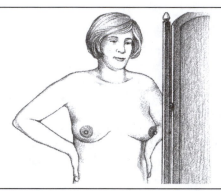
>
>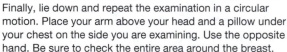
>
> Second, look at your breasts in a mirror, first with your arms at your sides, then with your arms extended over your head. Look for changes in appearance of the breasts, a swelling, dimpling of skin, or changes in the nipple.
>
> Finally, lie down and repeat the examination in a circular motion. Place your arm above your head and a pillow under your chest on the side you are examining. Use the opposite hand. Be sure to check the entire area around the breast.
>
>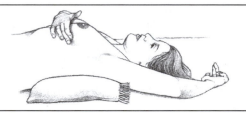

Adapted from *The Parent Manual,* Prepared Childbirth Association of Portland, Oregon. Illustrations by Marcia Smith.

develop. Most often, the lump will be caused by a plugged duct. See Chapter 14 for measures to treat a plugged duct.

If a lump does not move downward and begin to break up, it may be caused by a condition unrelated to breastfeeding. In this case, the woman is well advised to be examined by a physician to identify the cause of the lump. Lumps associated with **fibrocystic breast** change with the menstrual cycle, shrinking and becoming less noticeable after menstruation. Other types of benign cysts may also be present within the breast. A **galactocele,** which is caused by the closing or blockage

of a milk duct, contains a thick, creamy milklike substance that may be discharged from the nipple when the cyst is compressed. It can be aspirated, and some are removed surgically to prevent them from refilling. Stevens and colleagues (1997) found that eight galactoceles resolved spontaneously. This suggests that surgical intervention may not always be required. The presence of a galactocele is compatible with breastfeeding. If surgery is required, it can be done without suspending breastfeeding.

One type of nontender breast lump is an **intraductal papilloma,** a benign tumor within a duct. It is usually associated with a spontaneous bloody discharge from one breast. Please note that trauma is the most frequent cause of bloody discharge, intraductal papilloma is the next, and fibrocystic breast is slightly less frequent. After serious disease is ruled out and either the discharge stops or the involved duct is surgically removed, breastfeeding may continue.

If the lump is due to a malignancy, breastfeeding may need to be discontinued because it is not compatible with the treatments for breast cancer. Often, an infant will refuse to nurse from a cancerous breast (Saber, 1996). You will want to explore breast rejection by the baby whenever a lump is found. However, be careful not to confuse long-term rejection with temporary refusal to nurse for several feeds due to a plug of milk being expelled, or rejection due to conditions in the infant. If the physician locates a lump and wishes to perform a biopsy to rule out cancer, this can be done under local anesthesia without an interruption in breastfeeding. In many cases, lumps are benign and breastfeeding can continue without interruption. Mothers need to be aware that there is a small risk that a milk **fistula** may develop as a result of a biopsy. This may result in milk leaking from the biopsy incision site. Healing of the site may then require temporary interruption of breastfeeding in that breast (Schackmuth, 1993).

SUMMARY

Although breasts may vary from one woman to another in size and appearance, the basic anatomy of the breast makes it possible for the vast majority of women to nurture their babies in the manner in which nature intended. The mammary gland is an intricate system of sensory nerves that trigger milk production, and connective tissue that supports and contains fatty tissue as well as milk-producing and milk-transporting tissues. The blood carries proteins, fats, sugar, and other substances needed for lactation to the breast. The breast takes raw material from blood to create nutrients for the infant. This nutrition is transported through a system of lobuli and ducts that travel to the nipple and is released through several nipple pores. If a woman has undergone breast surgery that damaged the nerves or severed the ducts, her ability to breastfeed may be compromised.

Although puberty triggers the development of functional breast tissue, it is hormonal changes during pregnancy that produce the majority of growth toward lactogenesis. The areola undergoes changes in size and color, and the Montgomery glands become more pronounced. Throughout the 9 months of pregnancy, the breast experiences lactogenesis, transforming into a state of milk production and secretion. Estrogen, progesterone, prolactin, and oxytocin all play a role in altering the hormonal balance to stimulate milk production and release. This balance of hormones can be affected by stress and fatigue, and mothers may need to learn measures to lower stress and stimulate milk letdown.

REFERENCES

Alexander J et al. Randomised controlled trial of breast shells and Hoffman's exercises for inverted and non-protractile nipples. *Br Med J* 304:1030–1032; 1992.

Baird E. Keeping a milk supply after radiation therapy. *Rental Roundup* 6(1):1–2; 1989.

Blaikeley et al. Breastfeeding—factors affecting success. *J Obstet Gynaecol Br Emp* 60:657–659; 1953.

De Coopman J. Breastfeeding after pituitary resection: Support for a theory of autocrine control of milk supply? *J Hum Lact* 9:35–40; 1993.

Deutinger M and Deutinger J. Breastfeeding after aesthetic mammary operations and cardiac operations through horizontal submammary skin incision. *Surg Gynecol Obstet* 176:267–270; 1993.

Hallock G. Prediction of nipple viability following reduction mammoplasty using laser Doppler flowmetry. *Ann Plast Surg* 29:457–460; 1992.

Higgins S and Haffty B. Pregnancy and lactation after breast-conserving therapy for early stage breast cancer. *Cancer* 73:2175–2180; 1994.

Hill P and Humenick S. The occurrence of breast engorgement. *J Hum Lact* 10:79–86; 1994.

Hytten F and Baird D. The development of the nipple in pregnancy. *Lancet* 1:1201–1204; 1958.

Ikegami H et al. Relationship between the methods of treatment for prolactinomas and the puerperal lactation. *Fertil Steril* 47:867–869; 1987.

Inch S. Antenatal preparation for breastfeeding. In Einkin M and Keires M (eds). *Effective Care in Pregnancy and Childbirth*. Oxford: Oxford University Press; pp 335–342; 1989.

Ing R et al. Unilateral breastfeeding and breast cancer. *Lancet* 2:124–127; 1977.

Kesaree N et al. Treatment of inverted nipples using a disposable syringe. *J Hum Lact* 9:27–29; 1993.

Lawrence R. *Breastfeeding: A guide for the medical profession*. St. Louis, MO: Mosby; 1999.

MAIN Trial Collaborative Group. Preparing for breast feeding: Treatment of inverted and nonprotractile nipples in pregnancy. *Midwifery* 10:200–214; 1994.

Marshall D et al. Breast feeding after reduction mammoplasty. *Med J Aust* 159:428–429; 1993.

Neifert M et al. The influence of breast surgery, breast appearance, and pregnancy-induced breast changes on lactation sufficiency as measured by infant weight gain. *Birth* 17:31–38; 1990.

Saber A et al. The milk rejection sign: A natural tumor marker. *Am Surg* 62:998–999; 1996.

Schackmuth E et al. Milk fistula: A complication after core breast biopsy. *Am J Roentgenol* 161:961–962; 1993.

Stevens K et al. The ultrasound appearances of galactocoeles. *Br J Radiol* 70:239–241; 1997.

Waller H. *The Breasts and Breastfeeding.* London: Heinemann Medical Books; 1946.

Widstrom A and Thingstrom-Paulsson J. The position of the tongue during rooting reflexes elicited in newborn infants before the first suckle. *Acta Paediatr* 82:281–283; 1993.

Wilde C. Autocrine regulation of milk secretion by a protein in milk. *Biochem J* 305:51–58; 1995a.

Woolridge M and Fisher C. Colic, overfeeding, and symptoms of lactose malabsorption in the breast-fed baby: A possible artifact of feed management? *Lancet* ii:382–384; 1988.

▼

BIBLIOGRAPHY

Brucker M and Scharbo-DeHaan M. Breast disease: The role of the nurse-midwife. *Breastfeeding Review* 18:342–350; 1993.

Daly S and Hartmann P. Infant demand and milk supply, Part 1: Infant demand and milk production in lactating women. *J Hum Lact* 11:21–26; 1995.

Daly S and Hartmann P. Infant demand and milk supply, Part 2: The short term control of milk synthesis in lactating women. *J Hum Lact* 11:27–37; 1995.

Harris L et al. Is breast feeding possible after reduction mammaplasty? *Plast Reconstr Surg* 89(5):836–839; 1992.

Matthews MK. Developing an instrument to assess infant breastfeeding behavior in the early neonatal period. *Midwifery* 4:154–165; 1988.

Matthews MK. Mothers' satisfaction with their neonates' breastfeeding behaviors. *JOGNN* 20(1):49–55; 1991.

McGeorge D. The "Nipplette": An instrument for the non-surgical correction of inverted nipples. *Br J Plast Surg* 47:46–49; 1994.

Mulford C. The mother-baby assessment (MBA): An "Apgar score" for breastfeeding. *J Hum Lact* 8:79–82; 1992.

Slavin J et al. Nodular breast lesions during pregnancy and lactation. *Histopathology* 22:481–485; 1993.

Soderstrom B. Helping the woman who had breast surgery: A literature review. *J Hum Lact* 9:169–171; 1993.

Stutte P et al. The effects of breast massage on volume and fat content of human milk. *Genesis* 10:22–24; 1988.

Tay C et al. Twenty-four hour patterns of prolactin secretion during lactation and the relationship to suckling and the resumption of fertility in breastfeeding women. *Hum Reprod* 11:950–955; 1996.

Uvnas-Moberg K and Eriksson M. Breastfeeding: Physiological, endocrine and behavioral adaptations caused by oxytocin and local neurogenic activity in the nipple and mammary gland. *Acta Paediatr* 85:515–530; 1996.

Vorherr H. *The Breast, Morphology, Physiology, and Lactation.* New York: Academic Press; 1974.

Widdice A and Thingstrom-Paulsson J. The effects of breast reduction and breast augmentation surgery on lactation: An annotated bibliography. *J Hum Lact* 9:161–167; 1993.

Wilde C et al. Breast-feeding: Matching supply with demand in human lactation. *Proc Nutr Soc* 54:401–406; 1995b.

7

MATERNAL HEALTH AND NUTRITION

In order to develop good eating practices, parents need a basic understanding of nutrition and its effect on health. You can play an active part in making this information available and advising breastfeeding mothers about their own nutrition. Prenatal and postpartum breastfeeding and parenting classes offer an excellent opportunity to discuss nutrition. Proper nutrition is especially important to a woman during pregnancy and can also have an impact on her breastfeeding. You can offer guidance to mothers in the selection and preparation of foods, and can help them understand the nutritional factors which may cause them to feel hungry or fatigued.

COUNSELING WOMEN REGARDING THEIR NUTRITIONAL NEEDS

Nutritional education in the United States is alarmingly lacking. Public schools teach the importance of the **food pyramid**. However, they do not review nutritional quality of food effectively in terms of selection and preparation. According to the Center for Science in the Public Interest, school lunch programs need to be upgraded in terms of quality and desirability of the foods served. Many communities nationwide are actively working to bring about such changes in their schools. Although it is perhaps impractical to suggest that schools serve only fresh low-processed foods, present practices fail to provide a good model for students to carry into adult life. In many cases, formal nutrition education ends in grade school, at a time when children do not have enough control over their own diets to put the information into practice.

Although your primary role is to assist women with breastfeeding, giving nutrition information is also an important element in your counseling. As a lactation consultant, you can encourage parents to assume responsibility for their own health care and that of their children. Because health and well-being are closely related to nutrition, education in this area helps parents make responsible decisions.

Pregnancy and lactation are times when women are especially receptive to nutrition education. During these peak periods of interest, women want to provide their babies with the best nourishment possible. Many wish to have children without a significant change in their own body image. Some mothers in your care may be well educated nutritionally, so you will need to determine a mother's nutritional awareness before offering suggestions. For some, this may be a time when they recognize the close relationship between what they eat and how they feel. Whatever the reasons, this time can be considered a teachable moment—a time when a woman is most receptive to learning about nutrition. Tapping into the mother's motivating interests can influence a change in her eating habits.

NUTRITIONAL ISSUES IN PREGNANCY AND LACTATION

Nutrition awareness is an integral part of sound prenatal care. The nutritional status of the mother before pregnancy and her nutritional intake during pregnancy are important elements of a healthy pregnancy. There is a difference of opinion, however, concerning the degree of impact nutrition has on the pregnant woman and her fetus. Virginia A. Beal of the University of Colorado School of Medicine states, "If a woman has been well-nourished throughout her life, her intake during pregnancy, unless very different, is likely to have relatively little effect on the course of her pregnancy or the health and size of her baby. If she is poorly nourished during her growing years and enters pregnancy without reserves, her diet during pregnancy becomes crucial" (Beal, 1971).

The Bacon Chow study of nutritional supplementation for pregnant and lactating women showed no difference in birth weight or height between children of supplemented and unsupplemented mothers (Adair, 1985). On the other hand, the Brewers found that adequate nutrition is crucial, resulting in healthier babies and shorter labors with fewer complications (Brewer, 1977). Additionally, the roles of nutritional status and diet are masked by a number of confounding variables. Among them are income, health, education, lifestyle, fertility, and individual adaptations in activity level. Although nutrition is just one determinant of outcome, it is a significant one that can be modified.

Maternal **malnutrition**, defined here as inadequate nutrition due to improper diet, can restrict healthy fetal growth by reducing the number or size of cells, including brain cells. Severe malnutrition, due to critically low nourishment, can contribute to fetal death. Clearly, fetuses can be adversely affected by the mother's compromised nutritional status. Proper nutritional intake, based on a well-planned diet, is necessary during pregnancy to produce healthy, full-term babies.

You can encourage mothers to eat well in order to provide for the optimum growth and development of their babies as well as to keep their bodies in prime condition for labor, delivery, and lactation. Michaelsen found a positive association between weight gain during pregnancy and fat concentration in the mother's milk. The study suggested that if **fat stores** laid down in pregnancy are minimal, milk fat content might be decreased. However, no parameters were developed to assess the minimum level of weight gain that is acceptable (Michaelsen, 1994).

Not only does nutrition education affect the outcome of pregnancy and lactation, it can determine food patterns of the woman's entire family for years to come. The American diet is typically high in fats, calories, and empty calorie foods such as sugar and other **simple carbohydrates**. These foods may be present in unsuspected amounts in the diet and have little nutritive value except calories. Eating large amounts of sweet foods in place of more nutritious foods can contribute to weight gain. It can also prevent women from getting the vitamins, minerals, and other nutrients their bodies need. This can result in women of any socioeconomic level becoming malnourished. Although such women may be ingesting more than enough calories and are often overweight, they are not receiving a healthful balance of nutrients. These women enter pregnancy at a substantial nutritional disadvantage. If they continue their previous dietary practices, they risk jeopardizing their health or that of their babies. Many of these women may not receive adequate nutrition information from their caregivers. You can help foster an awareness in women of their eating practices and the influence those practices have on their health.

Concern for good nutrition does not end with the birth of the baby. Sound nutrition practices will continue to enhance the well-being of the entire family. The breastfeeding mother needs to be made aware of the effect her diet has on her own health and breastfeeding. She needs sufficient amounts of high-quality foods to produce vitamin-rich milk. This approach will ensure the optimum growth of her infant and still enable the mother to maintain a positive nutritional status for herself. An inadequate diet or irregular eating pattern can affect how a mother feels and acts, and how she views herself and the world. This factor, in turn, can negatively influence milk production and release, as well as her ability to cope with her baby and other family members and friends.

Lactation consultants have noted a higher incidence of sore nipples among poorly nourished women. Thus, a responsible part of counseling is making sure that lactating women have the opportunity and the necessary information to improve their health through nutrition. Because poor dietary habits are widespread and continually promoted by the advertising of nutritionally empty calorie foods, most mothers can benefit from sound practical suggestions. Becoming familiar with basic nutrition principles and, more specifically, food practices of the women in your care will help you understand the influences on their diet. This will provide you with some insight into helping them institute changes.

The nutrition information that you give to mothers needs to be based on sound, accurate principles. It should not reflect particular preferences or dietary practices. Many nutrition books promote fad diets and unproven theories that can be detrimental to a woman's health, especially that of a breastfeeding mother. By limiting yourself to basic nutrition information, you can minimize confusion and possible conflict for the woman, and help her apply the information to her eating practices. Some of your advice may be in conflict with her physician's present practices. Therefore, basing your advice on sound, well-documented nutrition information can give you the opportunity to educate the physician as well as the woman.

▼ The Food Pyramid

Foods with similar nutrient content are conveniently grouped together in the United States Department of Agriculture's (USDA) Food Pyramid (Fig. 7.1). The pyramid shows how much of each food group should be present in the diet relative to its size on the pyramid. The top of the pyramid—the smallest number of servings—contains fats, oils, and sweets. The next level contains milk, yogurt, cheese, meat, poultry, fish, dry beans, eggs, and nuts. The third level contains vegetables and fruit, and the bottom level—the largest number of servings—contains bread, cereal, rice, and pasta. Every person's total daily food intake needs to contain a variety of foods from each group. Although each meal may not

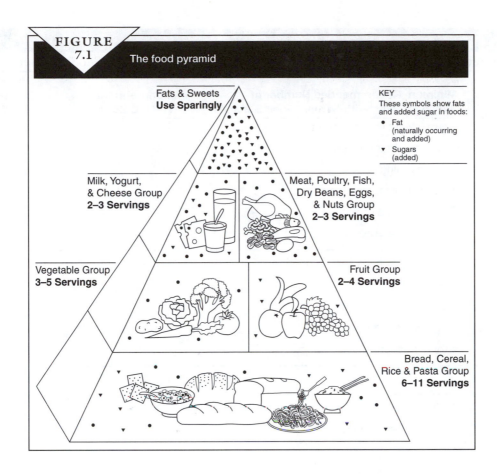

FIGURE 7.1
The food pyramid

Fats & Sweets
Use Sparingly

KEY
These symbols show fats
and added sugar in foods:
● Fat
(naturally occurring
and added)
▼ Sugars
(added)

Milk, Yogurt,
& Cheese Group
2–3 Servings

Meat, Poultry, Fish,
Dry Beans, Eggs,
& Nuts Group
2–3 Servings

Vegetable Group
3–5 Servings

Fruit Group
2–4 Servings

Bread, Cereal,
Rice & Pasta Group
6–11 Servings

contain all the pyramid groups, the total daily intake should be well balanced among them to provide a nutritious, healthful diet. The pyramid food groups are especially helpful in planning daily food choices for meals. They can serve as a guide for evaluating diet and determining if a person is eating enough of the right foods. The food pyramid represents the minimum number of daily servings recommended for the nonpregnant woman or for the pregnant or lactating woman. Young adolescents who have not completed their growth cycle and women who are very active will require additional servings in each group to meet their energy needs. Refer to Table 7.1 for specific menu selections based on the food pyramid.

▼ The Basic Nutrients

A basic understanding of nutrients and their functions in the body is necessary for realizing the importance of good nutrition. Good nutrition is achieved by eating all of the nutrients required by the body in proper quantities. The six nutrients—carbohydrates, fats, proteins, vitamins, minerals, and water—all have their own specific functions and relationship to the body. They must be present in proper quantities to maintain good health and a feeling of well being.

A woman needs an increased amount of most nutrients during pregnancy. This requirement increases even more as the infant nears term. When lactation is initiated, the woman's body becomes more efficient in its use of energy. This results in a gradual reduction of the number of calories required. As shown in Table 7.2, her protein needs also decrease during lactation, while vitamin and mineral **reference daily intake (RDI)** varies only slightly. A pregnant or lactating woman should have at least three well-balanced meals and two snacks per day, chosen from the food pyramid and distributed throughout the day. You can offer suggestions for high-quality foods that supply needed nutrients without excessive calories. You can also encourage women to read food labels carefully. The information on labels can help them make better decisions on the right foods for their family. Labels with nutritional information will provide the details they need in order to plan a well-balanced diet.

Carbohydrates

Carbohydrates are the main source of energy for all body functions and muscular exertion. They also help regulate protein and fat metabolism. Carbohydrates are needed in sufficient quantity so the body can avoid relying on protein as an energy source. This allows protein to perform other important body functions. Snacks high

TABLE 7.1

Menu Suggestions That Implement the Recommendations in the Food Pyramid

Food group	Minimum Recommended Number of Servings Daily (With Sample Food Servings)	Nonpregnant (1900 Calories)	Pregnant or Lactating (2200 Calories)
Milk or milk products	1 cup low fat milk or yogurt	2	3
	1½ oz. cheddar cheese		
	1 cup pudding		
	1¼ cups low fat ice cream		
	2 cups cottage cheese		
	1 cup tofu (soybean curd)		
Meats and meat substitutes	Cooked lean meat, fish, or poultry	5–7 ounces	7 ounces
	Cheddar cheese		
	½ cup cottage cheese		
	1 cup dried beans or peas		
	4 tbsp. peanut butter		
Eggs		1	1–2
Fruits	(Include vitamin C rich choice)	2–4	3–4
	½ cup cooked or juice		
	1 cup raw		
	1 medium-sized fruit		
Vegetables	(Choose from dark leafy and starch vegetables. Variety is recommended)	3–5	4–5
	½ cup cooked		
	1 cup raw		
Grains	(Whole grain, fortified, or enriched)	6–11	9–11
	1 slice bread		
	1 cup ready-to-eat cereal		
	½ cup cooked cereal, pasta, or grits		

Data from The Food Pyramid: How to make it work for you. *Consumer Reports on Health*, September, 1996; Charbonneau, K. "Nutrition Continuum." International Journal of Childbirth Education 8:16–18, 1993.

in **simple carbohydrates,** that is, mostly sugar, cause a sudden rise in blood sugar level. The level then drops again rapidly and can create a craving for more food. When consumed in the absence of nutritional foods, simple carbohydrate foods may cause fatigue, dizziness, nervousness, or headache. The **complex carbohydrate** foods are preferable because they contain important vitamins and minerals. Complex carbohydrates take longer to digest and do not stimulate a craving for more foods. Foods in this category include vegetables, fruits, whole grain cereals, rice, breads, and crackers. Raw fruits and vegetables, and whole grain breads and cereals, will also provide needed fiber.

Fats

Fats are the most concentrated source of energy in the diet. They act as carriers for the fat-soluble vitamins A, D, E, and K. Fats prolong the process of digestion by slowing down the stomach's emptying. This creates a

TABLE 7.2

Nutrient and Vitamin Chart

Key Nutrient	RDI for Ages 23–50	Important Sources	Important Functions
Water and liquids	N 4 C P 6–8 C L 8+ C	Water, juice, milk.	Carries nutrients to and waste products away from cells. Provides fluid for increased blood and amniotic fluid volume. Helps regulate body temperature and aids digestion. Comments: Often neglected. Is an important nutrient.
Protein amino acids	N 50 g P 60 g L 64 g	Animal: Meat, fish, eggs, milk, cheese, yogurt. Plant: Dried beans and peas, peanut butter, nuts, whole grains and cereals, soy milk, meat substitutes.	Constitutes part of the structure of every tissue cell, such as muscle, blood, and bone. Supports growth and maintains healthy body cells. Constitutes part of enzymes, some hormones and body fluids. Helps form antibodies that increase resistance to infection. Builds and repairs tissues, helps build blood and amniotic fluid. Supplies energy. Comments: Fetal requirements increase by about ⅓ in late pregnancy as the baby grows.
Minerals			
Calcium	N 800–1200 mg P 1200 mg L 1200 mg	Animal: Milk, cheese, yogurt, egg yolk, whole canned fish, ice cream. Plant: Whole grains, almonds, filberts, green leafy vegetables.	Combines with other minerals within a protein framework to give structure and strength to bones and teeth. Assists in blood clotting. Functions in normal muscle contraction and relaxation, and normal nerve transmission. Helps regulate the use of other minerals in the body. Comments: Fetal requirements increase by about ⅔ in late pregnancy.
Phosphorus	N 1000 mg P 1200 mg L 1200 mg	Animal: Milk, cheese, lean meats.	Helps build bones and teeth. Comments: Calcium and phosphorus exist in a constant ratio in the blood. An excess of either limits utilization of calcium.
Iron	N 18 mg P 30–60 mg L 18+ mg	Animal: Liver, red meats, egg yolk. Plant: Whole grains, leafy vegetables, nuts, legumes, dried fruits, prune prune and apple juice.	Aids in utilization of energy. Combines with protein to form hemoglobin, the red substance in blood that carries oxygen to and carbon dioxide from the cells. Prevents nutritional anemia and its accompanying fatigue. Increases resistance to infection. Functions as part of enzymes involved in tissue respiration. Provides iron for fetal storage. Comments: Fetal requirements increase tenfold in final 6 weeks of pregnancy. Supplement of 30–60 mg of iron daily recommended by National Research Council. Continued supplementation for 2–3 months postpartum is recommended to replenish iron.
Zinc	N 15 mg P 20 mg L 25 mg	Animal: Meat, liver, eggs and seafood, especially oysters.	A component of insulin. Important in growth of skeleton and nervous system. Comments: Deficiency can cause fetal malformation of skeleton and nervous system.
Iodine	N 150 μcg P 175 μcg L 200 μcg	Animal: Seafood. Plant: Iodized salt.	Helps control the rate of body's energy use, important in Thyroxine production. Comments: Deficiency may produce goiter in infant.

(continued)

TABLE 7.2 (CONTINUED)
Nutrient and Vitamin Chart

Key Nutrient	RDI for Ages 23–50	Important Sources	Important Functions
Magnesium	N 400 mg P 450 mg L 450 mg	Plant: Nuts, cocoa, green vegetables, whole grains, dried beans, peas	Co-enzyme in energy and protein metabolism, enzyme activator, tissue growth, cell metabolism, muscle action. Comments: Most is stored in bones. Deficiency may produce neuromuscular dysfunctions.
Fat-Soluble Vitamins			
Vitamin A	N 800 RE P 1000 RE L 1200 RE	Animal: Butter, whole milk, cheese, fortified lowfat milk, liver Plant: Fortified margarine, green and leafy vegetables, orange vegetables, fruits	Assists formation and maintenance of skin and mucous membranes that line body cavities and tracts, such as nasal passages and intestinal tract, thus increasing resistance to infection. Essential in development of enamel-forming cells in gum tissue. Helps bone and tissue growth and cell development. Functions in visual processes, thus promoting healthy eye tissues and eye adaptation in dim light. Comments: Is toxic to the fetus in very large amounts. Can be lost with exposure to light.
Vitamin D	N 5 μcg P 10 μcg L 10 μcg	Animal: Fortified milk, fish liver oils Plant: Fortified margarine, sun on skin	Promotes the absorption of calcium from the digestive tract and the deposition of calcium in the structure of bones and teeth. Comments: Toxic to fetus in excessive amounts. Is a stable vitamin.
Vitamin E	N 8 mg P 10 mg L 13 mg	Vegetable oils, leafy vegetables, cereals, meat, eggs, milk	Tissue growth, cell wall integrity, red blood cell integrity. Comments: Enhances absorption of Vitamin A.
Water-Soluble Vitamins			
B Vitamins and folic acid	N 400 μcg P 800 μcg L 600 μcg	Liver, green leafy vegetables, yeast	Hemoglobin synthesis, involved in DNA and RNA synthesis, co-enzyme in synthesis of amino acids. Comments: Water-soluble vitamins are interdependent on each other. Deficiency leads to anemia. Can be destroyed in cooking and storage. Supplement of 200–400 μcg/day is recommended by the National Research Council. Oral contraception use may reduce serum level of folic acid.
Niacin	N 13 mg P 15 mg L 18 mg	Pork, organ meats, peanuts, beans, peas, enriched grains	Coenzyme in energy and protein metabolism. Comments: Stable; only small amounts lost in food preparation.
Riboflavin	N 1.2 mg P 1.5 mg L 1.7–1.9 mg	Animal: Milk products, liver, red meat Plant: Enriched grains	Aids in utilization of energy. Functions as part of a co-enzyme in the production of energy within body cells. Promotes healthy skin, eyes, and clear vision. Protein metabolism. Comments: Severe deficiencies lead to reduced growth and congenital malformations. Oral contraceptive use may reduce serum concentrations.

TABLE 7.2 (CONTINUED)
Nutrient and Vitamin Chart

Key Nutrient	RDI for Ages 23–50	Important Sources	Important Functions
B1- Thiamin	N 1.0 mg P 1.4 mg L 1.5 mg	Pork, beef, liver, whole grains, legumes	Co-enzyme in energy and protein metabolism. Comments: Its availability limits the rate at which energy from glucose is produced.
B6 Pyrodoxine	N 1.6 mg P 2.2 mg L 2.1 mg	Unprocessed cereals, grains, wheat germ, bran, nuts, seeds, legumes, corn	Important in amino acid metabolism and protein synthesis. Fetus requires more for growth. Comments: Excessive amounts may reduce milk production in lactating women.
B12	N 2.0 µcg P 2.2 µcg L 2.6 µcg	Animal: Milk, cheese, eggs, meat, liver, fish Plant: Fortified soy milk, cereals meat substitutes	Assists in the maintenance of nerve tissue. Coenzyme in protein metabolism, important in formation of red blood cells. Comments: Deficiency leads to anemia and central nervous system damage. Is manufactured by microorganisms in intestinal tract. Oral contraceptive use may reduce serum concentrations.
Vitamin C	N 60 mg P 80 mg L 100 mg	Citrus fruits, berries, melons, tomatoes, chili peppers, green vegetables, potatoes	Tissue formation and integrity, "cement" substance in connective and vascular substances, increases iron absorption. Comments: Large doses in pregnancy may create a larger than normal need in infant. Benefits of large doses in preventing colds have not been confirmed.

L, lactating; N, nonpregnant; P, pregnant; RDI, reference daily intake.
From Worthington-Roberts B and Williams SR. *Nutrition in Pregnancy and Lactation,* St. Louis, MO, Times Mirror/Mosby College Publishing; 1989 and *www.nal.usda.gov.*

longer lasting sensation of fullness after a meal. Fatty acids, which give fats their different flavors, textures, and melting points, are available in either a saturated or unsaturated form. Saturated fatty acids come primarily from animal sources such as meat, milk products, and eggs. Unsaturated fatty acids are derived from vegetable, nut, and seed sources. A proper diet should contain a greater amount of unsaturated fats than of saturated fats.

Proteins

Many parts of the body are made up of protein, among them muscles, tissues, and hormones. Protein is the major source of building material for all internal organs, as well as for muscles, blood, skin, hair, and nails. Proteins are needed for the formation of hormones which, among numerous other functions, control sexual development, and the formation of milk during lactation. They may also be used as a source of heat and energy. However, this is necessary only if fats and carbohydrates are not present in sufficient amounts to perform that function.

Proteins are made up of combinations of 22 building blocks called amino acids. The human body can synthesize 14 of these amino acids. The remaining eight must be supplied in the diet and in the correct proportions in order for the body to properly synthesize proteins. Foods containing all of the essential amino acids are called complete, and those lacking or extremely low in any one of the essential amino acids are called incomplete. Most meats and dairy products are **complete protein** foods, whereas most vegetables and fruits are **incomplete protein** foods. When foods are combined carefully, those that are weak in an essential amino acid will be balanced by those that are adequate in the same one. An incomplete protein food can be combined with others to make a complete protein complement.

The body is constantly building and repairing tissues. At times of stress, such as surgery, hemorrhage, or prolonged illness, it is necessary to consume extra protein in order to meet the body's requirements for this function. The average woman requires 45 to 50 g of protein daily, depending on her weight and activity level. However, that same woman needs 60 g during pregnancy and 66 during lactation.

Vitamins

Although vitamins have no caloric or energy value, they are essential to the regulation of daily body functions. Vitamins convert fat and carbohydrates into energy and help form bone and tissue. Generally, the body cannot synthesize vitamins. Therefore, they need to be supplied in the diet or in dietary supplements. Fat-soluble vitamins (A, D, E, and K) are stored in the body's fatty tissues. **Water-soluble vitamins** (the B vitamins and vitamin C) are not stored by the body and need to be replenished daily. Table 7.2 lists the functions of each vitamin and its relationship to pregnancy and lactation.

If mothers consider their foods to be inadequate in vitamin and mineral content, they may take prescribed or self-administered supplements. These can be valuable as an addition to the average diet and also in special circumstances such as anemia, food intolerance, or allergies. However, supplements should not be used to replace the proper intake of vitamin and mineral rich foods. They can be helpful as supplements, not substitutes, for good nutrition. Encourage women to consult their physician before taking supplemental vitamins and minerals during pregnancy or lactation.

Folic acid is especially important to the pregnant woman in preventing anemia, and can be obtained from leafy green vegetables and whole grains. The U.S. Public Health Service advocates folic acid supplements during the childbearing years for all reproductive-aged women, in order to help prevent neural tube defects (**spina bifida**) (Charbonneau 1993; Nutrition Action, 1992). During lactation, increased levels of water-soluble vitamins are recommended because levels of these vitamins in the mother's milk can be affected by her intake (Jelliffe, 1978).

Minerals

Minerals contribute to a person's overall mental and physical well-being. They are involved in maintaining physiologic processes, strengthening skeletal structures, and preserving the vigor of the heart, the brain, and the muscle and nervous systems. They are also important in the production of hormones and help maintain the delicate water balance essential to the proper functioning of mental and physical processes. Minerals must be supplied by the diet. A varied and mixed diet of animal and vegetable origin that meets energy and protein needs will typically furnish adequate minerals. Specific minerals and their functions appear in Table 7.2. Additional discussion is presented in the following sections concerning calcium, iron, and salt because of their special importance during pregnancy and lactation.

Calcium and Iron

Calcium and iron are often the most commonly deficient minerals in the diet. Low levels of iron can affect the oxygen-carrying capacity of the blood, causing the woman to feel tired constantly, even after adequate rest. Calcium is an important dietary mineral, particularly during pregnancy and lactation. Its absorption and retention increase during pregnancy and, to a lesser degree, during lactation. However, women who lactate are not more prone to osteoporosis than those who have never been pregnant or have not lactated. Studies show that calcium mobilizes from the mother's bones during lactation, with a postweaning recovery of bone mass (Specker, 1991.) Also, the mother's reproductive history, including lactation, is not a long-term indicator of bone mineral density (Kritz-Silverstein, 1992). In spite of this reassuring information, the fact remains that if one does not consume enough calcium in the diet, the body will take what it needs from the bones. For this reason, adequate calcium intake needs to be discussed with mothers, particularly those younger than 25 years of age who are still experiencing an increase in bone content of calcium (Lipsman, 1985).

Mothers who do not care to drink milk, or who cannot tolerate milk or are allergic to it, can obtain calcium through the sources listed in Table 7.3. Women who avoid all milk products to minimize infant allergies must also compensate for the other nutrients available in milk—protein, vitamins, and calories—through other foods. Women who do not eat enough calcium-rich foods are advised to take calcium supplements. Calcium carbonate is considered to be the safest supplement. Bone meal is not recommended because several brands contain high levels of lead. Dolomite is also a poor choice because it may contain lead or other toxic metals. Experts say that there are no significant side effects from taking a supplement of between 500 and 1000 mg/day. This amount of calcium can cause problems only in people with **sarcoidosis** or a few other diseases (Nutrition Action, 1982). In a 1994 consensus statement issued by the National Institutes of Health (NIH), "Optimal Calcium Intake", it is recommended that pregnant or lactating women consume 1200 to 1500 mg of calcium daily (Nutrition Action, 1996). Women need to be informed that they do not have to drink milk in order to make milk.

Salt

In order for the fetus to remain healthy, placental growth and development must be proportionate to the infant's growth. As a woman's pregnancy progresses, the placenta needs much more blood flowing through it to work efficiently. During the course of a typical pregnancy, the woman's blood volume must increase by more than 40 percent to meet this need. Salt usually

TABLE 7.3
Good Sources of Calcium

Food	Calcium (mgs per serving)
Yogurt, plain (8 oz)	415
Cheddar cheese (2 oz)	408
Sardines, drained (3 oz)	372
Milk, skim or low-fat protein-fortified (8 oz)	352
American cheese (2 oz)	348
Yogurt, fruit flavored (8 oz)	345
Milk, whole, low-fat or skim (8 oz)	297
Watercress (1 cup chopped)	189
Chocolate pudding, instant (½ cup)	187
Collards (½ cup cooked)	179
Buttermilk pancakes (3–4″)	174
Pink salmon, canned (3 oz)	167
Tofu (4 oz)	145
Turnip greens (½ cup cooked)	134
Kale (½ cup cooked)	103
Shrimp, canned (3 oz)	99
Ice cream (½ cup)	88
Okra (½ cup cooked)	74
Rutabaga, mashed (½ cup cooked)	71
Broccoli (½ cup cooked)	68
Soybeans (½ cup cooked)	66
Cottage cheese (½ cup)	63
Bread, white or whole wheat (2 slices)	48

causes the body to retain fluid in the bloodstream. Pregnancy is one condition in which the body actually requires *more* salt in order to function well.

In the past, physicians traditionally encouraged women to limit weight gain during pregnancy and placed restrictions on salt intake in an attempt to control weight. Experts now agree that such routine salt restriction during pregnancy, just as with calorie restriction, is unphysiologic and unfounded (Worthington-Roberts, 1989). A low-salt, low-calorie diet during pregnancy overlooks the salt-conserving mechanisms of the body and can bring about the very conditions it seeks to prevent: high blood pressure, excess weight gain, and edema. It limits the normal expansion of blood volume, which, in turn, can limit the growth of the placenta, de-

velop areas of dead placental tissue, or cause the placenta to begin to separate from the wall of the uterus before it should (**abruptio placenta**). Excessive salt restriction and weight restriction during pregnancy impose an unnecessary risk on the mother and her fetus, and should be avoided.

When a pregnant woman experiences swelling in her legs and feet, her physician may place tight restrictions on her salt intake. Dr. Leon Chesley concluded after 40 years of research that normal swelling, or physiologic edema, is a sign of health in well-nourished pregnant women, and not a **pathologic** condition (Chesley, 1975). Joyce Vermeersch, an assistant professor at the University of California, further states that "a mild degree of edema is physiological in pregnancy and the measures commonly used to prevent it impose an unnecessary risk" (Worthington-Roberts, 1989). Therefore, in most pregnancies, the use of diuretics is unnecessary and dangerous. When normal swelling becomes uncomfortable, it may help to wear flat open shoes, minimize conventional chair sitting by sitting tailor style, lie with the feet elevated several times a day, and eat a balanced diet with sufficient salt intake. Excessive salt intake for anyone, including pregnant women, is not recommended. Rather, a positive nutritional approach, whereby the woman is evaluated on an individual basis instead of being placed on a blanket salt-restricted diet, is the best approach. Most pregnant women can continue to consume the same amount of salt as that recommended for the general population.

If excessive swelling occurs, the pregnant woman can be referred to her physician for a complete medical evaluation. Swelling is understandably increased when a pregnant woman is carrying twins. Coupled with rigid weight control, salt restriction, and diuretic therapy, a twin pregnany can become high risk, resulting in premature birth and lower birth weights. When mothers of twins meet their increased nutritional needs during pregnancy, refrain from taking diuretics, and eat sufficient salt to taste, they usually give birth at term to infants of normal birth weight.

Water

Water is the most abundant and by far the most important nutrient in the body. It is responsible for and involved in nearly every body process. Most foods contain water that is absorbed by the body during digestion. Fruits and vegetables are especially good sources of chemically pure water. The average adult female body contains 50 to 55 percent water (approximately 30 quarts), losing about two quarts daily through perspiration and excretion.

A pregnant or lactating woman needs to consume additional water in order to supply her fetus or infant with adequate fluids. The woman's consumption of additional water-containing foods as part of her normal increase in diet, as well as her natural sense of thirst, usually provides the additional water she needs. Sometimes, lactating women fail to respond to their increased thirst. Remind them to drink to satisfy their thirst. Many mothers find it convenient and easy to remember if they drink something every time they nurse their baby. During both pregnancy and lactation, a woman needs about six to eight cups of fluids a day to ensure that her body has enough fluid to function and to avoid constipation. Table 7.2 advises that a breastfeeding woman consume eight or more cups of fluid a day. However, this consumption would be dictated largely by thirst.

There is no data to support the suggestion that milk volume can be increased by increasing the mother's fluid intake. In fact, women who consume excessive amounts of fluid actually produce less milk and their babies gain less weight (Dusdieker, 1985). Restricting fluids has not been shown to decrease milk volume (Illingworth, 1986). "When fluids are restricted, the mother will experience a decrease in urine output, not in milk" (Lawrence, 1999). Mothers can monitor the adequacy of fluid intake by observing their urine. Except for the first morning void, the mother's urine should be clear to light yellow. If her urine appears more concentrated, she may increase her fluid intake throughout the day. These findings, which support decades of similar studies, demonstrate that women should be advised to drink when they are thirsty and to heed their body's cues. Drinking to satisfy thirst usually provides the mother with all of the fluids she needs.

◆ Food Selection

Wise selection of foods is an important factor in good nutrition. Giving considerable thought to grocery shopping helps in the selection of foods with the highest nutritive values. During pregnancy, many women become more conscious of the foods they eat. They can be encouraged to continue their emphasis on nutrition during lactation. This may lead to gradual improvement in the eating habits of the entire family. Fresh unprocessed foods are the most nutritious and most desirable choice, and food served directly after being purchased or picked is the most flavorful and nutritious. In addition, proper food storage helps preserve its nutritional quality.

Home gardening is the most desirable, although women can also be encouraged to look for fresh, crisp foods when shopping. Wilting indicates a lack of freshness and improper storage, which result in a loss of vitamins. Also, removing the skin of fresh fruits and vegetables robs them of much of their nutrients and fiber. Encourage mothers to select foods that are grown free, or with a minimum amount, of pesticides and

heavy metals—such as lead and mercury—that could be stored in their fatty tissue and later enter into their milk. They can do this by limiting the intake of freshwater fish and animal fats, and by washing all fruits and vegetables thoroughly.

◆ Reading Food Labels

Nutrition-conscious consumers can look for labeling that states the product is organic. Package labels also offer information on the recommended allowances of nutrients provided in foods. The Food and Nutrition Board of the National Academy of Sciences has established the RDI for essential nutrients healthy people need at different ages, at given weights, and under certain conditions such as pregnancy or lactation. However, these recommendations do not usually appear on food labels. RDIs, as defined by the USDA, are calculated according to the highest RDI levels and are used solely for the purpose of food labeling. RDIs are often presented both in grams and percentages. For example, two-thirds cup of shredded wheat cereal contains 3 g of protein, or 4 percent of the RDIs for protein. Because RDIs are not calculated specifically for pregnant or lactating women, a woman in her childbearing years will more likely find the measurement in grams more helpful in planning meals to suit her individual needs.

◆ Food Additives and Processing

There is a growing awareness today of the effects food additives and processing can have on a person's health. The nutritional quality of foods can be altered by chemical additives that color the food, enhance flavor, or preserve freshness. Although some of these changes may improve the quality, the benefits of each ingredient must be weighed against its possible harmful effects. Labels identify the foods and additives present in a product, with ingredients listed in descending order of quantity. When ingredients in several foods are compared, the most nutritious food has fewer highly refined or artificial ingredients at the beginning of the list. As a rule of thumb, women can purchase the best quality foods by selecting only those that have no highly refined foods or additives listed as the first three ingredients. Although it may not always be practical to purchase such foods, you can encourage parents to work toward this goal.

When selecting foods with no labels, such as fresh fruits and vegetables, women need to be aware that these can be altered by handling and preserving techniques as well. They may contain additives that are not obvious to the consumer. Mushrooms may be bleached, and other vegetables may be treated with fungicides to retard mold growth. Some fresh foods, such as peppers, cucumbers, and tomatoes, are waxed to preserve freshness during long transport and storage times. Other foods, such as some oranges, are colored to enhance their visual appeal. When they are available, fresh foods that have not been tampered with are a better choice. The consumer can ask her grocer to obtain such food treatment information from his suppliers.

Often the methods used to treat foods are beneficial because they allow foods to be stored or shipped so that they are available to the consumer throughout the year. It is nearly impossible for the consumer to avoid purchasing treated foods. By washing, soaking, or peeling foods that have been treated externally, the consumer can reasonably avoid the consumption of undesirable ingredients. In most cases, pesticide residues can be reduced by washing the food with water and mild dish detergent. A 1992 report on pesticides from the Environmental Working Group is available on the Internet at *www.ewg.org.*

Effect of Processing on Nutritional Value

Processing of foods can also change their nutritional value, again either favorably or unfavorably. They may be changed from their natural state before being purchased, through bleaching, removal of fiber, soaking, drying, heating, canning, or freezing. Frozen food is a better choice than canned, because the freezing process depletes a lower percentage of nutrients than does canning. There are nutritional differences among canned foods as well. Fruits canned in heavy syrup contain many more empty calories than those canned in natural fruit juices. Whole grain products are richer sources of vitamin E, vitamin B_6, folic acid, phosphorus, magnesium, and zinc than are enriched refined products. Some foods, such as enriched breads or cereals, are fortified to replace nutrients that are removed during processing. Other foods, such as iodized salt, are fortified to provide nutrients that are needed by the general population and are otherwise difficult to obtain.

Some forms of processing can be especially beneficial. For instance, popcorn that is popped is in a more digestible state than in its natural form. Home processing can also alter a food's natural state. Canning or freezing of fruits and vegetables make it possible to store them safely for longer periods of time. The consumer needs to be aware of the benefits and the disadvantages of various methods of processing and try to select those foods processed by methods that provide the most nutrients at an affordable price.

Cooking food for as short a time and in as little liquid as possible helps preserve nutrients. Stir frying and pressure cooking accomplish this. Steaming is preferable to boiling, because the nutrients are not lost in the water needed for boiling, and steaming cooks food in less time.

Raw food is even more desirable, because some vitamins are destroyed by cooking. Raw spinach, for example, contains more B vitamins than cooked spinach. Some foods such as meats may contain harmful bacteria and need to be cooked thoroughly before being served.

▼ Causes of Hunger and Fatigue

Because food consumption is usually regulated by hunger, understanding the causes of hunger may help a mother plan and control her selection of foods. Hunger can be activated by such things as an empty feeling in the stomach, by discussing or seeing an appealing food, or by a drop in the body's blood sugar level. Foods are absorbed by the body at varying rates and affect the blood sugar in different ways. It is, therefore, possible to feel hungry even after consuming a large amount of calories. For example, refined sugar is absorbed directly and quickly. This causes the blood sugar to rise and fall rapidly, resulting in hunger soon afterward. More complex carbohydrates like potatoes and grains are converted by the body into sugar. Although they enter the bloodstream more slowly than when sugar is eaten by itself, the blood sugar still rises and fades rapidly.

Proteins and fats, by contrast, are digested more slowly than carbohydrates. Blood sugar rises slowly and steadily, remains sustained for a longer period of time, and falls slowly. So, although many foods will result in a full stomach, low blood sugar levels will continue to cause hunger and lack of energy unless adequate protein and fat are included in the diet.

A breakfast consisting primarily of such refined carbohydrate foods as presweetened cereal, doughnuts, sweet rolls, pancakes, or waffles will cause the blood sugar to rise rapidly and then swoop downward. Two or three hours later, the person will feel hungry and in need of another lift. This syndrome is so common among devotees of the typical American diet that its corollary, the midmorning coffee break, has become an American institution. Coffee, tea, and sweet rolls, all of which temporarily elevate blood sugar levels, are consumed midmorning by millions of Americans to compensate for the effect of their high-sugar breakfasts.

Encourage mothers to include a sufficient amount of protein in their breakfasts in order to avoid midmorning and midafternoon fatigue. Breakfast should include about one-fourth of the required daily calories and protein in order to provide a feeling of well-being throughout the day, as well as the highest degree of efficiency in terms of attentiveness, performance, and endurance (Iowa, 1976). Peanut butter on toast, cottage cheese, hard cheese, yogurt, and milk are all quick sources of protein that do not require much preparation. High-quality protein foods will keep the mother's blood sugar level stable so that she will feel better both mentally and physically. Again, advise mothers to be mindful of serving foods from the food pyramid to ensure a healthful diet.

OFFERING NUTRITION ADVICE TO BREASTFEEDING WOMEN

What can a breastfeeding mother eat? Anything she wants! Qualify this with "in moderation" and "nutritious," and you have an easy, simple rule to share with mothers. When you have a solid understanding of nutrition and its impact on pregnant and lactating women, you can incorporate nutrition advice into your counseling and educate women about the basic elements of proper nutrition. However, after a woman accepts what she has learned about nutrition, it is yet another step for her to realize that what she actually eats may conflict with her new beliefs. For example, many of us know that it is important to eat breakfast, yet we continue to skip this essential meal. The women in your care need to learn how to restructure their routines relating to foods. Where they shop, what they buy, how they plan meals, and what they keep on hand for snacks all affect their eating habits.

Nutrition education can be a positive experience for a woman and, it is hoped, promote a continued interest in further education. Suggestions that result in an immediate improvement may catch her interest. For instance, women who are sensitive to the effects of caffeine will find that cutting out caffeinated beverages before bedtime helps them sleep better. Take care not to burden women with irrelevant information or unrealistic goals, such as cooking tips for women who eat out frequently, suggesting expensive foods to a low-income family, or suggesting that a working mother avoid convenience foods.

Some women fear they cannot breastfeed because they do not eat well enough. Good nutrition need not become a barrier to breastfeeding. You can help mothers see the strengths in their diets and how small changes can lead to big improvements. They will learn how both mother and infant will be better off, and that the human body is very flexible and can produce substantial milk out of many combinations of foods.

Diet Improvement

You can tactfully investigate a woman's diet practices by asking about her usual eating habits. However, general inquiries such as "Are you eating well?" will not give you much information about what and how the mother

eats. Few women would answer "No" to such a question! Open-ended questions or statements such as, "What have you eaten today?" or "It sounds like you haven't had a chance to eat breakfast yet," will provide you with more specific information.

In addition to becoming aware of what foods a woman is eating, it may also be helpful for you to understand why she chooses certain foods and what factors influence her choices. Her eating pattern will vary according to her body's requirements and her activity level, and to how these factors affect her appetite. Hunger may lead to eating as often as every 2 hours to only two meals a day. Nonfood stimulants or suppressants may also affect her appetite. Caffeine and tobacco tend to suppress the appetite, whereas marijuana promotes indiscriminate nibbling of food. Small amounts of alcohol can stimulate the appetite. However, when large amounts are consumed, the empty calories of alcohol take the place of more nutritious foods, often resulting in nutritional deficiencies. Both over-the-counter and prescription medications can affect appetite, either suppressing or stimulating it, depending on the components in the drug.

Food preferences clearly affect a woman's food selection. She will most often choose those foods that appeal to her, that are a part of her cultural heritage, and with which she is familiar. When you suggest diet changes to a woman, it is therefore important to consider her food preferences. She will use your suggestions only if they are appealing to her. The woman's understanding of nutrition will also affect her eating habits. You can influence her choices by providing accurate nutritional information. This will often help the woman avoid fad diets and improve poor eating patterns such as skipping meals.

The woman's attitudes about eating affect her food practices significantly. She may eat impulsively, using food to try to satisfy other needs. The woman who is especially conscious of her appearance may ignore her hunger in order to lose weight, or she may be conscientious about her eating practices in order to look and feel her best. Some overweight and underweight women may not see themselves as others do and therefore are not motivated to change their eating habits. A woman may eat in a desire to please someone who has prepared food for her, or she may eat with someone after having prepared food for them, without really being hungry or needing nourishment at that time.

The woman's living situation and lifestyle affect the types of food that are available to her and the regularity of meals. Women with limited incomes, particularly those on assistance programs, may have a narrow selection of foods from which to choose. When new parents are living with their relatives or in a cooperative arrangement with others, the foods they eat and the methods of preparation may be determined by those in charge. Work and school schedules often dictate whether family members share regular meals together and where those meals are eaten—at home, in restaurants, at fast food chains, from vending machines, or as bagged lunches at work. Even for the highly motivated woman, these outside influences can make it difficult for her to obtain the well-balanced diet she needs for lactation.

The person who does the shopping and cooking greatly influences the nutritional value of foods consumed by the family. The type of store and frequency of shopping determine the variety and quality of the foods, as does refrigerator and freezer space. When offering suggestions for diet improvement, take these factors into consideration so that they are practical for the woman to adopt. For example, suggesting that a woman make several casseroles at once and freeze them for later use is fine, provided that she has the freezer space. Women without such conveniences may benefit more by your suggestions on how to prepare quick, nutritious meals from canned foods.

A few women in your care may have health conditions that require special diet practices. These may include food allergies or intolerances, **diabetes**, hypertension, anemia, ulcers, or weight problems. When these conditions exist, you can help the woman work within the guidelines suggested by her physician in order to plan a diet that is suitable for lactation. Referral to a dietician may also be helpful.

After you gain a general idea of the woman's eating patterns and the kinds of food she typically eats, you can begin recommending diet changes. If she usually eliminates breakfast and eats mostly empty calories the rest of the day, as a first step you can suggest a quick protein food such as peanut butter on toast and a glass of milk for breakfast. An additional suggestion of whole wheat bread may be premature at this point, so help her change one step at a time, making sure she understands the purpose for each change. A realistic goal is one of diet improvement in the direction of three well-balanced meals a day with snacks as needed. If such changes are made gradually, the family may be more receptive and the woman will not feel she has had to change her entire lifestyle to accommodate pregnancy and breastfeeding.

Practical Suggestions for Diet

As you discover a mother's food practices, you can begin helping her realize the positive results of diet improvement. Women may become interested in learning about nutrition when they are shown how they will feel better or how their lives will become easier with sound nutrition practices. Some areas you might encourage a pregnant woman to consider are doing the best thing for her infant, having a healthy pregnancy, maintaining a safe weight during pregnancy, and losing weight more easily after delivery.

The pregnant woman can also be encouraged to begin working on good eating habits by learning the relationship of nutrition to the way she feels during her pregnancy. If she experiences morning sickness and nausea, you might suggest that she eat a cracker before getting out of bed. This can be followed by a high protein breakfast and continued access to simple and healthy foods throughout the day, to avoid an empty stomach and the return of nausea. It may also help to open a window or to turn on a fan to remove food odors. Encourage the woman to eat small frequent meals, avoid fatty foods, and drink plenty of liquids. She may also need to avoid highly spiced and especially rich foods. For constipation, you can suggest that a woman exercise regularly, drink plenty of fluids, and eat a sufficient amount of fiber in the form of fresh fruits and vegetables, whole grains, nuts, seeds, and bran, and that she avoid refined foods. After the baby arrives, you can help her understand how a good diet will help overcome problems with a fussy baby, recurring breast problems (mastitis or soreness), depression, and lack of energy. You can use the woman's problem or concern as a way of encouraging her to change her eating habits.

Suggestions that mention specific foods are easy for people to accept and adapt to their own eating practices. Instructions such as, "You need 65 g of protein a day," must be translated by the woman into a food practice. You can eliminate this step and give her the food practice itself, suggesting specific foods that provide protein. For example: "How about keeping a couple of containers of yogurt on hand for those mornings when you don't feel like making breakfast."

After the woman has accepted one change, she will be more receptive to further change. You may move a woman only a short way on the spectrum of food attitudes during the time she is in your care. Even the slightest improvement is worth your efforts.

Learning to read labels will help women avoid nutritionless fillers like corn syrup, sugar, and modified food starch, as well as large quantities of chemical preservatives and additives. Advise them to limit their use of fats that contain cholesterol and to use vegetable oils instead. All the vitamins and minerals necessary to a balanced diet may be obtained more easily by selecting a variety of foods from the food pyramid and in forms as near to their natural state as possible. For example, they can use whole wheat rather than white bread, bake with whole wheat flour (mixed half and half with unbleached flour), use whole grain cereals and crackers, and use brown rice rather than polished, instant, or converted rice. See Table 7.2 for other suggestions.

Because many vitamins are water soluble, vegetables should be cooked in a minimal amount of water, tightly covered, and until just tender. Cooking vegetables in their skins further helps preserve nutrients. Vegetable water can be saved to be used in making soups and gravies. It is also recommended that something raw be served at every meal, such as carrots, celery, peppers, cauliflower, broccoli, spinach salad, cabbage, cucumbers, grapefruit sections, apple slices, or fresh pineapple.

When canned fruits are purchased, selecting those that are canned in juice in place of those canned in heavy syrup will help reduce sugar intake. One hundred percent fruit juices are superior to fruit drinks or other sweet beverages that are high in sugar. Homemade popsicles can be made using real fruit juice, providing a nutritious substitute for commercial popsicles, which contain high levels of sugar. Some other nutritious snack ideas include a bran muffin with cream cheese, cheese with crackers, yogurt dip with raw vegetables, fresh fruit, custard, popcorn, cottage cheese and fruit, and a hard boiled egg.

Giving forethought to meals during pregnancy can help the woman's meal planning for the first days or weeks after the baby arrives. Stocking up on staples in the last few weeks of pregnancy can also prevent repeated trips to the store when she is home with her newborn. In addition, she can prepare meals and freeze them ahead of time to be reheated on days when time is at a premium.

Shopping wisely can help limit spending and enable families to purchase high-quality foods at a lower cost. Encourage mothers to compare prices, purchase less expensive cuts of meat, and select nonbrand name items in place of brand names when they are comparable in quality.

When shopping at retail stores, mothers can purchase larger quantities of foods, which usually have a lower price per unit. Taking advantage of store specials and coupons are other ways of minimizing cost, as well as limiting the purchase of convenience foods, which generally cost more than individual ingredients. Suggestions for diet improvement are summarized in Table 7.4.

Substances to Limit or Avoid

A pregnant or lactating woman needs to use caution in taking over-the-counter and prescription drugs. Advise her to consult her physician before taking anything. Women do not always have control over the selection of their caregiver, as in the case of a group practice or emergency care. This makes it even more important that the lactating mother have a clear understanding of the substances she can and cannot consume. You may be an important source for this information. The mother needs to make certain that her caregiver is aware that she is breastfeeding before prescribing a medication. See the section in Chapter 8 entitled "Properties of Human Milk" for a more complete discussion of drugs and social toxicants and their relationship to human milk.

Nicotine and Tobacco

Cigarette smoking should be avoided because of its connection with a higher incidence of pregnancy disorders and its retarding effect on fetal growth, even when the woman's food intake is increased (Naeye, 1980). The effects of passive smoke inhalation on the breastfed baby are of great concern. The baby ingests much more

TABLE 7.4	
Suggestions for Diet Improvement	
Practices	**Suggestions for Mothers**
Meal Planning	◆ Plan meals in advance, preferably on a weekly or monthly basis.
	◆ Include all food pyramid groups daily.
Shopping	◆ Prepare shopping list according to meal plans.
	◆ Read labels carefully.
	◆ Select fresh, high quality foods.
	◆ Limit purchase of convenience foods.
Cooking Practices	◆ Use preparation methods which preserve nutritive quality—steaming, stir frying, boiling for short periods in small amount of liquid.
	◆ Remove fatty portion from meats before cooking or by broiling, boiling, or draining off fat.
Eating Practices	◆ Plan regular family meals and nutritious snacks.
	◆ Select foods which provide a well-balanced diet when eating away from home.
	◆ When psychological factors cause a desire to eat, substitute another activity or choose nutritious low calorie foods.

nicotine from smoke in the air than he can from nicotine in the mother's milk. Nicotine levels in the milk are dependent on the number of cigarettes smoked and the amount of time between cigarettes.

Mothers who smoke should be advised to quit. If the mother is unable to quit, she can be encouraged to cut back as much as possible, to smoke away from the baby, and after feeds rather than before them in order to limit the baby's exposure. It is important to provide the mother with information regarding smoking and breastfeeding. There is evidence of reduced milk production in smokers. Heavy smoking can also lead to nausea and **vomiting** in the baby. Babies of mothers who smoke should be weighed more frequently to monitor their weight. Smoking reduces the volume and fat content of milk. It also increases the risk of sudden infant death syndrome, upper and lower respiratory infections, and asthma.

Alcohol

A safe level of alcohol consumption for breastfeeding women has not been determined. However, it is known that alcohol enters the bloodstream and quickly migrates to the milk. Alcohol is metabolized from human milk at about the same rate as it is metabolized from the body—1½ to 2 hours per ounce of absolute alcohol. Occasional alcohol use timed around breastfeeds has not been reported in the research to have any harmful effects on the breastfed infant. Moderate amounts of alcohol consumed over a period of time by the nursing mother may slow brain growth in her child. Large amounts delay brain growth even more dramatically and limit parental effectiveness. Excessive amounts of alcohol consumed by the mother can cause life-threatening conditions in both the fetus and the breastfed infant. Alcohol consumption by the breastfeeding mother is also discussed in Chapter 8.

Caffeine

The American Academy of Pediatrics has stated that up to 5 cups of coffee per day is acceptable in lactating women. However, caffeine is transmitted to the infant through the mother's milk and is not easily eliminated from the body by very young infants. Infants who are particularly susceptible may experience fussiness or excessive wakefulness. Additionally, it has been reported that regular coffee drinkers have a lower **hemoglobin** and **hematocrit** with lowered human milk iron (Munoz, 1988).

Allergens

There is some evidence that a fetus and young breastfed infant can be sensitized to **allergens** in utero and through breastfeeding. When a baby is born to parents with allergic manifestations, he has a greater possibility of developing the same allergies. Researchers have found that maternal avoidance of such allergen foods as cow's milk, eggs, and fish during late pregnancy and lactation provides the potential for a lower incidence of allergy (Lovegrove, 1994; Sigurs, 1992). Most foods are acceptable in the mother's diet unless they are known to cause allergic reactions in the mother or father or are being consumed in excessive amounts. Consult Chapter 8 for a more detailed discussion of substances found in human milk.

▼ Special Nutrition Programs

Some of the innumerable diets on the market today are specifically designed for pregnant women. The food suggestions in the diets that appear here will be helpful to meal planning and can be adapted to the woman's taste preferences by using the quantities in the food pyramid in Table 7.1 as a guideline. Frequently, new mothers wish to shed extra pounds from the pregnancy as soon as possible after giving birth. Breastfeeding plays a role in that process, and often, the mother will seek advice in losing weight safely while breastfeeding. Because of the prevalence of vegetarianism, the subject is discussed in detail to educate you about the practice and to provide specific suggestions for you to use when counseling vegetarian mothers. Also, because high-quality foods are often highly priced, many women will benefit from the special suggestions for planning low-cost meals.

Pregnancy and Lactation Diets

Breastfeeding in and of itself appears to offer the mother assistance in her postpartum weight loss. Kramer and colleagues (1993) studied breastfeeding and nonbreastfeeding mothers in the first 6 months postpartum. They noted larger reductions in hip circumference and greater weight loss at one month postpartum when mothers breastfed. At six months the changes were similar in all the groups studied regardless of infant feeding method.

Dewey and her colleagues (1993) examined breastfeeding duration up to 24 months and found that in the first 3 months, breastfeeding mothers do not lose weight more rapidly than their formula-feeding counterparts. However, between months 3 and 6, there is a significantly better weight reduction when the mothers continue breastfeeding. Between months 1 and 12, their research shows an average weight loss of 2 kg more in breastfeeding mothers than in formula-feeding mothers. They also noted a reduction in fat over the triceps area in breastfeeding mothers between months 9 and 12 that was not seen in formula-feeding mothers.

Presenting this information to breastfeeding women early postpartum or even prenatally may offer them a realistic picture of the normal postpartum course. Weight loss is not meant to happen quickly. It occurs gradually and is enhanced by the normal course of breastfeeding. Weight loss, particularly in the postpartum period, can be a significant issue for women. Rutishauser and Carlin (1992) found that women above the normal range for **body mass index (BMI)** at 1 month postpartum tended to stop breastfeeding sooner than those in the normal range. Aside from the correlation between excess weight and premature weaning, no other reason for this weaning could be found. Because Dewey's study does not show a significant weight loss in the first three months postpartum, it is highly possible that you will be contacted regarding postpartum weight loss possibilities and how to enhance the process.

It is important for the health of both the mother and infant that a woman be well educated about nutrition during pregnancy, that she establish good eating practices during this time of growth, and that she carry these healthful habits through the period of lactation. One of the most effective ways of encouraging such healthful eating habits is to provide specific food suggestions to accompany the teaching of the basic principles of nutrition. Translating the number of servings required from the food pyramid into meals with the proper number of calories may seem like a difficult task, especially to a new mother. You can help the mother eliminate that step by offering her the sample meal plans in Table 7.5. They contain the proper number of calories and all the necessary nutrients to support the infant's growth and the mother's well-being. The elimination of most sweets from these diets and the substitution of more nutritious selections have resulted in very generous amounts of food.

The specific foods listed in the sample meal plans are suggestions for diet planning. Substitutes can be made to suit an individual woman's preferences. Other modifications may also be made in the diet, such as grouping the foods into smaller, more frequent meals. For example, the lunchtime apple could be eaten as a midmorning snack. In addition to the fluids suggested, the woman will want to drink water according to her thirst.

A pregnant woman who is carrying two or more babies may need to increase her food intake significantly. Also, with added pressure from the babies on her abdomen, she may feel more comfortable eating smaller, more frequent meals. One way she could do this is by skipping the cereal at breakfast and eating only two ounces of meat at dinner. She can then have a morning snack consisting of one slice of bread or four crackers with 1 oz of meat or meat substitute. A woman who is

nursing twins also needs extra calories (approximately 500) in order to produce enough milk for her second baby and support her own body functions. She can obtain these additional calories by adding foods at meal or snack times or by increasing serving sizes. For example, an 8-oz glass of milk with a peanut butter and jelly sandwich on two slices of whole wheat bread could fulfill her increased caloric requirement.

Vegetarian Diets

Vegetarianism, although not new, is becoming of increasing interest to many people today. Vegetarian diets date back to the second millennium B.C. Today, however, because of philosophical, ecological, health, and economic reasons, the desire to reduce individual consumption of cholesterol and the rising cost of meats, vegetarianism is being practiced by many families. It is, therefore, very likely that you will come into contact with pregnant and lactating women who are on various forms of a vegetarian diet. There are several types of vegetarian diets, which are classified in Table 7.6 by the types of foods that are permitted.

A well-balanced vegetarian diet, or one that is modified to include fish or chicken, can easily supply the pregnant or lactating woman with the necessary nutrients to support her body functions as well as provide for the healthy growth of her baby. Indeed, this type of diet can be credited with the survival of the majority of the world's population. The rice and bean combination has been a staple in China, India, Africa, and South America for centuries. In some ways, a balanced vegetarian diet may be more healthful than a meat-based diet. More volume and fiber are consumed with fewer calories and fats, thereby aiding digestion and decreasing the likelihood of accumulating excess weight.

The breastfeeding mother should inform her physician before beginning a vegetarian diet. Maintenance of lactation while consuming a vegetarian diet can be managed, provided that all the basic principles of sensible vegetarian eating are followed carefully. Appropriate extra sources of calories, protein, and calcium must be clearly defined. The key to successful management of a vegetarian diet is the planning of combinations of foods that will provide the eight essential amino acids. Without the proper balance of amino acids, the body is unable to synthesize the proteins necessary for building tissues. A poorly managed vegetarian diet, or one that is severely restrictive in terms of the types of foods permitted, can be seriously deficient in protein. This problem may result in inadequate growth of the fetus and breastfed infant, as well as inadequate nourishment of the mother. A basic understanding of nutrition, careful meal planning, and selective food shopping are prerequisites for a woman on a vegetarian diet.

TABLE 7.5

Sample Meal Plan

	Sample Menu One			Sample Menu Two	
Breakfast	Cereal, honey nut cornflakes + skim milk 4 oz	156 calories	Breakfast	1 English muffin	134 calories
				Peanut butter, 2 tablespoons	188 calories
	Fruit juice (100%), apple 6 oz	84 calories		Jelly	54 calories
				Skim milk 8 oz	86 calories
Snack	1 medium banana	138 calories	Snack	4 rye crackers	90 calories
				Low-fat swiss cheese 1 oz	50 calories
				Orange juice (100%) 6 oz	78 calories
Lunch	Sliced turkey (low fat)	47 calories	Lunch	Bowl chicken vegetable soup	166 calories
	Whole wheat bread, 2 slices	140 calories		4 saltine crackers	50 calories
	Low-fat mayonnaise, 1 tablespoon	68 calories		Apple	65 calories
	Lettuce	4 calories		Skim milk 8 oz	86 calories
	Tomato slice	20 calories			
	Vegetable juice 6 oz	35 calories			
Snack	Low fat or nonfat yogurt 1 cup	210 calories	Snack	¼ cup raisins	129 calories
Dinner	Hamburger (extra lean ground beef or ground turkey)	213 calories	Dinner	Broiled chicken 3 oz	175 calories
		193 calories		Broccoli ½ cup	22 calories
	Whole grain bun	113 calories		Rice, brown ½ cup	109 calories
	Tomato slice, lettuce, onion	34 calories		Dinner roll	75 calories
	Spinach and tomato salad	26 calories		Spinach and tomato salad w/low-fat dressing	26 calories
	w/low-fat dressing	20 calories			20 calories
	Skim milk 8 oz	86 calories		Skim milk 8 oz	86 calories
Snack	3 low-fat graham crackers	1165 calories	Snack	½ cup nonfat ice cream	110 calories
	Skim milk 8 oz	86 calories			
TOTAL		1,645 calories	TOTAL		2,093 calories

Source: Medela, Inc., Rental Roundup, Vol. 10, Number 1, Winter 1993. http://www.nutribase.com

Many vegetarians become well versed in nutrition through years of practice. They may have a high level of knowledgeable about balanced diets. Some may believe that they are knowledgeable and yet do not actually understand or may be misinformed about the basics of a healthful vegetarian diet. If you encounter a woman whom you believe needs help with her diet, you may be able to motivate her to make changes by explaining the effect that her diet has on her well-being and on her baby's growth. You can build on the woman's present knowledge of nutrition to help her understand what additional foods she needs. Open-ended questions will help you learn about her knowledge of nutrition and how she plans her meals.

Refer to Table 7.2 for plant sources that provide specific nutrients. With this table, you can offer the mother suggestions for selecting nonanimal foods to fulfill her nutrient needs. Specific food suggestions are usually the most helpful to women. Combinations of nuts and bread or crackers with nut spreads or tofu (soybean curd) spreads are good snack foods. Calcium needs can be met by large quantities of green leafy vegetables, broccoli, almonds, molasses, tofu, soy milk, and soy protein. Eggs and dairy products, if acceptable to the woman, can meet both the protein and calcium needs. The requirement for vitamin D can be met through exposure to sunlight and yeast. Green leafy vegetables, nuts, and legumes can satisfy iron requirements. Some suggestions for combining vegetables and grains to make complete protein casseroles are presented in Table 7.7.

Be watchful for any severe vegetarian regimens such as the zen macrobiotic diet, fruitarianism, or any restricted diet or arbitrarily adopted pattern that may be harmful to a woman's pregnancy or lactation. These diets tend to be unbalanced, emphasizing one specific food group while neglecting others, at the expense of needed proteins, vitamins, minerals, and calories.

Because vitamin B_{12} is available only from animal sources, women on vegetarian diets—particularly strict vegan diets—may be deficient in this vitamin. Even mothers with low consumption of animal foods may be at risk for deficiency (Allen, 1994). Levels of vitamin B_{12} are similar in both **serum** and human milk, and a low intake by the mother leads to low intake in her milk. Be alert for signs in the 4- to 8-month-old infant that suggest a deficiency. These signs include anemia, growth failure, neurologic delay, tremors, and excess skin pigmentation. Kuhne and colleagues (1991) suggest that vitamin B_{12} supplementation during pregnancy and lactation is essential when the mother's diet limits or excludes sources of the vitamin. These supplements should be prescribed by a caregiver who is knowledgeable of the woman's diet. Because animal products are a good source of vitamin B_{12}, many vegetarian women are often deficient in this vitamin and can benefit from supplementing their diets with up to 4 mg/day.

Low-Cost Foods

Women who are concerned about proper nutrition, and who cannot afford the high cost of some more nutritional foods, can employ cost-saving methods in purchasing, storing, and preparing foods for their families. Advance meal planning; the use of menus, food store advertisements, and coupons; and a well-written shopping list are all ways to control grocery shopping costs. Through comparison shopping, women can pay close attention to unit pricing labels and purchase store brand name items, which are generally the same quality as popular brand names at substantially lower prices. Some convenience foods may be higher priced. In these cases, women can purchase individual items and make their own dishes. Larger size packages are usually lower priced per serving and are practical only if adequate storage is available. Proper storage and careful menu planning will help minimize food waste, an often overlooked factor in food costs.

Some inexpensive sources of protein are listed in ascending order of cost in Table 7.8. Families who enjoy steak can purchase a beef chuck roast and slice it to half the thickness, making two steaks. When marinated and cooked with care, this type of meat can be an appealing

---

TABLE 7.6
Classification of Vegetarian Diets

Type of Vegetarian Diet	Types of Foods Permitted
Vegan	Foods from plant sources only. (No animal products are consumed.)
Lacto-vegetarian	Milk and milk products, such as cheese and ice cream, in addition to plant foods.
Ovo-vegetarian	Plant foods plus eggs.
Lacto-ovo-vegetarian	Plant foods, dairy products, and eggs.
Fruitarian	Fruits, nuts, olive oil, and honey.

Reprinted, by permission of *The New England Journal of Medicine*, Vol. 299, 317–323, 1978.

TABLE 7.7				
Complete Protein Casseroles				

Directions: Choose one ingredient from each of the five columns in the table. Mix together ingredients from the first four columns. Pour into a greased 2-quart casserole dish and bake 30 minutes at 375°F. Top with one choice from column five and bake 15 minutes longer at 325°F. Salt to taste. Serve with bread and a salad.

Grain: 2 cups cooked	Beans: 1 cup cooked	Sauce: 1 can soup and ¾ cup water	Vegetables: Vegetables: to make 1½ cups	Toppings: to make 3 to 5 tablespoons
Brown rice.	Soybeans.	Cream of tomato soup.	Browned celery and green onions.	Wheat germ.
Macaroni, enriched or whole wheat.	Dried lima beans.	Cream of potato soup.	Mushrooms and bamboo shoots.	Slivered almonds.
Corn.	Dried whole or split peas.	Cream of mushroom soup.	Browned green pepper and garlic.	Fresh whole wheat bread crumbs.
Spaghetti, enriched or whole wheat.	Kidney beans.	Cream of celery soup.	Cooked green beans.	Sesame seeds.
White rice, converted.	Lentils.	Cheddar cheese soup.	Cooked carrots.	Chopped peanuts.
Noodles, enriched, or whole wheat.	Garbanzos (chickpeas).	Cream of pea soup.	Brown onion and pimento.	Sunflower seeds.

Reprinted by permission of Nutrition Services, Allegheny County Health Department.

substitute for higher priced cuts of beef. Many inexpensive meats and meat substitutes can be combined with other foods into a casserole or other main dish. With some creativity, the family may never realize that they are eating a low-cost meal!

In addition to these suggestions, you can direct the woman to a local health or welfare office for nutrition assistance. WIC provides supplemental foods and nutrition counseling to pregnant and postpartum women, breastfeeding mothers, and children from birth to age 5 years if they meet basic requirements of income or nutritional risk. If you are counseling a low-income woman, you can discreetly suggest this option for acquiring the nutrition she will need during pregnancy and lactation. Other U.S. assistance programs available are the Food Stamp Program and Aid to Families with Dependent Children. Lactation consultants outside of the United States can check with their local health authority for similar programs.

Weight Loss and Exercise

Reducing the amount of calories by 300 will help the breastfeeding woman achieve a gradual loss of the excess weight that has accumulated during pregnancy. She can substitute skim milk for whole milk and unsweetened yogurt for other dessert-type foods. The use of lean meat, fewer eggs, and less cheese will serve to cut down on fats and thereby decrease calorie consumption. She may wish to add more foods if she begins losing weight too rapidly, if she becomes easily fatigued, or if her baby does not seem to be satisfied at the breast. Additional low-calorie fluids will be needed to replace the fruit juice snack that has been eliminated.

Several researchers have addressed the concern over the safety of maternal dieting while breastfeeding. Butte and colleagues (1984) found that in well-nourished women, a modest reduction in caloric intake allowed for gradual weight reduction and for continued

TABLE 7.8

Inexpensive Sources of Protein

Food	Market Price per Unit	Cost of 20 g of Protein
Beans, dry	.69 per lb.	.15
Beef liver	.89 per lb.	.21
Eggs, large	1.15 per doz.	.30
Chicken, whole fryer	.99 per lb.	.37
Milk, whole	1.31 per half gal.	.37
Turkey, whole	1.09 per lb.	.37
Peanut butter	1.59 per lb.	.28
Pork, picnic	1.39 per lb.	.44
Tuna, canned, light chunk	.75 per 6 ½ oz.	.33
Beef, ground	1.29 per lb.	.32
Cheese, cheddar	3.99 per lb.	.44
Beef chuck roast	1.49 per lb.	.49
Pork sausage	2.79 per lb.	1.32
Bacon, sliced	2.79 per lb.	1.50

Market prices (in U.S. dollars): Millersburg, Pennsylvania, December, 1997.

appropriate infant growth. Dusdieker (1994) noted that well-nourished, healthy women can safely lose up to 1 lb (0.45 kg) per week. In her study, Dusdieker found that milk production continued to show appropriate increases, with no decrease in fat, that allowed for appropriate infant growth. Dewey and McCrory (1994a) further note that this amount of weight loss is appropriate after lactation is established, cautioning that the caloric intake should not go below 1800 kcal/day. Further caution against liquid diets and diet medications is given.

In addition to advising breastfeeding women about weight loss, you can share information with the mother regarding exercise. Moderate, regular exercise is a part of any healthy lifestyle and should be incorporated into the postpartum period. Dewey and colleagues (1994b) note that exercising as many as four to six times per week, beginning six to eight weeks postpartum while breastfeeding, is safe for most women. They also found that infant acceptance of postexercise mother's milk was not a problem in most cases. You can encourage the mother who is considering either a change in diet or exercise to discuss her plans with her physician or midwife before or at her postpartum checkup.

▼ Group Instruction in Nutrition

Example is the best teacher, so any refreshments that are served at meetings and classes should always be nutritious. You can encourage healthful snacking and eating habits either by bringing nutritious refreshments yourself or by requesting that volunteers bring specific foods to be served. Nutritious snacks might include natural fruit juices, fresh fruit, raw vegetables and dip, wholesome cookies and breads, cheese and crackers, and other snacks suggested in this chapter. Figure 7.2 suggests topics on nutrition that can be used by a mother-to-mother support group.

▼ SUMMARY

You can be a positive force in helping women to improve nutrition for themselves and their families. Educating them about their nutritional needs and the effects of their nutrition on their health and the way they feel will help influence dietary changes. Offering practical food suggestions rather than theoretical dietary requirements makes it easier for women to initiate these changes. Pregnancy and lactation are milestones in a woman's life

FIGURE 7.2   Nutrition topics for group meetings

There are many interesting and entertaining ways to present nutrition information during group discussions. It is hoped that those listed below will interest mothers in nutrition and help them understand how it relates to their daily food selection and preparation.

◆ At a discussion on the "First Days of Breastfeeding," you can emphasize good nutrition as a necessity for pregnant women and new mothers. Avoid overwhelming mothers with health food ideas. Stress two or three basic points, and explain why they are important.
◆ Diet recall: Ask mothers to record everything they have eaten that day. Have them analyze their diets according to food groups, or ask them to hand in their recall lists anonymously for the group to analyze. Look for foods that supply specific nutrients such as protein, vitamin C, iron, calcium, and so on.
◆ At a discussion on "Starting the Baby on Solid Foods," present a buffet of homemade infant foods including finger foods for mothers to sample. For comparison, also provide a taste of the same food prepared commercially.
◆ To highlight a nutrition discussion, serve several complete protein dishes made with meat substitutes and show several milk servings in nutritionally equal amounts (milk, cheese, yogurt, sesame seeds, soy products, and so on).
◆ Approach an old topic with a new point of view. For example, the health benefits of breastfeeding, delaying solid foods, and how to introduce solid foods, can be approached from the perspective of avoiding food intolerances and entitled "Food Intolerances and Healthier Babies."
◆ Have a recipe swap asking everyone to bring a nutritious snack and recipe for all to sample and enjoy.
◆ The National Dairy Council has many other good teaching aids and games for teaching nutrition at meetings.

when she is most receptive to nutrition counseling. Give mothers the information and support they need to avoid impurities in their milk and preserve their babies' health. Be available to advise mothers on special diet regimens they may be considering. Help families integrate sound nutrition into their lifestyles gradually to increase the likelihood that these practices will continue to benefit family members for years to come.

REFERENCES

Adair, Pollitt. Bacon Chow study. *American Journal of Clinical Nutrition*; May 1985.

Allen L. Vitamin B12 metabolism and status during pregnancy, lactation and infancy. *Adv Exp Med Biol* 352:173–186; 1994.

Beal VA. Nutritional studies during pregnancy: Dietary intake, maternal weight gain and size of infant. *J Am Diet Assoc* 58:321; 1971.

Charbonneau K. Folic acid and neural tube defects. *Int J Childbirth Education* 8:42–44; 1993.

Chesley L. *Testimony to U.S. Food and Drug Administration*. Rockville MD: Bureau of Drugs, OB Gyn Advisory Committee; July 17, 1975.

Dewey K et al. A randomized study of the effects of aerobic exercise by lactating women on breastmilk volume and composition. *N Engl J Med* 330:449–453; 1994b.

Dewey K and McCrory M. Effects of dieting and physical activity on pregnancy and lactation. *Am J Clin Nutr* 59(supp): 446s-453s; 1994a.

Dewey KG et al. Maternal weight-loss patterns during prolonged lactation. *Am J Clin Nutr* 58:162–166; 1993.

Dusdieker L et al. Is milk production impaired by dieting during lactation? *Am J Clin Nutr* 59:833–840; 1994.

Dusdieker LB et al. Effect of supplemental fluids on human milk production. *J Pediatr* 106:207; 1985.

Fukushima Y et al. Consumption of cow milk and egg by lactating women and the presence of B-lactoglobulin and ovalbumin in breastmilk. *Am J Clin Nutr* 65:30–35; 1997.

Illingworth PJ et al. Diminution in energy expenditure during lactation. *Br Med J* 292:437; 1986.

Iowa Breakfast Studies, Cereal Institute, Inc., Schaumburg, Illinois, p. 13; 1976.

Jelliffe DB and Jelliffe EFP. *Human Milk in the Modern World*. Oxford: Oxford University Press; 62; 1978.

Kramer FM et al. Breastfeeding reduces maternal lower-body fat. *J Am Diet Assoc* 93:429–433; 1993.

Kritz-Silverstein D. Pregnancy and lactation as determinants of bone mineral density in postmenopausal women. *Am J Epidemiol* 136:1052–1059; 1992.

Lappe FM. *Diet for a Small Planet*. Ballantine Books Mass Market Paperback; New York; 1992.

Lawrence R. *Breastfeeding: A Guide for the Medical Profession*. St. Louis, MO: Mosby; 1999.

Liebman B. *Folic acid for all*. Nutrition Action Healthletter 19(10):4; December, 1992.

Lipsman S et al. Breastfeeding among teenage mothers: Milk composition, infant growth and maternal dietary intake. *J Pediatr Gasteroenterol Nutr* 4:426; 1985.

Lovegrove JA et al. The immunological and long-term atopic outcome of infants born to women following a milk-free diet during late pregnancy and lactation: A pilot study. *Br J Nutr* 71:223–238; 1994.

Michaelsen K et al. The Copenhagen Cohort study on infant nutrition and growth: Breast-milk intake, human milk macronutrient content, and influencing factors. *Am J Clin Nutr* 59:600–611; 1994.

Munoz LM et al. Coffee consumption as a factor in iron deficiency anemia among pregnant women and their infants in Costa Rica. *Am J Clin Nutr* 48:645–651; 1988.

Naeye RL. Cigarette smoking and pregnancy weight gain. *The Lancet* 1(8171):765–766; April, 1980.

Prentice A. Calcium requirements of breast-feeding mothers. *Nutr Rev* 56:124–130; 1998.

Rutishauser L and Carlin J. Body mass index and duration of breastfeeding: A survival analysis during the first six months of life. *J Epidemiol Community Health* 559–565; 1992.

Sigurs N et al. Maternal avoidance of eggs, cow's milk and fish during lactation: Effect on allergic manifestations, skin-prick tests and specific IgE antibodies in children at age 4 years. *Pediatrics* 89:735–739; 1992.

Specker BL. Changes in calcium homeostasis over the first year postpartum: Effect of lactation and weaning. *Obstet Gynecol* 78:56–62; 1991.

Worthington-Roberts B and Taylor LE. *Nutrition During Pregnancy and Breastfeeding*. Chicago, Budlong Press Co.; 1981.

▼ BIBLIOGRAPHY

Brewer S and Brewer T. *What Every Pregnant Woman Should Know. The Truth About Diets and Drugs in Pregnancy.* New York: Random House; p. 76; 1977.

Butte N et al. Effect of maternal diet and body composition on lactation performance. *Am J Clin Nutr* 39:296–306; 1984.

Center for Science in the Public Interest. Good sources of calcium and vitamin D. *Nutrition Action* 13; 1982.

Iowa Cereal Institute, Inc. *Iowa Breakfast Studies.* Shaumburg, Illinois; 13; 1976.

Kuhne T et al. Maternal vegan diet causing a serious infantile neurological disorder due to vitamin B12 deficiency. *Euro J Pediatr* 150:205–208; 1991.

Liebman B. Calcium and Vitamin D. *Nutrition Action Healthletter* 23(3):6–7; 1996.

Liebman B. Fraud or find? *Nutrition Action Healthletter* 24(7):8–11; 1997.

Mennella JA and Beauchamp GK. Maternal diet alters the sensory qualities of human milk and the nursling's behavior. *Pediatrics* 88(4):737–44; Oct 1991.

Motil K et al. Lean body mass of well-nourished women is preserved during lactation. *Am J Clin Nutr* 67:292–300; 1998.

Mughal M et al. Florid rickets associated with prolonged breast feeding without vitamin D supplementation. *Br Med J* 318:39–40; 1999.

Spurr G et al. Increased muscular efficiency during lactation in Colombian women. *Eur J Clin Nutr* 52:17–21; 1998.

Tinkle M. Folic acid and food fortification: Implications for the primary care practitioner. *Nurse Pract* 22:105–114; 1997.

Worthington-Roberts BS et al. Nutrition in Pregnancy and Lactation. St. Louis, MO; The CV Mosby Company; 1989.

8

PROPERTIES OF HUMAN MILK

Human milk is a marvelous substance that is more than just nutrition for the child. Initially, the breast secretes a protein rich substance, colostrum, that provides the infant with antibodies and other factors to protect him against disease. Colostrum is exactly what the newborn needs, both in amount and composition, during this transitional time in his life. During the first days after birth, colostrum mixes with increasing quantities of more mature milk to form transitional milk. It then is replaced totally by mature human milk (Viverge, 1990). The composition of human milk is ideally suited to the human infant. Its components are studied continually, and despite efforts by the manufacturers of artificial baby milk substitutes, no parallel can be found to this perfect infant nutrition.

COLOSTRUM: THE EARLY MILK

Colostrum may be secreted prenatally and up to 10 days postpartum. It is a thick, sticky, rich-looking substance, yellowish in color and concentrated with protein suited to early rapid growth of the newborn. Colostrum is actually the residual mixture of materials present in the mammary glands and ducts, which started production at about 120 days gestation. This substance is mixed with the newly formed milk, and is the thick, clear to golden yellow fluid that the infant receives.

Colostrum contains approximately 57 kcal/100 ml (17 kcal/oz). In the first 24 hours, an infant takes approximately 7 to 14 ml per feeding. This increases over the next 36 hours until intake is approximately 500 ml in a 24-hour period by day 5 or 6. Compared with mature milk, colostrum is richer in sodium, potassium and chloride, protein, fat-soluble vitamins, and minerals. It also contains less fat and lactose than mature milk (Jelliffe, 1978; Wagner, 1996). Although it contains less fat, the amount present is the required level and balance of the essential fatty acids required by the newborn (Ronneberg, 1992).

Colostrum is a baby's first immunization against many bacteria and **viruses.** It contributes to the infant's

health as artificial baby milk cannot, which makes it the ideal first food for infants. Colostrum plays an important role in protecting the infant against infection. It contains many living cells which engulf and digest disease organisms. Colostrum aids in rapid gut closure, or resistance of the baby's intestinal wall to penetration by disease organisms and **antigens.** This means that the infant who receives colostrum is less likely to develop disease and infantile allergies.

Colostrum contains many antibodies, which are biologic as well as chemical substances produced by the body in response to a threat by a particular microbial invader called an antigen. The mother's system produces antibodies to all the diseases to which she has already acquired relative **immunity.** The mother passes many antibodies to her fetus via the placenta and to her newborn via colostrum and human milk.

Three specific antibodies that are highly concentrated in colostrum and human milk are immune globulin A (IgA), immune globulin G (IgG), and immune globulin M (IgM). An immune globulin, or **immunoglobulin,** is a group of proteins that provides immunity. Of these immunoglobulins, IgA occurs in the highest concentrations in colostrum and human milk and is the most biologically active. **Secretory IgA** is obtained only through mother's milk and is not produced by the baby until approximately 6 months of age. Secretory IgA is not present in artificial baby milks.

The infant receives most of his circulating antibodies from the placenta. The very high levels of IgA and other antibodies in colostrum provide further protection to his gastrointestinal tract against organisms that might otherwise begin to invade it. Colostrum facilitates the establishment of bifidus **flora** (normal bacteria and other microbes) in the digestive tract. The bifidus flora promotes the growth of beneficial bacteria and facilitates the passage of meconium. Studies indicate that newborns who are fed fresh human milk—which also contains these protective agents, although in lower concentrations—develop an intestinal flora that is quite unlike the flora of infants receiving boiled human milk or formula (Wilkinson, 1976).

Some **pathogens** (disease agents) against which colostrum provides protection are polio, Coxsackie B virus, several staphylococci, and *Escherichia coli,* the intestinal bacteria that can cause serious intestinal, urinary, and other infections in infants. Health professionals have found colostrum so effective in preventing disease that they have given it successfully to premature infants, older children, and teenagers whose immune systems were not functioning or who had **metabolic** disorders (Arnold, 1995).

In addition to providing disease protection and superior nutrition during the infant's first days of life, the ingestion of colostrum produces a laxative effect that results in the elimination of meconium from the infant's bowels. Meconium is a thick, black, sticky substance that is present in the newborn infant's first stools. Stimulating bowel function is necessary for the infant's body to begin excreting waste products effectively. This elimination can be a critical factor in reducing the severity of jaundice. It is reassuring to a mother to know that her newborn is indeed receiving nourishment, as well as other important health benefits, and is not starving or merely subsisting until her milk production increases and changes to mature milk. The removal of colostrum by the infant also stimulates further production of colostrum and milk, thereby providing an additional benefit. If any water or artificial feeds are given, colostrum's effects are diluted. Additionally, a baby's kidneys are not meant to handle large volumes of fluid and are put under stress by additional water. Breastfed newborns do not need water.

TRANSITION TO MATURE MILK

The color and consistency of human milk vary according to the type of milk and specific additives in the mother's diet. Transitional milk is produced from approximately 7 to 10 days to 2 weeks postpartum and then gives way to mature milk. Mature human milk is secreted in two forms, approximately one-third foremilk and two-thirds hindmilk. The foremilk, which is low in fat and therefore has a thin appearance, collects in the lactiferous sinuses and is readily available to the infant at the beginning of each feed. As the baby's suckling stimulates the nipple, oxytocin is released to activate letdown. The milk is then squeezed out of the alveoli, and the rush of milk washes the fat from the walls of the ducts and ductules. This process results in hindmilk, which is much higher in fat and thus richer looking than foremilk (Smith, 1978).

Appearance of Mature Milk

If a mother expresses some of her milk into a container, she may be alarmed at its watery appearance. It may be that the mother has never seen human milk or milk that is not homogenized, or that she has expressed only foremilk, which is low in fat. Also, milk expressed in the morning and other times when the supply is more plentiful, is usually more dilute. If the mother expresses milk in the early afternoon after nursing or at the end of a feed when the fat content is high, she can observe the thicker consistency of her milk.

Human milk often appears bluish and may take on other colors as well. The typical bluish cast of human milk is caused by the presence of **casein,** a component of the proteins in milk. A greenish color may be due to additives in vitamin or iron supplements taken by the mother or, in rare cases, stagnant milk from a plugged duct. Excessive amounts of vitamin A, either in foods or as a supplement, may color the milk yellow. Black milk can result from use of the drug minocycline (Hunt, 1996). It is helpful to inform a mother to expect these variations so that she will not be concerned unnecessarily.

MILK VOLUME

For a variety of reasons, mothers may worry about the amount of milk they produce. Others may ask the mother if she has enough milk whenever the baby cries. Many times this question arises when a mother needs to express milk for missed feeds. She may wonder if her supply is greatest at a specific time of day, and whether she can express milk between feeds and still maintain an adequate amount of milk for her baby. Milk is most plentiful in the morning hours, especially immediately after the mother awakens. She can express milk at that time and throughout the day without decreasing the amount of milk available to her baby.

The volume of milk is dependent on regular removal of milk from the breast, whether it be through nursing, manual expression or pumping. It also depends on the degree of drainage at each feed or pumping session. Volume is not decreased because of supplemental milk removal. Rather, it will probably increase because of more frequent removal of milk from the breast. Minor variations may occur, either in the volume produced by each breast, on different days, or in response to the infant's suckling pattern. Milk volume is most dependent on the baby's removal of milk from the breast. Babies have the ability to self-regulate their feeds to meet their individual needs for optimal growth (Woolridge, 1990). They determine their supply on a feed-to-feed basis through the amount of milk they remove. Removal of milk at one feed signals the amount of milk available at the next feed. (Daly, 1993).

Although milk volume is most dependent on regular milk removal from the breast, it is to a much lesser extent influenced by the mother's nutrition and on her water intake. In communities with poor nutrition, milk volumes can be low. However, lactation ceases totally only in cases of extremely malnourished mothers. In parts of the world with seasonal food shortages, daily output may drop by 4 to 8 oz (Jelliffe, 1978). It is known that when a woman's diet includes the reference daily intake (RDI) of all nutrients, there is no significant decrease in milk volume. This helps explain why worldwide, under varied nutritional conditions, women are able to nourish their babies so that their growth patterns are very similar to the baby of a well-nourished mother. The actual point at which milk volume decreases or ceases has not been determined (Hambraeus, 1978).

COMPOSITION OF HUMAN MILK

The composition of human milk continually changes throughout lactation as the child grows and even during any given day or feed. The many components in human milk—fat, protein, lactose, vitamins, minerals, and so on—are being studied continually. All have their specific function in ensuring optimum nourishment of the human infant.

Human milk constantly changes to meet the needs of the growing child from the first few days of colostrum to mature milk beyond the second year. The milk is high in immunoglobulins and protein during the first several weeks postpartum, yielding to a relatively dilute state by the first month. In the later months of lactation, the fat content decreases. From 6 to 12 months of age, three-quarters or more of the infant's major nutrient needs can still be met by human milk. During the second year, the output of human milk is equivalent to at least one 8-oz glass of milk daily. Thus, human milk is still valuable to the toddler's diet in both quantity and composition.

Protein and fat content are considerably higher at the end of a feed, with four to five times as much fat and one and a half times as much protein than at the beginning. Nearly one-sixth of the calories are consumed between the 11th and 16th minute. Therefore, it is important that no limits be placed on the amount of time the baby is at each breast (Hall, 1997). Although as much as 80 to 90 percent of the volume can be consumed in the first 4 minutes, when the baby is feeding effectively (Lucas, 1979). The major portion of high-fat milk is obtained after that time. In order for the baby to

obtain important fats, proteins, and calories, it is recommended that the mother continue to nurse until the baby decides his needs are met and ends the feed.

Clearly, human milk provides an appropriate change in composition to meet the child's needs. It varies in sensory qualities as well. Human milk provides the exclusively breastfeeding infant with richly changing experiences in taste and odor that are not provided to the artificially fed infant, whose formula tastes and smells the same all the time. Mennella (1991) even noted in her research that babies demonstrated a preference for garlic-flavored milk.

Calories

Colostrum contains 17 kcal/oz. By 2 weeks, the average caloric content of mature human milk is 20 kcal/oz. At around 4 months, the caloric content is about 26 kcal/oz. Variations in caloric content of mature milk are a result of variations in fat. If a feed is not long enough for the infant to receive the fatty hindmilk, he may receive only half the calories available. In severely malnourished mothers, both volume and fat may be lower. However in the vast majority of women, this is not an issue. The caloric content of human milk is ideally suited to the human infant, so much so that formula companies design their products around the average calories found in human milk.

Fat

In human milk, fat provides 50 to 55 percent of the infant's energy needs. It is the main source of fat-soluble vitamins and essential fatty acids needed for growth and development of the infant's central nervous system. Fat is the most variable of all constituents in human milk. The amount of available fat is dependent on maternal body fat stores (Allen, 1991; Martin, 1993; Nommsen, 1991). In fact, Michaelsen (1994) found that maternal fat stores laid down during pregnancy are easier to mobilize for lactation than other fat stores in the mother's body. If the mother is severely malnourished (which is usually not an issue in developed countries), the level of fat in her milk will be lowered. Within a feed, the fat content will change as the feed progresses. The longer a baby nurses, the higher the fat content of the milk becomes during that feed. (Daly, 1993a). Should a mother's milk fat content be lowered, Tyson (1992) found that the baby will stay at the breast longer in order to gain a higher fat yield that is comparable to the baby whose mother's milk fat is adequate. This further illustrates the importance of baby-led feeds (Perez-Escamilla, 1995).

Short-chain, medium-chain, and long-chain fatty acids are very important. Linoleic and linolenic acids, essential fatty acids, have significance in the quality of myelin laid down. One study showed that multiple sclerosis is rare in countries where breastfeeding is common (Dick, 1976). It was postulated that the development of **myelin** in infancy is critical to preventing degradation later. Arachidonic acid (AA) from linoleic acid and docosahexaenoic acid (DHA) from linolenic acid are essential for development of visual acuity (Ballabriga, 1994; Carlson, 1996; Farquharson, 1995).

The amount of fat a breastfed infant receives depends on the length of time spent suckling at the breast. Hindmilk contains four times the amount of fat present in foremilk and is obtained in the later part of the feed only after sufficient suckling time. A baby who is not gaining sufficient weight may not be nursing long enough at each feed or frequently enough throughout the day and night. If a baby is removed from one breast too early, before receiving the fatty hindmilk, he will fill up on foremilk from both breasts. This could lead to colicky behavior and poor nourishment. Fat content decreases after 5 or 6 months and also is lower when the letdown reflex is inhibited.

Carbohydrates

Lactose is present in human milk in high levels (7 percent) and represents almost all of the carbohydrate in the milk (Jelliffe, 1978). Lactose provides 40 to 45 percent of the energy. Lactose concentration increases by approximately ten percent over the first six months of lactation (Allen, 1991; Coppa, 1993). It is specific for newborn growth and performs three unique functions that benefit the infant. Lactose enhances calcium absorption, thereby helping prevent rickets. It helps supply energy to the infant's brain. Also, it helps check the growth of harmful organisms in the infant's intestine. Lactose is essential to development of the central nervous system.

Lactose is the major sugar in mammalian milk and is found nowhere else in nature. It is generally recognized as being the most constant among mothers of all the constituents in human milk. It remains constant throughout the day and despite dietary changes (Jelliffe, 1978). Lactose is slowly digested so that there is a steady release of glucose into the bloodstream. Sucrose, the sugar often used in milk substitute formulas such as soy, is sweeter and splits rapidly, resulting in a high peak of glucose in the infant's bloodstream. It is also thought that sucrose plays a significant role in tooth decay, whereas lactose does not (Tonk, 1965). Additionally, the ramifications of feeding an infant a food without lactose, such as soy formula and milk-based lactose-free formula, have not been studied.

Protein

All animal species have growth and development needs that determine their milk composition. Within the animal kingdom, human milk contains the least amount of protein, which results in the slowest rate of growth. The distribution of specific proteins in human milk is ideally suited to the growth of the human infant. It enables him to use the proteins with extremely high efficiency. Colostrum contains about three times more protein than does mature milk. The protein content of human milk seems to remain relatively constant regardless of the mother's nutritional status or dietary practices. Protein in human milk is easily digested and well absorbed.

Manufacturers of artificial baby milk substitutes have attempted to adjust their products to equal the protein content of human milk as closely as possible. Infant formula, however, lacks certain proteins found in human milk, such as **lactoferrin.** It also is not completely used by the infant, with some amino acids being passed in the stool. Cow's milk curd is tough and rubbery, whereas the curd of human milk is soft, small, and less compact, making it easier for the infant to digest. The **whey** (clear fluid when milk stands) to-casein (curds) ratio changes throughout lactation from 90:10 in early milk to 60:40 in mature milk and to 50:50 in late lactation. The ratio in formula varies depending on the manufacturer. Wagner (1996) notes that ratios in Carnation Good Start are 100:0. In Enfamil, ratios are 60:40, and in Similac, ratios are 28:18.

Lactoferrin, the iron-binding protein in whey, inhibits the growth of iron-dependent bacteria (E. coli) in the gastrointestinal tract. This protects the baby against gastrointestinal (GI) infections. Lactoferrin renders intestinal iron unavailable to pathogens in the baby's gut, thus protecting him from such infections as salmonella, *E. coli,* and *Candida albicans.* Giving iron supplements to newborns may saturate the lactoferrin, thus allowing proliferation of *E. coli.* Protection from lactoferrin is not present if the baby receives any other type of feeding.

Another whey protein found in human milk is lysozyme. One of the over 20 active enzymes present in human milk, lysozyme provides an **antimicrobial** factor against *enterobacteriaceae* and gram-positive bacteria. Human milk also contains eight essential amino acids. One example, taurine, is important for vision and general development, and improves fat absorption in preterm infants.

Vitamins

Generally, all vitamins are available in human milk in sufficient quantities (note the discussion of vitamin D in the next section). Excessive doses of vitamin B_6 (300 to 600 mg/day) can reduce milk production. Strict lacto-ovo-vegetarians may be deficient in vitamin B_{12}, which can result in megoblastic anemia and neurologic malfunction in the newborn (see the discussion of vegetarian diets in Chapter 7.) Colostrum is particularly rich in vitamin E and human milk levels are also high. Since a deficiency in vitamin E in infancy can result in anemia, breastfeeding is a preventive measure against anemia in infancy. Vitamin D and vitamin K are discussed below.

Vitamin D

Vitamin D has been found to be present in the water-soluble portion of human milk, as well as in the fatty portion, in sufficient amounts to meet the infant's needs (Lakdawala, 1997). Notably, a low incidence of rickets is found in full-term breastfed infants who are not supplemented with vitamin D. This offers strong evidence that babies who are breastfed exclusively do not require vitamin D supplements, provided that the mother's supply of vitamin D is adequate and the baby receives sufficient sunlight (American Academy of Pediatrics [AAP]).

Specker (1985) suggests that in order to maintain adequate levels of vitamin D in exclusively breastfed babies at risk for vitamin D deficiency, the babies should be exposed to sunlight for 30 minutes per week wearing only a diaper or 2 hours per week if fully clothed without a hat. Lactation consultants need to be particularly aware of the circumstances that increase the risk of vitamin D deficiency. Darkly pigmented skin, living in a cold climate, residing in an inner city home, and maternal vegetarian diet or restricted diet are all potential risk factors. Make sure that mothers in these situations are made aware of ways to meet their babies' vitamin D needs (Bhowmick, 1991). Also, babies in day care centers often do not go outside during the day. Many times it is dark in the morning when they are dropped off and dark at night when they are picked up.

Vitamin K

Vitamin K is present in small amounts in human milk and provides the infant with that essential vitamin. Additionally, the infant is protected by vitamin K from fetal stores and the **prophylactic** dose given at birth until he receives sufficient milk from his mother and his intestine matures enough to manufacture its own. Vitamin K is routinely given to newborns either by intramuscular (IM) injection or oral dose to promote blood clotting. There has been much debate regarding the use of prophylactic vitamin K given to the newborn. It raises the question of whether human milk is sufficient in any instance to provide adequate vitamin K for the newborn. Some question why supplemental doses of vitamin K are necessary, and if so, how they are most effectively given.

A 1991 study of infant clotting factors noted that babies fed human milk were not at a greater risk for bleeding than those fed infant formula. In this study, both the breastfed and artificially fed groups of babies received an intramuscular dose of vitamin K at birth, (Greer, 1991).

Increasing the lactating mother's dietary intake of vitamin K has thus far been shown to not increase the amount present in her milk. Therefore, a vitamin K source other than human milk is currently recommended (Canfield, 1991; Pietschnig, 1993). At the present time, there is no screening method to identify those babies at risk for hemorrhagic disease. However, Cornelissen (1992) has identified a substance, found in the blood of 3-month-old breastfed babies who were given oral vitamin K at birth, which occurs only with vitamin K deficiency. In light of the possibility of a rare but real risk of a fatal disease and no identifying indicator of risk, the current practice of giving a prophylactic dose of vitamin K appears to be the best way to offer generalized protection to newborns.

There is some debate about the use of intramuscular injection versus an oral dose of vitamin K to the newborn. Cornelissen's study comparing oral and intramuscular vitamin K **prophylaxis** showed that babies receiving oral vitamin K shortly after birth demonstrated a need for a repeated oral dose in order to prevent vitamin K deficiency after 1 month of age. On the other hand, the oral dosing is much less distressing to the newborn than an injection, which also carries the risk of nerve damage. Certainly, more study is needed on the relationship of vitamin K and breastfeeding.

▼ Minerals

The mineral balance in human milk is more favorable to the baby's needs than that in cow's milk. Human milk has a lower percentage of minerals and minimizes the load on the baby's immature kidneys. The calcium in human milk is absorbed much more efficiently (Rudloff, 1990). In fact, the higher ratio of phosphorus to calcium that is present in cow's milk can interfere with calcium absorption. Owing to this factor, artificially fed infants are more likely to develop late neonatal **hypocalcemia** than their breastfed counterparts (Specker, 1991). Also, under stress situations such as hot weather or diarrhea, the higher mineral content of a cow's milk–based infant formula is a significant contributor to dehydration.

The higher solute load of infant formulas may require additional water intake by the infant to expel the solutes. The thirst induced by this type of food is often misinterpreted as hunger, with more formula being given to the baby instead of the water he needs. Babies who are breastfed exclusively require no water supplements—not even in hot climates—because there is little waste to be flushed through the kidneys (Ashraf, 1993). Increased feeds will satisfy the need for more fluids when it is hot. The higher weight gains in infants who are fed artificial baby milk may be caused by a greater retention of sodium and water. Likewise, a relatively sudden change from breastfeeding to bottle feeding can be accompanied by a rapid gain in weight due to water retention associated with increased body sodium (McCance, 1975).

Iron

During the final 6 to 8 weeks of pregnancy, a healthy nonanemic mother lays down iron stores to provide her baby with enough iron through her milk for the first few months postpartum. Blood from the umbilical cord also contributes iron that the infant stores in his liver. Although iron is present in human milk in small quantities, the level is sufficient to meet the iron requirements of the exclusively breastfed full-term infant until he is approximately 6 months old (Aggett, 1989, McMillan, 1976; Pizarro, 1991). A premature infant may need iron supplementation because he may not have received a sufficient quantity of iron in utero.

The iron in human milk is absorbed more efficiently than that of cow's milk, partially because of the high vitamin C level present in human milk. 60 percent of iron in human milk is absorbed by the baby, compared with only 4 percent of iron in artificial baby milk. The infant does not begin to deplete his own iron stores until 4 to 6 months after birth or even later. Because lactoferrin loses its ability to inhibit the growth of bacteria when saturated with iron (Bullen, 1972), routine supplementation of iron is questionable and in fact, may, be detrimental to the breastfed infant.

The healthy infant's hemoglobin is high at birth (18 to 20 g/dl) and decreases rapidly as the infant's body adjusts to extrauterine life. Hemoglobin is the portion of the red blood cell that carries oxygen to all parts of the body. At 4 months of age, the typical range is between 10.2 and 15 g/dl. Over this same period, there is also a change in the type of hemoglobin, from a fetal type to an adult type, which is more efficient in delivering oxygen to the tissues. Therefore, although the actual grams of hemoglobin decrease, the efficiency of each gram increases as this change takes place.

Fluoride

Breastfed infants have fewer dental caries and better dental health. Conclusive studies have shown that during the development of primary and secondary teeth, fluoride supplements ingested by the infant reduce cavities by 50 to 60 percent. In communities with fluoridated drinking water, breastfed babies receive fluoride through their mother's milk. If the family's water supply contains less than 0.3 ppm (parts per million) of fluoride, infant fluoride supplementation is recommended after the age of 6 months (AAP, 1995; Institute of Medicine, 1991). Babies who receive supplementary fluoride may occasionally exhibit allergic reactions, described by mothers in the form of fussiness, irritability, refusal to take the fluoride, and spitting it up (Jelliffe 1978). Excessive fluoride may cause dental mottling, a form of discoloration (Vorherr, 1974).

▼ Other Constituents

Human milk contains over 200 known components, including the trace elements copper, zinc, manganese, silicon, aluminum, and titanium. The complete significance of these components has not been determined and needs further investigation. Zinc deficiency in infancy can cause failure to thrive and skin **lesions**. In the inherited zinc deficiency disorder **acrodermatitis enteropathica**, human milk can be life saving due to the increased bioavailability of the zinc, whereas cow's milk formula has no effect (Lawrence, 1994).

More than 20 human milk enzymes have been identified, as well as prolactin and steroid hormones (Lawrence, 1999). One enzyme, **lipase**, is essential for the digestion of fat so that it is available to the infant as energy. Another enzyme, **amylase**, is important for carbohydrate digestion (Dewit, 1993). Artificial baby milk lacks these digestive enzymes.

One portion of human milk that is being investigated is the presence of nitrogen compounds. An example of a nonprotein nitrogen that is relatively absent in cow's milk are nucleotides. Nucleotides are an integral part of the immune system. They act as the host defense against bacteria, viruses, and parasites, as well as various malignancies.

Still under study are **prostaglandins**, bile salts, and epidermal growth factors. Epidermal growth factor—found in colostrum, and preterm and term human milk—has been shown to promote the growth of intestinal cells in culture. It is speculated that such growth also occurs in living infants. In preterm babies, the implications of this possibility are significant in helping their guts mature more efficiently. Artificial baby milks do not contain this growth factor (Ichiba, 1992; Koldovsky, 1989).

Not only does human milk contain a vast number of components, studies of specific components show how each mother's milk differs slightly due to individual genetic codes. In other words, each breastfed infant receives a totally unique product! The **oligosaccharides** in human milk are one example of this (Coppa, 1993). The major elements in human milk are compared in Table 8.1 with those present in cow's milk.

TABLE 8.1

Comparison of Components in Human Milk and Cow's Milk

Component	Human Milk	Cow's Milk
Water (ml/100 ml)	87.1	87.2
Energy (Cal/100 ml)	60–75	66
Total solids (g/100 ml)	12.9	12.8
Protein (%)	0.8–0.9	3.5
Fat (%)	3–5	3.7
Lactose (%)	6.9–7.2	4.9
Ash (minerals) (%)	0.2	0.7
Protein (% of total protein)		
Casein	40	82
Whey	60	1.8
Ash, major components per liter		
Calcium (mg)	340	1170
Phosphorus (mg)	140	920
Sodium (mEq)	7	22
Vitamins per liter		
Vitamin A (IU)	1898	1025
Thiamin (μg)	160	440
Riboflavin (μg)	360	1750
Niacin (μg)	1470	940
Vitamin C (mg)	43	1.1

HEALTH BENEFITS OF HUMAN MILK

Human milk is a species-specific first food that offers appropriate nutrition for the child as well as health protection to support his developing immune system. The mother affords her child the specific protection he needs for the environment in which they live, both in terms of allergens and infection protection. Human milk further protects the infant through its packaging. It does not spoil, the temperature is always correct, it cannot be mixed incorrectly, there are no omissions of components, and there are no product recalls! Research is continually uncovering new health benefits of human milk both for the newborn and older child.

Immunologic Properties

Perhaps the most spectacular advantage of human milk over commercially prepared infant formula is its protection to the infant against disease. Human milk contains a wide variety of soluble, cellular, and **humoral** factors that protect the infant against a host of diseases. The infant is protected against bacterial infections, viral infections, protozoa, and allergies (Ahmed, 1992; Morrow, 1992; Ruiz-Palacios, 1990). These factors are identified in Table 8.2, Table 8.3, and Table 8.4.

Human milk protects the infant and also the breast by providing anti-infective agents and by minimizing inflammation (Hennart, 1991; Koutras, 1989). It also protects against infections outside the GI tract, such as upper and lower respiratory infections, as well as some chronic childhood diseases (Cunningham, 1979; Piscane 1994a, Wright, 1989). There has been evidence for protection against diseases in later life such as Crohn's disease, juvenile diabetes, childhood lymphoma, multiple sclerosis, and heart disease (Davis, 1988; Koletzko, 1989; Mayer, 1988; Piscane, 1994b).

Although human milk is not sterile, it contains a number of anti-infective agents that maintain a very low bacterial level within the fluid for many hours. It can destroy bacteria in the infant's GI tract before they affect

TABLE 8.2

Antibacterial Factors Found in Human Milk

Factor	Shown in Vitro to Be Active Against
Secretory IgA	*E. coli* (also *pili*, capsular antigens, CFA1), *C. tetani, C. diphtheriae, K. Pneumoniae, S. mutans, S. sanguins, S. mitis, S. agalactiae, S. salvarius, S. pneumoniae, C. burnetti, H. influenza. H. pylori, S. flexneri, S. boydii, S. sonnei, C. jejuni, N. meningitidis, B. pertussis, S. dysenteriae, C. trachomatis,* Salmonella (6 groups), *Campylobacter flagelin, S. flexneri* virulence plasmid antigen, *C. diphtheriae* toxin, *E. coli* enterotoxin, *V. cholerae* enterotoxin, *C. difficile* toxins, *H. influenza* capsule, *S. aureus* enterotoxin F, *Candida albicans*
IgG	*E. coli, B. pertussis, H. influenza* type b, *S. pneumoniae, S. agalactiae, N. meningitidis,* 14 pneumoccocal capsular polysaccharides, *V. cholerae* lipopolysaccharide, *S. flexneri* invasion plasmid–coded antigens, major opsonin for *S. aureus*
IgM	*V. cholerae* lipopolysaccharide
IgD	*E. coli*
Free secretory component*	*E. coli* colonization factor antigen I (CFA1)
Bifidobacterium bifidum	Enteric bacteria
Growth factors (oligosaccharides, glycopeptides)	
Other Bifidobacteria growth factors (alpha-lactoglobulin, lactoferrin, sialyllactose)	
Factor-finding proteins (zinc, vitamin B$_{12}$, folate)	Dependent *E. coli*
Complement C1-C9 (mainly C3 and C4)	Killing of *S. aureus* in macrophages
Lactoferrin*	*E. coli, E. coli*/CFA1, *Candida albicans*
Lactoperoxidase	Streptococcus, Pseudomonas, *E. coli, S. typhimurium*
Lysozyme	*E. coli,* Salmonella, *M. lysodeikticus,* growing *Candida albicans* and *Aspergillus fumigatus*
Unidentified factors	*S. aureus, B. pertussis, C. jejuni, E. coli, S. typhimurium, S. flexneri, S. sonnei, V. cholerae, L. pomona, L. hyos, L. icterohaemorrhagiae, C. difficile* toxin B, *H. pylori*
Nonimmunoglobulin (milk fat, proteins)	*C. trachomatis,* Y. *enterocolitica*
Carbohydrate	*E. coli* enterotoxin, *E. coli, C. difficile* toxin A
Lipid	*S. aureus, E. coli, S. epidermis, H. influenzae, S. agalactiae*
Ganglioside GM$_1$	*E. coli* enterotoxin, *V. cholerae* toxin, *C. jejuni* enterotoxin, *E. coli*
Ganglioside GM$_3$	*E. coli*
Phosphatidylethanolamine	*H. pylori*
Sialyllactose	*V. cholerae* toxin, *H. pylori*
Mucin (milk fat globulin membrane)	*E. coli* (S-fimbrinated) sialyloligosaccharides on sIgA(Fc) *E. coli* (S-fimbrinated) adhesion
Glycoproteins (receptor-like) + oligosaccharides	*V. cholerae*
Glycoproteins (mannosylated)	*E. coli*

TABLE 8.2 (CONTINUED)

Antibacterial Factors Found in Human Milk

Factor	Shown in Vitro to Be Active Against
kappa-Casein*	*H. pylori, S. pneumoniae*
Casein	*H. influenza*
Glycolipid Gb$_3$	*S. dysenterae* toxin, shigatoxin of shigella and *E. coli*
Fucosylated oligosaccharides	*E. coli* heat-stable enterotoxin, *C. jejuni, E. coli*
Analogues of epithelial cell receptors (oligosaccharides)	*S. pneumoniae, H. influenza*
Milk cells (macrophages, neutrophils, B and T lymphocytes)	By phagocytosis and killing: *E. coli, S. aureus, S. enteritidis*
	By sensitised lymphocytes: *E. coli*
	By phagocytosis: *Candida albicans*[†,‡], *E. coli*
	Lymphocyte stimulation: *E. coli*, K antigen, tuberculin
	Spontaneous monokines: simulated by lipopolysaccaride
	Induced cytokines: PHA, PMA + ionomycin
	Fibronectin helps in uptake by phagocytic cells.

*Factors found at low level in human milk can be antibacterial at higher levels, eg. secretory leukocyte protease inhibitor (antileukocyte protease) has antibacterial *(E. coli, S. aureus)* and antifungal (growing *C. albicans* and *A. fumigatus*) activity.

[†]Fungi.

[‡]Contain fucosylated oligosaccharides.

From Proceedings of Breast Milk and Special Care Nurseries: Problems and Opportunities Conference. August 1995. Melbourne. Copyright J. T. May and Australian Lactation Consultants Association Victorian Branch, 1995. Updated August, 1998. Reprinted by permission of Department of Microbiology, La Trobe University, Bundoora Victoria 3083, Australia.

the infant. Milk components also coat the GI tract, thus preventing other offending organisms and molecules from entering the infant's system. Many researchers have reported a lower incidence of infection present in breast-fed babies (Bertotto, 1991 to 1993; Chen, 1988; Chiba, 1987; Cleary, 1991; Popkin, 1990; Udall, 1990).

At birth, the infant is suddenly exposed to a variety of microorganisms to which the mother is already immune. She passes this immunity to her baby, both across the placenta before birth, and through her colostrum and milk after birth. Furthermore, if a new microorganism is introduced into the environment, the mother will most likely produce appropriate antibodies and pass those antibodies to the baby by means of her milk. In addition to this internal mechanism, it seems that the breast itself also produces antibodies to the organisms passed into it by the suckling infant. In response to the organisms, the mammary gland produces immunoglobulins locally and passes them to the infant in the mother's milk, thereby protecting him from the harmful effects of disease organisms.

The presence of IgA in colostrum and human milk serves to protect the gastrointestinal tract of the infant against penetration by organisms and antigens. It is probably the most important of the antiviral defense factors and is at its highest level immediately after birth. IgA continues to remain at a significant level for at least 6 or 7 months. Colostrum and human milk also contain living white cells—lymphocytes and **macrophages**—that engulf and digest bacteria and synthesize IgA and other protective substances.

Growth factors enhance the infant's development and maturation of the immune system, the central nervous system, and organs such as skin. Digestive enzymes **lactase** and lipase, and many other important enzymes, protect babies born with immature or defective enzyme systems. Lactase is necessary for converting lactose into simple sugars that can be assimilated easily by the infant. A deficiency in lactase, which generally occurs as a result of diminishing activity of intestinal lactase after weaning, can result in **lactose intolerance**. A person who is lactose intolerant is unable to digest milk sugar (lactose). The condition is more prevalent in adults and is rarely found in children under 3 years of age. As discussed earlier, lactose helps prevent rickets, and aids calcium absorption and brain development.

The breastfed infant is protected by the enzyme lysozyme, which breaks up bacteria in the bowel. The

TABLE 8.3

Antiviral Factors Found in Human Milk

Factor	Shown in Vitro to Be Active Against
Secretory IgA	Polio types, 1, 2, 3. Coxsackie types A9, B3, B5, echo types 6, 9, Semliki Forest virus, Ross River virus, rotavirus, cytomegalovirus, reovirus type 3, rubella varicella-zoster virus, herpes simplex virus, mumps virus, influenza, respiratory syncytial virus, human immunodeficiency virus, hepatitis C virus, hepatitis B virus, measles.
IgG	Rubella, cytomegalovirus, respiratory syncytial virus, rotavirus, human immunodeficiency virus, Epstein-Barr virus.
IgM	Rubella, cytomegalovirus, respiratory syncytial virus, human immunodeficiency virus.
Lipid (unsaturated fatty acids and monoglycerides)	Herpes simplex virus, Semliki Forest virus, influenza, dengue, Ross River virus, Japanese B encephalitis virus, sindbis, West Nile, human immunodeficiency virus, respiratory syncytial virus, vesicular stomatitis virus.
Non-immunoglobulin macromolecules	Herpes simplex virus, vesicular stomatitis virus, Coxsackie B4, Semliki Forest virus, reovirus 3, poliotype 2, cytomegalovirus, respiratory syncytial virus, rotavirus.
alpha2-macroglobulin (like)	Influenza haemagglutinin, parainfluenza haemagglutinin.
Ribonuclease	Murine leukaemia.
Haemagglutinin inhibitors	Influenza, mumps.
Mucin (glycoprotein/lactadherin)	Rotavirus
Chondroitin sulphate (-like)	Human immunodeficiency virus
Secretory leukocyte protease inhibitor (colostrum levels)	Human immunodeficiency virus, *Bifidobacterium bifidum*, Rotavirus
sIgA + trypsin inhibitor	Rotavirus
Lactoferrin	Cytomegalovirus, human immunodeficiency virus, respiratory syncytial virus, herpes simplex virus type 1, hepatitis C
Milk cells	Induced interferon: virus, PHA, or PMA and ionomycin
	Induced cytokine: herpes simplex virus, respiratory syncytial virus.
	Lymphocyte stimulation: rubella, cytomegalovirus, herpes, measles, mumps, respiratory syncytial virus.

Factors found at low levels in human milk, known to be antiviral at higher levels:

 prostaglandins E2, F2 alpha (parainfluenza 3, measles)

 gangliosides GM1-3 (rotavirus, respiratory syncytial virus)

 heparin (cytomegalovirus, respiratory syncytial virus)

 glycolipid Gb4 (human B19 parvovirus)

From Proceedings of Breast Milk and Special Care Nurseries: Problems and Opportunities Conference. August 1995. Melbourne. Copyright J. T. May and Australian Lactation Consultants Association Victorian Branch, 1995. Updated August, 1998. Reprinted by permission of Department of Microbiology, La Trobe University, Bundoora Victoria 3083, Australia.

bowels are also protected by lactoferrin, an iron-binding protein, which acts together with specific antibodies to inhibit the growth of *E. coli*, the major cause of bowel infection in infants. If a baby receives too much iron, through supplements or enriched foods, the effectiveness of this protein will be significantly diminished (Bullen, 1972).

The growth of undesirable organisms such as *E. coli* can also be discouraged by the **bifidus factor,** a carbohydrate. The bifidus factor is present in high concentrations in both colostrum and human milk. Human milk contains seven times as much of this factor as does cow's milk. The bifidus factor works with the low pH of the stool to help special bacteria grow in the infant's intestine and prevent other harmful bacteria from growing.

TABLE 8.4	
Antiparasite Factors Found in Human Milk	
Factor	**Shown in Vitro to Be Active Against**
Secretory IgA	*Giardia lamblia*
	Entamoeba histolytica
	Schistosoma mansoni (blood fluke)
	Cryptosporidium
	Toxoplasma gondii
	Plasmodium falciparum (malaria)
IgG	*Plasmodium falciparum*
Lipid (free fatty acids and monoglycerides)	*Giardia lamblia*
	Entamoeba histolytica
	Trichomonas vaginalis
	Giardia intestinalis
	Eimeria tenella (animal coccidiosis)
Unidentified	*Trypanosoma brucei rhodesiense*

From Proceedings of Breast Milk and Special Care Nurseries: Problems and Opportunities Conference. August 1995. Melbourne. Copyright J.T. May and Australian Lactation Consultants Association Victorian Branch, 1995. Updated July, 1996. Reprinted by permission of Department of Microbiology, La Trobe University, Bundoora Victoria 3083, Australia.

Otitis Media

One of the most common infant infections, otitis media, or middle ear infection, has been shown to occur with increased frequency in the absence of breastfeeding. Aniansson (1994) observed this link and noted that the first episode of otitis media occurs earlier in children who are weaned before 6 months of age. In this study, both mixed feeds and the absence of human milk in the diet increased the risk of infection.

The best protection against otitis media appears to be exclusive breastfeeding for at least 4 months (Duncan, 1993). Even after weaning, the protection against otitis media afforded by human milk is at work. Sassen (1994) noted that even 4 months after breastfeeding stopped, the risk of otitis media was lower. A study by the **Centers for Disease Control and Prevention (CDC)** states that "when compared with exclusively breastfed infants, infants who received only formula had an 80 percent increase in their risk of developing diarrhea and a 70 percent increase in their risk of developing an ear infection" (Scariati, 1997).

Necrotizing Enterocolitis and Sepsis

Human milk has been shown to decrease the risk of the occurrence of **necrotizing enterocolitis (NEC)**. NEC is characterized by inflammation of the intestinal wall, often causing the tissue to die. It is frequently associated with prematurity, respiratory disease, and early enteral feeds of formula in premature babies (Lucas, 1990). NEC is said to occur in 2 to 7 percent of premature babies (Buescher, 1994; Udall, 1990). Lucas found that NEC is 6 to 10 times more likely to occur in artificially fed babies than those fed human milk exclusively. Among babies born after 30 weeks' gestation, the risk was 20 times higher for the artificially fed babies. He further noted that NEC was three times more likely to occur in babies receiving mixed feeds than those receiving feeds of human milk alone (Dugdale, 1991; Lucas, 1990).

Because the actual cause of NEC is not well understood, the role human milk plays in protection is unclear as well. It is speculated that secretory IgA and possibly the phagocytic cells play a role in protection (Buescher 1994; Udall, 1990). Should a mother be unable initially to provide enough of her own milk for feeds, researchers suggest that the protection against NEC is found with pasteurized **donor milk** as well (Dugdale, 1991; Lucas, 1990).

Another protection offered by human milk to hospitalized babies is a decreased incidence of **nosocomial** (hospital-acquired) **sepsis**. Researchers at George Washington University Hospital found that even though babies who were fed expressed human milk were colonized with bacteria like those in formula-fed babies, they had a significantly lower incidence (El-Mohandes, 1997).

Protection from Maternal Antigens

Protection from human milk extends beyond that against common childhood illnesses and illnesses of the mother. It protects the infant in his immediate environment as well. Whenever a mother contracts an infection, whether it be a cold, fever, or more serious illness, her body responds by producing antibodies in her milk that help protect her breastfed baby. Although some viruses may be transmitted through human milk, the presence of antibodies to counteract them offsets the potential harm to the baby. In fact, there is evidence that milk responds to and remembers for years specific infections it has encountered. Asian mothers in the United Kingdom showed antibodies to pathogens they had encountered in their home countries several years earlier (Nathavitharana, 1994).

Often, a more likely mechanism of disease transmission from mother to baby is through close contact such as touching, and through close mouth and nose contact—and not through the mother's milk. Subsequently, when the mother contracts an illness, it is likely that her baby has already been exposed to it through contact with her during her most contagious period. Therefore, the most effective treatment for the infant would be to continue breastfeeding while receiving any necessary medication. The mother could also decrease the infant's exposure to the disease by careful handwashing before contact with her baby and, in extreme cases, by wearing a mask over her nose and mouth.

A breastfeeding mother who develops a cold or fever need not worry about infecting her baby through her milk. Encourage her to practice good hygiene and to limit facial contact with her baby during the infectious period. Advise her to rest and follow the treatment plan prescribed by her physician in order to return to good health quickly and not compromise her milk production.

The response to immunizations found in breastfed babies varies somewhat in the research. Scheifele (1992) reports that breastfed and artificially fed infants have similar levels of protection after immunization. Both Azzari (1990) and Hahn-Zoric (1990) report a better immune response to **immunizations** in infants fed human milk.

Other Immunologic Factors

There are countless other factors yet to be identified that aid in the protection of the human infant from disease. Ongoing research is continually uncovering these protective factors. **Mucins** found in human milk have been linked to protection against bacterial infections, including such severe illnesses as neonatal sepsis and meningitis (Schroten, 1992, 1993). Mucins in human milk have also been linked to protection against rotavirus, an acute GI infection (Yolken, 1991). Oligosaccharides in human milk demonstrate protection against urinary tract infections in both the child and the mother (Coppa, 1990; Piscane, 1992). Human milk also has been shown to contain three essential thyroid hormones that are totally lacking in cow's milk and conventional infant formulas. These hormones may be responsible for preventing hypothyroidism, masking diagnosis, and protecting the baby until he is weaned.

In light of what has already been learned about human milk, the AAP (1997) recommends that all mothers breastfeed their infants for 1 year, both for the psychological value afforded the breastfeeding mother and infant and for the protection against disease received by the maturing infant. Research from developed countries sometimes concludes that breastfeeding is not important to protection from infection for babies in wealthy nations (Bauchner, 1986; Rubin, 1990). However, these studies are flawed both by methodological problems and improper grouping of partially breastfed and exclusively breastfed babies. Breastfeeding advocates need to be aware of the critiques and counter-arguments (Cunningham, 1988; 1990, 1991).

▼ Allergy Protection

The infant's GI tract develops more quickly when he is fed human milk, thus preventing foreign proteins from entering his system. Nutrients such as zinc and the long-chain polyunsaturated fatty acids aid in the development of the infant's immune response. Giving babies even a single feeding of artificial baby milk in the first days of life can increase the rates of allergic disease. All formulas, including soy formulas, carry a risk of allergy (Ellis, 1991; Saylor, 1991).

Cow's milk is the most common food allergen in infants. Three-fourths of cow's milk allergies begin in the first 1 to 2 months of life (Jelliffe, 1978). Cow's milk formulas do not contain the antibodies necessary to protect the infant's intestines. For sensitive infants, the foreign protein of cow's milk passes through the infant's intestinal wall and causes allergic reactions. These reactions may manifest themselves as colic-like behavior, diarrhea, vomiting, malabsorption, **eczema**, ear infections, or asthma.

Symptoms of allergy are more prevalent in infants fed cow's milk-based formula than in breastfed infants, presumably because of cow's milk. In a group of children followed for 17 years in Finland, evidence of reduced allergy in the breastfed group was still apparent at age 17 (Saarinen, 1995). There is also the possibility that other food antigens cause allergy responses in these infants because solid foods are frequently started at an earlier age in formula-fed infants. "In infants at risk of developing allergies, exclusive breastfeeding until four to six months and a delayed introduction of foods other than milk significantly reduces, at least up to 12 to 36 months of age, the incidence of atopic symptoms, especially eczema, and of gastrointestinal symptoms attributable to cows' milk as compared to feeding infant formulae based on cows' milk or soya protein" (European Society of Pediatric Gastroenterology and Nutrition, 1993).

There are almost no antibodies in the immature intestine of a newborn infant, leaving the wall of the intestine susceptible to invasion by foreign proteins. Human milk contains high levels of antibodies, especially IgA, which are thought to provide an antiabsorptive protection on the lining of the infant's intestine. This shields the surface from the absorption of foreign protein as well as from bacterial invasion.

Researchers Jakobsson and Lindberg of the University of Lund in Malmo, Sweden, studied a group of breastfed infants with infantile colic, most of whom had a family history of allergic disease. With the speculation that the colic was being caused by cow's milk proteins transmitted from mother to baby through her milk, each mother was put on a diet free of cow's milk protein. The colic disappeared promptly in three-quarters of the infants (Jacobsson, 1978). An infant is rarely, if ever, allergic to his mother's milk. However, he may show allergic symptoms in response to foods ingested by the mother and passed through her milk (Clyne 1991; Maeda, 1993). The allergens would pass through the mother's milk, causing reactions such as spitting, vomiting, gas, diarrhea, colic-like behavior, or skin rash.

For any infant, with or without allergic tendencies, human milk is best able to protect him until his intestinal tract and immune system mature (Renz, 1991). In one case study, babies who were breastfed exclusively for 6 months were no longer susceptible to eczema, food allergy, or asthma, despite an hereditary risk of such ailments (Saarinen, 1979). Breastfeeding does not totally eliminate food allergies. However, it greatly reduces their incidence or delays their onset.

Human Milk for the Premature Infant

Physicians are increasingly aware that human milk is important to the premature infant. The milk of women who deliver prematurely has special properties that are particularly beneficial to the premature infant (Gross, 1980). Such milk contains higher concentrations of sodium, chloride, and nitrogen, as well as immunopro-

tective factors. This may be of great significance for the immature GI tract of the preterm infant. Human milk can help prevent NEC, a common illness in premature infants. Additionally, preterm infants who are fed human milk, including mature donor milk, have better neurodevelopment than their artificially fed counterparts (Lucas, 1994). Human milk is also associated with higher intelligence quotient (IQ) scores during childhood (Lucas, 1992). It is for all of these reasons that many physicians recommend that the premature infant be fed his mother's milk whether or not the mother had planned to breastfeed.

There remains much debate about the special needs of premature babies. At issue is whether a supplement to the infant's own mother's milk is necessary. Much emphasis is given to keeping up with the missed intrauterine growth through increased protein and energy in the preterm diet. Optimal brain growth is often not considered (Ebrahim, 1993). The composition of human milk and how it relates to the preterm's needs is not yet well understood (Beijers, 1992). Extra nutrients often are added to the mother's milk before it is given to her baby, depending on his particular needs.

Human milk has the ideal protein balance for babies who weigh 1500 g or more (about 3 lbs, 5 oz). However, for those who weigh less than 1500 g, and especially those under 1000 g (a little over 2 lbs), the mother's milk is not considered adequate as her baby's sole source of nutrition. Supplements of protein, calcium, and potassium phosphate may be needed in these cases. If they are not supplemented, these infants may experience fractures of the long bones during rapid growth phases. Supplements are not without concern, however. Quan (1994) found that some additives, particularly cows' milk–based infant formulas, have an adverse effect on the anti-infective properties of human milk. This effect was not seen in his study with soy-based infant formulas nor with **human milk fortifier.**

IMPURITIES IN HUMAN MILK

Some impurities, owing to their molecular weight or binding capacity, are excluded from the mother's milk. However, in many cases, substances are secreted into the milk in low concentrations and pose no danger to the infant. When a substance does pass into the milk, the infant's GI tract often offers protection by not absorbing or altering it. The infant may still experience some adverse effects, however, from contaminants that come through the milk and are not altered or eliminated by his GI system. Drugs ingested by the mother can travel through her milk to the baby, as can social toxicants such as tobacco, caffeine, alcohol, marijuana, and other mood-changing drugs. **Environmental contaminants** may also be present in the mother's milk and passed on to her baby. When impurities are present in the mother's milk, whether it be from medication, social toxicants, or environmental contaminants, the most important consideration is the effect a particular substance has on the breastfeeding infant.

Drugs and Contaminants

Much concern and confusion exist when a lactating woman consumes medication or social toxicants, or when she is exposed to environmental contaminants. Not long ago, it was thought that if a woman was breastfeeding she should take no drugs, and if she needed medication, she should not breastfeed. Since then, as the benefits of breastfeeding have been studied more fully, a more rational approach has been taken toward drugs and breastfeeding. Until recently, little has been known about the potential dangers of social toxicants and environmental contaminants. A problem also

exists when there is little definitive information available about a particular drug in question.

A legitimate evaluation of medical information must go beyond personal observation and stand the test of scientific criticism. The effectiveness of a drug or treatment should be compared with other treatments and its safety determined after large numbers of observations over long periods of time. The burden of proof rests with the researcher—the one who is recommending giving a particular drug or treatment—especially if it involves a substance that is not well established in medical practice.

Critical Reading of Drug Studies

Many review articles have been written both in lay and professional publications that are helpful in providing background information on lactation and impurities in human milk. When reading such articles, you will need to give careful consideration to how the studies were conducted and what conclusions are being drawn. See Figure 8.1 for factors to consider when reading literature about drugs.

FIGURE 8.1   Factors to consider in drug literature

Factor	Comments
Newness of the data	There is much case reporting of drugs used in nursing pairs that provides newer data, whereas original data regarding drugs in human milk were published between 1920 and 1960.
Human versus animal data	Animal data may or may not apply to human lactation. The peer review process will assist in determining this relevance.
Completeness of screening	The reader should always look for whether the researcher mentions studying metabolites of the particular drug in question. If metabolites were not studied, justification is needed. Usually, researchers will justify that within their study. Consulting a pharmacologist will help you understand the significance and quality of a study about drugs.
Isolated cases	Much of the original data about a particular substance may be based on only one or two case reports, with insufficient controls. This results because ethics prevent experiments on humans. Clinicians are left to make decisions without complete data to guide them. If a mother needs a medication and wants to continue breastfeeding, physicians sometimes allow it, monitor it and then write up the experience to share with colleagues. Such case reports have no control but the medical community has at least a small amount of information instead of none. One cannot conclude universal safety from one case report. However, physicians who support breastfeeding even in difficult circumstances may be less reluctant to try a drug instead of stopping breastfeeding.
Sampling technique	Older studies may show random sampling of milk rather than samples based on drug peak and **trough levels**. Trough is the lowest blood or milk level achieved by the drug during its dosing period. Women who are given gentamicin, for instance, are tested every three days or so to see what the highest and lowest levels of the drug are in the blood. This is done by testing an hour after a dose and an hour before the next dose is due. The timing of testing is different in different drugs. Some drugs have a narrow safety range, so it is important to keep the dose within that range. Although newer research is less problematic in this area, it is still important that you consider this when reading such research.
Personal correspondence	Although much personal correspondence is useful, the reader should be aware that the data may not be available for public inspection and could be biased. Often, personal correspondence is research in progress that lends support to the article at hand.
Speculation	Speculation by the author of the original article may be interpreted as fact after several review articles have been written. This can be a problem, and readers should always beware of speculation.

Effect of Contaminants on the Breastfeeding Infant

Almost any substance that is present in the mother's blood will also be present in some amount in her milk. The degree to which a substance is excreted into the mother's milk and its possible effects on the infant are important considerations when reviewing the advisability of a particular substance. In determining risk to the infant, consideration should be given to whether or not the medication is used in pediatric medicine. It is also important to note that a medication considered safe during pregnancy is not necessarily safe during lactation. As Lawrence explains, "during pregnancy, the maternal liver and kidney are serving as detoxification and excretion resources for the fetus via the placenta, whereas during lactation the infant has to handle the drug totally on his own once it has reached his circulation" (Lawrence, 1999).

The mother needs to consider whether she really needs the medication and if it will pass into her milk and be absorbed in the baby's GI tract. Also, most important of all, can the infant safely be exposed to the substance as it appears in her milk? These are all difficult questions to answer. Understanding a little about the characteristics of a substance may help illustrate the dilemma of both physician and mother when the need for a medication arises. See Figure 8.2 for the factors that influence the complex process by which a substance passes from the mother's bloodstream into her milk and the amount that eventually reaches the infant.

FIGURE 8.2   Considerations for infant's potential exposure to substances secreted in human milk

Factors to consider

- Size of the molecules in the substance.
- Solubility of the substance in water or fat (diffuses more easily into milk).
- Binding capacity of the substance with protein.
- pH of the substance.
- The milk/plasma ratio.
- Route of administration (oral, **intramuscular, intravenous**).
- Short or long-acting version of the drug.
- Activity or inactivity of components of the substance.
- Rate of detoxification in the mother's system.
- Whether the substance accumulates in the mother's system.
- Duration of use.
- Time substance is ingested relative to the feed.
- Number of days postpartum when substance is consumed.
- Age and size of the infant (premature, fullterm, older baby).
- Amount of milk the infant consumes (exclusively breastfed or supplemented).
- Absorption of the substance in the infant's gut.
- Safety in giving the substance to the infant directly.

The effect of any substance on the breastfed infant is of primary importance when maternal medication is indicated or when the mother consumes a substance such as caffeine or tobacco. There are many factors that influence the level of a substance found in the infant's bloodstream. Some are related to the infant; others are based on characteristics of the drug itself.

The amount of human milk a baby consumes is directly related to the amount of a substance he will receive through the milk. A baby who is being supplemented with artificial baby milk or solid foods will receive a lesser amount of a substance than an infant who is breastfed exclusively. The volume of milk consumed is less and may be diluted by the supplemental food in the infant's system. The baby's age and size will also be factors. A premature infant **assimilates** food, drugs, and other impurities received through the mother's milk differently than does a full-term infant or older baby. An older and larger baby may be able to metabolize a substance more effectively, and therefore, it will have less effect on his system. The baby's age will also determine his ability to **detoxify** a substance with his liver and excrete it in the urine or stool. Because an infant's liver is immature in the early days postpartum, it may be difficult for him to excrete even small amounts of a substance. A drug that depends on the liver for detoxification could pose a risk if not metabolized effectively by an immature liver.

If a substance is particularly resistant to being destroyed in the infant's GI system, it would pose a danger to the infant as it accumulates to toxic levels. On the other hand, drugs that must be administered by injection because of their ineffectiveness when taken orally, that is, those destroyed in the infant's GI tract, may reduce the infant's systemic absorption of the drug but could cause GI symptoms such as diarrhea. Some substances compete for protein-binding sites, displacing other toxic substances that then can migrate to other parts of the body. Sulfadiazine, an antibacterial agent, may displace bilirubin and cause it to flow freely in the infant's blood during the first weeks postpartum, thereby increasing the risk of jaundice for the baby.

Giving Advice about Medications

According to the AAP, among the drugs on which information is available, few are contraindicated in breastfeeding (AAP 1994). Generally, only 1 to 2 percent of a dose crosses into the mother's milk (Bagatol, 1989). A breastfeeding mother still needs to use caution in taking any medication. She should always consult the baby's physician before taking any prescription drug, over-the-counter medication, or supplemental vitamins. When her physician prescribes medication, the mother can remind him that she is breastfeeding and confirm the drug's advisability.

Generally, if a drug was safe during pregnancy, it is likely to be safe during lactation. During pregnancy, the mother's system excretes the drug; however, exposure during lactation requires the infant to handle the drug on his own. Also, although a drug may be safe both for the fetus and for the breastfeeding infant, it could affect the mother's letdown reflex, milk production, or milk secretion.

Concern often arises about over-the-counter medications, including pain relievers, cough medicines, cold remedies, suppositories, antacids, diarrhea remedies, and the like. Because these medications are more accessible than prescription drugs, there is a greater possibility that they will be consumed. Thus, you may receive calls questioning their potential risk to the infant and to breastfeeding. Many cold remedies contain antihistamines to dry up nasal secretions. Although some mothers may worry that these agents will also reduce their milk supply, this has never been proved scientifically. However, antihistamines may enter human milk and could produce sedation in the infant. Thus, it is better to use nonsedating antihistamines.

Any person taking over-the-counter medications needs to exercise caution in taking drugs and other substances when there is the possibility of interaction among prescription drugs, over-the-counter medications, and vitamins. Mothers are encouraged to discuss such concerns with their baby's physician to determine the safety in taking an over-the-counter drug. Physicians need to be informed of the mother's present consumption of drugs, vitamins, or other substances before prescribing any additional medication.

Minimizing Effects of Medications

When drugs are present in the mother's milk, they may affect milk production, or secretion. Some will lower production, and others may serve to stimulate it. They can also cause reactions in the infant. The mother can watch for unusual changes in her baby's behavior, feeding and sleeping patterns, fussiness, lethargy, rash, vomiting, or diarrhea.

There are a number of ways in which a mother can minimize the effects of drugs in her milk, either in terms of selection of a less offensive drug or with respect to the mother's schedule for taking the drug. Medications can be scheduled to ensure that the least amount of drug possible gets into the milk. Because of the usual absorption rates and peak levels of most drugs, the mother will want to take the medication immediately after nursing or 3 to 4 hours before the next feed. Depending on the drug, breastfeeding may be avoided when the drug is at its peak level in the milk. Keeping in mind that the fat content of milk changes and is highest at midday, a fat-soluble drug could be taken at bedtime, when the baby usually does not feed as often.

Advise mothers to avoid using medications with long plasma half-life, because this form is more difficult for the infant to eliminate and could, over time, build up to higher concentrations in the infant's plasma. It usually requires enzyme action in the liver in order to be metabolized, thus increasing the possibility of accumulation of the drug in the infant. When possible, the physician can be asked to choose a drug that produces the least amount in the milk and has the least potential for causing problems. If a mother must take a medication that has been untested for safety during lactation, she can weigh her options with her baby's physician. You can also provide her with information from a source such as Hale's *Medications and Mother's Milk*. See Table 8.5 for the safety of various drugs.

The Lactation Consultant's Role Regarding Medications

You can work most effectively with mothers by assuming the role of facilitator in sharing information and pointing out options. You will often be contacted by mothers with questions and concerns about the possible effects a medication will have on breastfeeding. Your role as a facilitator is to encourage the mother to be an active health consumer and to take the responsibility for making decisions and taking specific action. In this role, you can help the mother pose questions and stimulate her thinking so that she will explore the facts and base her decisions on accurate and sound information. It is important that all drug information be presented objectively and not in a manner that appears to be recommending or advising the mother about the safety of a particular medication.

It is extremely important that you use caution in how you share drug information with a mother. You run the risk of placing yourself in a vulnerable legal position if you deviate from the facts or attempt to interpret the information. When a mother expresses doubt or fears to you concerning a medication, you can be an objective listener and encourage her to think through all of the options available to her. In exploring the options, you first can obtain information from the mother to clarify her situation and then consider the following points:

◆ Does she feel she really needs the drug, or can she choose an alternative course that would not involve drugs?

◆ Can other safer drugs or procedures be substituted?

◆ Do the benefits of the drug to the mother outweigh possible risk to the baby?

◆ Does exposure to the drug pose less risk to the baby than the use of an artificial baby milk?

◆ Would another medical opinion be helpful?

TABLE 8.5
Medications for the Breastfeeding Mother

◆ Breastfeeding contraindicated.	◆ Anticancer drugs (antimetabolites).
	◆ Radioactive substances (stop breastfeeding temporarily).
◆ Continue breastfeeding: Side effects possible; monitor the baby for drowsiness.	◆ Psychiatric drugs and anticonvulsants.
◆ Continue breastfeeding: Use alternative drug, if possible.	◆ Chloramphenicol, tetracyclines, metronidazole.
	◆ Quinolone antibiotics (e.g., ciprofloxacin).
◆ Continue breastfeeding: Monitor baby for jaundice.	◆ Sulphonamides, dapsone.
	◆ Sulfamethoxazole + trimethoprim (co-trimoxazole).
◆ Continue breastfeeding: Use alternative drug (may inhibit lactation).	◆ Estrogens (including estrogen-containing contraceptives).
	◆ Thiazide diuretics.
	◆ Ergometrine.
◆ Continue breastfeeding: Safe in usual dosage. Monitor baby.	◆ Most commonly used drugs.
	◆ Analgesics and antipyretics: Short courses of paracetamol, acetylsalicylic acid, ibuprofen; occasional doses of morphine and pethidine.
	◆ Antibiotics: Ampicillin, amoxacillin, cloxacillin and other penicillins. Erythromycin.
	◆ Antituberculars, antileporotics (see dapsone earlier).
	◆ Antimalarials (except mefloquine, anthelminthics, antifungals.
	◆ Bronchodilators (e.g., salbutamol), corticosteroids, antihistamines, antacids, drugs for diabetes, most antihypertensives, digoxin.
	◆ Nutritional supplements of iron, iodine, and vitamins.

Source: Breastfeeding and Maternal Medication, Recommendations for Drugs in the Eight WHO Model List of Essential Drugs, Division of Diarrhoeal and Acute Respiratory Disease Control, UNICEF/WHO, 1995. Printed with permission.

Again, it is essential that you present these options in an objective manner and that you not give the impression of recommending or advising. You can encourage the mother to consult her physician regarding these questions and to share any concerns she may have. The example in Table 8.6 may help clarify your role with mothers about a drug question.

Locating Drug Information

Use only drug information that is obtained from well-documented sources. When presenting this information to mothers, read the facts to her exactly as they appear on the page, citing the reference for the information. As a lactation consultant, you are not medically qualified to interpret the data and, therefore, must confine yourself to the facts only. If you have a personal experience or opinion that conflicts with the research, take care not to share this with a mother. When you share studies and research in an appropriate manner, mothers can use the information to make informed decisions.

You will want to become acquainted with the various drug groups and their potential risks and benefits. When you share information with a mother about a particular drug, you often will need to determine the drug's generic name in order to locate it in a drug listing. Information about the advisability of taking a drug during breastfeeding needs to be obtained from a reliable source. Two recommended sources are *Medications and Mother's Milk* by Hale (1999) and *Drugs in Pregnancy and Lactation* by Briggs, Freeman, and Yaffe (1998).

	TABLE 8.6	
	Responding To A Mother's Question About A Drug	
Mother	**Consultant**	**Comments**
I have a sore throat, what can I take for it?	Gee, that must really bother you. What have you done for it?	Begin with emotional support. Gather information.
I haven't done anything yet because I wanted to find out what is safe.	There are a number of things you could do for it; why don't you call your physician and see what he suggests.	As a lactation consultant you cannot give information unless the mother asks about a specific drug.
(Saw her doctor who prescribed "xyz" medicine.) My doctor prescribed "xyz." Is that safe when I'm breastfeeding?	I'm not qualified to advise you on the safety of any drugs. I can share research results with you. The generic name of this drug is "abc" and it *is* excreted in human milk. The effects are. . . . This data came from . . .	You give referenced facts only, and read directly from the information source.
Is there another drug I can take that is *not* excreted in my milk?	I'm not qualified to tell you that. You could call to remind your doctor that you're breastfeeding and ask if there is something else which is safer. Explain where your information came from (cite reference again). If another drug is prescribed, feel free to call me and I'll see if I have any information about it.	You cannot suggest an alternative drug. However, you can encourage the mother to question her physician about the advisability of the drug prescribed. If the physician does not prescribe a safer drug and instructs the mother to wean, the mother has the option of asking for a consultation with another physician.

▼ Social Toxicants

Social mood-changing toxicants—such as tobacco, coffee, tea, alcohol, marijuana and other drugs—are used in varying degrees in most cultures. It is important to recognize that the use of recreational drugs is not an issue of class, race, or economics. Mothers need to be cautioned about substances that can negatively affect the quality or quantity of their milk.

Nicotine and Tobacco

The breastfeeding mother who smokes cigarettes occasionally to moderately, probably affects her baby more by the smoke the baby inhales than by the small amount of nicotine present in her milk. Children whose parents smoke in the home have a greater susceptibility to respiratory ailments than do children of nonsmokers (Lenfant, 1980; Wright, 1991). Second-hand cigarette smoke exposure has also been linked to increased incidence of otitis media (Owen, 1993). Mothers and other members of the babies' households need to be discouraged from smoking at all. If the mother chooses to continue smoking, advise her to not smoke in the baby's presence. She can time her breastfeeding to minimize the baby's exposure in her milk, smoking after a feed rather than just before it. It is noteworthy that smoking is not just an issue with breastfeeding. Babies who are fed artificial baby milks are also exposed to a myriad of undesirable chemicals without the protective benefits of human milk (Minchin, 1991; Newman, 1990).

Nicotine in the mother's milk can cause fussiness, diarrhea, shock, vomiting, rapid heart rate, and restlessness in the breastfed infant. The mother may also experience a decrease in milk production due to a lowered prolactin level, leading to poor infant weight gain. Twenty cigarettes daily can lead to relatively high levels of fat-soluble nicotine in the mother's milk, which can be harmful to the baby and cause vomiting and nausea. It can also diminish the mother's milk secretion, lower the fat concentration in her milk, or inhibit her letdown reflex if the mother smokes immediately before feeding her baby (Hopkinson, 1992; Vio, 1991). Because any of these factors could be a cause of slow weight gain, mothers of slow-gaining babies should be asked if they smoke. Those who smoke should be advised to quit or to reduce the amount of cigarettes they smoke. Smoking cessation programs, such as the use of a nicotine patch and chewing gum for nicotine withdrawal, can be used by nursing mothers (Hale, 1998). The nicotine level is about one-third that of cigarettes.

In order to continue nursing safely, mothers who are on such a program cannot smoke in addition to the nicotine patch or chewing gum because this would further increase the baby's level of exposure to nicotine. Mothers who smoke should be told that they will need twice the usual intake of vitamin C because smoking interferes with the body's ability to use that vitamin (Pelleteir, 1970).

Caffeine

Caffeine is present in coffee, tea, cola, and chocolate—substances often consumed in large quantities in Western culture. Breastfeeding mothers can safely ingest moderate amounts of these foods. However, they should watch for signs in their babies, such as wakefulness, hyperactivity, and colic-like behavior. Such symptoms may indicate an excessive amount of caffeine in their milk. Because an immature digestive system takes longer to eliminate caffeine from the body, newborn and premature babies are particularly susceptible to caffeine's effects.

Breastfeeding infants have been shown to react to their mothers' consuming six to eight servings of caffeinated beverage daily. Symptoms disappeared within 1 week after caffeine was discontinued (Rivera-Calimlim, 1987). As many as five cups of coffee daily may be acceptable (Ryu, 1985). However, the amount of caffeine present in human milk varies dramatically from mother to mother and according to the timing of ingestion. Some women appear to have low absorption and efficient metabolism and excretion, so that levels of caffeine in their milk remain low. Therefore, each mother-infant pair is unique with respect to caffeine response. Acceptable levels of ingestion for the mother depend on her baby's individual reaction.

Table 8.7 identifies the most common sources of caffeine. Women should be cautioned about high intake of herbal tea as a substitute for caffeinated drinks. Herbal teas may contain active ingredients that can be secreted into human milk and cause toxic effects. For instance, cathartics such as buckhorn bark and senna may result in cramps and diarrhea in the infant. Camomile tea may sensitize the infant to ragweed pollen and cause an allergic reaction (Abramowicz, 1979).

Alcohol

Alcohol rapidly enters a woman's bloodstream, and subsequently her milk. A safe level of alcohol consumption has not been defined for the breastfeeding mother. It is known that alcohol achieves the same level in the mother's milk that it does in blood (Silva, 1993). Alcohol consumption can cause sleepiness in the infant and affect the infant's development and linear growth. A 1989 study found that infants of mothers who con-

sumed the equivalent of four drinks daily had psychomotor scores one standard deviation below the mean (Little, 1989).

The baby's response to alcohol present in human milk has also been noted. Mennella (1991) found that babies consumed less milk after mothers ingested an alcoholic beverage. In addition, excessive amounts completely block the release of oxytocin and prevent letdown from occurring. Excessive alcohol consumption can also limit parental effectiveness and result in life-threatening conditions in the breastfed infant.

Generally, the consumption of one or two drinks socially is not a contraindication for breastfeeding. A mother may ask when it is safe to nurse again after having consumed alcohol. She can be told that she can breastfeed when she feels normal again, that is, when the effects of the alcohol have worn off. By this time, plasma levels will be quite low (Hale, 1998).

Drugs of Abuse

Substance abuse is of grave concern to neonatologists, who see an increasing number of infants suffering from the damaging effects of drug exposure. Generally, breastfeeding mothers should be advised to avoid all drugs of abuse. The AAP Committee on Drugs (1994) considers drugs of abuse to be contraindicated during breastfeeding. These drugs include amphetamines, cocaine, heroin, marijuana, and phencyclidine hydrochloride (angel dust). Drugs of abuse are hazardous both to the breastfeeding infant and to the health of the mother. Although you can educate a mother and warn her about harmful practices, you cannot take responsibility for her actions. If she chooses to ignore your advice, you can remind her of the potential danger to her baby and urge her to tell her baby's physician about the substance she is using.

Marijuana can have a direct effect on the mother's ability to produce sufficient quantities of milk. However, no untoward effects have been found in breastfed babies when their mothers use marijuana (Hale, 1998). Heroin passes to the infant through the mother's milk. It can cause increased sleepiness and poor appetite, resulting in an undernourished baby. An uncoordinated and ineffective suckling reflex may also result from heroin ingestion. Tremors, restlessness, and vomiting are other effects on the infant.

Cocaine is a powerful central nervous stimulant. Effects of cocaine intoxication are irritability, jitteriness, and tremors in the infant, as well as increased heart and respiratory rate. Cocaine has a plasma half life of about 30 minutes. It is metabolized and excreted slowly over a prolonged period. Even after the effects of cocaine have subsided, the mother's milk is likely to contain significant quantities of benzoecgonine, the inactive metabo-

TABLE 8.7

Common Sources of Caffeine

Product	Caffeine in Milligrams	Product	Caffeine in Milligrams
Hot Drinks		**Soft Drinks (cont.)**	
Coffee (16 oz) Starbucks	550	Diet Dr. Pepper	37
Coffee (12 oz) Starbucks	375	Pepsi Cola	37
Coffee (8 oz) Starbucks	250	Royal Crown Cola	36
Coffee, non-gourmet (8 oz)	136	Diet Rite Cola	34
Maxwell House (8 oz)	110	Diet Pepsi	34
Coffee, instant (8 oz)	95	Coca-cola	34
Caffe Latte or Cappuccino Starbucks	70	Sunkist Orange	0
Espresso, double (2 oz) Starbucks	70	7-Up	0
Coffee, decaf (16 oz) Starbucks	15	Diet 7-Up	0
Coffee, decaf (8–12 oz) Starbucks	10	RC-100	0
Coffee, decaf, nongourmet (8 oz)	5	Diet Sunkist Orange	0
Espresso, decaf (1 oz) Starbucks	5	Patio Orange	0
Tea, leaf or bag (8 oz)	50	Fanta Orange	0
Tea, green or instant (8 oz)	30	Fresca	0
Tea, bottled (12 oz)	15	Hires Root Beer	0
Tea, decaf (8 oz)	5	**Pain Relievers (standard dose)**	
Chocolate, dark, bittersweet, or semi-sweet (1 oz)	20	Excedrin	130
Chocolate milk mix (1 oz)	5	Anacin	65
Cocoa or hot chocolate (8 oz)	5	Midol	65
Water, caffeinated (Edge20) (8 oz)	70	Plain aspirin (any brand)	0
Nonprescription Stimulants (standard dose)		**Diuretics (standard dose)**	
Caffedrine Capsules	200	Aqua-Ban	200
NoDoz Tablets, maximum strength	200	Pennathene H20ff	200
Vivarin Tablets, maximum strength	200	Pre-Mens Forte	100
NoDoz, regular strength	100	**Cold Remedies (standard dose)**	
Soft Drinks		Coryban-D	30
Mountain Dew	55	Triaminicin	30
Mello Yello	51	**Weight-control Aids (daily)**	
Tab	44	Dexatrim	200
Shasta Cola	42	Dietac	200
Dr. Pepper	38	Prolamine	280
		Dristan	32

*As tested by Consumers Union for the October 1981 issue of Consumer Report. Formulations can change.
Sources: Consumers Union of United States, Inc., Mount Vernon, NY 10550—reprinted by permission of *Consumer Reports*, October 1981; Caffeine: The Inside Scoop, Nutrition Action Newsletter, December 1996.

lite of cocaine. Urine samples for both the mother and infant are likely to test positive for cocaine metabolites for a week or more. Hale (1998) states that, "Significant secretion into breastmilk is suspected with a probable high milk:plasma ratio. A number of case reports in the literature clearly indicate the transmission of maternal cocaine to the infant via milk with significant agitation in the breastfeeding infant resulting." The mother should be advised to pump and dump her milk for 24 hours to be safe. In one extreme case, an infant died because his mother had applied cocaine topically to her nipples and then breastfed.

Regardless of the pharmacologic effects or safety to the infant, there is also concern about the mother's ability to care for her infant when she is abusing drugs. A 1992 study showed that mothers intending to breastfeed were found to be more likely to decrease or stop their substance abuse (Frank, 1992). Given the number of risks, both known and unknown, mothers should be educated whenever possible about the dangers of using such drugs both prenatally and while breastfeeding. They also need to recognize the dangers involved due to the inhibition of effective parenting skills while under the influence of these drugs.

Breast Implants

In recent years, the issue involving silicone breast implants and perceived risks to the breastfeeding infant made media headlines. There was one report describing a connection between an infant's esophageal swallowing dysfunction and having been breastfed (Levine, 1994). This controversial study involved a small, selective group of infants and did not apply the same standards to the control group as the study group. There have been no reports of swallowing dysfunction. The study also did not take into account the large amount of data available that demonstrate significant health benefits afforded the child through breastfeeding (Williams, 1994).

Berlin, in his commentary to this study (1994), noted that the compound used in breast implants, polydimethylsiloxane (PDMS) has not been found in the few samples of milk from mothers with implants. He also noted that Mylicon drops, frequently recommended for infant colic, contain PDMS. They have been used for decades with no reports of side effects. Berlin suggests that there should be no contraindication to breastfeeding with silicone implants based on this one study. Greater amounts of silicone are found in other substances, such as cow's milk formulas!

The author of these controversial studies was an expert witness for the plaintiffs in a lawsuit against Dow Corning. Some of the mothers in these studies were the plaintiffs in the class action litigation. Levine has since retracted his study, and it has been debunked.

Environmental Contaminants

Mothers can actively avoid the ingestion of social toxicants, as discussed earlier. They may not, however, have such control over exposure to contaminants in their environment. DDT has been a concern for years. Restrictions on its use have resulted in a decline in the levels of DDT in human milk since 1950 (Jelliffe, 1978). In May 1973, polybrominated biphenyls (PBB) were accidentally introduced into animal feed in Michigan, resulting in residents ingesting PBBs through milk, beef, eggs, and other farm-animal products (Finberg, 1977). PBBs and PCBs (polychlorinated biphenyls) are strongly resistant to chemical breakdown, which has led to pollution of the environment. Because biphenyls are primarily deposited in fat, which is excreted through milk, traces of PBB and PCB have been found in human milk and passed onto the breastfeeding infant. Although possible long-term effects are not known, there was no evidence of short-term toxicity in the doses that Michigan infants experienced (Rogan, 1980).

In a study conducted at the Piedmont Mother's Milk Bank in Raleigh, North Carolina, it was found that 85 percent of the women studied had trace amounts of PCBs in their milk. All women had DDT in trace amounts. However, in following the babies over a 4-year period, no adverse effects were found in their health or development. Because the benefits of breastfeeding far outweigh the possible dangers, mothers generally are not discouraged from breastfeeding because of exposure to environmental contaminants (Berlin, 1989; Frank, 1993; Gladen, 1988; Gladen, 1991; Jacobson, 1990; Jacobson, 1993).

Studies continue on environmental pollutants and their effects on humans—more specifically for this discussion, their effects on the breastfed infant. Analysis of available data leads to the conclusion that there is no firm scientific basis for advising against breastfeeding. However, many women are breastfeeding after returning to work, and women are increasingly involved in jobs that may expose them to such chemical pollutants as lead, mercury, cadmium, pesticides, plastics, or chemicals. Mothers need to be made aware of these contaminants in the same way they are made aware about drugs and alcohol. The physician, suspicious that an illness in a child might be caused by a contaminant in the mother's milk, might also ask about occupational exposures.

Mothers are not entirely at the mercy of the environment, however. They can actively attempt to reduce their exposure to contaminants. The guidelines that follow will help reduce the potential for chemical pollutants in the mother's milk.

Guidelines to Reduce Exposure

◆ Limit the use of domestic sprays such as pesticides and household cleaners.

◆ Limit consumption of freshwater fish because chemical wastes are washed into lakes and streams and concentrated there.

◆ Avoid fatty meats and remove excess fat.

◆ Thoroughly wash or peel fresh fruits and vegetables.

◆ Avoid crash diets that release accumulated toxic substances stored in body fat.

◆ Avoid occupations involving possible exposure to chemicals.

◆ Avoid permanently moth-proofed garments that may contain dieldrin, a chemical which is absorbed through the skin.

Mothers sometimes inquire about having their milk tested. This is not recommended unless the physician sees signs of chronic illness in the mother or baby due to chemical exposure. Such tests are expensive and must be repeated over several weeks to be conclusive.

▼
Guidelines for Counseling a Mother about Impurities

The following guidelines will help you when you are counseling a mother concerning the potential for impurities in her milk. They are presented both as a reminder to you of the proper procedures concerning these questions and as a guide for you to use while you are talking to a mother. The guidelines apply to any of the substances that may contaminate a mother's milk. They are most important when discussing medications with a mother.

Recommendations for Advising Mothers About Contaminants

◆ Give well-documented facts in an objective manner.

◆ Make a mother aware of her options concerning potential impurities.

◆ Urge a mother to seek her physician's advice and share her concerns openly.

◆ Urge a mother to remind her physician that she is breastfeeding.

◆ Cite references for facts that you give a mother.

◆ Suggest ways a mother can minimize the effects of drugs.

◆ Advise a mother to avoid unnecessary consumption of or exposure to contaminants.

What to Avoid When Advising Mothers About Contaminants

◆ Refrain from giving personal opinions.

◆ Do not attempt to interpret drug information for a mother.

◆ Do not advise a mother about a drug's safety.

◆ Do not indicate to a mother that you disagree with advice from her physician, or other medical resource, unless you are medically trained.

◆ Avoid recommending a drug substitute to a mother.

◆ Do not suggest that a mother refuse a drug when it is needed.

◆ Avoid encouraging a mother to go against her physician's advice.

▼
DIFFERENCES BETWEEN HUMAN MILK AND INFANT FORMULA

Breastfed babies are shown to be healthier than those who are raised on artificial baby milk substitutes. As demonstrated earlier, human milk embodies a host of immunologic agents that protect the infant against infections and allergens until his own defenses are developed more fully. In addition, research is demonstrating increasingly that infant feeding can affect the immune system for life (Hamosh, 1996). The personalized characteristics of each woman's milk provide her own baby with nourishment that is ideally suited to his specific needs for health and growth. Additionally, donor milk is always the best alternative for a baby whose own mother is unable to breastfeed or provide her own milk.

During and after World War II, cow's milk formula came to be the routine source of infant nutrition in the United States and other developed countries. This resulted from a growing reliance on scientific achievements and new technology, together with decreasing knowledge and skills about breastfeeding initiation and support, especially in Western hospitals.

America is one of the largest markets for infant formula, with much of it subsidized by the taxpayer via the WIC program. Infant formula manufacturers promote their products with a theme that "Breastmilk is best ... but ... our product is closest to mother's milk." Try as they might, these companies can never replicate all the bioactive, immunologic, and nutritional properties, not to mention the other health benefits of human milk (Goldman, 1998; Hamosh, 1996; Hanson, 1998).

Risks of Artificial Baby Milk

Artificial baby milk feeding has been referred to as one of "the largest uncontrolled in vivo experiments in human history" (Minchin, 1998). Studies show that artificial feeding of infants carries with it serious risks for infants, young children, and their mothers (Akre, 1989; Cunningham, 1990). In 1981, an awareness of these dangers prompted the World Health Organization to adopt the *International Code of Marketing of Breastmilk Substitutes*. The code attempts to restrict the unethical marketing and promotion of foods and drinks such as infant formula used to feed babies inappropriately, as well as all associated paraphernalia, such as bottles and teats. When the World Health Assembly considered the code, the United States cast the lone dissenting vote, which stirred a wave of controversy throughout the world. In 1994, the United States finally approved the code.

The United States is not immune to the dangers of infant formula. The potential dangers of misuse are dramatic in any impoverished community with substandard conditions and low educational levels. Incorrect and inadequate use of infant formula account for about one million deaths each year worldwide (Walker, 1992, 1993). Some of these deaths occur even in affluent communities with access to clean water and education, and in highly specialized intensive care nurseries, as it is intrinsically hazardous to deprive any infant of its mother's milk (Lucas, 1990).

Deficiencies in Infant Formula

Artificial baby milk can contain micronutrients or macronutrients in either excessive or deficient amounts. It may also be completely lacking in essential elements or contain contaminants. Infant formulas are deficient in essential fatty acids that are important to proper brain development and visual acuity. See Table 8.8 for the levels of essential fatty acids in popular infant formulas. Note that C20 and C22, both long-chain polyunsaturated fatty acids that are needed for brain development, are absent in infant formula. Recent attempts to add these fatty acids have led to other concerns, such as the effect on infant growth. No current formula has replicated human milk's complex fatty acid pattern, even after adding fats derived from a variety of sources including fish heads, egg yolks, or genetically engineered marine algae. Vitamin D, which is toxic in high doses, has been shown to be excessive in many formulas. Some formulas have been found to be deficient in chloride. Any artificial baby milk that contains high levels of iodine could affect neonatal thyroid function.

Infant and Maternal Health Risks

In its *Summary of the Hazards of Infant Formula*, and later in *Summary of the Hazards of Infant Formula: Part 2*, the International Lactation Consultant Association (ILCA) provides a partial comprehensive review of the risks associated with artificial feeding (Walker, 1992, 1998). For instance, IQ levels may be eight points lower

---

TABLE 8.8

Unsaturated Fatty Acids in Human Milk and 8 Commercial Infant Formulas

Fatty Acid	Human Milk	Enfamil	ProSoBee	SMA	Nutramigen	Similac	Isomil	Gerber	GoodStart
C16 1n-9	35.0	14.2	14.2	39.4	39.4	16.1	16.1	16.1	33.0
C20 1n-9	0.8	—	—	—	—	—	—	—	—
C18 2n-5	11.8	25.0	25.0	13.0	13.0	34.2	34.2	32.7	20.1
C22 2n-6	0.1	—	—	—	—	—	—	—	—
C18 3n-3	0.7	2.5	2.5	1.0	1.0	4.8	4.8	6.3	2.1
C20 3n-6	0.3	—	—	—	—	—	—	—	—
C20 4n-6	0.4	—	—	—	—	—	—	—	—
C22 4n-6	0.05	—	—	—	—	—	—	—	—
C20 5n-3	0.05	—	—	—	—	—	—	—	—
C22 5n-3	0.05	—	—	—	—	—	—	—	—
C22 6n-3	0.2	—	—	—	—	—	—	—	—

From Nettleton JA. Are N-3 fatty acids essential nutrients for fetal and infant development? *J Am Diet Assoc* 93:58–64; 1993.

TABLE 8.9		
Health Risks Associated with Artificial Feeding		

Health risk as identified in studies	Ratios Reported in Studies	
	Not breastfed	Breastfed
Infants are hospitalized more often.	15:1	10:1
Infants get sick more often and when sick they are more sick.	21:8	
Infants are more likely to get certain childhood cancers.	6:1	8:1
Gastroenteritis is more common in infants.	6:1	
Infants are more likely to suffer from ulcerative colitis and Chron's Disease.	3:1	
Infants have more bronchitis and pneumonia.	5:1	2:1
Infants are more likely to die from SIDS.	3:1	5:1
Premature infants are more likely to develop necrotizing enterocolitis (NEC).	20:1	
Infants are more likely to develop juvenile diabetes (*require insulin each day*).	2:1	7:1
Women are at a greater risk for breast cancer.	2:1	
Women are at a greater risk for ovarian cancer.	1.6:1	

in formula-fed babies than in breastfed babies. One bottle of formula can change the gut flora for 3 weeks. It also sensitizes the baby to cow's milk protein and can provoke an allergy later in the first year if the baby is exposed again to cow's milk. Women who do not breastfeed have an increased risk of developing osteoporosis. Table 8.9 shows some of the ratios reported in studies of infants who are fed artificial baby milk compared with those who are breastfed (Walker 1992, 1993).

Infants who are fed soy formula receive the equivalent of 6 to 11 times the dose of isoflavones. That is enough to change menstrual patterns in women who are fed soy. Although no studies have sought to look at outcomes of such exposure in infants who are fed soy formula, parents should be aware of the relatively high levels of isoflavones their infants will receive (Liebman, 1998). There may be additional hormonal effects from other estrogen-mimicking compounds known as **phthalates,** which are found in various plastics that infants can be exposed to, often by artificial feeding (Densley, 1996).

Dangers in Preparation

Aggressive marketing of infant formula, together with modeling of its use in wealthy countries where infant mortality is generally low, has contributed to a massive shift away from breastfeeding. This change has occurred both in developed countries and among women in developing countries who cannot use artificial baby milk safely and whose babies become ill and malnourished. In communities where the mother cannot afford to buy sufficient quantities of infant formula, she may attempt to stretch her supply by diluting it. She also may have no access to refrigeration, clean water, or adequate waste facilities. Additionally she may not understand directions well enough to mix the infant formula properly. Mixing errors are not confined to the less educated population. One college-educated father failed to read mixing directions carefully and fed his newborn concentrated infant formula.

Even when formula is mixed according to the directions on the can, there may be wide variations in the final composition of the product. This is partly because the composition of formula in the can cannot be totally standardized when the milk from which it is made varies from season to season. It is also because the powder can pack down in the can over time, so that a scoop of powder can contain a greater or lesser quantity by weight.

Even in communities with acceptable water supplies, there are concerns about the water with which powdered or concentrated formula is mixed. Artificially fed infants are at a greater risk for lead intoxication from lead received through the water source. Some formulas have been found to be contaminated with aluminum. A bacteria that can cause sepsis and meningitis is a frequent contaminant in powdered formula. If parents fail to wash the formula can and the can opener, residue from pesticides and animal droppings present in the warehouse may enter the formula. Babies are susceptible to methemoglobinemia from nitrate containing water. Also, oral water intoxication resulting in seizures is becoming more common in the United States when water is used to dilute or substitute for expensive formula.

Impact on the Family

The use of artificial baby milks can have an adverse impact on all members of a family. The family of a baby who is not breastfed will experience the economic burden of purchasing infant formula and equipment needed for artificial feeding. The financial burden imposed on families in the United States for the purchase of infant formula and feeding devices alone can be in excess of $1400 annually (Breastfeeding Support Consultants, 1998). Where people are poor, families could spend as much as 100 percent of their cash income for these products if they were to use them appropriately. In an attempt to stretch their supply of formula, parents may dilute it or supplement their baby's diet with inappropriate foods such as coffee, tea, sugared fruit drinks, and soy milks. The women and family members often go hungry if money is spent on artificial formula and on medications to deal with the sickness it brings. Such malnutrition can have serious long-term effects.

Women who do not breastfeed experience an earlier return of fertility, which results in shorter birth intervals, maternal depletion, and a higher number of pregnancies over their life span, often resulting in an earlier maternal death. They are at increased risk for developing premenopausal breast cancer and ovarian cancer, together with osteoporosis in later life. Families also have the increased cost of medical expenses that are incurred when the baby lacks the health protection of human milk. Formula-fed infants are more likely to be sensitized to cow's milk and to receive whole cow's milk at an earlier age than are breastfed infants. This bovine protein sensitivity can lead to serious malabsorption problems even in affluent communities. The family's time and convenience are affected also, because the infant formula must always be carried in sufficient quantity along with its paraphernalia to prepare and feed it. The preparation of the infant formula by the mother or other family member includes the time to shop, store, prepare, and clean up—all time taken away from interacting with the baby.

Impact on the Community

The community's burden from the use of artificial baby milks is far reaching. The production and packaging consume valuable land and resources. Production errors, such as contamination and mishandling, create a burden on society as a whole as well as on the individual child. Once packaged, the distribution process takes additional resources for fuel and contributes to environmental pollution. Even the disposal of waste products such as infant formula tins taxes the environment. Research is also burdened by the ever-increasing need to improve the infant formulas. This drains time and resources that could be used productively for unavoidable health concerns, or indeed, used to help women breastfeed and to make safe

human milk available for infants whose mothers cannot provide it.

The community is further affected by the fact that health care workers' time must be spent on educating parents in the proper use of infant formula—purchasing, storing, following complicated directions, keeping records in case of a recall, and the like. As previously noted, many errors, omissions, and purposeful rationing occur with the use of infant formulas. The consequences are subtle as well as not-so-subtle harm to the child. Parents' time is spent caring for those children who are acutely and chronically ill due to the lack of human milk. This leads to an increase in the spending of health care dollars—a burden passed along to the consumer.

Informing Parents of the Risks of Artificial Feeding

As discussed previously, there are clear and substantial differences between human milk and artificial baby milk. Human milk is far superior to any substitute. Formula is deficient in many of the constituents that are essential for optimum infant growth and health. Artificial feeding is not without its risks to infants, young children, mothers, and their families. Yet, parents are not informed of these hazards and the media promotes human milk substitutes as the social norm (Hawkins, 1994; Sawatski, 1994). In order for parents to be responsible health consumers, they need all the facts. You can assist parents in acquiring necessary information so that they can make an informed choice about infant feeding.

Choosing and Preparing An Artificial Baby Milk

A mother may find herself in a situation where she is not able to breastfeed or to feed her own milk to her baby. If she is not a candidate for or does not wish to use donor human milk, she will need education regarding the use of human milk substitutes. When choosing a human milk substitute, the family history must be considered with respect to allergies and problems with past use of such substitutes. The allergy history of the entire family—siblings, parents, and other close blood relatives—needs to be considered. Symptoms of those allergies need to be investigated. Because of these cautions, the choice of human milk substitute must be made in conjunction with the baby's physician.

The mother further needs to consider her family's financial circumstances and storage facilities when deciding to purchase a formula, which is either ready-to-feed, concentrated, or powdered. The possibility of substances such as lead, nitrites, sodium, fluoride, bacteria, and parasites in the water is another consideration. Careful attention to expiration dates and label instructions are important as well. Some clinicians advise mothers to write down the lot number of each can in a notebook in the event of a recall or class action lawsuit. Care must be given during preparation to use clean or sterile utensils, because the baby will not be receiving the infection protection from human milk. The tins need to be thoroughly washed because they are exposed to quite a bit of handling from factory to consumer. Advise mothers to open the can from the bottom because the bottom is less susceptible to pesticide sprays than the top (Kutner, 1996).

Advise that the mother or other caregiver hold the baby in the same way for the feeding as for breastfeeding. This facilitates eye contact and social interaction, and prevents aspiration of the milk substitute. Consideration must be given to the length of time the substitute is left at room temperature and how long it may be stored in the refrigerator after the tin is opened. Parents often mix several bottles at one time. They need to understand that artificial baby milk substitute is an **inert** substance. Unlike human milk, it does not contain anti-infective properties to fight bacteria. Formula mixed from concentrate must be discarded after 48 hours, and formula mixed from powder must be discarded after 24 hours. Formula that has been removed from the refrigerator must be discarded after 1 hour (Barger, 1997). When a feed is finished, any unused portion must be discarded immediately to prevent the baby from receiving any contaminated milk substitute.

▼

SUMMARY

Human milk is the perfect nutrition for the human infant. Health benefits to the infant resulting from the immunologic properties of the mother's milk are irrefutable. Human milk is specific to the infant's age and undergoes a transition from colostrum to mature milk to meet the infant's changing needs. Researchers continue to uncover new-found benefits of the many components in this rich and complex substance. Caregivers have a responsibility to promote the use of human milk for all babies. The AAP has translated this responsibility into strong statements in support of breastfeeding through the first year of a child's life. Artificial baby milks are not an equivalent substitute for mother's milk.

▼

REFERENCES

AAP, Fluoride Supplementation for Children: Interim Policy Recommendation (RE9511), *Pediatrics* 95:777, 1995.

Abramowicz M. Toxic reactions to plant products sold in health food stores. *Medical Letter on Drugs and Therapeutics* 21(7):1–3; 1979.

Addy DP. Infant feeding: A current view. *Br Med J* 1(6020):1268–1271; 1976.

Aggett P et al. Iron for the suckling. *Acta Paediatr Scand* 361 (Suppl): S96–S102; 1989.

Ahmed F et al. Community-based evaluation of the effect of breastfeeding on the risk of microbiologically confirmed or clinically presumptive shigellosis in Bangladeshi children. *Pediatrics* 90:406–411; 1992.

Akre J. "Infant feeding: The physiological basis." *WHO Bulletin Supplement* 67; 1989.

Allen J et al. Studies in human lactation: Milk composition and daily secretion rates of macronutrients in the first year of lactation. *Am J Clin Nutr* 54:69–80; 1991.

Aniansson G et al. A prospective cohort study on breastfeeding and otitis media in Swedish infants. *Pediatr Infect Dis J* 13:183–188; 1994.

Arnold L. Use of donor milk in the treatment of metabolic disorders. *J Hum Lact* 11:51–53; 1995.

Arnold RR et al. A bacteriocidal effect for human lactoferrin. *Science* 197:263–264; 1977.

Ashraf R et al. Additional water is not needed for healthy breast-fed babies in a hot climate. *Acta Paediatr* 82:1007–1011; 1993.

Azzari C et al. Modulation by human milk of IgG subclass response to hepatitis B vaccine in infants. *J Pediatr Gastroenterol Nutr* 10:310–315; 1990.

Ballabriga A. Essential fatty acids and human tissue composition: An overview. *Acta Paediatrica Suppl* 402:63–68; 1994.

Barger J and Kutner L. Teaching parents safe formula feeding. *Clinical Issues in Lactation* 2(2):1–2; 1997.

Bauchner H et al. Studies of breastfeeding and infections: How good is the evidence? *JAMA Assoc* 256:887–892; 1986.

Beijers R. Composition of premature breast-milk during lactation: Constant digestible protein content (as in full term milk.) *Early Hum Dev* 29:351–356; 1992.

Berlin C. Silicone breast implants and breastfeeding. *Pediatrics* 93:547–549; 1994.

Bertotto A et al. Memory T cells in human breast milk. *Acta Paediatr Scand* 80:98–99; 1991.

Bertotto A et al. Mycobacteria-reactive T cells are present in human colostrum from tuberculin-positive mothers but not tuberculin-negative mothers. *Am J Reprod Immunol* 29:131–134; 1993.

Bhowmick S et al. Rickets caused by vitamin D deficiency in breastfed infants in the southern United States. *Am J Child Dis* 145:127–130; 1991.

Buescher S. Host defense mechanisms of human milk and their relations to enteric infections and necrotizing enterocolitis. *Clin Perinatol* 21:247–262; 1994.

Bullen JJ et al. Iron-binding proteins in milk and resistance to *Escherichia coli* infection in infants. *Br Med J* 69:69–77; 1972.

Canfield L et al. Vitamin K in colostrum and mature human milk over the lactation period—a cross sectional study. *Am J Clin Nutr* 53:730–735; 1991.

Carlson S et al. Visual acuity and fatty acid status of term infants fed human milk and formulas with and without docosahexaenoate and arachidonate from egg yolk lecithin. *Pediatr Res* 39:882–888; 1996.

Chen Y et al. "Artificial feeding and hospitalization in the first 18 months of life." *Pediatrics* 81:58–62; 1988.

Chiba Y et al. Effect of breast feeding on responses of systemic interferon and virus-specific lymphocyte transformation in infants with respiratory syncytial infection. *J Med Virol* 21:7–14; 1987.

Cleary T et al. Human milk secretory immunoglobulin A to Shigella virulence plasmid-coded antigens. *J Pediatr* 118:34–38; 1991.

Clyne P and Kulczycki A. Human breast milk contains bovine IgG. Relationship to infant colic? *Pediatrics* 87:439–444; 1991.

Coppa G et al. Preliminary study of breastfeeding and bacterial adhesion to urocpithelial cells. *Lancet* 335:569–571; 1990.

Coppa G et al. Changes in carbohydrate composition in human milk over 4 months of lactation. *Pediatrics* 91:637–641; 1993.

Cornelissen E et al. Effects of oral or intramuscular vitamin K phrophylaxis on vitamin K 1, PIVKA-II, and clotting factors in breastfed infants. *Arch Child Dis* 67:1250–1254; 1992.

Cunningham A. *Breastfeeding, Bottlefeeding & Illness: An Annotated Bibliography 1990.*

Cunningham A et al. Breast-feeding and health in the 1980s: A global epidemiologic review. *J Pediatr* 118:659–666; 1991.

Cunningham A. Morbidity in breastfed and artificially fed infants. *J Pediatr* 95:685–689; 1979.

Daly S et al. Degree of breast emptying explains changes in the fat content but not fatty acid composition of human milk. *Exp Physiol* 78:741–755; 1993a.

Daly, S et al. The short-term synthesis and infant-regulated removal of milk in lactating women. *Exp Physiol* 78:209–220; 1993b.

Davis M et al. Infant feeding and childhood cancer. *Lancet* 2:365–368; 1988.

Dewit, O et al. Breastmilk amylase activities during 18 months of lactation in mothers from rural Zaire. *Acta Paediatr* 82:300–301; 1993.

Dick G. The etiology of multiple sclerosis. *Proc R Soc Med* 69:611; 1976.

Dugdale A. Breast milk and necrotising enterocolitis. *Lancet* 337:435; 1991.

Duncan B. et al. "Exclusive breastfeeding for at least 4 months protects against otitis media." *Pediatrics* 91:867–872; 1993.

Ebrahim G. Feeding the preterm brain. *J Trop Pediatr* 39:130–131; 1993.

El-Mohandes A et al. Use of human milk in the intensive care nursery decreases the incidence of nosocomial sepsis. J Perinatol 17:130–134; 1997.

Ellis L and Picciano M. Bioactive and immunoreactive prolactin variants in human milk. *Endocrinology,* 136:2711–2720; 1995.

European Society of Paediatric Gastroenterology and Nutrition Committee on Nutrition. Comment on antigen-reduced infant formulae. *Acta Paediatr* 82:317; 1993.

Farquharson J et al. "Effect of diet on the fatty acid composition of the major phospholipids of infant cerebral cortex." *Arch Dis Child* 72:198–203; 1995.

Finberg L. PBBs: The ladies' milk is not for burning. *Journal of Pediatrics,* 90(3):511; 1977.

Frank D et al. Cocaine and marijuana use during pregnancy by women intending and not intending to breast-feed. *J Am Diet Assoc* 92:215–216; 1992.

Frank, J and Newman J. "Breastfeeding in a polluted world: uncertain risks, clear benefits." *Can Med Assoc J* 149:33–37; 1993.

Gladen B et al. Development after exposure to polychlorinated biphenyls and dichlorodiphenyl dichloroethene transplacentally and through human milk. *J Pediatr* 113:991–995; 1988.

Goldman AS. The immunological system in human milk: the past—a pathway to the future. In Woodward WH, Draper HH, (eds). *Advances in Nutritional Research.* Plenum Press; 1998; p 106.

Greer F et al. Vitamin K status of lactating mothers, human milk and breastfeeding infants. *Pediatrics* 88:751–756; 1991.

Gross SJ et al. Nutritional composition of milk produced by mothers delivering preterm. *Journal of Pediatrics* 96(4): 641–644; 1980.

Hahn-Zoric M et al. Antibody responses to parenteral and oral vaccines are impaired by conventional and low protein formulas as compared to breast-feeding. *Acta Paediatr Scand* 79:1137–1142; 1990.

Hale T. *Medications and Mother's Milk.* Pharmasoft Publishing; 1998 Amarillo, TX, p. 165.

Hall B. Changing composition of human milk and early development of appetite control, *Keeping Abreast—Journal of Human Nurturing,* 12:3; 1997.

Hambraeus L et al. Nitrogen and protein components of human milk. *Acta Paediatr Scand* 67(5):561; 1978.

Hamosh M. Breastfeeding: Unravelling the mysteries of mother's milk. *Medscape Womens' Health;* 1996.

Hanson L. Breastfeeding provides passive and likely long-lasting active immunity. *Ann Allergy Asthma Immunol* 5:178–180; 1998.

Hawkins N. Potential aluminum toxicity in infants fed special infant formula. *J Pediatr Gastroenterol Nutr* 19:377–381; 1994.

Hennart P et al. Lysozyme, lactoferrin and secretory immunoglobulin A content in breastmilk: Influence of duration of lactation, nutrition status, prolactin status, and parity of mother. *Am J Clin Nutr* 53:32–39; 1991.

Hunt, M et al. Black breast milk due to minocycline therapy. *Br J Dermatol* 134:943–944; 1996.

Ichiba H et al. Measurement of growth promoting activity in human milk using a fetal small intestinal cell line. *Biol Neonate* 61:47–53; 1992.

Jacobson J and Jacobson S. A 4-year follow up study of children born to consumers of Lake Michigan fish. *J Great Lake Res* 19:776–783; 1993.

Jacobson J et al. Effects of in utero exposure to polychorinated biphenyls and related contaminants on cognitive functioning in young children. *J Pediatr* 116:38–45; 1990.

Jakobsson I and T Lindberg. Cows's milk as a cause of infantile colic in breast-fed infants. Lancet 2(8087):437–439; 1978.

Jelliffe DB and EFP Jelliffe. *Human Milk in the Modern World*. New York Oxford University Press; 1978.

Koldovsky O. Is breastmilk epidermal growth factor biologically active in the suckling? *Nutrition* 5:223–225; 1989.

Koletzko S et al. Role of infant feeding practices in development of Crohn's disease in childhood. *Br Med J* 289:1617–1618; 1989.

Koutras, A and Vigorita, V. Fecal secretory immunoglobulin A in breast milk versus formula feeding in early infancy. *J Pediatr Gastroenterol Nutr* 9:58–61; 1989.

Kutner L. Lactation Management Course, Breastfeeding Support Consultants Center for Lactation Education; 1996.

Lakdawala DR and EM Widdowson. Vitamin D in human milk. *Lancet* 1(8044):167–168; January 22, 1997.

Levine J and Ilowite N. Scleroderma-like esophageal disease in children breastfed by mothers with silicone breast implants." *JAMA* 271:213–216; 1994.

Little R, et al. Maternal alcohol use during breast-feeding and infant mental and motor development at one year. *N Engl J Med* 321:425–430; 1989.

Lonnerdale B. Effects of maternal nutrition on human lactation. In Hamosh M. and Goldman AS, (eds). *Human Lactation 2: Maternal and Environmental Factors.* New York: Plenum Press; 1986; pp 301–323.

Lucas A et al. Pattern of milk flow in breastfed infants. Lancet, 2(8133):57–58; 1979.

Lucas A. Breastmilk and neonatal NEC. *Lancet* 336: 1519–1523; 1990.

Lucas A et al. Breastmilk and subsequent intelligence quotient in children born preterm. *Lancet* 339:261–264; 1992.

Lucas A et al. A randomised muticentre study of human milk versus formula and later development in preterm infants. *Arch Dis Child* 70:F141–F146; 1994.

Maeda S. et al. The concentration of bovine IgG in human breast-milk measured using different methods. *Acta Paediatr* 82:1012–1016; 1993.

Martin J et al. Dependence of human milk essential fatty acids on adipose stores during lactation. *Am J Clin Nutr* 58:653–659; 1993.

Mayer E et al. Reduced risk of insulin-dependent diabetes mellitus (IDDM) among breastfed children. *Diabetes* 37:1625–1632; 1988.

McCance JA and E Widdowson FM. Hypertonic expansion of the extracellular fluids. *Acta Paediatrica* 46:337; 1975.

McMillan JA et al. Iron sufficiency in breast-fed infants and the availability of iron from human milk. *Pediatrics* 58(5):686–691, 1976.

Mennella J and Beauchamp G. Maternal diet alters the sensory qualities of human milk and the nursling's behavior. *Pediatrics* 88:737–744; 1991.

Mennella J and Beauchamp G. The transfer of alcohol to human milk. *N Engl J Med* 325:981–985; 1991.

Meny R et al. Codeine and the breastfed neonate. *J Hum Lact* 9:237–240; 1993.

Michaelsen KF et al. The Copenhagen cohort study on infant nutrition and growth: Breastmilk intake, human milk macronutrient content and influencing factors. *Am J Clin Nutr* 59:600–611; 1994.

Minchin M. Breastfeeding Matters: What we need to know about breastfeeding. Alma Publications, Victoria, Australia, p. 360, 1998.

Minchin M. Infant formula: A mass, uncontrolled trial in perinatal care. *Birth* 14:1; 1987.

Minchin, M. Smoking and breastfeeding: An overview. *J Hum Lact* 7:183–188; 1991.

Morrow A. Protection against infection with *Giardia lamblia* by breast-feeding in a cohort of Mexican infants. *J Pediatr* 121:363–370; 1992.

Nahas GG. Marijuana. *JAMA*, 233(1):79; 1975.

Nathavitharana K et al. IgA antibodies in human milk: Epidemiological markers of previous infections. *Arch Dis Child* 71:F192–F197; 1994.

Newman J. Drugs and breastmilk (Letter to the Editor). *Pediatrics* 86:148; 1990.

Nommsen L. et al. Determinants of energy, proteins, lipid and lactose concentrations in human milk during the first 12 months of lactation: The DARLING study. *Am J Clin Nutr* 53:457–465; 1991.

Pelleteir O. Cigarette smoking and vitamin C. *Nutrition Today* 5(3):12–15: Autumn, 1970.

Pietschnig B et al. "Vitamin K in breastmilk: No influence of maternal dietary intake." *Eur J Clin Nutr* 47:209–215; 1993.

Pisacane A et al. Breastfeeding and urinary tract infection. *Euro J Pediatr* 151:789–790; 1992.

Pisacane A et al. Breastfeeding and multiple sclerosis. *Br J Med* 308:1411–1412; 1994a.

Pisacane A et al. Breastfeeding and acute lower respiratory infection. *Acta Paediatr* 83:714–718; 1994b.

Pizarro F et al. Iron status with different infant feeding regimens: Relevance to screening and prevention of iron deficiency. *J Pediatr* 118:687–692; 1991.

Popkin B et al. Breastfeeding and diarrheal morbidity. *Pediatrics* 86:874–882; 1990.

Renz, H et al. Breast feeding modifies production of sIgA cow's milk-antibodies in infants. *Acta Paediatr Scand* 80:149–154; 1991.

Rivera-Calimlim L. The significance of drugs in breast milk. *Clin Perinatol* 14:51; 1987.

Rogan W. The sources and routes of childhood chemical exposures. *J Pediatr* 97(5):861–865; 1980.

Ronneberg R and Skara B. Essential fatty acids in human colostrum. *Acta Paediatr* 81:779–783; 1992.

Rudloff S and Lonnerdal B. Calcium retention from milk-based infant formulas, whey-hydrolysate formula, and human milk in weanling rhesus monkeys. *Am J Child Dis* 144:360–363; 1990.

Ruiz-Palacios G et al. Protection of breast-fed infants against *Campylobacter* diarrhea by antibodies in human milk. *J Pediatr* 116:707–713; 1990.

Ryu J. Effect of maternal caffeine consumption on heart rate and sleep time of breastfed infants. *Deve Pharmacol Ther* 8:355–363; 1985.

Saarinen U and Kajosaari M. Breastfeeding as prophylaxis against atopic disease: Prosepective follow-up study until 17 years old. *Lancet* 346:1065–1069; 1995.

Saarinen UM et al. Prolonged breast-feeding as prophylaxis for atopic disease. *Lancet* 2(8135): 163–166; 1979.

Sassen M. et al. Breastfeeding and acute otitis media. *Am J Otolaryngol* 15:351–357; 1994.

Sawatzki G. et al. Pitfalls in the design and manufacture of infant formulae. *Acta Paediatr* 402(Suppl):40–45; 1994.

Saylor J and Sami L. Anaphylaxis to casein hydrolysate formula. *J Pediatrics* 118:71–74; 1991.

Scheifele D. et al. Breastfeeding and antibody responses to routine vaccination in infants. *Lancet* 340:1406; 1992.

Silva DA et al. Ethanol pharmacokinetics in lactating women. *Braz J Med Biol Res* 26:1097–1103; 1993.

Smith G et al. Breastfeeding and infant nutrition. *Am Fed Proc* 92; 1978.

Specker B et al. Low serum calcium and high parathyroid hormone levels in neonates fed "humanized" cow's milk-based formula. *Am J Dis Child* 145:941–945; 1991.

Tonk G. Relation of diet to variation of dental caries. *J Am Dent Assoc* 70:394–403; 1965.

Tyson J et al. Adaptation of feeding to a low fat yield in breast-milk. *Pediatrics* 89:215–220; 1992.

Udall J. Gastrointestinal host defense and necrotizing enterocolitis. *J Pediatr* 117 (Suppl):S33–S34; 1990.

Vio F et al. Smoking during pregnancy and lactation and its effects on breastmilk volume. *Am J Clin Nutr* 54:1011–1016; 1991.

Viverge D et al. Variations in oligosaccharides and lactose in human milk during the first week of lactation. *J Pediatr Gastroenterol Nutr* 11:361–364; 1990.

Vorherr H. Drug excretion in breast milk *Postgrad Med*, 56(4):97–103; 1974.

Wack R et al. Electrolyte composition of human breast milk beyond the early postpartum period. *Nutrition* 13:774–777, 1997.

Wagner C et al. Special Properties of Human Milk. *Clin Pediatr* 35:283–293; 1996.

Walker M. A fresh look at the risks of artificial infant feeding. *J Hum Lact* 9:97–107; 1993.

Walker M. Summary of the hazards of infant formula: Part 2. Raleigh NC; International Lactation Consultants Association; 1998.

Walker M. Summary of the hazards of infant formula. Raleigh NC; International Lactation Consultants Association; 1992.

WHO/UNICEF. *Breastfeeding Management and Promotion in a Baby-Friendly Hospital*. UNICEF, New York 1993.

Wilkinson B et al. Stool bacteria and low birth weight in infants: Changes with milk formula, *Pediatr Res* 10:361; 1976.

Williams A. Silicone breast implants, breastfeeding and scleroderma. *Lancet* 343:1043–1044; 1994.

Woolridge MW et al. Do changes in pattern of breast usage alter the baby's nutrient intake? *Lancet* 336:395–397; 1990.

▼

BIBLIOGRAPHY

American Academy of Pediatrics Committee on Drugs. The transfer of drugs and other chemicals into human milk. *Pediatrics* 93:137–150, 1994.

American Academy of Pediatrics. The Transfer of Drugs and Other Chemicals into Human Milk. *Pediatrics* 93:137–150; 1994.

American Academy of Pediatrics. Breastfeeding and the Use of Human Milk. *Pediatrics* 100:1035–1039, 1997.

Angier N. Mother's milk found to be potent cocktail of hormones. *New York Times* B5; May 24, 1994.

Arnold L. Human milk for premature infants: An important health issue. *J Hum Lact* 9:121–123; 1993.

Batagol R. *Drugs and Breastfeeding*. London; British National Formulary; 1994.

Batagol R. Drugs and breastfeeding. *Breastfeeding Review* 14:13–20; May, 1989.

Berlin C. Drugs and chemicals: Exposure of the nursing mother. *Clin Pharmacol Ther* 36:1089–1097; 1989.

Blackwell A and Salisbury L. Administrative petition to relieve the health hazards of promotion of infant formulas in the U.S. *Birth and the Family Journal* 8(4):290; 1981.

Breastfeeding Support Consultants (BSC): *Infant Feeding Costs.* Chalfont, Pennsylvania; 1998.

Briggs G, Freeman R, Yaffe S, *Drugs in pregnancy and lactation;* Baltimore: Williams & Wilkins; 1998.

Calvo E et al. Iron status in exclusively breast-fed infants. *Pediatrics* 90:375–379; 1992.

Chang Y et al. Hypocalcemia in nonwhite breast-fed infants. *Clin Pediatr* 31:695–698; 1992.

Chasnoff I et al. Cocaine intoxication in a breast-fed infant. *Pediatrics* 80:836–838; 1987.

Cunningham A. Studies of breastfeeding and infections. How good is the evidence? A critique of the answer from Yale. *J Hum Lact* 4:54–56; 1988.

Davis M. Review of the evidence for an association between infant feeding and childhood cancer. *Int J Cancer* (Suppl 11):29–33, 1998.

Densley B. Phthalates in formula: A report. *ALCA Galaxy* 7(3):34–37; 1996.

Ebrahim G. Breastmilk endocrinology. *J Trop Pediatr* 42:2–4; 1996.

Ellis M et al. Anaphylaxis after ingestion of a recently introduced hydrolyzed whey protein formula. *J Pediatrics* 118:74–77; 1991.

Genze, Boroviczeny O et al. Fatty acid composition of human milk during the first month after term and preterm delivery. *Eur J Pediatr* 156:142–147; 1997.

Gessner B et al. Nutritional rickets among breast-fed Black and Alaska native children. *Alaska Med* 39:72–74, 1997.

Grover M. et al. Effect of human milk prostaglandins and lactoferrin on respiratory syncytial virus and rotavirus. *Acta Paediatr* 86:315–316; 1997.

Grulee CG et al. Breast and artificial feeding. *JAMA,* 103(10):735; 1934.

Hansen B and Moore L. Recreational drug use by the breast-feeding woman. Part I: Illicit drugs. *J Hum Lact* 5:178–180; 1989.

Harvard Medical School, Department of Continuing Education. Evaluating medical information. Harvard Medical School Health Letter 7(1):6; 1981.

Haschke F et al. Iron nutrition and growth of breast- and formula-fed infants during the first nine months of life. *J Pediatr Gastroenterol Nutr* 16:151–156; 1993.

Heiskanen K et al. Risk of low vitamin B_6 status in infants breast-fed exclusively beyond six months. *Pediatr Gastroenterol Nutr* 23:38–44; 1996.

Hey B. Tap-water supply safety questioned. AAP News, 11(11):1; 1995.

Hillman S. Mineral and vitamin D adequacy in infants fed human milk or formula between 6 and 12 months of age. *J Pediatr* 117 (Suppl):S134–S141; 1990.

Hopkinson J et al. "Milk production by mothers of premature infants: Influence of cigarette smoking." *Pediatrics* 90:934–938; 1992.

Horwood L & Fergusson D. Breastfeeding and later cognitive and academic outcomes. *Pediatrics* 101:1; 1998.

Howard C and Lawrence, R. Breast-feeding and drug exposure. *Obstet Gynecol Clin North Am* 25:195–217, 1998.

Institute of Medicine (National Academy of Sciences). *Nutrition During Lactation.* Washington, D.C., National Academy Press; 1991.

Irvine C et al. The potential adverse effects of soybean phytoestrogens in infant feeding. *N Z Med J* 108:208–209; 1995.

Ito S et al. Prospective follow-up of adverse reactions in breast-fed infants exposed to maternal medication. *Am J Obstet Gynecol* 168:1393–1399; 1993.

Ito S et al. Maternal noncompliance with antibiotics during breastfeeding. *Ann Pharmacother* 27:40–42; 1993.

Jensen RG. *The Lipids of Human Milk*, CRC Press, Boca Raton, FL; 1989

Kacew S. Adverse effects of drugs and chemicals in breastmilk on the nursing infant. *J Clin Pharmacol* 33:213–221; 1993.

Kramer MS. Does breastfeeding help protect against atopic disease? Biology, methodology, and a Golden Jubilee of controversy. *J Pediatr* 112:181–190; 1988.

Krugman S and Law P. Breastfeeding and IQ (letter). *Pediatrics* 103:193–194; 1999.

Kuhne T et al. Maternal vegan diet causing a serious infantile neurological disorder due to vitamin B_{12} deficiency. *Eur J Pediatr* 150:205–208; 1991.

Lanting C et al. Neurological condition in 42-month-old children in relation to pre- and postnatal exposure to polychlorinated biphenyls and dioxin. *Early Human Dev* 50:283–292; 1998.

Lawrence RA. Breastfeeding: A guide for the medical profession. St. Louis MO; Mosby; 1999.

Lebenthal E ed. *Testbook of Gastroenterology and Nutrition in Early Infancy.* 2nd ed., Raven Press, chapter by Goldman & Goldblum.

Lenfant C and Liu BM. Passive smokers vs voluntary smokers. *N Engl J Med,* 302(13):742; 1980.

Liebman B. The soy story. *Nutrition Action Healthletter* 25:6; 1998.

Lin T et al. Longitudinal changes in Ca, Mg, Fe, Cu and Zn in breast milk of women in Taiwan over a lactation period of one year. *Biol Trace Element Res* 62:31–41, 1998.

Lucas A et al. Randomized outcome trial of human milk fortification and developmental outcome in preterm infants. *Am J Clin Nutr* 64:142–151; 1996.

Lucas A and Cole T. Breastmilk and neonatal necrotising enterocolitis. *Lancet* 336:1519–1523; 1990.

Malpas T et al. Neonatal abstinence syndrome following abrupt cessation of breastfeeding. *N Z Med J* 112:12–13, 1999.

Marano H, Breast or bottle. New evidence in an old debate, *New York Magazine*, 59–60, October 29; 1979.

Mennella J. Infants' suckling responses to the flavor of alcohol in mothers' milk. *Alcoholism: Clin Exp Res* 21:581–585; 1997.

Nahas GG et al. Inhibition of cellular mediated immunity in marijuana smokers. *Science*, 193:419; 1974.

Nettleton JA. Are N-3 fatty acids essential nutrients for fetal and infant development? *J Am Diet Assoc*, 93:58–64; 1993.

Nutrition Action Newsletter. Caffeine: The inside scoop. December, 1996.

Nysenbaum AN et al. Sucking behavior and milk intake of neonates in relation to milk fat content. *Early Human Dev* 6:205–213; 1982.

Oldaeus G et al. Extensively and partially hydrolyzed infant formulas for allergy prophylaxis. *Arch Dis Child* 77:4–10; 1997.

Ortega R et al. Influence of smoking on vitamin E status during the third trimester of pregnancy and on breastmilk-to-tocopherol concentrations in Spanish women. *Am J Clin Nutr* 68:662–667, 1998.

Ortega R et al. Ascorbic acid levels in maternal milk: Differences with respect to ascorbic acid status during the third trimester of pregnancy. *Br J Nutr* 79:431–437, 1998.

Owen M. et al. Relation of infant feeding practices, cigarette smoke exposure, and group child care to the onset and duration of otitis media with effusion in the first two years of life. *J Pediatr* 123:702–711; 1993.

Perez-Escamilla R et al. Maternal anthropometric status and lactation performance in a low-income honduran population: Evidence for the role of infants. *Am J Clin Nutr* 61:528–534; 1995.

Quan R et al. The effect of nutritional additives on anti-infective factors in human milk. *Clin Pediatr* 34:325–328; 1994.

Quinsex P et al. The importance of measured intake in assessing exposure of breast-fed infants to organochlorines. *Eur J Clin Nutr* 438–444; 1996.

Rubin D et al. Relationship between infant feeding and infectious illness: A prospective study of infants during the first year of life. *Pediatrics* 85:464–471; 1990.

Rubow S et al. The excretion of radiopharmaceuticals in human breast milk: Additional data and dosimetry, *Eur J Nucl Med* 21:144–153; 1994.

Sample J et al. Breast milk contamination and silicone implants. Preliminary results using silicon as a proxy measurement for silicone. *Plast Reconstr Surg* 102:528–533, 1998.

Sankaran K et al. A randomized, controlled evaluation of two commercially available human breast milk fortifiers in healthy preterm neonates. *J Am Diet Assoc* 96:1145–1149; 1996.

Scariati P et al. A longitudinal analysis of infant morbidity and the extent of breastfeeding in the U.S. *Pediatrics* 99(6) E5–7; 1999.

Schroten H et al. Inhibition of adhesion of S-fimbriated *E. coli* to buccal epithelial cells by human skim milk is predominantly mediated by mucins and depends on the period of lactation. *Acta Paediatr* 82:6–11; 1993.

Schroten H et al. Inhibition of adhesion of S-fimbriated *Escherichia coli* to buccal epithelial cells by human milk fat globule membrane components: A novel aspect of the protective function of mucins in the nonimmunoglobulin fraction. *Infect Immun* 60:2893–2899; 1992.

Schulte P, Minimizing alcohol exposure of the breastfeeding infant. *J Hum Lact* 11(4) 317–319; 1995.

Scott FW. Cow milk and insulin-dependent diabetes mellitus: Is there a relationship? *Am J Clin Nutr* 51:489–491; 1990.

Setchell K et al. Exposure of infants to phytoestrogens from soy-based infant formula. *Lancet* 350:23–27; 1997.

Silverdal S et al. Protective effect of breastfeeding on invasive *Haemophilus influenzae* infection: A case-control study in Swedish preschool children. *Int J Epidemiol* 26:443–450; 1997.

Specker B et al. Sunshine exposure and serum 25-hydroxyvitamin D concentrations in exclusively breastfed infants. *J Pediatr* 107:372–376; 1985.

U.S. Department of Health and Human Services, Breastfeeding, Public Health Service, Health Services Administration; Bureau of Community Health Services, Rockville, Maryland; 1979.

Voepel-Lewis T et al. Evaluation of simethicone for the treatment of abdominal discomfort in infants. *J Clin Anesth* 10:91–94; 1998.

WHO. The use of essential drugs: Technical Report Series 796. Geneva, Switzerland; WHO; 1990.

Wright A et al. Breastfeeding and lower respiratory tract illness in the first year of life. *Br J Med* 299:946–949; 1989.

Wright A et al. Relationship of parental smoking to wheezing and nonwheezing lower respiratory tract illness in infancy. *J Pediatr* 118:207–214; 1991.

Yolken R et al. "Human milk mucin inhibits rotavirus replication and prevents experimental gastroenteritis." *J Clin Invest* 90:1984–1991; 1992.

PRENATAL CONSIDERATIONS

Parents face many choices regarding the care of their new babies. Among them are lifestyle choices that can vary greatly in their consequences. Some choices, such as dress or daily routines, have little or no impact on the health of the child. However, health care choices directly impact the health and well-being of children in both short-term and long-term ways. Examples of health care choices include the use of a car seat, immunizations, and breastfeeding. Just as there are serious risks to the child of parents who choose not to use a car seat or immunize, so it is with choosing not to breastfeed. Breastfeeding, however, may involve lifestyle choices and adjustments as well. Parents may, therefore, benefit from your guidance in blending breastfeeding into their lives.

The health care profession has an obligation to provide true informed consent to women and their families prenatally. An understanding of the consequences of not breastfeeding is essential for them to make an informed decision. Lactation consultants can look for ways to reach women prenatally in order to give parents the opportunity to make an informed feeding decision. Contacting local groups that offer prenatal classes, childbirth educators, obstetrician's offices, and family practice groups who provide obstetric care is an excellent start. If sound breastfeeding education is unavailable, you might wish to provide breastfeeding classes to your clients. You might also provide breastfeeding updates to physicians, nurses and other caregivers who see prenatal women.

MAKING THE DECISION TO BREASTFEED

A belief in breastfeeding is the underlying motivator in a woman's infant feeding decision. Although brochures can increase information, they have little influence on the incidence of breastfeeding. The choice is affected most by a positive attitude toward breastfeeding prior to pregnancy (Coreil, 1988). Generally, experience shows that the woman most likely to breastfeed is in her mid to upper 20s. She is college educated, white, married, and in the middle income level. Statistically, black and teen mothers are the least likely to breastfeed. A woman is more likely to breastfeed if she has received positive in-

formation about breastfeeding and if she views breastfeeding as a natural extension of birth (Rentschler, 1991).

Factors That Influence a Woman's Decision to Breastfeed

Many societal barriers are in place that, at best, fail to recognize breastfeeding as the natural way to nourish babies. At worst, barriers openly discourage breastfeeding. In prenatal contact with mothers, it is important that the caregiver be aware of these concerns and address them with clients. You can help women verbalize and address the conflicting feelings that sometimes are involved in the decision to breastfeed (Kitzinger, 1992). Separation of generations, frequent relocation, and lack of breastfeeding as the cultural norm can leave new mothers with little confidence in their ability to breastfeed or little understanding of how the process works. Few women have breastfeeding role models. You can help women recognize the important contribution they make to society in their role as a mother and nurturer of the next generation.

Bottle feeding as the model in Western culture affects professionals and lay persons alike. When media and advertising portray the breast as a sexual object, they ignore the importance of breasts for infant feeding. Much of the health care system bases routines, policies, education, and even the facility's architectural layout on artificial feeding. Although the maxim *breast is best* is freely spoken, many infant feeding messages imply equality between human milk and artificial baby milk. When such mixed signals are sent to parents, they add to the parents' confusion.

Research suggests that close to half of women make their infant feeding choices before pregnancy, and as many as half will make the decision during pregnancy (Dix, 1991). A small focus group revealed that breast and bottle feeders had the same goals regarding infant feeding. However, they differed in their perception of barriers to breastfeeding, most significantly embarrassment and inconvenience (Marchand, 1994). During prenatal teaching, it would help to ask women to name their goals and specifically to discuss these two perceived barriers.

Influence From Other People

Significant people in a woman's life can exert a substantial influence over her decision to breastfeed. Women are more likely to breastfeed if other family members have either breastfed or are supportive of breastfeeding. Having friends and other acquaintances who breastfeed provides additional role models. Additionally, the support of the baby's father plays a pivotal role in her decision. Likewise, she will be influenced greatly by the attitude and knowledge level of her caregivers. These latter two areas of influence are discussed more completely below.

Influence From the Baby's Father

One of the strongest influences on the breastfeeding decision in the United States is that of the child's father. Pregnant women frequently say, "But if I breastfeed, my husband won't be able to feed the baby." Fathers want to be involved in caring for their infant, and they often see feeding as an important interaction. In a qualitative study, 14 fathers identified the process of postponing feeding the baby as a significant issue (Gamble, 1993). These mens' experiences can form the basis for your prenatal education of parents.

A 1994 study by Littman noted that the father's approval of breastfeeding was the single most statistically significant indicator of whether or not women in the study breastfed. A study conducted by Freed (1992a) among expectant mothers revealed that women do not always correctly predict the attitudes of the father regarding breastfeeding. Lactation consultants can encourage more discussion by couples and more sharing of information with fathers. Freed (1992b) also found that among an indigent population, lack of support for breastfeeding by a significant other was the most important predictor of bottle feeding. This is further evidence for the importance of including fathers in education. See Chapter 17 for ways fathers can be involved with their babies.

Influence From the Caregiver

Caregivers exert a tremendous influence on a parent's choice of infant feeding. Frequently, knowledgeable professionals are unaware of or may even openly dispute the normalcy of breastfeeding in spite of evidence to the contrary (Walker, 1992). The approach taken with women can turn them in the direction of breastfeeding. A positive approach assumes that all pregnant women intend to breastfeed unless they indicate otherwise. Asking, "Do you plan to breastfeed?" or

"How do you plan to feed your baby?," implies equality between human milk and its substitutes. When the caregiver asks, "How can I help you with breastfeeding?," it conveys the caregiver's belief in the superiority of breastfeeding. If the woman indicates that she does not plan to breastfeed or if she seems uncertain, it provides an opportunity to discuss concerns or misconceptions. Caregivers can help instill in women a belief in their ability to breastfeed and an understanding of its superiority over artificial baby milk. It's all a confidence game! And the mother's confidence is determined in large part by her caregivers.

Issues That Influence the Decision to Breastfeed

A variety of issues may also affect a woman's decision to breastfeed. Almost all women know that breastfeeding is best for the baby. A woman who chooses to breastfeed may be motivated by the health and nutrition benefits for her and her baby. She may be concerned about the increased risk to her baby of substituting artificial milks. Breastfeeders perceive breastfeeding as more convenient. Interestingly, women who choose to bottle feed tend to perceive breastfeeding as less convenient, perhaps associating it with a loss of freedom. They believe that if they bottle feed, someone else can feed the baby and they will be able to resume outside activities earlier than if they breastfeed. Among low-income women, other factors identified as barriers to the decision to breastfeed include modesty, privacy, work or school conflicts, lack of confidence, and lifestyle issues such as diet, stress, and inadequate sleep (Bryant, 1993).

Another culturally evident trend in the infant feeding decision mirrors trends in the management of labor and birth. Women often fear being totally responsible for their baby's weight gain and health, much as they fear embracing the responsibility of laboring and birthing. Women describe a need to have **epidural anesthesia** or a need to have their physician deliver the baby. After birth they may reject the next step of motherhood—breastfeeding—for fear of failure. This may also be influenced by the need for control in one's life. Women who view control as a priority are more likely to rely on bottle feeding in an effort to achieve this. Fear of failure may be due to the woman's lack of confidence that her body could produce a superior product that will provide sufficient food for her baby.

Customs in the home environment may influence a woman to feed her baby artificially if it is what everyone else in her culture does. Her knowledge of infant care or lack of knowledge about breastfeeding may cause her to believe that it will not fit into her lifestyle. Commercial messages about human milk substitutes and bottle feeding may be so strong that she is convinced that there is little difference between breastfeeding and artificial feeding. An aversion to her breasts being touched may make it emotionally painful for her to breastfeed. Such an aversion is common in women who are survivors of sexual or physical abuse. Many times, the woman may not even be aware of the past abuse. The act of birth and breastfeeding may be the trigger that releases memories. See Chapter 18 for a discussion of sexual abuse survivors.

In discussing infant feeding with pregnant women, the risks of *not* breastfeeding provide a sound basis for informed decision making. You can also point out that a breastfeeding mother need not purchase special equipment or incur daily expenses of infant formula. Her only special need is one extra nutritional snack per day to maintain milk production. While breastfeeding, the mother has a free hand to attend to other needs or enjoyments such as reading, snacking, and helping other children. Because breastfeeding can be done virtually anywhere, travel and other activities are more convenient. Give mothers examples of how breastfeeding can be done modestly in front of others. Mothers are also pleased to find that their breastfed baby's stools and spit-up have a less offensive odor than those of formula-fed babies; the stools also do not stain clothing.

▼ Realistic Expectations Regarding Breastfeeding

Fear of instilling guilt is not an acceptable excuse for failing to inform women of the potentially negative outcomes of formula use. When compared with breastfeeding, bottle feeding falls far short. Bottle feeders often choose this approach because of a perceived disagreeable aspect of breastfeeding. You can help a mother develop realistic expectations about breastfeeding by acquainting her with some of the realities. In the early days of breastfeeding, she may experience a degree of breast fullness and nipple tenderness. Because of the more frequent feeds required by a breastfed baby, she will need to be available to her young baby for nourishment. It is important that you not minimize a mother's concerns regarding these issues. You can encourage her to consider that this is the normal, expected postpartum course. Remind her, too, of the many immunologic, emotional, and financial benefits of breastfeeding.

Help the woman see that there are ways of decreasing discomforts and minimizing inconveniences. Address her specific concerns by offering her ways of coping and including her baby in her activities. This type of support may be all she needs to build her confidence and help her overcome perceived obstacles. Learning how to fit breastfeeding into their lifestyle will be the first of many accommodations parents will make as they blend their new child into their family.

Misconceptions That Influence the Mother's Decision to Breastfeed

There are a number of misconceptions about breastfeeding that may cause a woman to choose not to breastfeed. You can help dispel these misconceptions and increase the pregnant woman's confidence in her decision to breastfeed. Below is a list of some common misconceptions.

The baby will be too dependent if he breastfeeds.
Breastfed babies actually seem to display more independence because their needs are met. See Chapter 11.

Breastfeeding is too time consuming.
There is actually less work involved in breastfeeding than in bottle feeding. This frees the mother's time that can be spent with her baby and other family members. See Chapter 17.

My mother didn't have enough milk, so maybe I won't either.
Each well-nourished woman produces the amount of milk her own baby needs. The breastfeeding experience of the woman's mother has no bearing on her own ability to breastfeed. Women who attempted to breastfeed between 1930 and 1970 received little effective advice or support from their physicians to enable them to breastfeed. See Chapter 1.

Maybe my milk won't agree with my baby.
Each mother's milk is ideally suited to her own baby. Breastfed babies rarely experience negative reactions to their mother's milk. Conversely, babies may develop an intolerance to cow's milk. See Chapter 8.

My breasts are too small to breastfeed.
The size of a woman's breasts is determined by the amount of fatty tissue, not functional breast tissue, and so size has no bearing on her ability to produce sufficient milk. See Chapter 6.

I am too high-strung to breastfeed.
Breastfeeding can actually be calming to a high-strung woman because of the hormones activated by nursing. The added skin contact with the baby can also have a calming effect on a mother. See Chapter 6.

If I breastfeed, my diet will be too restricted.
Breastfeeding babies generally can tolerate the same foods the mother can tolerate. The only foods a breastfeeding mother may need to restrict are those that seem to produce signs of intolerance in her baby. See Chapter 7.

If I have a cesarean birth, I won't be able to breastfeed.
Mothers who deliver by cesarean birth are able to breastfeed. The type of birth a mother experiences has no effect on her ability to breastfeed. See Chapter 10.

Breastfeeding will drain my energies too much.

All mothers find caring for a newborn infant tiring, regardless of feeding method. Breastfeeding allows a mother to relax during feeding times. This permits her to get even more rest than a mother who bottle feeds her baby. A mother can recoup her energies by making it a practice to rest while her baby is sleeping. Breastfeeding seems to be nature's way of ensuring that the mother gets the rest she needs in the postpartum period. See Chapter 7. The formula feeding mother spends more time purchasing and preparing formula. See Chapter 8.

Breastfeeding mothers lose their figures and get sagging breasts.

The sagging in a woman's breasts is caused by pregnancy and loss of muscle tone as women age, not by breastfeeding. See Chapter 6. The caloric demands of breastfeeding can actually help mothers control their weight. See Chapter 7.

Artificial baby milk is just as healthy as human milk.

There are substantial differences between infant formula and human milk. Human milk is a live substance that provides immunities and antibacterial properties. See Chapter 8 for a detailed discussion about the properties and health benefits of human milk.

Breastfeeding is essentially an alternative to infant formula.

Breastfeeding is much more than human milk. It is a dynamic process, a bonding relationship between a mother and her baby. Breastfeeding involves people, not simply infant food. See Chapter 3.

Mothers who plan to return to work most likely will have to wean before they return.

Mothers who are separated from their babies, whether for a return to work, school, or other activity, have many options. They can express milk to be fed to the baby or provide formula for the baby during the separation. Unrestricted breastfeeding at times when the mother and baby are together will help maintain milk production. See Chapter 22.

▼ Conditions That Contraindicate Breastfeeding

It is a rare circumstance in which a mother may not breastfeed her baby. Sheehan's syndrome, as discussed in Chapter 6, prevents the mother from producing any milk. Long-term drug therapy that requires a substance or treatment that would be dangerous to the infant, such as with lithium, rules out breastfeeding. Severe illness in the mother, such as unresolved congestive heart failure or chemotherapy treatment of cancer, may contraindicate breastfeeding. A mother can breastfeed after she has received at least 2 weeks of treatment for active tuberculosis (Lawrence, 1997). Women who test positive for the human immunodeficiency virus and live in a developed country with a sanitary water supply are advised not to breastfeed in certain circumstances. See Chapter 23 for a discussion of these conditions.

▼ PREPARATION FOR BREASTFEEDING

Women throughout the world have breastfed their babies for centuries without the aid of recent scientific knowledge and devices. Many modern women, however, benefit from education about breastfeeding techniques and preparation for breastfeeding. Although women historically have nurtured their babies primarily with their own milk, the past several decades have experienced an increase in the popularity of bottle feeding and a decline in breastfeeding. Consequently, fewer family members are knowledgeable enough about breastfeeding to offer the mother the practical information and support she needs in order to breastfeed. The educational process and the mother's active participation in planning for her breastfed baby are effective means of preparing the mother psychologically for breastfeeding. Her self-confidence will increase, enabling her to overcome any common discomforts and obstacles she may experience that are associated with nursing her baby.

▼ Learning about Breastfeeding

A woman who plans to breastfeed will benefit from learning about it early in her pregnancy. The earlier she receives information, the more likely it is that she will breastfeed for a substantial period of time. The woman's attentiveness and retention of the information may be greater in the later months of her pregnancy, as she gets closer to her delivery date. Keeping this in mind, you may want to focus early discussions on the decision-making process. You can then discuss the practical aspects of breastfeeding management closer to the time she will deliver.

One way for pregnant women to obtain such information is through attending a prenatal breastfeeding class. They may also wish to begin attending meetings of a community support group for breastfeeding mothers, such as those offered by La Leche League and Nursing Mothers Council. These meetings can enhance women's confidence and increase their knowledge of breastfeeding. They also provide an opportunity for mothers to share common interests with others in the community.

Through contact with the woman during her pregnancy, you can discuss her individual goals for breastfeeding. What is her vision of breastfeeding in her everyday life? How important are feeding issues to her and her partner? What do they expect breastfeeding to be like? Answers to these questions may provide a foundation for their breastfeeding education. Give the mother information that will help blend breastfeeding into her life. Help her identify the aspects of breastfeeding education that will be useful to her personally. This leads to the development of useful strategies that she may apply postpartum. It will also help form an effective relationship between you and the mother (Pridham, 1993).

See Figure 9.1 for questions that may be helpful in gathering the information necessary to assess a woman's need for education and support related to breastfeeding. Note that, when possible, questions are open ended to encourage more descriptive information in the mother's response.

In order to prepare for breastfeeding, the women in your care can educate themselves in several ways. By obtaining factual information from literature, classes, and meetings, they will be able to develop a firm base for proper management of breastfeeding. This will help them avoid or minimize problems. A woman can familiarize herself with baby care and breastfeeding by associating with mothers of young babies and occasionally caring for infants during her pregnancy. In this way, she will develop proficiency in handling babies. She will also build confidence in her mothering abilities, which will enable her to overcome worries she may encounter when her own baby arrives. Attending childbirth classes and practicing relaxation techniques can enhance a woman's awareness of her body and help her learn ways of overcoming tension and discomfort. The information and skills she obtains during pregnancy will be especially useful to her when she and her baby go through the trial and error period of establishing a comfortable breastfeeding routine.

Breastfeeding Classes

A large part of breastfeeding teaching can be done through group instruction. Breastfeeding classes are an important part of your practice. Through classes, you are able to reach large numbers of women at various stages. Class content is determined by the purpose of the class. Ideally, breastfeeding discussions are incorporated into the couple's childbirth classes. Early in the series, couples benefit from a discussion that helps them make the decision regarding infant feeding. After the decision has been made, a discussion of expectations and getting off to a good start with breastfeeding is helpful. After the baby has been born and is breastfeeding, parents benefit from the support and information provided in a postpartum class.

Guidelines For Teaching a Breastfeeding Class

The most important rule in teaching a parent class is to keep it simple. If you are fortunate to have more than a couple of hours for parent classes, dividing your teaching into three separate classes, as described later, will give short frequent feeds of information to parents. Most of what is accomplished during the prenatal period is in the area of attitude and expectations. Parents may remember little of the particulars for establishing breastfeeding. They will, however, recall the impressions they gained in class regarding the health benefits and ease of breastfeeding, as well as the risks of not breastfeeding. These perceptions will reinforce their decision after the baby has been born. Teach parents that the only rule in breastfeeding is that there are no rules! Basically all that is required is that the baby gain weight appropriately and the mother is comfortable in the process. Encourage parents to trust their instincts and to respond to their baby's cues.

Identify the teachable moment for class participants, and tailor your teaching methods to adult learners. During a prenatal class, parents may be so focused on their anticipated delivery that it will be difficult to see beyond that point. Use activities that will involve them actively in order to enhance their learning. Recognize that much of what they learn prenatally may be lost, so you will want to rein-

FIGURE 9.1 Questions about breastfeeding to ask pregnant women

Assessing a woman's need for breastfeeding education

◆ How does she feel about the prospect of breastfeeding?
◆ What practical knowledge does she have about breastfeeding?
◆ What prior experience or exposure does she have to breastfeeding?
◆ How many friends or relatives have breastfed?
◆ What reading has she done on breastfeeding? What videos has she seen?
◆ Has she attended a breastfeeding information class?
◆ Is she attending prepared childbirth classes?
◆ What has her physician discussed with her about breastfeeding?
◆ What has she done to prepare for breastfeeding?
◆ Has she checked for inverted nipples?
◆ What has she learned about breast care?
◆ What clothing does she have that will allow her baby easy access to her breast?
◆ What arrangements has she made for help at home?
◆ Does she plan to have rooming-in, if she is delivering in a hospital?
◆ Is she interested in attending group discussions with other breastfeeding mothers?
◆ What are her specific questions or concerns?

force learning with handouts on specific issues. Visual aids such as other breastfeeding parents and short videotapes may also be effective. Help parents focus on the positive aspects of breastfeeding and regard it as a learning process for both the mother and the baby. Help couples recognize that should any problems arise, they are resolvable.

Infant Feeding Class

Advertising a class as an infant feeding class rather than a breastfeeding class will make it clear that the class is open to everyone. Because fathers are instrumental in the mother's decision to breastfeed, be sure to encourage their participation as well as the mother's. Clearly relate the desire for them to attend the class. You may help some undecided couples choose breastfeeding. In this class, you can dispel any misconceptions the couples may have and address information they will need for making their decision. Discuss the health benefits of breastfeeding for both the mother and the baby, as well as the convenience, economics, and ease of travel. Often, couples express a concern that fathers will be left out if the mother breastfeeds. Help them recognize the importance of the father's participation in making the decision to breastfeed, and discuss ways he can be involved with the baby (as discussed in Chapter 17). Addressing the short-term and long-term risks of not breastfeeding will also be useful.

Prenatal Breastfeeding Class

In a prenatal class, you can address issues that will help parents prepare for establishing breastfeeding. Identify cues and behaviors of babies as these relate to feeding. Point out to parents that babies communicate through distinct cuing before, during, and after feeds. Help them identify how these cues can enable them to understand and best meet their babies needs (Delight, 1991). See Chapter 11 for a discussion of infant feeding cues.

FIGURE 9.2 Sample outline for a prenatal breastfeeding class

  I. Welcome and introductions (5 minutes)
  II. Risks to mother and baby of not breastfeeding (class discussion—15 minutes)
  III. What is infant formula? (15 minutes)
    A. Its use and overuse (lecture and discussion)
    B. What our culture says about formula (class discussion)
    C. What our culture says about breasts (class discussion)
  IV. How were we fed? (15 minutes)
    A. Our parents and grandparents did their best at that time (lecture and discussion)
    B. Guilt for us and those around us (lecture)
    C. How guilt helps us (lecture)
BREAK (10 minutes)
  V. Our babies (10 minutes)
    A. Speaking their language (lecture)
      1. Sleep states
      2. Feeding cues
    B. What the baby human *needs* (discussion and lecture)
      1. Relating baby's nutritional needs and growth to adult eating patterns
      2. Relating baby's nighttime needs to the adult
  VI. Breastfeeding basics (30 minutes)
    A. Milk supply (lecture)
      1. Milk removed is replaced
      2. Getting started, rooming-in and the first week
      3. How to know baby is getting enough
      4. Feeding diary
    B. Positions for mom and baby (lecture and video)
      1. Basics: How to achieve good position and why it is important
      2. Options
      3. Comfort
    C. Attachment and suckling (lecture and video)
      1. Why it is important
      2. Works with good position
      3. Steps to a good latch
      4. Normal suckling
  VII. Breastfeeding myths you may hear (lecture and discussion—10 minutes)
  VIII. How to find breastfeeding help and why you may need it (lecture—10 minutes)

Used by permission of Debbie Shinskie.

Use visual examples to demonstrate the usual positions mothers use for holding their babies for feeding. Give parents dolls to practice the positions. Show them through videos and slides how to recognize when their baby has a good latch and is positioned well at the breast. Explain how latch is the key to milk transfer and to avoiding nipple soreness. Help parents learn how to determine if their baby is receiving enough milk, and discuss milk production in the context of supply and demand. Help them learn to watch for other signs of good intake, such as audible swallows and the number of wet diapers and stools. Provide them with a feeding diary that may be used for the first 2 weeks of breastfeeding to identify the appropriate number of feeds, voids, and stools. Characterize the first 2 weeks as a learning time for both the mother and baby. Explain the importance of eating when hungry and drinking when thirsty without strict dietary regimens. Encourage mothers to rest with their babies to facilitate recovery after childbirth. All of these issues will help parents achieve a smooth transition to initiating breastfeeding. See Figure 9.2 for a sample outline of a prenatal breastfeeding class.

Postpartum Breastfeeding Class

You may want to have a separate postpartum class to give mothers support and information after delivery of the baby. Pregnant women can be encouraged to attend this class as well. It might even be developed into a mother-to-mother support group in which pregnant women will have an opportunity to talk with breastfeeding mothers and to see babies breastfeed. At this time, you can discuss what the new parents might expect in the next several months. Help them anticipate typical infant behavior, growth spurts, crying, and teething. Discuss planning of activities, breastfeeding in public, and returning to work or school. You may also want to address the topic of complementary foods and weaning at this time. Allow some time for group problem solving and prevention of problems such as engorgement, plugged ducts, and mastitis. Review the importance of exclusive breastfeeding and the question of supplementing with infant formula. Make sure that mothers know where they can go for help with questions or concerns. See Figure 9.3 for a sample outline for a postpartum breastfeeding class.

Prenatal Breast Care

During pregnancy, hormones act on the breast to prepare it for lactation. The skin stretches and becomes more pliable in order to accommodate internal breast development. The nipple and areola enlarge and are protected by increasing pigmentation. The Montgomery glands are thought to lubricate the nipple and areola, protecting the keratin from drying out and flaking off. Near the beginning of the third trimester, the mother can determine whether her nipples will need any assis-

---

FIGURE 9.3   Sample outline for a postpartum breastfeeding class

I. Welcome and introductions (5 minutes)
II. Breastfeeding's continued importance (lecture and discussion—15 minutes)
   A. Review of risks of not breastfeeding
   B. AAP breastfeeding recommendations
III. Growing baby milestones and issues (lecture and discussion—20 minutes)
   A. Growth spurts
   B. Crying
   C. Sleep
   D. Baby's new abilities
   E. Teething
IV. New parents' issues (lecture, discussion and video—20 minutes)
   A. Resuming activities, prioritizing and not overdoing
   B. Ideas for including baby
   C. Staying healthy—rest, diet, and exercise
BREAK (10 minutes)
V. Returning to work or school (lecture, hands-on, and discussion—30 minutes)
   A. Options
   B. Planning ahead—talk with employer, prioritize needs
   C. How you will feed baby in your absence
   D. Pumps and other devices
   E. Troubleshooting and realistic expectations
VI. The family table and weaning (lecture and discussion—10 minutes)
VII. Where to find breastfeeding help (lecture—10 minutes)

Used by permission of Debbie Shinskie.

tance for a good latch. She can do this by performing the pinch test described in Chapter 19. A nipple that protrudes when stimulated makes it easiest for the baby to get a good mouthful of breast tissue. A nipple that remains flat or inverts may require assistance to improve latch. The last trimester is the best time for the woman to manipulate flat or inverted nipples because the skin has gained elasticity and stretches more easily than earlier in her pregnancy.

Nipple Correction

When a woman has flat or inverted nipples, it must first be established that intervention is appropriate or necessary. A woman with a history of prematurity or a tendency toward miscarriage or severe false labor should discuss with her physician the advisability of nipple preparation, breast foreplay, or intercourse. Such stimulation may trigger oxytocin release, which can cause the uterus to contract and induce labor.

Mothers need to know that some babies breastfeed on an inverted nipple without any difficulty. However, some babies will have difficulty with an inverted nipple that does not stimulate the baby's palate in a way that elicits his response. When correction is indicated, a woman may want to wear breast shells during the first few weeks of breastfeeding. Breast shells exert gentle pressure around the nipple, making the skin more pliable and the breast easier to grasp. When the infant suckles on the breast, this process further increases skin elasticity. An inverted syringe may also be used to pull out the nipple before a feed. See Chapter 19 for a discussion of breast shells and the use of an inverted syringe.

Colostrum During Pregnancy

Some sources may recommend that a woman express colostrum prenatally. However, this is not advised for several reasons. Nipple stimulation may induce labor in some women. Because colostrum acts as a barrier to bacteria and virus, removing it could also leave the breast susceptible to invasion and possible infection. It is not known whether colostrum is continually produced with consistent quantities of each component or whether the quality changes as it is removed. Removing colostrum prenatally may, therefore, deprive the baby of that essential food, both in terms of quantity and quality.

Infrequently, there are women whose breasts become uncomfortably full with colostrum. These women can gently express only to the point of comfort. If they experience leaking, they can gently blend the colostrum into the areola. If colostrum causes the bra to stick to the nipple, moistening the bra with warm water before attempting to remove it will prevent skin irritation.

Practices to Avoid

Despite information to the contrary, some expectant women may mistakenly believe that they should rub their nipples with a towel to toughen them. In light of our knowledge of how the keratin layer is built up, rubbing of any kind damages breast tissue and should not be practiced. Mothers also will want to avoid wearing tight bras and other clothing that binds the breasts. Such localized pressure on breast tissue can cause discomfort and result in plugged ducts. Advise women to

◆ avoid the use of soap or other drying agent on the nipples and areola.

◆ avoid the use of plastic liners in breast pads.

◆ avoid the use of artificial lubricants unless they are needed.

◆ avoid the use of lubricants that do not allow the skin to breathe or that must be washed off. Read labels on lotions or creams carefully.

◆ refrain from expressing colostrum prenatally.

◆ refrain from rubbing the nipples with a towel or washcloth.

◆ refrain from wearing tight, restrictive clothing.

▼ Practical Planning Suggestions

An expectant woman also can prepare her family, home, and wardrobe for breastfeeding. Suggest that she plan a quiet place in her home for feeds. She will want to consider initial sleeping arrangements for the baby, as well as clothing in her wardrobe that will accommodate breastfeeding. You can also encourage her to arrange household help for her first weeks home with her newborn. These plans and preparations, as well as learning about breastfeeding management, can be instrumental in building the woman's confidence.

Planning a Nursing Area

A few simple arrangements in the home will help the mother get a comfortable start with breastfeeding. The mother may wish to consider planning a particular space that will be convenient for feeds. She will want a quiet spot where she can relax undisturbed for 20 to 30 minutes at a time. Whether she decides to nurse in a chair or on a sofa or bed, she will want several pillows available for support so that she is able to relax and find a comfortable position. A comfortable chair with armrests will assist the mother in supporting her baby during feeds. A footstool will enable her knees to be high enough to provide additional support. Placing a small table within arm's reach will provide a place for a beverage, snack, reading materials, and any other items she may need. Just as planning for and arranging the nursery helps a woman prepare mentally for the arrival of her baby, planning a cozy nursing corner can help the breastfeeding mother feel confident and prepared for feeding her newborn at home.

Clothing Suggestions

Many representations of breastfeeding women show their upper chest area uncovered. In truth, a mother need not expose so much of her chest while feeding her baby. Breastfeeding can be done discreetly, with little of the woman's body visible. The mother can choose clothing that will cover her upper torso and allow her baby easy access to the breast. Her lower chest and abdomen will be covered by her breastfeeding infant.

The wardrobes of most women already include many items suitable for breastfeeding. Very few clothing purchases are necessary. One type of clothing is a loose-fitting item that can be opened midway. Two-piece outfits, blouses, pullovers, sweaters, and dresses with front or side openings are ideal. Blouses that button in the front can be unbuttoned from the bottom for good coverage. During feeds the mother can drape any exposed area of the breast with an open sweater, jacket, blanket, or diaper. Dark-patterned materials hide spots caused by milk leakage, and natural fiber materials are the most comfortable. Synthetic materials are less desirable because they tend to hold in moisture and do not allow the skin to breathe. Half slips make breastfeeding less cumbersome for some mothers, and other mothers adapt full slips by altering the straps. For nighttime feeds, the mother can select front-opening gowns, pajamas, or special nursing nightgowns with layered bodices.

Selecting a Nursing Bra

The mother can select a nursing bra during her last trimester of pregnancy. At that time, she will wear about the same size as when she will be breastfeeding (after the initial fullness subsides). She will want a bra that provides support and does not bind. Underwires and elastic around the cups can prevent sufficient drainage by pressing on milk ducts, and therefore, these items should be avoided. For the same reason, the seams of the bra need to be situated well past the front of the breast, toward the underarm. Suggest that the mother try on bras for proper fit before making a purchase and that she buy only one bra initially. After she wears the new bra for a while she can decide whether it meets her needs before purchasing another one.

Bra cups should be made from cotton or a cotton-polyester blend. Breast pads, handkerchiefs, or diapers can be placed inside the bra to absorb leaking. A bra with simple cup fasteners will allow easy access to the breast. The mother can try on the bra and practice unfastening and fastening the cup several times to decide whether she will be able to manage it easily with one hand. Velcro fasteners, although convenient, are sometimes noisy. This may attract attention when breastfeeding in public, and may make the mother uncomfortable. The mother will want to try a variety of bras and decide which type best fits her needs.

Planning for Help at Home

Expectant parents often receive offers of help for the first several weeks after delivery. They will want to clarify the roles of potential helpers before accepting any offers of assistance. Perhaps the father can arrange vacation time for several days while the mother and baby get settled in at home. Household chores can be handled by family and friends who offer to help so that the postpartum mother can relax, rest, and care for her baby. It is important that helpers understand that the parents will be caring for and bonding with their baby. The helpers can perform household tasks, run errands, and ensure that the mother is well rested and well nourished. Dana Raphael devotes an entire book, entitled *Breastfeeding: The Tender Gift*, to the topic of a helper for the mother. She offers practical suggestions for parents in determining what they would like the role of their helper to be. Marshall Klaus, in his book *Mothering the Mother*, describes the role of the **doula** in labor and delivery. The Greek word *doula* refers to an experienced woman who helps other women either during the birth process or in the early postpartum period. Many times, a doula extends her services to the postpartum period as well, assisting the mother at home.

Sleeping Arrangements

Parents will need to consider sleeping arrangements for their breastfed baby, especially for the early weeks. Nighttime feeds can be made easy by keeping the baby in the parents' bed or in a separate bed in the same room. In this way, the mother needs to make only minor adjustments for the baby to latch on. Limiting disruptions will make it more likely that both mother and baby will quickly return to sleep. The practice of cosleeping is increasing in the middle classes in the United States. If parents do not wish for the baby to remain in their bed, they might place an extra bed or mattress on the floor in the baby's room. When the baby falls asleep after nursing, the mother can return to her own bed and leave him undisturbed on the mattress (depending on his age and degree of mobility). Some mothers prefer a rocking chair in the baby's room for nighttime feeds. See Chapter 11 for further discussion of cosleeping and other sleep issues.

PHYSICIAN FOR MOTHER AND BABY

Women will need to select a physician for both themselves and their baby. In the United States, choice of physician is largely dictated by the insurance company that provides coverage for the mother and child. Most likely, they will have established a relationship with a gynecologist before pregnancy. They can consider whether that same physician will meet their needs regarding prenatal care and birth. Perhaps an even more important decision is that of selecting a physician for the care of the baby. This is especially an issue for a woman who plans to breastfeed. She will want to know that her baby's physician will support her plans and provide appropriate advice.

Factors to Explore in Selecting a Physician

When selecting a physician, whether it is for care of the mother or the baby, there are many things parents may want to investigate before making their choice. Parents need to be comfortable and secure in their decision, and have confidence in their physician's ability. It is of equal importance that the parents and physician are able to develop an adult working relationship. Parents want a physician who is willing to listen, respond to questions, and demonstrate flexibility in decisions. Their goal is to form a partnership with their physician to develop a health plan that will result in the most favorable outcome.

Background

Parents can check the physician's credentials and background by contacting the local hospital, requesting information from the physician's receptionist, or calling the county medical society. They may also question friends who use this physician's services. The Directory of Medical Specialists, available in any public library, will indicate whether the physician has graduated from a fully accredited medical school. Parents may also want to ask whether the physician is board certified and what his hospital standings are. These items can reflect his qualifications and professional standing.

Continuing Education

Parents can check books around the physician's office to see if they are recently published and appear to have information about breastfeeding management. They can ask about continuing education in breastfeeding and other activities such as teaching at a nearby hospital or medical school.

Hospital Affiliation

Parents will want to know if the physician is affiliated with a facility that they would consider using. Is it family centered? Have they heard positive reports from people who have used the facility, including women who have breastfed?

Accessibility

The physician should be easily accessible for scheduled visits and emergencies. Many parent questions can be answered by the nurse, nurse practitioner, or receptionist, who may have been educated to handle phone consultation. However, when there is a pressing medical concern, parents have the right, after describing a problem to the nurse, to talk directly with the physician. They also will want to choose one who, when not on duty, is covered by someone who is acceptable to them. They can ask how much time the physician allots for office visits, whether there is a specific telephone hour, and the physician's promptness of return calls.

Standing Orders

Most physicians have standing orders that apply to all patients under that physician's care. These are orders that the nursing staff follow unless they are directed otherwise. Parents will want to learn this particular physician's standing orders relative to breastfeeding and postpartum care in the hospital. Such orders may concern the administration of certain medications, routine water bottles for infants, or other practices that parents may want to discuss with the physician before delivery.

The nursing staff also have special instructions, referred to as **nursing protocol**, in all areas including breastfeeding. Parents will want to be alert to the possibility of scheduled feeding times, routine use of nipple shields or pacifiers, or routine supplementation with water bottles for all babies. If the mother and physician develop a plan that is different from the standing orders or nursing protocol, advise that they put this in writing, and that it be signed by both the parents and physician. Copies can be kept by the parents, the physician, and hospital personnel. This will help ensure that the parents' wishes are observed.

Relationship With the Patient

Parents will want a physician who genuinely listens to patients, gives understandable explanations, welcomes questions, and returns calls. Will the physician openly discuss alternatives and welcome a second opinion? What is the physician's position regarding prepared childbirth and breastfeeding? Parents may want to talk to friends who use this physician's services, discussing his or her strengths and weaknesses.

Recommending Physicians

If you are asked by a woman to recommend a physician, it is advisable to give the names of at least three physicians, when possible. This provides the woman with a choice of physicians to suit her personality and her needs. It also helps ensure that the breastfeeding women in your community will work with a variety of physicians. This increases the physicians' practical experience with management of breastfeeding. Also, it helps you remain objective in making recommendations and contacts with the medical profession.

In addition to the physicians' names, you can be prepared to give women as much factual information as is practical about each physician and at the same time, avoid any personal opinions. You may want to keep an accurate updated file on physicians, including office hours, call hours, practices related to breastfeeding, and standing orders for the hospital and office procedures. You can provide mothers with pertinent questions to ask a prospective physician. You may also use your information about physicians to help prepare mothers for their hospital experiences and pediatric group checkups. ("Dr. so-and so usually tells mothers to . . . at the first checkup. You may want to think about this before you go so that you can have any questions or concerns ready.") An informed and prepared mother is more likely to be satisfied with the outcome of her physician's visit. She is more likely to understand and follow recommendations, and less apt to need to call the physician back for clarification.

Questions to Ask the Baby's Physician

The choice of a baby's physician is an important decision for parents. Encourage them to give the selection careful consideration and investigation. They may choose either a pediatrician or family practice physician. Many parents place their baby's care under a physician who specializes in pediatrics. Suggest that the parents arrange a prenatal visit with the physician to discuss the following points.

- How soon after birth the first office visit will be scheduled.
- The number of times the physician expects to see the baby for health maintenance.
- The physician's staff privileges at the hospital where the baby will be delivered and, if none, would the physician give a referral to another pediatrician or family practitioner.
- Degree to which parents are encouraged to make nonmedical decisions such as feeding schedule, sleep patterns, supplemental foods, and weaning.
- Treatment of jaundice in the newborn.

- Viewpoint on circumcision.
- Hospital policy regarding delay of antibiotic ointment in the baby's eyes to enhance initial bonding between parents and baby.
- Policy on vitamin, iron, and fluoride supplements.
- Percentage of breastfeeding babies in the practice and the average duration of breastfeeding.
- Hospital policy regarding how soon the mother and baby can breastfeed after delivery.
- Hospital's encouragement of rooming-in.
- Breastfeeding protocol in the hospital.
- Policy on water and formula supplementation.
- Willingness to allow the mother to determine breastfeeding management.
- Management of breastfeeding problems.
- The person who answers breastfeeding questions.
- Whether there is a lactation consultant on staff.
- Whether mothers are referred to a lactation consultant if there is not one on staff.
- Criteria for starting solid foods.
- Criteria for weaning.
- Relationship with breastfeeding support groups in the community.

Working with the Physician

Make sure mothers know that it is never too late to discuss a concern with the physician. If she has second thoughts after a visit, suggest that she call her physician. While in the hospital, a mother may have questions for the physician that cannot wait until the scheduled rounds. She can ask the nursing staff to contact the physician. If the staff is busy, they may not get to this as quickly as the mother would like. She need not wait. She can place the call herself. When the mother and the physician have a plan, she can ask that the change be recorded on her or her baby's chart. Many times, physicians will be flexible when a mother explains her position and displays confidence and self-assurance.

If the mother decides to contact her physician with a concern, you can help her formulate her questions and clarify the physician's response. Ask the mother what the physician's exact words were, "you must . . ." or, "you can start solid foods now." Encourage her to share any confusion and to talk tactfully with her physician. Most physicians enjoy educating receptive parents. Encourage the mother to communicate to her physician her feelings about the importance of breastfeeding and appeal for support through difficulties.

When the Physician's Advice Seems Detrimental to Breastfeeding

You can offer suggestions to prepare a mother for dealing with a physician whose advice seems detrimental to breastfeeding. Provide her with a solid basis of information before she sees the physician. Giving her literature to take to her physician will help educate him or her about breastfeeding. Encourage the mother to work along with and inform her physician about the day-to-day management of lactation. If she is under the care of a medical team, suggest that she try to work with the physician who is the most supportive and knowledgeable about breastfeeding.

It is important that mothers understand that their physician's advice is simply that—advice. When a physician advises that a patient have his or her cholesterol checked, the patient can decide whether or not to act on the physician's advice. The physician cannot make the patient comply with the advice. Physicians advise; they do not command. Only when there is clear and definite danger for the child should there be any question that the parent must comply. Responsible parents can make responsible decisions regarding the care of their baby. This includes breastfeeding management decisions which are, for the most part, not medical in nature.

Working through Conflicts

Sometimes mothers encounter conflicts with their physicians. You can help the mother who has difficulty communicating with her physician by supporting her while being careful not to drive a wedge between the two of them. Prepare her before a visit by reminding her of typical breastfeeding management at her baby's present stage of development. Encourage the mother to prepare specific questions prior to office visits.

When seemingly detrimental advice is given, urge the mother to ask why the physician gave the advice and whether alternative treatment is possible. Help her work out solutions with her physician. Never encourage a mother to go against her physician's medical advice either openly or by implication. Help a mother adapt the physician's advice to breastfeeding if you can. If the physician insists that supplements or solid foods be given to the baby, you can help the mother accommodate it to her breastfeeding management. For instance, she may compromise by giving supplements after a breastfeed and limiting the quantity of the supplements. Suggest that she use a device for supplementing at the breast in order to adequately stimulate milk production. You might suggest that the mother ask for a trial period during which she can nurse more frequently in an effort to increase her milk production. Perhaps a checkup can be scheduled for a short time later and the decision about supplements postponed until then.

Asking for a Consultation

Often, a difficulty can be resolved if the mother asks for a consultation with another physician. It is not recommended that you suggest that a mother change physicians. This decision must be initiated by the parents. If a mother finds that she and her physician are always at odds and she wants to change, you can suggest the names of three local physicians. In this way, it does not appear that you are recommending a particular physician. Rather, you are providing several names and asking the mother to make the decision. If the mother is basically satisfied with her physician and only wants a consultation on a specific issue, she can ask her physician to arrange it with another physician whom she may name if she wishes. If you are asked, you can suggest a local physician whom you know to be qualified.

SUMMARY

You and other caregivers can be instrumental in helping parents in their decision to breastfeed. Parents are entitled to the facts that will enable them to make informed choices. Teaching and counseling parents prenatally will help them acquire this information at a time when they are considering a method of infant feeding. Help couples distinguish between breastfeeding facts and the myriad of misconceptions that cause confusion and concern. Provide practical suggestions prenatally regarding breast care and preparations at home. Be available to expectant parents who may need assistance in selecting a physician who is knowledgeable and supportive of breastfeeding. Consider offering a series of classes on breastfeeding to provide relevant information at key times. A prenatal class on infant feeding will help in the decision-making process. A later prenatal class on breastfeeding management will help parents prepare for their baby's arrival. Finally, a postpartum breastfeeding class will reinforce proper management and address any questions the parents may have as they continue breastfeeding. All of these early interventions will form a strong foundation for parents as they face hospital routines and policies regarding breastfeeding.

REFERENCES

Bryant C. Empowering women to breastfeed, *Int J Childbirth Education* 8:13–15; 1993.

Coreil J and Murphy J. "Maternal commitment, lactation practices, and breastfeeding duration." *JOGNN* 17:273–278; 1988.

Delight E et al. "What do parents expect antenatally and do babies teach them?" *Arch Dis Child* 66:1309–1314; 1991.

Freed G et al. "Accuracy of expectant mothers' predictions of fathers' attitudes regarding breast-feeding." *J Fam Pract* 37:148–152; 1922a.

Freed G et al. "Prenatal determination of demographic and attitudinal factors regarding feeding practice in an indigent population." *Am J Perinatol* 9:420–424; 1992b.

Gamble D and Morse J. "Fathers of breastfed infants: Postponing and types of involvement." JOGNN 22:358–365; 1993.

Klaus et al. "Maternal Assistance in Support in Labor: Father, Nurse, Midwife or Doula?" *Clinical Consultations in Obstetrics and Gynecology* 4; December, 1992.

Kitzinger J. "Counteracting, not reenacting, the violation of women's bodies: The challenge for perinatal caregivers." *Birth* 19:219–220; 1992.

Marchand L and Morrow M. "Infant feeding practices: Understanding the decision-making process." *Fam Med* 26:319–324; 1994.

Pridham K. "Anticipatory guidance of parents of new infants: Potential contribution of the Internal Working Model construct" *Image* 25:49–56; 1993.

Rentschler D. "Correlates of successful breastfeeding." Image 23:151–154; 1991.

Walker M. "Why aren't more mothers breastfeeding?" *Childbirth Instructor*, pp 19–24; Winter; 1992.

▼

BIBLIOGRAPHY

Auerbach K. "Breastfeeding promotion: Why it doesn't work." *J Hum Lact* 6:45–46; 1990.

Danner S. How do we influence the breastfeeding decision? Birth, 18(4):227–228; December, 1991.

Dix D. "Why women decide not to breastfeed" *Birth* 18:222–225; 1991.

Edwards M. "Group process: A tool for dynamic change." *Int J Childbirth Education*, 32–35; May, 1990.

Hanson S. "Adding pizazz to childbirth education." *Int J Childbirth Education* 8:11–12; 1993.

Hoelscher J. "Making breastfeeding user friendly." *Int J Childbirth Education* 8:30–31; 1993.

Izatt S. Breastfeeding counseling by health care providers. *J Hum Lact* 13:109–113; 1997.

Jordan P and Wall V. "Supporting the father when an infant is breastfed." *J Hum Lact* 9:31–34; 1993.

Jordan P and Wall V. "Breastfeeding and fathers: Illuminating the darker side." *Birth* 17:210–213; 1990.

Kaufman K and Hall L. "Influences of the social network on choice and duration of breastfeeding in mothers of preterm infants." *Res Nurs Health* 12:149–159; 1989.

Lawrence R. *Breastfeeding: A guide for the medical profession,* Mosby, St. Louis, MO; 1999.

Lawrence R. Roundtable: The breastfeeding decision/will it become American to breastfeed? *Birth*, 18(4):226–227; Dec 1991.

Leff E et al. Maternal Perceptions of Successful Breastfeeding, *J Hum Lact* 10(2) 99–104; 1994.

Littman H et al. "The decision to breastfeed" *Clinical Pedatrics* 214–219; April, 1994.

March of Dimes/National Foundation. Adolescent Pregnancy, Leaders Alert Bulletin, White Plains, New York; March, 1980.

Raphael D. *Breastfeeding: The Tender Gift.* New York; Schocken Books; 1976.

Ryan Alan et al. Recent declines in breastfeeding in the United States, 1984–1989, *Pediatr*, Vol 88, No 4; October, p 719; 1991.

St. Clair P and Anderson N. "Social network advice during pregnancy: Myths, misinformation, and sound counsel." *Birth* 16:103–108; 1989.

Vojta E. "Perfectly yours: A tool for teaching the benefits of breastfeeding." *J Hum Lact* 5:176; 1989.

Weissinger D. A breastfeeding teaching tool using a sandwich analogy for latch-on. *J Hum Lact* 14:51–56; 1998.

10

HOSPITAL PRACTICES THAT SUPPORT BREASTFEEDING

Contributing Author: Jan Barger

Hospital practices have a direct influence on a mother's breastfeeding experience. The establishment of breastfeeding is enhanced in an environment that is supportive and accepting, and builds the mother's self-confidence. Institutional routines need to reflect a belief in breastfeeding as the norm and facilitate sound breastfeeding management. Policies must be evidence based, rather than based on "just in case" scenarios, personal experience, or tradition. Developing hospital policies related to breastfeeding that are based on the Ten Steps to Successful Breastfeeding (WHO/UNICEF, 1989) is the first step in providing a supportive environment.

The *Ten Steps to Successful Breastfeeding* that form the basis of this discussion state that every facility providing maternity services and care for newborn infants should

1. Have a written breastfeeding policy that is routinely communicated to all health care staff.
2. Train all health care staff in skills necessary to implement this policy.
3. Inform all pregnant women about the benefits and management of breastfeeding.
4. Help mothers initiate breastfeeding within a half-hour of birth.
5. Show mothers how to breastfeed and how to maintain lactation, even if they should be separated from their infants.
6. Give newborn infants no food or drink other than breastmilk unless medically indicated.
7. Practice **rooming in**—allow mothers and infants to remain together—24 hours a day.
8. Encourage breastfeeding on demand.
9. Give no artificial teats or pacifiers (also called dummies or soothers) to breastfeeding infants.
10. Foster the establishment of breastfeeding support groups, and refer mothers to them on discharge from the hospital or clinic.

SETTING THE STAGE PRIOR TO BIRTH

Many women view caregivers as authority figures. The caregiver's opinions are valued because of their exten-

sive training and experience, and their attitudes about breastfeeding greatly influence the mother's own attitude and, indirectly, the quality of her breastfeeding. A hospital that is baby friendly fosters a climate of acceptance and support for breastfeeding mothers through supportive policies and health care professionals.

Establishing Supportive Breastfeeding Policies

STEP ONE OF THE TEN STEPS

Have a written breastfeeding policy that is routinely communicated to all health care staff.

One of the first responsibilities of the lactation consultant at a hospital may be to develop breastfeeding policies. Such policies will improve the quality of care given to breastfeeding mothers and decrease obstacles that hamper the smooth initiation of breastfeeding. Developing a set of breastfeeding policies that are based on current scientific knowledge will help eliminate a lot of unnecessary and intrusive interventions that negatively impact the initiation of breastfeeding. Policies reflect what we do and procedures describe how we do it. (Procedures are discussed in later sections.) Policies do not need to be extensive. In fact, they will be followed more closely if they are kept to the minimum number that cover the salient points. Policies are read during staff orientation periods and often left in policy books to be referred to only when there is a specific question. Posting policies where they can be reviewed frequently by the staff will facilitate improved compliance.

Policies need to be communicated to all health care staff who come into contact with breastfeeding mothers and infants. This extends beyond the nursing staff on the mother-baby unit. It includes physicians, ancillary staff, patient care technicians, and administrative staff of all units that care for mothers and babies. Staff in the neonatal intensive care unit (NICU), labor and delivery, pediatrics, and to a certain extent, the emergency room and medical-surgical units have contact with breastfeeding mothers.

▼ Teaching Breastfeeding Management to Staff

▼ STEP TWO OF THE TEN STEPS

Train all health care staff in skills necessary to implement this policy.

After policies are in place and communicated, procedures for implementation are necessary. Another job of the lactation consultant is to educate the health care staff in how to implement the breastfeeding policies. Understanding the rationale and scientific basis behind the policies will increase acceptance by both the medical and nursing staff. Training in basic breastfeeding management, such as positioning and latch, as well as how to evaluate a feed effectively and when and how to supplement infants, will free up the lactation consultant to concentrate on more difficult cases. It also ensures that mothers will get appropriate and consistent help when the lactation consultant is not available. See Chapter 24 for further discussion of staff education.

▼ Educating Pregnant Women

▼ STEP THREE OF THE TEN STEPS

Inform all pregnant women about the benefits and management of breastfeeding.

All women need to know about the benefits and management of breastfeeding. This will help them make an informed decision about how they will feed their infant. It also helps dispel any myths the mother may have. Many hospitals offer prenatal breastfeeding classes. If one does not exist in your hospital, you can initiate one. Or, you can work in cooperation with childbirth education classes to ensure that information about breastfeeding is included in every class. This approach will reach some women who may not otherwise receive it. Working with obstetric and family practice physicians and prenatal clinics will ensure they are including correct and consistent information about breastfeeding during prenatal visits.

▼ LABOR AND DELIVERY PRACTICES THAT SUPPORT EARLY BREASTFEEDING

A woman's labor and delivery experience can affect early breastfeeding and whether or not she will breastfeed her baby for a long period of time. It is very difficult to superimpose normal postpartum breastfeeding over interventionist labor and delivery practices. Policies that routinely separate mothers and babies and interfere with the process of breastfeeding are not in the best interest of mothers and babies and need to be changed. A mother needs a warm, reassuring, and caring atmosphere that supports her goals and helps her develop the self-confidence that will enable her to be comfortable with making decisions concerning her baby.

▼ Provide Labor Support

A 1991 study showed that women who had been supported during labor were more likely to be breastfeeding at 6 weeks than those who were not supported. Although support specific to breastfeeding was offered, the women also believed that they had coped well and thus were more confident. This self-confidence carried over to their feelings about mothering and breastfeeding (Hofmeyer, 1991).

Ideally, hospitals encourage laboring women to have an experienced labor support person, often referred to as a doula, with them throughout the entire labor and delivery. This results in a need for fewer medications, less anesthesia, and fewer complications. Babies are more alert and responsive after an unmedicated birth, and they are better able to begin breastfeeding within 1 to 2 hours after birth.

The presence of a doula during labor and birth provides the laboring woman with continuous physical, emotional, and informational support. The doula does not replace the baby's father or other support person chosen from among the mother's family or friends. Rather, the doula is an enhancement to the mother's support system. She is experienced in the use of comfort measures that will decrease the pain of labor without using medications or anesthesia. Furthermore, she provides ongoing support in a manner different from that of the baby's father.

Women are more effective than men in supporting women during labor, regardless of how loving and supportive the man desires to be. Studies show that the presence of a doula results in fewer interventions for the mother and baby. It can reduce the overall cesarean birth rate by 50 percent, the length of labor by 25 percent, pitocin use by 40 percent, pain medication by 30 percent, the need for **forceps** by 40 percent, and requests for epidural anesthesia by 60 percent (Klaus, 1992).

▼ Limit Interventions

The use of medications, anesthesia, and other interventions during the labor and birth process can affect early breastfeeding and influences whether a baby is breastfed for a long period of time. It can be difficult to achieve normal and optimal postpartum breastfeeding management after a labor and delivery that involved interventions. Policies that routinely separate mothers and babies interfere with breastfeeding and are unnecessary.

Non-Essential Routine Interventions

Between the years 1975 and 1982, the United States experienced the peak of the natural childbirth movement. During that same time period, the breastfeeding initiation rate increased from 25 percent to 62 percent. This was followed by more than a decade during which medical interventions in birth increased by more than 50 percent—interventions such as medications, epidural anesthesia, intravenous drugs, electronic fetal monitors, and cardiac monitors. During the same period, breastfeeding initiation declined from 62 percent to 51 percent. Between 1991 and 1997, the breastfeeding initiation rate rose from 51 percent to 62.4 percent.

Labor and birth are normal biologic processes that need to be treated as such. The events that surround birth clearly have an impact on breastfeeding (Hofmeyer, 1991; Matthews, 1989). Traditionally, American hospitals have evolved to rely on an increased use of technology. In order for breastfeeding to get off to a good start, the routine use of technology surrounding birth must be limited. Mothers need to be given an opportunity and assistance to put the baby to breast within 1 hour of birth unless there is a clearly identifiable and justifiable reason for intervention.

Medications Used in Labor

Medications that the mother receives during labor may cause babies to become drowsy and to have difficulty suckling. They may also make mothers less responsive to their babies. It is best to avoid these drugs when possible. Caregivers need to acquaint themselves with techniques that are least likely to interfere with breastfeeding, such as the use of support persons, walking, bathing, birthing balls, and the like (Bond, 1992).

Analgesia

Mothers frequently are given analgesia such as nalbuphine, alphaprodine, butorphanol, and meperidine to reduce labor pain. Matthews, in a 1989 study, found that the babies of mothers who received Nisentil 1 to 3 hours before delivery took an average of 21.2 hours to establish effective breastfeeding. Only 66 percent were breastfeeding effectively by 24 hours. On the other hand, babies whose mothers received no central nervous system depressants in labor took only 11.8 hours to establish feeds, and 93 percent were breastfeeding effectively by 24 hours. Mothers who have been medicated during labor are more likely to leave the hospital without having established breastfeeding.

Epidural Anesthesia

At present, no studies exist that explore the effects of epidural anesthesia specifically on babies and their abilities to breastfeed. However, a 1992 study by Sepkoski noted that women who received epidural anesthesia in labor were given significantly more Pitocin in labor, had more forceps deliveries, and spent less time with their babies while in the hospital. The babies of these mothers had poorer behavioral outcome and recovery and less alertness and ability to orient over the first month of life. Also, they were less mature in their motor function. Furthermore, traces of bupivucaine, an anesthesia used in epidurals, have been found in the babies' **cord blood** and in the neonate's blood up to 3 days after delivery. Sepkoski suggests that the depressed performance of infants may be a direct result of the anesthetic on the neonatal central nervous system. A later study showed that mothers who receive epidurals during labor have an increased incidence of intrapartum fever. The baby may then also be worked up for sepsis, receive antibiotics, and be transferred to the NICU (Liberman, 1997). It has been noted that the earlier an epidural is given, the higher the risk of cesarean birth (Morton, 1994).

Other Interventions During Labor and Delivery

Medical interventions that are used frequently and routinely during labor and birth have been observed clinically to increase the risk of interference with breastfeeding. Many of these interventions result from the overuse of central nervous system depressants and epidural anesthesia. Women need to be empowered to birth their babies without the use of medications and anesthesia, and be given the support to do so.

Women who have had an **episiotomy** often find it difficult to get comfortable, particularly when they sit upright. An episiotomy also increases the risk of a fourth-degree laceration, which is a tear through the rectal mucosa. If the mother is not comfortable when she is sitting, it is difficult for her to relax enough to focus on getting the baby positioned well at the breast. Because pain can inhibit the mother's milk ejection reflex, she may also need more analgesia, which can be transferred in small doses to the infant.

Hospital staff may be inclined to put a baby to breast immediately after deep suctioning and visualization of the larynx, in an attempt to soothe him. However, this practice can have disastrous consequences for breastfeeding. Some babies appear to associate breastfeeding with the pain that preceded their first experience at the breast and to react negatively whenever put to breast.

Forceps and **vacuum extraction** both carry an increased risk of bruising and sensitivity to the infant's head. This problem will limit the ways in which he can be held comfortably for early breastfeeds. Bruising also increases the risk of jaundice, thereby causing sleepiness and a lack of interest in feeding.

Pitocin, used to induce or stimulate labor, has an antidiuretic effect. Edema may result, particularly in extremities such as the breast and nipple tissue. The result may be "meaty" and "flat" nipples. It will be difficult for the infant to latch on until the edema is relieved, generally in about 3 days. Lactation consultants have noted that women who receive many liters of IV fluids in conjunction with epidurals and pitocin seem to experience a delay in milk production which may be due to edema in the breast.

Babies often are placed in radiant warmers because of their inability to regulate their own temperatures. However, warmers are unnecessary if the mother and baby are allowed to remain together in skin-to-skin contact. Clinical observation shows that babies who are snuggled skin to skin with their mothers kangaroo style warm faster, stay warm longer, and have less risk of dehydration than babies placed under radiant warmers (Christensson, 1992). Skin-to-skin contact allows for the maintenance of adequate temperature without increased fluid loss. The infant's nose is near the mother's skin, and thus, the infant breathes warm, humidified air, rather than dry hospital air. The heat from the mother's body is humidified, unlike the dry air from artificial warmers. This finding was supported by a study from Nepal showing that the mother's body successfully prevents hypothermia in the newborn (Johanson, 1992).

The longer a mother waits to initiate breastfeeding, the more likely she will be to feed her baby infant formula in the first few days of life. Kurinji (1991) reports that "this implies that hospital staff and routines, centered around a formula-feeding mode, can by suggestion influence maternal-infant feeding behavior. These nonverbal hospital routines may be responsible for the observed differences in exclusive breastfeeding rates between hospitals." The routines cited include delayed first feeding, rising cesarean birth rate, decreased mother-baby contact, and feeding on a schedule. The labor and delivery staff can preserve and protect breastfeeding by removing these obstacles. Avoiding the need for an episiotomy and other technologic assistance increases comfort for the mother and her baby.

Promote Bonding

Expectant parents have experienced 9 months of anxious waiting, and finally, their baby arrives. Ideally, they will be able to spend the initial moments with their baby, hugging, smiling, loving, and nursing. They will flourish in their transition to parenthood in a supportive environment that enables them to begin their new family in privacy—an environment that is both baby-friendly and mother-friendly.

The Moments Immediately After Birth

When an infant leaves the comfortable secure confines of his mother's womb, he finds himself in an unfamiliar and perhaps unsettling environment. When he is placed in the comfort of his mother's arms, he is warmed by her body heat and can nuzzle at her breast. Bonding between the mother and her baby is strongest in the first 1 or 2 hours. It is enhanced even further with skin-to-skin contact. A newborn's rooting and sucking reflexes are particularly strong in the first hour or two after an unmedicated delivery. The mother's normal body bacteria will colonize her baby's body—but only if she is the first person to hold him rather than a nurse, physician, or others. Keeping the mother and baby together will accomplish all of this.

Soon after birth, the infant is observed, assessed, and given an Apgar score—which evaluates the baby's heart rate, respiratory effort, body tone, grimace and color—with a score ranging from 0 to 10. The Apgar score will indicate his overall state of health and assists the caregivers in determining if any intervention is necessary. It is performed at 1 minute of life and again at 5 and 10 minutes of life. This need not interfere with bonding, however. It can be performed with no interference while the infant is held by his mother.

State laws require that all newborn infants' eyes be treated with an antibiotic to safeguard against the effects of sexually transmitted disease. This procedure, however, can be delayed to allow the parents and baby at least 1 hour of uninterrupted time together. Postponing antibiotic treatment of the baby's eyes allows eye contact and enhances bonding between the parents and baby.

The Bonding Process

John Kennell and Marshall Klaus (1976) popularized the term "bonding" in their book *Maternal-Infant Bonding*. They discuss many aspects of bonding or attachment and the consequences of separation on this process. Importance is placed on close physical contact between the mother and baby soon after birth, as well as the detrimental effects of routine hospital practices which separate them. Delayed contact following birth and strict feeding schedules, with the baby spending the majority of time in the nursery, were two practices found to discourage the development of attachment. The most favorable time to initiate bonding was found to be during the first minutes after birth, when the baby is alert and the parents are most eager to see and touch their baby.

The process of bonding begins with the first parent-infant contact in the hours following birth, and continues as parent and infant interact to form a unique lasting relationship. This close emotional tie develops through exchanging messages and feelings with all their senses—sight, touch, smell, taste, and sound. Parents often express attachment through touching, fondling, talking to, and kissing their babies while holding them face to face. Babies reciprocate through recognition of and response to the parents' overtures. They smile, follow their parents' image with their eyes, and show signs of contentment and acceptance. The skin and eye contact, the pattern of the parent speaking, and the baby responding, as well as other interchanges, are essential to building a loving relationship. Time spent together soon after birth encourages affectionate contact between parent and child throughout the child's formative years.

The Positive Results of Bonding

Studies cited by Kennel and Klaus (1982) showed that extended contact (contact beyond regular feeding times) between mother and baby during the first 3 days of life resulted in behavioral and developmental advantages for the child during the early years of life. Mothers who had extended contact showed a higher incidence of breastfeeding and more responsive behavior to their children, with more fondling and face-to-face contact. At 3 months, these mothers perceived their adaptation to their infants to be easier and expressed fewer problems with nighttime feeds, despite the fact that nighttime feeds lasted almost twice as long as those in the control group. When observed during a 10-minute play period at 3 months of age, early-contact babies and mothers smiled and faced one another more. At 5 years, the children had significantly higher I.Q.s and better-developed skills.

It is important to keep in mind that bonding encompasses the affectionate attachment of both mother and father to their newborn infant. Fathers find touching, fondling, and talking to their newborn babies pleasing and necessary to form close emotional ties. Interestingly, the father's fascination with his baby may be mixed with some jealousy about the more intimate relationship between the mother and her breastfeeding baby. It is the bonding and the building of love for the baby that helps the father adjust to the new family relationships.

Help Mothers Initiate Breastfeeding

STEP FOUR OF THE TEN STEPS

Help mothers initiate breastfeeding within a half-hour of birth.

Baby-friendly hospital procedures facilitate early breastfeeding for mothers and babies. Studies show that mothers who breastfeed immediately after birth breastfeed longer than mothers who must wait. A 1994 study revealed that mothers who took no medication in labor established effective breastfeeding within 6.4 hours, compared with 50.3 hours for those who breastfed immediately and received analgesia. Mothers who received no analgesia and whose first breastfeed was 1 hour or more after delivery took 49.7 hours to establish effective breastfeeding. Those whose first feed was delayed and who also received analgesia took 62.5 hours (Crowell, 1994). This finding has implications for mothers who leave the hospital at 48 hours. They may not yet have established effective feedings by the time of discharge.

There are many health advantages to the initiation of breastfeeding as early as possible. Mothers who breastfeed in the delivery room are likely to breastfeed longer than those who initiated breastfeeding 12 to 16 hours later (Sousa, 1974). Increased oxytocin secretion from suckling contracts the uterus more quickly and controls bleeding. Routine use of synthetic oxytocin is not necessary when mothers breastfeed after delivery. Colostrum clears meconium from the baby's gut and provides immunologic factors. Delaying the first bath allows for the **vernix** to soak into the baby's skin, lubricating and protecting it. It also prevents temperature loss, which could interfere with the first breastfeed.

Helping mothers maintain **hydration** during labor can support their early breastfeeding. Dehydration can deplete a woman's energy, which, in turn, may have a subtle impact on her birth and early feeding experiences. Women should be allowed to labor in any position they choose rather than required to labor lying down. When a woman labors while lying down, she may experience more difficulty during the second stage of labor due to the fact that gravity is not assisting her. Following a difficult second stage and delivery, she may experience further difficulty with the initiation of breastfeeding.

Let the Baby Lead the Way

It is unnecessary to hurry and force babies to breast. A mother and her unwrapped baby can be left alone to remain quietly in skin-to-skin contact until they both are ready to breastfeed. A warmed blanket placed over both of them will prevent heat loss. When the mother and baby are quietly kept skin to skin, the baby typically works through prefeeding behaviors such as bringing his hands to his mouth and making sucking motions. This is an excellent time to teach feeding cues and encourage mothers to respond to them. See Chapter 11 for a discussion of infant feeding cues.

A 1987 study by Widstrom, and repeated by Righard and Alade in 1990, showed that babies who were left on their mother's abdomen undisturbed would accomplish breastfeeding on their own. They would crawl up the mother's abdomen, search out the nipple, latch on, and suckle—all within about 1 hour of the birth. Babies who were left with their mother for 20 minutes, and then taken to another part of the delivery room to receive eye drops and be washed, dried, suctioned, and so on had a great deal of difficulty remembering what to do.

Widstrom advises that suckling and feeding develop in a predictable and organized way after birth. Nutritive sucking can be affected adversely when drugs that depress the central nervous system are given to the mother in labor. Mothers who were given medication in labor (pethidine, in this case) had babies who could not suck correctly. None of the babies who both were taken away from their mothers after 20 minutes and whose mother's were given pethidine during labor, were able to latch onto the breast in the delivery room. According to Widstrom, it takes an average of 55 minutes for most babies to move to the breast, attach, and begin to suckle. To facilitate this process, hospital practices need to allow mothers and babies to stay together for at least 2 hours with no interference.

Help with the First Breastfeed

Birth attendants can help this natural process described by Widstrom by placing the baby in skin-to-skin contact with the mother's abdomen or chest immediately after birth and covering both the mother and baby with a warm blanket. The mother can make the breast available close to the baby's mouth and allow him to lick and explore the breast. A caregiver should be available to help with attachment if the baby wishes to breastfeed yet has not started spontaneously within 1 hour. The mother can initiate the rooting reflex by gently stroking her baby's mouth area with her nipple. In response, her baby will turn toward the nipple and open his mouth. (The rooting reflex is described further in Chapter 11.) The early moments of bonding can be further supported by keeping mothers and babies together as they leave the delivery area (if they are to be in a different room for their postpartum stay).

Breastfeeding After a Cesarean Delivery

Cesarean delivery does not preclude early breastfeeding. A mother who has delivered surgically can breastfeed as soon as the repair is completed and she has been moved to the recovery room. Occasionally, a mother may receive general anesthesia for the cesarean delivery. In this case, she may breastfeed as soon as she is awake and able to respond. Use of general anesthesia does not rule out breastfeeding.

You can help the mother who has undergone cesarean delivery find a comfortable position for breastfeeding. Lying on her side with her baby placed next to her will help avoid incisional pain in the first hours. It also permits breastfeeding even if the mother's head must remain down after spinal anesthesia. Pillows can be placed under the top knee, supporting her abdomen, and behind her back. Another position is for the mother to lie flat with the baby lying on top of her. When she feeds in a sitting position, a pillow can be placed over the surgical incision to cushion it from the pressure of the baby's body. Additional pillows can be placed under her knees to provide support. She might also hold her baby along the side of her body, with the arm closest to the breast, tucking her baby under her arm (known as a **clutch hold** or **football hold**). A positive experience with the initiation of breastfeeding helps normalize the postpartum experience for mothers, who may feel a sense of failure or disappointment that they were not able to give birth vaginally.

CREATING A SUPPORTIVE POSTPARTUM CLIMATE

Treating women as individuals, and understanding their lifestyle and previous experiences regarding breastfeeding and parenting, helps facilitate their learning. Mothers and caregivers must have realistic expectations for the early days of breastfeeding. Both need to understand that while breastfeeding is meant to be instinctive, it often requires learning and practice to accomplish. In the early hours and days especially, encourage mothers to be flexible and patient. First-time breastfeeding mothers are novices, as are their babies. They need time and patience to adjust to one another's idiosyncracies as they learn to work together as a team. The mother may feel awkward and clumsy at times. In an accepting atmosphere, her awkwardness will not deter her from continuing. A relaxed and supportive climate will encourage her to seek help, to laugh at any missteps, and to help her baby learn to breastfeed effectively.

Taking time to instruct the mother and showing a willingness to listen to her concerns will demonstrate to her the importance of breastfeeding. This, in turn, will encourage her to put forth extra effort to continue, ultimately making the caregiver's role easier and more rewarding. Quality time spent instructing each mother is paid back tenfold through her assuming responsibility for her baby's care and for her decisions. Your efforts in teaching and supporting the mother will produce long-term health benefits for both mother and baby.

▼ Eliminate Negative and Unnecessary Practices

In order to dispel anxiety of the unknown, the pregnant woman can learn as much as possible about the hospital's routines and procedures so that she will know what to expect during her stay. A hospital setting may produce varying degrees of interference for the mother. She will experience continual interruptions from an array of people entering her room at any hour of the day and night. Her obstetrician will visit her daily to check on her progress. The pediatrician may come to her room to examine her baby or to report to her daily about her baby's progress. The nursing staff will enter her room periodically throughout the day and night to check her baby, monitor her temperature and blood pressure, examine any incisions and intravenous line, check her uterus and breasts, provide medications and snacks, fill her water pitcher, and change her bed linens. Dietary personnel will bring meals and later pick up empty trays and menus. Housekeeping personnel will clean her bathroom daily and dust the room. A representative from the baby photo company may stop by and take the baby for pictures, while someone else comes in to get information for the birth certificate. Other interruptions may occur from members of maintenance, television services, volunteer services and clergy—not to mention friends and relatives who come for a personal visit. And these interruptions will be doubled if she is sharing her room with another new mother! You can help mothers limit interference by encouraging them to request that visitors wait until they are at home to visit.

Routines that limit interruptions are a positive contribution to breastfeeding. Routines that inhibit mother-infant interaction, practices that imply possible failure, and incorrect problem solving can all influence both short-term and long-term breastfeeding. Such practices are often dictated by tradition and misinformation. With some exceptions, the degree of knowledge regarding breastfeeding management is relatively low among the general population of nurses and physicians (Anderson, 1991). Breastfeeding advice may derive from personal experience or misconceptions rather than fact-based information. In the absence of sound knowledge of breastfeeding practices, erroneous and incorrect advice can lead to a bumpy start for the mother and baby.

Give Nothing But Mothers' Milk

STEP SIX OF THE TEN STEPS

Give newborn infants no food or drink other than breast-milk, unless medically indicated.

There is clear evidence that breastfeeding infants do not need supplemental water (DeCarvalho, 1981). Newborns who breastfeed frequently from birth, every 2 to 3 hours or in response to feeding cues, never need water and seldom need an artificial substitute. Routine use of glucose water or formula for breastfeeding babies should be discouraged. Their use may set up long-term allergies and implies to the mother that her milk alone may not be sufficient. This undermines her confidence in her ability to provide adequate nourishment for her baby. Infant formulas or water, or both, are often incorrectly introduced to supplement colostrum. The misconception that colostrum is insufficient for total nourishment needs to be corrected. The only time breastfeeding babies should receive any type of supplement is in the rare instance of a specific medical need. In the event of a medical need for supplemental food, the supplement should be offered in small amounts and only after a breastfeed. Supplements should not be given routinely and should never be left with a mother without specific instructions for their use.

Acceptable Medical Reasons for Supplements

In light of the many concerns related to the use of artificial baby milk, it is important to note that on rare occasions, exceptions may arise. For the vast majority of babies, human milk is their normal and expected source of nourishment and protection. However it is crucial that you be aware of those situations in which human milk may need to be supplemented, either by the mother's expressed milk, donor human milk, or an artificial baby milk. There are also rare situations in which breastfeeding must be avoided altogether. The 1997 AAP statement, for instance, says that untreated active tuberculosis, human immunodeficiency virus (HIV)–positive status of the mother, a small number of drugs (mostly cancer chemotherapy agents), and illegal drugs should contraindicate breastfeeding. Human T-cell lymphocytic virus type 1 (HTLV-1) is usually a contraindication as well.

The debate regarding preterm infants and their nutritional needs, as previously discussed, may continue for some time. The need for human milk fortifiers is under study, even in preterm infants who weigh as much as 1850 g. The scientists agree that more study is needed to determine clearer recommendations (Lucas, 1996;

Sankaran, 1996). Babies who experience hypoglycemia that does not improve through increased breastfeeding need to receive additional human milk by an alternate means such as cup, dropper, or spoon until breastfeeding is established. If a baby is in a situation in which he is experiencing acute water loss, such as with **phototherapy** for jaundice, supplementation of expressed milk may be required if increased breastfeeds are not able to meet his needs. Babies with certain inborn errors of metabolism, such as **phenylketonuria**, need supplementation to breastfeeds. Infants with **galactosemia** are unable to breastfeed altogether.

In rare instances, the baby may be able to breastfeed but the mother is not. If the mother experiences a severe illness, such as psychosis, **eclampsia**, or shock, breastfeeding and expressing mother's milk may be postponed. In countries with sanitary conditions and a safe water supply, HIV-positive mothers are advised to not breastfeed. Should a mother need to take certain medications such as cytotoxic, radioactive, or antithyroid (other than propylthiouracil) drugs, she will be unable to breastfeed while the drug levels to which the baby is exposed are harmful to him. This may necessitate temporary interruption of breastfeeding while the mother expresses her milk to maintain milk production. Also, the mother could wean totally and feed her baby donor milk or infant formula (WHO/UNICEF, 1993). See Chapter 23 for further discussion of circumstances that require supplementation.

Give No Artificial Teats to Infants

STEP NINE OF THE TEN STEPS

Give no artificial teats or pacifiers (also called dummies or soothers) to breastfeeding infants.

A baby suckles differently on an artificial nipple than on the breast, so the use of bottles and pacifiers can cause considerable confusion for some babies. Although some babies may not be confused when given an artificial nipple, they may prefer the smaller, longer, rigid latex or silicone nipple, which fits in their mouth like their fingers. Baby-friendly hospitals avoid the use of bottles unless there is an indication that supplements are medically indicated. And even then, if the need for **supplementary feeds** arises, an alternate feeding method is used, rather than a bottle with an artificial nipple. (Alternate feeding methods are discussed in Chapter 19.) If the mother is not rooming in with her baby, she can ask that the baby be brought to her when he is hungry and at frequent intervals. She can also instruct the nursery to bring her baby to her during the night for feeds.

Restrict the Use of Nipple Shields

A nipple shield is another type of artificial teat, which is placed over the mother's nipple. Hospital personnel may give a mother a nipple shield to protect a sore nipple or to help the baby pull out a nipple that is difficult to grasp. Use of a nipple shield is not an appropriate intervention for nipple soreness. Sore nipples usually occur due to poor positioning, which can easily be corrected. The nipple shield should not be given to the mother as a quick fix for a baby who cannot latch on. Because use of a nipple shield can interfere with milk production, it is vital that it not be used without specific guidelines and careful clinical supervision and informed consent. Furthermore, it should not be used before the mother's milk has increased enough in volume so that milk can actually flow through it. See Chapter 19 for guidelines on the use of a nipple shield. A nipple shield should be used only as a last resort—after all other alternatives have been tried.

Place No Restrictions on Feeds

Baby-friendly hospitals place no rules or restrictions on feedings. Most hospitals will state that they encourage breastfeeding in response to feeding cues. However, in facilities in which babies are kept in the nursery for most of the day, babies are customarily fed on a schedule of every 3 or 4 hours, or when they cry. Feeding a baby on such a rigid schedule or ignoring his natural feeding cues does not help the mother learn how to respond to those cues, and often does not allow the baby to begin feeding before he is frantic. Additionally, when feeds are delayed or rigidly scheduled, milk production is slowed and mothers experience increased breast engorgement.

Feeding restrictions also cause an increase in the incidence of jaundice and hypoglycemia in the baby (DeCarvalho, 1985; Varimo, 1986). Clinicians refer to this as "lack of breastfeeding jaundice," indicating that the jaundice is a result of the mismanagement of breastfeeding. If the mother finds herself governed by a rigid schedule, she may not be breastfeeding often enough to stimulate milk production or satisfy her baby. Many hospitals maintain a 3- or 4-hour schedule depending on the baby's birth weight. In this case, the mother can ask her baby's physician to order a 3-hour feeding schedule regardless of the baby's birth weight. Baby-friendly hospitals place no rules or restrictions on feedings and keep babies with their mothers.

Promote Practices That Support Breastfeeding

An integral element of an accepting atmosphere is a strong set of protocols that will enable the mother and baby to establish breastfeeding smoothly. Baby-friendly practices encourage the mother to be with her infant. This practice transmits a belief in the mother's ability to breastfeed and provides sound principles of breastfeeding management. Mothers and babies remain together from the moment of birth, followed by rooming in for the remainder of the hospital stay.

▼ STEP SEVEN OF THE TEN STEPS

Practice rooming in—allow mothers and infants to remain together—24 hours a day.

Encourage Rooming In

Rooming in is a component of family-centered maternity care that is an option available in most hospitals (Fig. 10.1). Parents may need to make prior arrangements for this accommodation and may require a private or semiprivate room. Rooming in provides maximum opportunity for the mother and infant to interact. Keeping the baby with the mother in her room increases the mother's self-confidence in handling her baby. She learns to recognize hunger cues and can feed her baby as frequently as he desires. It is also reassuring for the mother to have her baby close, rather than in the nursery where she cannot see and respond to him. Encourage rooming in as soon as the mother can care for her baby. If feasible, having a support person stay with the mother on the postpartum unit will facilitate earlier rooming in.

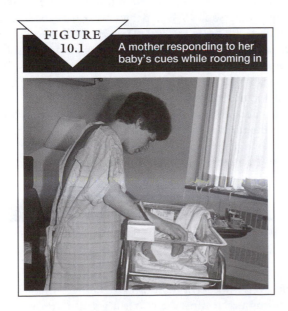

▼ FIGURE 10.1   A mother responding to her baby's cues while rooming in

Variations in Rooming In Policies

The availability of the various types of rooming in arrangements varies from one hospital to another. Prenatally, through childbirth education classes and their prenatal care providers, parents need to be informed of the rooming-in options open to them. They can then locate a hospital that will meet their needs. Twenty-four–hour rooming in allows the baby to stay with the mother at all times. Some hospitals allow the baby to remain with the mother during the day except when she is sleeping or showering, with the baby taken to the nursery at night. Other hospitals require that the baby also return to the nursery during visiting hours. Flexible rooming in permits the mother to have her baby in her room and to take him to the nursery if the need arises.

Many mothers find that flexible rooming in, beginning from the moment of birth, is the most desirable arrangement. It offers new parents the chance to get acquainted with their baby and learn to care for him before assuming sole responsibility at home. It also allows the mother with older children an opportunity to get to know her new baby before returning home and dividing her time between her new baby and her other children.

Benefits of Rooming In to Breastfeeding

Hospital practices alone do not determine how long breastfeeding continues. However, there is clear evidence for the correlation between rooming in and longer breastfeeding duration (Lindenberg, 1990; Nylander, 1991). Positive effects are found especially when the rooming in is accompanied by guidance for the mother (Perez-Escamilla, 1992). In a 1991 study, parents who knew their babies' abilities were better able to notice them (Delight, 1991).

Rooming in offers physical and emotional benefits to the entire family. It promotes bonding and immediate relief of fussiness and hunger, and incorporates the baby into the family unit immediately after birth. The frequent feeds made possible by this arrangement reduce breast engorgement and encourage early milk production in the breastfeeding mother. Mothers who room in with babies and take no pain or sleep medications sleep just as well as mothers who take medication and leave their babies in the nursery (Keefe, 1988).

Mothers who room in and care for their babies around the clock have babies who are better breastfeeders. The babies have a less disorganized cry, startle less frequently, and feed more often than babies cared for in central nurseries. Optimal feeding occurs when the baby gives cues such as mouthing and hand-to-mouth activity (Anderson, 1989). Rooming in enables mothers to recognize and respond to their babies' hunger cues.

A 1990 study found that babies who room in have more frequent feeds and greater weight gain. The authors suggest that because rooming in promotes caregiver response, the infant experiences less crying and movement, thereby conserving energy (Yamauchi, 1990). It is clear that keeping mothers and babies together during their hospital stay promotes learning and enhances the mother's self confidence. In this baby-friendly environment, the mother learns feeding cues and breastfeeding techniques in a setting where she can have her questions answered and her techniques evaluated (Anderson, 1989). Mothers are also able to provide antibodies to the microbes in the vicinity. If a baby is kept in a nursery with its own set of pathogens, the mother's milk will not reflect this.

Leaving Babies to Cry in the Nursery

Centralized nurseries with babies cared for by nursing staff most of the 24 hours are still present in many hospitals. It is not uncommon for several babies to be found crying in the nursery at any given time. Gene Cranston Anderson (1989) advises that "the belief that newborn infants need to cry is not true." In healthy, full-term infants, an adequate functional reserve is present in the lungs after the first breath. The lungs are as fully expanded at 30 minutes after birth as they are at 24 hours. Newborns who are allowed to self-regulate their care by being cared for by their mothers cry less than those whose care is controlled externally by hospital staff. In the first hour after birth, newborns in Anderson's study whose feeds were time controlled cried for 10 minutes, startled 12 times, and cried for 38 minutes during the first 4 hours. Babies who self-regulated their care cried less than 1 minute in the first hour after birth. They did not startle and they cried only 2 minutes during the first 4 hours after birth. Sucking pressures were four times as strong, and blood pressure averaged 10 mm/Hg (millimeters of mercury) lower than babies who were under time-controlled care. Blood glucose levels stay higher when babies do not cry. Crying uses up glycogen stores and drops glucose levels.

STEP EIGHT OF THE TEN STEPS

Encourage breastfeeding on demand.

Teach Mothers Feeding Cues

Encouraging breastfeeding on demand implies that the mother respond to her baby's feeding cues. There is a clear relationship between the baby's feeding schedule and the establishment of sound breastfeeding management. The ideal schedule allows the baby to nurse whenever he demonstrates feeding cues. This is one of the most important ways in which breastfeeding can get off to a good start. It ensures the early establishment of milk production through frequent breast stimulation

and milk removal. Feeding in response to feeding cues encourages bonding between the mother and baby and helps avoid milk stasis, which can lead to problems such as breast engorgement or plugged ducts.

Hospital policies that reflect responding to the baby's cues will help mothers learn to recognize their baby's hunger cues. Newborns become hungry anywhere from every 1½ to 3 hours, and sometimes sooner. They may feed every 1 to 1½ hours three or four times and then sleep for 4 or 5 hours. Observing the number of feeds in 24 hours rather than timed intervals between feeds is more normal for the infant and mother. It is important to remember and teach mothers that babies go to the breast and demonstrate feeding cues for reasons other than just hunger. They may be hungry or thirsty. They may be uncomfortable or need to suckle for comfort. Also, they may need to pass gas or have a bowel movement. Breastfeeding is not just another method of feeding a baby. It is a relationship that needs to be nurtured. Mothers may assume that they do not have enough milk if the baby wants to go to the breast so frequently. It is important to help them understand how to know their baby is getting enough to eat, and that nurturing is an important component of breastfeeding.

Breastfeeding during the night is essential for establishing milk production. Whenever a baby wakes at night, he should be breastfed, not offered pacifiers, water, or an artificial substitute. Many mothers make up missed sleep by napping during the daytime. Frequent feeds day and night encourage early milk production and decrease uncomfortable breast fullness.

Some understand demand feeding to mean feeding the baby when he cries. However, most babies show feeding cues (see Chapter 11) such as mouthing and hand-to-mouth activity, for up to 30 minutes before sustained crying (Anderson, 1989). Babies who have been crying have difficulty breastfeeding. They are unable to organize themselves to focus on feeding. Crying compromises and disorganizes their suck, and sucking strength drops. Pediatrician William Sears (1993) suggests that "crying is good for the lungs like bleeding is good for the veins". Parents need to learn how to respond to their baby's cues before he reaches the crying stage.

Show Mothers How to Breastfeed

STEP FIVE OF THE TEN STEPS

Show mothers how to breastfeed and how to maintain lactation, even if they should be separated from their infants.

Help every mother initiate breastfeeding, either directly or through educating the maternity staff to provide such education. Nurses often cite lack of time as a barrier to adequate lactation assistance (Patton, 1996). However, time taken by the maternity staff for the early initiation of breastfeeding will help the mother establish sound breastfeeding management. She will avoid difficulties that would require additional staff time later in problem solving. Policy needs to reflect that every breastfeeding mother receive basic instruction in breastfeeding management and that a knowledgeable caregiver be present for the first feed to assist and answer questions.

Recognize that some mothers may need no help. Although mothers may require help in getting started breastfeeding, many have an important need for privacy during feeds. Provisions need to be made for breastfeeding mothers to feed their babies in a quiet, uninterrupted setting. Hospital rooms need to provide privacy and a comfortable chair for breastfeeding mothers. There should also be comfortable accommodations in the nursery for mothers who wish to breastfeed their babies there.

Being a novice at breastfeeding, the infant may have difficulty in his initial attempts or he may be a natural pro. Many newborns sleep most of the time. It is not uncommon for an infant born in the hospital to show little interest in nursing the first few times the mother brings him to breast. A breastfeeding baby may lose up to 7 percent of his birth weight during the first week. Generally he will regain birth weight by 10 days to 2 weeks. It is important that the mother be aware of this pattern so that she does not become concerned by his initial weight loss. An infant who enjoys unrestricted access to the breast may experience little or no weight loss.

Teach Breast Care

Teaching mothers appropriate breast care will help them avoid the discomfort of nipple soreness. Healthy skin contains sufficient moisture to keep it soft and pliable. When the baby nurses, there is additional moisture on the breast from the mother's milk and the baby's saliva. Following a feed, the mother can keep her breast skin healthy by leaving her breasts exposed to the air until the moisture has dissipated. She can pat her nipples dry with a soft cloth or, if she is wearing a bra, leave her bra flap down for a short time to remove excessive moisture. Air drying is especially important if the mother plans to apply a lubricant to her nipples. The lubricant will trap moisture unless the nipples are thoroughly dry before application.

The nipples require no treatment unless they are tender or sore. The healthy nipple needs no special attention other than observing practices that will preserve the health of the skin. Avoiding any drying agents, such as soap and shampoo, from touching the nipples will help keep them from chafing. Standing in the shower and allowing the water to stream over the breasts provides sufficient cleansing. If the mother's nipples are sore or tender, she can shield them from the direct spray of water, by either turning her back to the shower or covering her breasts with her hands.

Provide Effective Discharge Planning

Many women will begin breastfeeding with no prior reading or instruction. Some may not even have made the decision to breastfeed until the baby arrives. You may need to guide a new mother in making this decision and help her examine its benefits. After the decision is made, it cannot be assumed that a mother will automatically know what to do, even if she has learned about breastfeeding previously. Once she is caring for her baby, a review of breastfeeding techniques will help her relate to the information more readily than she did before the baby arrived.

The postpartum period is a time in the mother's parenting experience when she is eager to listen and learn what to do—a teachable moment. The postpartum nursing staff must be prepared to provide this vital information to new mothers. Before hospital discharge, the mother will need to understand basic breastfeeding management and how to assess her baby's needs. Learning about typical patterns of feeding and breastfeeding milestones will help her know what to expect. This will help prevent problems and aid her in continuing to breastfeed for as long as she desires.

A variety of infant care matters tend to become breastfeeding issues if the mother is unaware of the typical pattern for newborns. A baby who has a fussy period in the late afternoon may be exhibiting typical newborn characteristics. The mother may misinterpret it as a problem with her milk production and begin to question her ability to breastfeed. Often concerns related to sleep, crying, and sucking needs are associated with breastfeeding because of its unique nature. Providing anticipatory guidance regarding these normal concerns will help mothers to view them appropriately.

Provide Follow-Up Care

> **▼ STEP TEN OF THE TEN STEPS**
>
> Foster the establishment of breastfeeding support groups and refer mothers to them on discharge from the hospital or clinic.

A typical brief hospital stay leaves little time for teaching breastfeeding classes before the mother is discharged. Easy-to-read handouts and videos can help bridge this gap. At discharge, consider what the mother's immediate needs will be when she returns home. Help her plan realistically to meet her needs and her baby's needs. Some mothers will be able to arrange for help at home for several days, perhaps from a relative or through a postpartum doula service. However, the majority of mothers will need to manage on their own.

Mothers need referral to community resources such as an international board-certified lactation consultant (IBCLC), breastfeeding support group, and the local Women, Infants and Children (WIC) program if the mother qualifies. If there are no local breastfeeding support groups, it would be advantageous for a hospital to develop its own. A warm line can also provide support to mothers after they go home.

When mothers receive early contact and telephone follow-up from knowledgeable caregivers, there is a significant increase in the duration of breastfeeding (Bernard-Bonnin, 1989). Arrange to have one of the staff place a follow-up phone call at about 2 days after discharge. The baby should also have a weight check within 48 hours of discharge. Depending on the mother's insurance carrier, she may be able to receive a home visit at around day three. Suggest that mothers check with their insurance carrier to learn if this is covered by their insurance plan.

A 48-HOUR PLAN OF CARE FOR BREASTFEEDING MANAGEMENT IN THE HOSPITAL

In order to provide consistency of care, all postpartum staff need to have a clear understanding of the basics in breastfeeding management. An informed staff can give breastfeeding mothers the tools that will enable them to establish breastfeeding at home. You can assist the staff in developing a care map that will utilize the staff's time and talents efficiently.

Below is a care map for breastfeeding during a 48-hour hospital stay. It identifies for each hospital shift, specific responsibilities to the mother-baby dyad that will get breastfeeding off to the best possible start. Coordination of care and instruction will ensure that every breastfeeding mother receives the information she needs. This care map covers all areas in which the mother receives care, beginning with labor and delivery and continuing through postpartum care.

Labor and Delivery

After the birth, mothers can learn about positioning and management of the first feed. Show the mother the feeding cues her baby is exhibiting at this time. If the baby is not interested in feeding, he can be placed with the mother skin to skin. Keep the room quiet, dim the lights, and reduce stimulation. Postpone visitors for at least 1 hour so that the parents can have quiet time alone with their baby.

Hours 1 to 8

Review positioning and observe the baby's latch. Observe a breastfeed, pointing out to the mother the difference between a nutritive and non-nutritive suck. Review feeding cues (see Chapter 11) and put the baby to breast according to cues. Keep the baby with the mother. He may feed only once or several times during the first eight hours. If the baby has not fed at all by 10 to 12 hours after birth (including time spent in labor and delivery), initiate expression of milk either by pumping or manual expression.

Hours 9 to 16

Review basic nutrition with the mother, advising her to eat a normal healthy diet and to drink when she is thirsty. The baby should breastfeed two or more times during the next eight hours. If the baby is not breastfeeding, feed him expressed milk with an alternative feeding method such as a cup. Review risk factors for breastfeeding problems (Fig. 10.2) and take appropriate action.

Hours 17 to 24

The mother should now be able to demonstrate correct positioning and latch-on. Observe a feed, and ask the mother to point out nutritive and non-nutritive sucking. The baby should breastfeed two or more times during this time period, with a total of at least six feeds in the first 24 hours. If he still is not latching on, the mother should continue to express her milk two or three times during the shift and feed the milk to the baby. The lactation consultant needs to be notified.

Hours 25 to 32

Teach the mother the appropriate number of feeds, wet diapers and stools in a 24-hour period. Give her a breastfeeding diary and information on how to know when breastfeeding is going well, as well as warning signs (Fig. 10.3) that indicate a problem. Teach her how to prevent nipple soreness and engorgement, and when to call her lactation consultant. The baby should breastfeed two or more times during this shift.

Hours 33 to 40

Make sure the mother can position and latch the baby on by herself. Observe a complete feed, and document the findings. Teach the mother about her own nutritional requirements (to drink when thirsty, and eat when hungry), **cluster feeds**, role of the father, avoidance of artificial nipples, and hazards of formula use. Discuss cosleeping, and provide anticipatory guidance for the first few nights at home.

▼ Hours 41 to 48

By now, the mother should be able to observe nutritive sucking and swallowing during feeds. Teach her that crying is the last sign of hunger; that feeding cues are in place for 20 to 30 minutes before sustained crying, and that crying compromises and disorganizes the baby's suck. The infant should be latching on and feeding well. The mother should appear comfortable holding, dressing, and diapering her infant.

▼ Discharge

Make sure the mother understands the signs of adequate milk production (as described in Chapter 14). Give her contact information for community resources, including pump rental stations if necessary. Notify the baby's physician of any potential problems based on risk factors. Ask the mother to confirm when she will take her baby to the physician for a weight and skin color check.

▼ Baby Friendly Hospital Practices

You can be most helpful to the mother during her early postpartum days by being alert to the potential for any complications. Make sure that the mother understands

---

FIGURE 10.2   Red flags and risk factors for breastfeeding problems

Maternal Factors
- ☐ Gained less than 18 pounds during pregnancy
- ☐ Previous breast surgery or breast trauma
- ☐ Little or no breast change in size or color during pregnancy
- ☐ History of low milk supply or breastfeeding "failure" with previous infants
- ☐ Flat or inverted nipples or taut, tight breast tissue
- ☐ Primipara
- ☐ Epidural in labor
  - ☐ In place longer than 3 to 4 hours before delivery
  - ☐ Put in more than one time
  - ☐ Received more than one bolus of epidural medication
- ☐ Induction of labor with Pitocin
- ☐ Received excessive intravenous fluids; on Magnesium Sulfate; edema present in ankles that wasn't present before labor
- ☐ Pain medication in labor more than 1 hour before delivery
- ☐ Breastfeeding initiated more than 1 hour after delivery
- ☐ Sore nipples throughout feed at time of discharge from hospital

Infant Factors
- ☐ Less than 37 weeks' gestation
- ☐ Weighs less than 7 pounds
- ☐ Male infant
- ☐ Vacuum or forceps used for delivery
- ☐ Baby has ankyloglossia (tongue tie) or cleft lip or palate, or both
- ☐ Fetal distress; meconium during delivery
- ☐ Insult to the oral cavity (laryngoscope and deep suctioning)
- ☐ Baby kept in nursery instead of with mother
- ☐ SGA or LGA
- ☐ Feeding restrictions placed on infant (timed feeds, NPO)
- ☐ Multiple bottles given during hospitalization
- ☐ Jaundice
- ☐ Sleepy, difficult to wake; doesn't give clear feeding cues
- ☐ Difficulty latching on consistently; has not established effective breastfeeding by hospital discharge
- ☐ 7% or greater weight loss at time of hospital discharge

All factors can contribute to problems with breastfeeding. Some are more significant than others. Multiple factors indicate that the dyad *must* be followed after discharge from hospital. The goal of this checklist is to identify potential dyads who may have problems establishing either an adequate milk supply or positive milk transfer. The health worker can work with them while they overcome their problems and in a manner that is both safe and supportive of the breastfeeding experience.

LGA, large for gestational age; SGA, small for gestational age.

Printed by permission of Jan Barger and Linda Kutner.

FIGURE 10.3
Warning signs that breastfeeding is not going well

Baby's birth date and time _____
Your baby will be 4 days old on _____
Baby's birth weight _____
Baby's discharge weight _____
Baby's first week weight _____
Baby's second week weight _____

Lactation Consultant's name _____

Telephone Number _____

WARNING SIGNS!

BREASTFEEDING IS GOING WELL IF:

✔ Your baby is breastfeeding at least 8 times in 24 hours.

✔ Your baby has at least 6 wet diapers every 24 hours.

✔ Your baby has at least 4 bowel movements every 24 hours.

✔ You can hear your baby gulping or swallowing at feeds.

✔ Your breasts feel softer after a feed.

✔ Your nipples are not painful.

✔ Breastfeeding is an enjoyable experience.

Remember! If you go home from the hospital in less than 48 hours, your baby should be seen by a physician 2 or 3 days after discharge and again at 10 days to 2 weeks of age. Generally, these visits are for physical assessments and color and weight checks. It is your responsibility to contact the clinic or doctor to schedule these visits, and to notify them and/or your board certified lactation consultant if at any time you feel breastfeeding isn't going just right for either you or your baby.

CALL YOUR BABY'S DOCTOR OR LACTATION CONSULTANT IF:

✔ Your baby is having fewer than 6 wet diapers a day by the 6th day of age.

✔ Your baby is still having meconium (black, tarry stools) on the 5th day of age or is having fewer than 4 stools by the 6th day of age.

✔ Your milk supply is full but you don't hear your baby gulping or swallowing frequently during breastfeeding.

✔ Your nipples are painful throughout the feed.

✔ Your baby seems to be breastfeeding "all the time."

✔ You don't feel that your milk supply has become full by the 5th day.

✔ Your baby is gaining less than ½ ounce a day, or has not regained his birth weight by 10 days of age.

Printed by permission of Breastfeeding Support Consultants.

the importance of sound breastfeeding management. Encourage her to view this as a period of learning and adjustment, and to not become discouraged by obstacles. If she receives conflicting advice from you and her other caregivers, you can help her make appropriate compromises and decisions. You can also lead discussions among the postpartum and newborn staff nurses about conflicting advice and the importance of explaining suggestions to mothers. You can support them through this transitional time and encourage them to look ahead to the more relaxed atmosphere of their own environment.

Baby-friendly hospitals undergo evaluation to determine the extent to which they promote and support breastfeeding, in other words, the degree to which they follow the *Ten Steps to Successful Breastfeeding*. This chapter has explained all ten steps within the context of the mother's hospital experience. Figure 10.4 presents the questions asked under each of the Ten Steps in the self-appraisal process. They are reprinted from the forms used by WHO and UNICEF to facilitate the process of hospital self-appraisal.

SUMMARY

The course of a mother's breastfeeding takes root in her experience during and immediately after her baby's birth. The initiation of breastfeeding can be affected by medications and other interventions in labor and delivery. Practices that interfere with breastfeeding need to be replaced with those that promote bonding, encourage breastfeeding within 1 hour of delivery, offer assistance with the first feed, and create a climate of acceptance. Such policies will encourage rooming in, responding to feeding cues, and preserving healthy breast and nipple tissue. It is important that the mother be provided with information about basic breastfeeding and anticipatory guidance to prepare her for milestones during breastfeeding. Finally, a sound breastfeeding policy and discharge guidelines will provide the framework necessary for preserving and protecting breastfeeding for women and infants.

FIGURE 10.4   Ten steps to successful breastfeeding: self-appraisal tool

Step 1. Have a written breastfeeding policy that is routinely communicated to all health care staff.

1.1 Does the health facility have an explicit written policy for protecting, promoting, and supporting breastfeeding that addresses all Ten *Steps to Successful Breastfeeding* in maternity services?

1.2 Does the policy protect breastfeeding by prohibiting all promotion of and group instruction for using breastmilk substitutes, feeding bottles, and teats?

1.3 Is the breastfeeding policy available so all staff who take care of mothers and babies can refer to it?

1.4 Is the breastfeeding policy posted or displayed in all areas of the health facility that serve mothers, infants, and/or children?

1.5 Is there a mechanism for evaluating the effectiveness of the policy?

Step 2. Train all health care staff in skills necessary to implement this policy.

2.1 Are all staff aware of the advantages of breastfeeding and acquainted with the facility's policy and services to protect, promote, and support breastfeeding?

2.2 Are all staff caring for women and infants oriented to the breastfeeding policy of the hospital on their arrival?

2.3 Is training on breastfeeding and lactation management given to all staff caring for women and infants within 6 months of their arrival?

2.4 Does the training cover at least eight of the Ten Steps?

2.5 Is the training on breastfeeding and lactation management at least 18 hours in total, including a minimum of 3 hours of supervised clinical experience?

2.6 Has the health care facility arranged for specialized training in lactation management of specific staff members?

Step 3. Inform all pregnant women about the benefits and management of breastfeeding.

3.1 Does the hospital include an antenatal care clinic or an antenatal inpatient ward?

3.2 If yes, are most pregnant women attending these antenatal services informed about the benefits and management of breastfeeding?

3.3 Do antenatal records indicate whether breastfeeding has been discussed with the pregnant woman?

3.4 Is a mother's antenatal record available at the time of delivery?

3.5 Are pregnant women protected from oral or written promotion of and group instruction for artificial feeding?

3.6 Does the health care facility take into account a woman's intention to breastfeed when deciding on the use of a sedative, an analgesic, or an anaesthetic (if any) during labor and delivery?

3.7 Are staff familiar with the effects of such medicaments on breastfeeding?

3.8 Does a woman who has never breastfed or who has previously encountered problems with breastfeeding receive special attention and support from the staff of the health care facility?

Step 4. Help mothers initiate breastfeeding within a half-hour of birth.

4.1 Are mothers whose deliveries are normal given their babies to hold, with skin contact, within a half-hour of completion of the second stage of labor and allowed to remain with them for at least the first hour?

4.2 Are the mothers offered help by a staff member to initiate breastfeeding during this first hour?

4.3 Are the mothers who have had caesarean deliveries given their babies to hold, with skin contact, within a half-hour after they are able to respond to their babies?

4.4 Do the babies born by caesarean delivery stay with their mothers with skin contact at this time, for at least 30 minutes?

Step 5. Show mothers how to breastfeed and how to maintain lactation, even if they should be separated from their infants.

5.1 Does nursing staff offer all mothers further assistance with breastfeeding within 6 hours of delivery?

5.2 Are most breastfeeding mothers able to demonstrate how to position and attach their babies correctly for breastfeeding?

5.3 Are breastfeeding mothers shown how to express their milk or given information on expression or advised of where they can get help, should they need it?

5.4 Are staff members or counselors who have specialized training in breastfeeding and lactation management available full-time to advise mothers during their stay in health care facilities and in preparation for discharge?

5.5 Does a woman who has never breastfed or who has previously encountered problems with breastfeeding receive special attention and support from the staff of the health care facility?

5.6 Are mothers of babies in special care helped to establish and maintain lactation by frequent expression of milk?

Step 6. Give newborn infants no food or drink other than breastmilk, unless medically indicated.

6.1 Do staff have a clear understanding of what the few acceptable reasons are for prescribing food or drink other than breastmilk for breastfeeding babies?

6.2 Do breastfeeding babies receive no other food or drink (other than breastmilk) unless medically indicated?

6.3 Are any breastmilk substitutes including special formulas that are used in the facility purchased in the same way as any other foods or medicines?

6.4 Do the health facility and all health care workers refuse free or low-cost supplies of breastmilk substitutes, paying close to retail market price for any? (Low-cost = below 80% open-market retail cost. Breastmilk substitutes intended for experimental use or "professional evaluation" should also be purchased at 80% or more of retail price.)

6.5 Is all promotion for infant foods or drinks other than breastmilk absent from the facility?

(continued)

FIGURE 10.4   Ten steps to successful breastfeeding: self-appraisal tool (CONTINUED)

Step 7. Practice rooming in allows mothers and infants to remain together—24 hours a day.

7.1 Do mothers and infants remain together (rooming-in 24 hours a day, except for periods of up to an hour for hospital procedures or if separation is medically indicated?

7.2 Does rooming in start within an hour of a normal birth?

7.3 Does rooming in start within an hour of when a caesarean mother can respond to her baby?

Step 8. Encourage breastfeeding on demand.

8.1 By placing no restrictions on the frequency or length of breastfeeds, do staff show that they are aware of the importance of breast-feeding on demand?

8.2 Are mothers advised to breastfeed their babies whenever their babies are hungry and as often as their babies want to breastfeed?

Step 9. Give no artificial teats or pacifiers (also called dummies or soothers) to breastfeeding infants.

9.1 Are babies who have started to breastfeed cared for without any bottle feeds?

9.2 Are babies who have started to breastfeed cared for without using pacifiers?

9.3 Do breastfeeding mothers learn that they should not give any bottles or pacifiers to their babies?

9.4 By accepting no free or low-cost feeding bottles, teats, or pacifiers, do the facility and the caregivers demonstrate that these should be avoided?

Step 10. Foster the establishment of breastfeeding support groups, and refer mothers to them on discharge from the hospital or clinic.

10.1 Does the hospital give education to key family members so that they can support the breastfeeding mother at home?

10.2 Are breastfeeding mothers referred to breastfeeding support groups, if any are available?

10.3 Does the hospital have a system of follow-up support for breastfeeding mothers after they are discharged, such as early postnatal or lactation clinic check-ups, home visits, telephone calls?

10.4 Does the facility encourage and facilitate the formation of mother-to-mother or health care worker-to-mother support groups?

10.5 Does the facility allow breastfeeding counseling by trained mother-to-mother support group counselors in its maternity services?

REFERENCES

American Academy of Pediatrics Committee on Fetus and Newborn. Hospital stay for healthy term newborns. *Pediatrics* 96(4):788–789; 1995.

Anderson E and Geden E. Nurses' knowledge of breastfeeding. *JOGNN* 20:58–64; 1991.

Anderson G. Risk in mother-infant separation postbirth. *Image* 21:196–199; 1989.

Bernard-Bonnin A et al. Hospital practices and breastfeeding duration: A meta-analysis of controlled trials. *Birth* 16:64–66; 1989.

Bond G and Holloway A. "Anaesthesia and breast-feeding—the effect on mother and infant." *Anaesth Intens Care* 20:426–430; 1992.

Christensson K et al. Temperature, metabolic adaptation and crying in healthy full-term newborns cared for skin-to-skin or in a cot. *Acta Paediatr* 81:488–493; 1992.

Crowell K et al. Relationship between obstetric analgesia and time of effective breastfed. *J Nurs Mid* 39(3):150–56; 1994.

DeCarvalho M. Effects of water supplementation on physiological jaundice in breastfed babies. *Arch Dis Child* 56:568–569; 1981.

DeCarvalho M et al. Fecal bilirubin excretion and serum bilirubin concentrations in breastfed and bottle fed infants. *J Pediatr* 107:786–790; 1985.

Delight E et al. What do parents expect antenatally and do babies teach them? *Arch Dis Child* 66:1309–1314; 1991.

Hofmeyer G et al. Companionship to modify the clinical birth environment: Effects on progress and perceptions of labour, and breastfeeding. *Br J Obstet Gyneacol* 98:756–764; 1991.

Johanson R et al. Effect of post-delivery care on neonatal body temperature. *Acta Paediatr* 81:859–863; 1992.

Keefe M. The impact of infant rooming-in on maternal sleep at night. *JOGNN* Mar/Apr, 122–126; 1988.

Kennell J et al. Continuous emotional support during labor in a U.S. hospital. *JAMA* 265:2197–2201; 1991.

Klaus M and Kennell J. *Mother-Infant Bonding* St. Louis, MO: C.V. Mosby Company; 1982.

Klaus et al. Maternal assistance in support in labor: Father, nurse, midwife or doula? *Clinical Consultations in Obstetrics and Gynecology* 4; 1992.

Klaus M et al. *Mothering the Mother*. Menlo Park, CA: Addison-Wesley Publishing Company; 1993.

Kurinij N and Shiono P. Early formula supplementation of breast-feeding. *Pediatrics* 88:745–750; 1991.

Liberman E et al. Epidural analgesia, intrapartum fever, and neonatal sepsis evaluation. *Pediatrics* 99(3):415–419; 1997.

Lindenberg C et al. The effect of early post-partum mother-infant contact and breast-feeding promotion on the incidence and continuation of breast-feeding. *Int J Nurs Stud* 27:179–186; 1990.

Lucas A et al. Randomized outcome trial of human milk fortification and developmental outcome in preterm infants. *Am J Clin Nutr* 64:142–151; 1996.

Morton SC et al, Effect of epidural analgesia for labor on cesarean delivery rate. *Ostet Gynecol* 83:1045–52; 1994.

Nylander G et al. Unsupplemented breastfeeding in the maternity ward: Positive long term effects. *Acta Obstet Gynecol Scand* 71:205–209; 1991.

Patton C et al. Nurses' attitudes and behaviors that promote breastfeeding. *J Hum Lact* 12:111–115; 1996.

Perez-Escamilla R et al. Effect of the maternity ward system on the lactation success of low-income urban Mexican women. *Early Hum Dev* 31:25–40; 1992.

Righard L and Alade M. Effect of delivery room routines on success of first breastfeed. *Lancet* 336:1105–1107; 1990.

Sepkoski L et al. The effects of maternal epidural anesthesia on neonatal behavior during the first month. *Dev Med Child Neurol* 32:1072–1080; 1992.

Sousa P. Paper delivered at International Congress on Pediatrics, Brazil; 1974.

Varimo P et al. Frequency of breastfeeding and hyperbilirubinemia. *Clin Pediatr* 25:112; 1986.

WHO/UNICEF. Protecting, promoting and supporting breastfeeding: A joint WHO/UNICEF statement. Geneva, Switzerland; 1989.

WHO/UNICEF. Breastfeeding management and promotion in a baby-friendly hospital: An 18-hour course for maternity staff. UNICEF, New York; 1993.

Widstrom AM et al. Gastric suction in healthy newborn infants. *Acta Paediatr Scand* 76:566–572; 1987.

Yamauchi Y and Yamanouchi I. The relationship between rooming-in/not rooming-in and breastfeeding variables. *Acta Paediatr Scand* 79:1017–1022; 1990.

BIBLIOGRAPHY

Anderson GC. Development of sucking in term infants from birth to four hours postbirth. *Res Nurs Health* 5:21–27; 1982.

Ansley-Green A. Glucose: A fuel for thought. *J Paediatr Child Health* 27:21–30; 1991.

Axelsson IG et al. Anaphylaxis and angioedema due to rubber allergy in children. *Acta Paediatr Scand* 77:314–316; 1988.

Barr RG and Elias MF. Nursing interval and maternal responsibility: Effect on early infant crying. *Pediatrics* 81(4):529–536; 1988.

Barros FC et al. Use of pacifiers is associated with decrease of breastfeeding duration. *Pediatrics* 95:497–499; 1995.

Blomquist HK et al. Supplementary feeding in the maternity ward shortens the duration of breastfeeding. *Acta Paediatr Scand* 83:1122–1126; 1994.

Bocar DL and Shrago LC. Pre-discharge breastfeeding assessment. *La Leche League Breastfeeding Abstracts* 9(1):1–2; 1989.

Buton KE and Gielen A et al. Women intending to breastfeed: Predictors of early infant experiences. *Am J Prev Med* 7:101–106; 1991.

Chen D et al. Stress during labor and delivery and early lactation performance. *Am J Clin Nutr* 68:335–344; 1998.

Cornbluth M et al. Hypoglycemia in infancy: The need for a rational definition. ACIBA Foundation discussion meeting. *Pediatrics* 85:834–837; 1990.

Crowell M et al. Relationship between obstetrical analgesia and time of effective breastfeeding. *J Nurs Mid* 30:150–155; 1994.

de Jong M et al. Randomised controlled trial of brief neonatal exposure to cows' milk on the development of atopy. *Arch Dis Child* 79:126–130; 1998.

deChateau P and Wiberg B. Long-term effect on mother-infant behaviour of extra contact during the first hour post partum. *Acta Paediatr Scand* 66:145–151; 1997.

Driscoll J. Breastfeeding Success and Failure: Implications for nurses. Clinical issues in perinatal and women's health nursing: Breastfeeding. *NAACOG* 3(4):565–569; 1992.

Eidelman A et al. Cognitive deficits in women after childbirth. *Obstet Gyn* 81(5):764–767; 1993.

Ellis DJ. The impact of agency policies and protocols on breastfeeding. Clinical issues in perinatal and women's health nursing: Breastfeeding. *NAACOG* 3(4):553–559; 1992.

Fort P et al. Breast and soy-formula feedings in early infancy and the prevalence of auto-immune thyroid disease in children. *J Am Coll Nutr* 9:164–167; 1990.

Gill NE et al. Transitional newborn infants in a hospital nursery: From first oral cue to first sustained cry. *Nurs Res* 33(4):213–217; 1984.

Glover, J. Supplementation of breastfeeding newborns: A flow chart for decision making. *J Hum Lact* 11(2):127–131; 1995.

Goldsmith R. Baby's first spring water. *Pediatrics* 90:281; 1992.

Gordon N et al. Effects of providing hospital-based doulas in health maintenance organization hospitals. *Obstet Gynecol* 93:422–426; 1999.

Host A et al. A prospective study of cow's milk allergy in exclusively breastfed infants. Incidence, pathogenetic role of early inadvertent exposure to cow's milk formula, and the characterization of bovine milk protein in human milk. *Acta Paediatr Scand* 77:663–670; 1988.

Host A. Importance of the first meal in the development of cow's milk allergy and intolerance. *Allergy Proc* 12:227–232; 1991.

Janson S and Rydberg B. Early postpartum discharge and subsequent breastfeeding. *Birth* 25:222–234; 1998.

Kirk EP et al. Vaginal birth after cesarean or repeat cesarean section: Medical risks or social realities? *Am J Obstet Gynecol* 162:1398–1405; 1990.

Laning CI and Touwen BC. Neurological differences between 9 year-old children fed breastmilk or formula as babies. *Lancet* 344:1319–1322; 1994.

Lewinski C. Nurses' knowledge of breastfeeding in a clinical setting. *J Hum Lact* 8(2):143; 1992.

Lie B and J Juul. Effect of epidural vs. general anesthesia on breastfeeding. *Acta Obstet Gynecol Scand* 67:207–209; 1988.

Lifschitz CH et al. Anaphylactic shock due to cow's milk protein hypersensitivity in a breastfed infant. *J Pediatr Gastroenterol Nutr* 7:141–144; 1988.

Lowe TJ. An investigation of the problems experienced with breastfeeding and the reasons for early breastfeeding failure among primiparous mothers. *Breastfeeding Review* 1(13): 73–74; 1988.

Maiman L et al. Improving pediatricians' compliance-enhancing practices: A randomized trial, *Am J Dis Child* 142: 773–779; 1988.

Matthews MK. The relationship between maternal labor analgesia and delay in the initiation of breastfeeding in healthy neonates in the early neonatal period. *Midwifery* 5:3–10; 1989.

Mulford C. Swimming upstream: Breastfeeding care in a non-breastfeeding culture. *JOGNN* 24(5):464–474; 1995.

National Center for Health Statistics. *Month Vital Stat Rep* 44(11S):15–16; 1996.

Neifert M et al. Nipple confusion: Toward a formal definition. *J Pediatr* 126:S125–S129; 1995.

Newman J. Breastfeeding problems associated with the early introduction of bottles and pacifiers. *J Hum Lact* 6:59–63; 1990.

Nissen E et al. Effects of maternal pethidine on infants' developing breast feeding behavior, *Acta Paediatr* 84:140–145; 1995.

Perry HM and LS Jacobs. Rabbit mammary prolactin receptors. *J Biol Chem* 253:1560; 1978.

Rajan L. The impact of obstetric procedures and analgesia/anaesthesia during labour and delivery on breastfeeding. *Midwifery* 10:87–103; 1994.

Righard L and M Alade. Sucking technique and its effect on success of breastfeeding. *Birth* 91:185–189; 1992.

Rubin R. Attainment of the maternal role. *Nurs Res* 16(3)237–245; 1957.

Ryan A et al. Duration of breast-feeding patterns established in the hospital. *Clin Pediatr* 29(2):99–107; 1990.

Sachdev HPS et al. Water supplementation in exclusively breastfed infants during summer in the tropics. *Lancet* 337:929–933; 1991.

Salariya EM et al. Duration of breastfeeding after early initiation and frequent feeding. *Lancet* 2:1141–1143; 1978.

Sankaran K et al. A randomized, controlled evaluation of two commercially available human breast milk fortifiers in healthy preterm neonates. *J Am Diet Assoc* 96:1145–1149; 1996.

Sears W. *The Baby Book*, Boston: Little, Brown; 1993.

Sepkoski C et al. Neonatal effects of maternal epidurals. *Dev Med Child Neurol* 36:375–376; 1994.

Snell B et al. The association of formula samples given at hospital discharge with the early duration of breastfeeding. *J Hum Lact* 8:67–72; 1992.

Sosa R et al. The effect of early mother-infant contact on breastfeeding, infection and growth. *Breastfeeding and the Mother*. Ciba Foundation symposium 45. Amsterdam: Elsevier, 179–193; 1976.

Stickler G et al. Is supplemental water necessary for breast-fed babies? *Clin Pediatr* 29:669; 1990.

Taylor P Malani J Brown D. Early suckling and prolonged breastfeeding. *Am J Dis Child* 140:51–54; 1986.

Thorp JA et al. Epidural analgesia in labor: An evaluation of risks and benefits. *Birth* 23:63–83; 1996.

Verronen P. Breast feeding: reasons for giving up and transient lactational crises, *Acta Paediatr Scand* 71:447–450; 1982.

Victora CG et al. Pacifier use and short breastfeeding duration: Cause, consequence, or coincidence? *Pediatrics* 99(3):445–453; 1997.

Waldenstrom U and Nilsson C. No effect of birth centre care on either duration or experience of breast feeding, but more complications: Findings from a randomised controlled trial. *Midwifery* 10:8–17; 1994.

Walker M. Management of selected early breastfeeding problems seen in clinical practice. *Birth* 16:3; 1989.

Walker-Smith JA. Cow-milk sensitive enteropathy: Predisposing factors and treatment. *J Pediatr* 121:111–115; 1992.

Wolf L and Glass R. Feeding and swallowing disorders in infancy. *Therapy Skill Builders* p 424; 1992.

Zoppi G et al. Respiratory quotient changes in full-term infants within 30 hours from birth before start of milk feeding. *Eur J Clin Nutr* 52:360–362; 1998.

11

INFANT ASSESSMENT AND BEHAVIOR

Contributing Authors: Jan Barger and Linda Kutner

When assessing the breastfeeding dyad, it is important to be aware of typical newborn reflexes and characteristics. A newborn's behavior is closely tied to breastfeeding. Babies signal to their mothers through feeding cues. In your interactions with mothers, you can point out these behaviors and interpret them for parents. Patterns of behavior, growth, sleeping, crying, and digestion vary from one baby to another. Certain anatomic presentations may also indicate the need for changes in your approach to assisting a mother.

▼ ASSESSMENT OF THE NEWBORN

It is important to obtain a complete history of the mother and infant as it pertains to breastfeeding. This will help you assess both members of the dyad for situations that may impact on the course of lactation. An assessment of the infant is generally recommended with any initial contact. This applies especially when there is any question of poor weight gain, food intolerance, irritability, lethargy, or sucking difficulties. Perform the assessment with the baby completely undressed. You will want to evaluate his posture, skin, head, oral cavity, clavicle, reflexes, color, elimination, and feeding cues he demonstrates. Ascertain if there are any areas on his body that cause pain or discomfort.

▼ Posture

Because babies prefer the fetal position, the posture of a healthy newborn is generally one of **flexion**. They hold their arms and legs in moderate flexion, with their fists closed and usually held near their face. When awake, the baby will resist having his extremities extended and may cry. Observing the baby's body tone will give you clues about potential problems. As the baby matures, he will remain in the fetal position less often, and will spend more time comfortably in semi-extension. When held in the **ventral** position, the infant will be on his abdomen,

draped over the hand of the examiner. A full-term infant will alternate between trying to bring his head up and putting it down again. At extreme positions, a baby's body tone may be too loose (hypotonic) or too rigid (hypertonic). Both are described in the following sections.

Hypotonia

The hypotonic baby may be described as the classic wet noodle. His extremities are in extension and there is little resistance to passive movement. The baby appears floppy, sluggish, flaccid, and perhaps even lazy, as illustrated in Figure 11.1. The hypotonic baby may have difficulty latching onto the breast, due to a weak suck. He may find it difficult to maintain intraoral negative pressure even on the examiner's finger. He frequently nurses with his shoulders elevated to just beneath his ears in an effort to support his neck and chin. In the ventral position, the hypotonic baby lays over the examiner's hand with his head hanging down, unable to bring it up. An infant who is premature or who has **Down syndrome** will show some degree of hypotonia. See Chapter 21 for a discussion on premature infants and Chapter 23 for a discussion on Down syndrome.

Hypertonia

The hypertonic baby is often in hyperextension, arching away from the breast and away from the mother (Fig. 11.2). The mother may report that he is difficult to comfort, pulls his head and face away from contact, and does not snuggle into her chest or neck. Rather, he prefers to lean back, away from her. Many of these babies cannot tolerate being handled and prefer to interact from a safe distance. They are often very alert and squirmy, and they will hold their head erect from a **prone** position or on the shoulder. When held in the ventral position, the hypertonic baby will be virtually straight, lifting both his head and buttocks, and maintaining them on a horizontal plane. A baby with neurologic damage may be hypertonic. See Chapter 23 for a discussion of neurologic disorders.

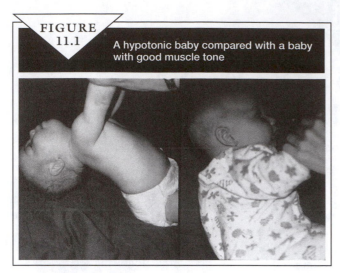

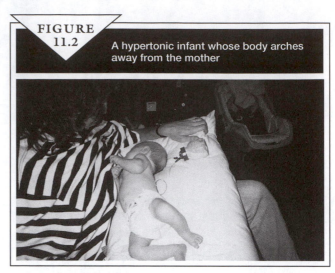

FIGURE 11.1	A hypotonic baby compared with a baby with good muscle tone

Printed by permission of Kay Hoover.

FIGURE 11.2	A hypertonic infant whose body arches away from the mother

Printed by permission of Linda Kutner.

▼ Skin

Healthy newborn skin is warm and dry, with a pink or ruddy appearance. The ruddiness is a result of increased concentration of red blood cells in the blood vessels, coupled with minimal **subcutaneous** (beneath the skin) fat deposits. **Acrocyanosis** (bluish tinge of the hands and feet) may be present after birth due to poor **peripheral** (referring to the outside surface or surrounding area of an organ or other structure) circulation, especially with exposure to cold. It should disappear after a few days.

Hydration

An evaluation of the **turgor** of the skin is an important part of checking for breastfeeding adequacy. Turgor is the normal strength and tension of the skin caused by outward pressure of the cells and the fluid that surrounds them. A good area on which to test skin turgor is on the baby's chest, abdomen, or thigh. When gently grasped between your finger and thumb, the skin should spring back to its original shape when you let go of the tissue. It should not have an indentation, fold, or wrinkled appearance. Loose skin that slowly returns to a position level with the tissue next to it is a sign of dehydration. A baby's skin may be dry, flaky, or peeling, especially by the end of the first or second week. This is normal, and not a sign of dehydration.

Skin Color

Skin color will vary depending on the baby's ethnic origin. If the newborn's bilirubin level increases significantly, it can be detected in his skin color. It is important to assess for jaundice in natural light. Blanch the skin by pressing with your index finger, and note the color when your finger is lifted. For a quick estimation, some care-

givers use a method referred to as the rule of fives, which roughly estimates bilirubin levels in the infant. Jaundice becomes visible in the sclera when the bilirubin level reaches about 5 mg/dl. As it progresses down the body, the bilirubin level will increase successively by approximately 5 mg/100 ml from the infant's face to his feet. Jaundice to the level of the shoulders correlates to 5 to 7 mg/dl; to the level of the umbilicus to 7 to 10 mg/dl; below the umbilicus to 10 to 12 mg/dl; and below the knees to >15 mg/dl. This progression is seen only when the bilirubin level is rising. When it begins to fall, the skin color fades gradually in all affected areas at the same time (Kramer, 1969). For a complete discussion regarding jaundice and its implications, see Chapter 20.

Erythema Toxicum

Erythema toxicum is a pink to red **macular** (raised) area with a center that is yellow or white. It has no apparent significance and requires no treatment. This is common on the newborn's trunk or limbs and is temporary. It appears 1 to 2 days after birth and usually disappears within 1 week.

Infant Acne

Infant acne resembles adolescent acne. It appears on the face, primarily on the nose, forehead, and cheeks. It changes when the baby is hot, cool, crying, or quiet. Infant acne starts at about 2 weeks of age and disappears at 8 to 10 weeks. This is a normal response to the maternal hormones of pregnancy.

Diaper Rash

Diaper rash appears as a reddened, small, pimple-like rash. It should respond to careful washing of the buttocks and use of a zinc oxide preparation. A diaper rash that does not go away with appropriate treatment may be caused by a yeast infection. A diaper rash caused by yeast occurs in patches and is generally characterized by a shiny red flat area. It is usually seen on the front of the infant's perineum and not around the rectum. If the skin is **excoriated** (chafed) or has **pustules** (blisters filled with pus), the infant needs to be seen by his physician to rule out a bacterial infection.

▼ Head

The newborn's head is large in proportion to the rest of his body. It is approximately one-fourth of his total body size. The skull bones are soft and pliable because they are not yet fused in order to allow for descent through the birth canal during second stage labor. After birth, the head may appear asymetric due to the overriding of skull bones. This is called **molding**.

Caput Succedaneum

Caput succedaneum is a collection of fluid between the skin and cranial bone of the newborn. It is usually formed during labor as a result of the presenting area of the head in the cervical opening. The longer the head is engaged, the greater the swelling may be. This condition occurs in 20 to 40 percent of vacuum extractions (Volpe, 1995). There may be red or bruised discoloration, and the baby may be sensitive to pressure on that area. The swelling begins to subside soon after birth.

Cephalhematoma

Cephalhematoma is swelling caused by the pooling of blood between the bones of the head and the **periosteum**, the covering of the bone. It may begin to form during labor and slowly become larger in the first few days after birth. As the blood is reabsorbed, the baby's bilirubin levels may increase. It will take about 6 weeks to resolve completely. Cephalhematoma is usually a result of trauma, often from forceps. Because the baby may be sensitive to touch on that area, the mother will want to avoid touching his head when she puts him to breast.

Fontanel

The fontanel is a space between the bones of an infant's skull that is covered by tough membranes. The anterior fontanel remains soft until the baby reaches about 18 months. The posterior fontanel closes at about two months. Increased brain pressure may cause a fontanel to become tense or bulge. If the infant is dehydrated, his fontanel may be soft and sunken when he is lying down.

Facial Asymmetry

Facial **asymmetry** may result from injury to the nerves due to birth trauma and may cause the baby's tongue to not be centered in his mouth. In this instance, the mother can be advised to center her nipple over the center of the baby's tongue rather than the center of his mouth. Facial asymmetry also occurs when the infant's face is wedged against his body or the uterus. The asymmetry will resolve over several days following birth.

Eyes

Jaundice in the white portion of the eye usually appears when the baby's bilirubin is above 5. Additionally, there may be swelling of the eyelids which will go down in a few days. Final eye color is achieved by 6 to 12 months of age.

▼ Oral Cavity

The oral cavity of a newborn is extremely sensitive. It is not necessary to perform an oral digital exam on all babies. However a visual inspection of the mouth is useful. Look for gum lines that are smooth and a palate that is intact and gently arched. The tongue should be able to extend over the lower **alveolar ridge** (gum line) and up to the middle of the baby's mouth when it is open wide.

Frenulum

The **frenulum** is the fold of skin under the tongue that checks or controls the tongue's motion. If the baby is unable to extend his tongue over the alveolar ridge, it may be due to **ankyloglossia**—a short frenulum (Fig. 11.3). A short or tight frenulum may cause a heart-shaped appearance to the tip of the tongue which can interfere with breastfeeding. Be especially alert to the possibility of a short frenulum as the cause of chronic nipple soreness. A short frenulum can make it difficult for the baby to stay attached to the breast during feeding and may result in poor weight gain.

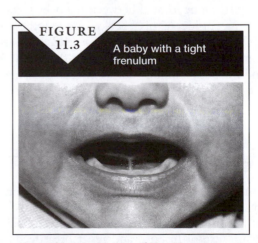

FIGURE 11.3 A baby with a tight frenulum

Printed by permission of Kay Hoover.

Buccal Pads

Buccal pads inside the cheeks (also called fatty pads or sucking pads) help decrease the space within the infant's mouth, which in turn can increase the negative pressure. This feature facilitates milk transfer. If the infant is malnourished or born preterm, the buccal pads may not be present. It may be necessary to position the infant at the breast in such a way that the mother can use her finger against the infant's cheeks to compensate for the lack of these fatty pads of tissue.

Palate

The palate is the roof of the mouth. It is divided into the hard palate and soft palate. The hard palate is in the front of the mouth, and the soft palate lies in line with the end of the upper alveolar ridge. The condition and shape of the palate can become an issue in breastfeeding. A high, arched or bubble palate may cause the mother's nipple to get "caught" in the groove and therefore not elongate as it should. This type of palate also makes it more difficult for the infant's tongue to compress the lactiferous sinuses adequately. Mothers who have infants with such palates often complain of nipple soreness and inadequate milk transfer.

When an infant has a cleft lip, it is immediately obvious to everyone. Frequently, infants with cleft lips also have cleft palates. Occasionally, an infant will have a cleft of the soft palate, which may escape initial diagnosis. Infants with a cleft palate may choke and gag while nursing, and milk may escape from the nose during the mother's letdown. Changing the infant's position while nursing is very helpful. See Chapter 23 for more information on breastfeeding management of infants with a cleft of the lip or palate, or both.

Thrush

Thrush is a yeast infection that often is characterized by white patches that cannot be removed without causing bleeding. It can be located between the baby's gums and lips, on the inside of his cheeks, and on the tongue. Thrush is caused by the organism *Candida albicans,* and is also referred to as **candidiasis**. Both the mother's nipples and the baby's mouth can be infected, making it imperative that both be treated at the same time. See the discussion in Chapter 14 of yeast as a cause of nipple soreness.

▼ Clavicle

A fractured clavicle is a fairly common birth trauma. It is usually identified when the baby is first examined. However, it may not be discovered until later. The baby may restrict the use of his arm and resist breastfeeding in a position that places pressure on the fractured area. For instance, a baby with a fractured left clavicle may be uncomfortable feeding at the right breast in the **cradle hold**. A fracture can be confirmed by x-ray study. Treatment consists of immobilizing the arm by pinning it in a t-shirt. A fractured clavicle heals quickly within about 3 weeks. After healing, there may be a callus on the clavicle, which will disappear as the baby grows.

▼ Reflexes

Reflexes seen in the newborn are present due to immaturity of the central nervous system. Essentially, they are a form of communication that tells us much about what the baby needs. Some reflexes are protective, such as blinking or gagging. Other reflexes indicate a need for more or different interaction. The **Moro** (or startle) reflex encourages more gentle handling of the baby. The grasp reflex is encouraging to parents, as they see their baby respond to them. Arching indicates a need for different positioning or a pause from activity (Fig. 11.4). If pressure is exerted on the back of the baby's head that pushes his face into a surface (i.e., against the breast during a feed) he may arch backward.

Pressure on the soles of the baby's feet will elicit spontaneous crawling efforts and extension of the baby's head. This is **Bauer's** response. When positioning the infant, be careful that his feet do not come into contact with the back or side of the couch or chair. This could cause him to extend away from the breast. A full term healthy newborn has many reflexes that aid his breastfeeding. At the forefront of these reflexes are rooting and sucking.

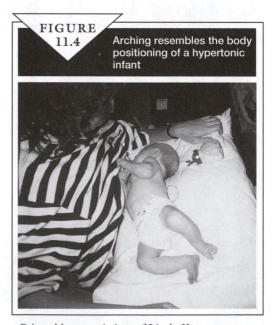

FIGURE 11.4 Arching resembles the body positioning of a hypertonic infant

Printed by permission of Linda Kutner.

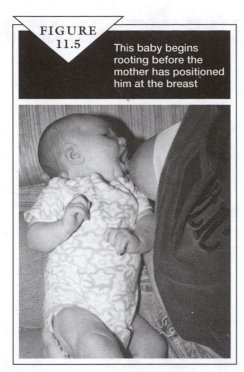

FIGURE 11.5 This baby begins rooting before the mother has positioned him at the breast

Printed by permission of Debbie Shinskie.

Rooting

Stroking the baby's cheek lightly will cause him to turn his head in the direction of the stimulus. His mouth will open, and his tongue will come forward. This is the rooting reflex, as illustrated in Figure 11.5. Gently touching the lower lip will cause his mouth to open. The mother can initiate the baby's rooting reflex by brushing her nipple against his cheek. This will cause him to turn toward her breast and facilitate latch-on.

Sucking

Any object will elicit sucking when it is placed far enough back into the baby's mouth to reach the juncture between the hard and soft palate. Infants will demonstrate two types of sucking. A high-flow nutritive suck is characterized by a long, deep suck-swallow-breathe pattern of about one suck per second. A low-flow non-nutritive suck of about two sucks per second is characterized by a light suck, almost a flutter, with short jaw excursions and little or no audible swallowing.

▼ DIGESTION

Babies are individuals, and each exhibits his own growth and activity patterns. Patterns of digesting food and expelling waste are just as individualized. You can help parents understand these characteristics and encourage them to observe and become familiar with their own baby's digestive patterns and special needs. A change in pattern can alert the mother to problems or illnesses before they become serious. If a mother notices a change, encourage her to look at her baby's overall pattern before contacting her physician. This will help her determine whether it is just one small change in his habits or a more extensive change.

Patterns of digestion need to be considered in relation to the baby's disposition, eating and sleeping patterns, and body temperature. Also, the mother should observe his skin color, changes in breathing, or other signs of illness such as glassy eyes or abdominal cramping. Three functions that occur during digestion—burping, spitting, and stooling—are discussed in the following sections.

▼ Burping

Breastfed babies need to be burped as regularly as those who are bottle fed. This is especially the case with babies who suck vigorously, causing them to gulp air. If the mother watches for feeding cues and feeds her baby before he becomes ravenous, crying can be reduced, resulting in less air in the baby's stomach. Burping will make the baby more comfortable because it decreases gas pains and reduces the possibility of spitting up. Air bubbles are interspersed throughout the milk. Gentle patting or rubbing will help them coalesce and rise to the top of the baby's stomach for a burp. If a baby consistently spits up after nursing, the mother may not be taking enough time to burp him and bring up air bubbles.

There are a number of ways in which a mother can burp her baby, and she can experiment to determine which works best for her. She can sit her baby in her lap, gently rocking him or rubbing his back with her hand. Another method is for the mother to hold her baby against her shoulder and massage or pat him in the middle of his back with a firm pressure from the bottom up. The mother can also lie her baby on his stomach across her lap, turning his head to one side so that his nose is free, and gently rub his back from the bottom up. It helps some babies to remain at a 45-degree angle after feeds to bring up air before being put down for sleep. A baby sling, or infant seat or swing will accomplish this. If the baby has been crying hard, he will need to be burped before being put to breast. If he is a frantic feeder, he will need to be nursed before he becomes ravenous in order to cut down on the amount of air he gulps.

▼ Spitting Up

The passage between the baby's stomach and mouth is very short. Additionally, the muscle valve at the upper end of the baby's stomach (the **cardiac sphincter**) is not as efficient as it will be later in life. Therefore, many

		TABLE 11.1		
		Birth and Feeding Documentation for Nine Breastfed Newborns		
Infant	**Delivery**	**Apgar**	**Comments**	
1	Vaginal	7–8	Moist lungs; O_2 for 2½ hours; all feeds GBF.	
2	Vaginal	8–9	Mother told, "Baby smells your milk and that is why he wants to nurse all the time. We could give him some formula." Mother refused.	
3	Cesarean	8–9	Circumcision day 2; won't wake to nurse after circumcision.	
4	Vaginal	8–9	No problems.	
5	Vaginal	8–9	Had three poor feeds in first 8 hours with no pumping; first GBF at 15 hours of age.	
6	Vaginal	8–9	First three feeds PBF; started mother pumping; GBF by 14 hours.	
7	Vaginal	8–9	35 weeks' gestation, male infant; isolette for 36 hours; started mother pumping 7 hours after feeds.	
8	Vaginal	8–9	Night nurse suggested infant could be hungry; cup fed formula two times in nursery.	
9	Cesarean	8–9	Breech; cup-fed formula two times; no reason stated in nurses' notes; cup fed two times in nursery at mother's request.	

GBF—good breastfeed PBF—poor breastfeed (See Chapter 5 for definitions.)
Data gathered at a North Carolina hospital, printed by permission of Linda Kutner, RN, BSN, IBCLC.

babies spit up quite often during the early months. Some infants spit up more than others. Frequent spitting could be a sign of overeeding or an overactive letdown reflex. It may be caused by the mother waiting too long between feeds. This produces an overabundance of milk at one time and can cause the baby to be overanxious and gulp air with the milk. Spitting can also be caused by mucus in the baby's stomach. This is more common directly after birth and whenever the baby is congested from an upper respiratory infection.

Although spitting is messy and inconvenient, it is not usually a cause for serious concern. There are ways in which a mother can attempt to lessen the chances of her baby spitting. Because the stomach opens to the esophagus on the left side, the mother can reduce her baby's spitting by lying him on his right side for sleep-

		TABLE 11.2			
		Intake and Output Patterns of Nine Breastfed Newborns in Hospital			
Infant	**Time of Birth**	**Birth Weight**	**Time of 1st Feed**	**Time of 1st Stool**	**Time of 1st Void**	**Total Feeds 1st 24 Hours**
1	10:37 pm	8 lb 2 oz	3 hours	3 hours	7 hours	7
2	12:37 pm	7 lb 6 oz	1½ hours	9½ hours	½ hour	8
3	8:18 pm	9 lb	3 hours	7½ hours	7½ hours	7
4	3:30 pm	8 lb 11 oz	¼ hour	1 hour	8 hours	8
5	6:23 pm	8 lb 15 oz	½ hour	2 hours	1 hour	6
6	11:01 am	7 lb 15 oz	1 hour	1 hour	2 hours	9
7	9:14 pm	6 lb 4 oz	1 hour	8 hours	1 hour	8
8	12:35 pm	7 lb 6 oz	1½ hours	9½ hours	½ hour	8
9	1:36 pm	8 lb 8 oz	1½ hours	8 hours	11 hours	8

Data gathered at a North Carolina hospital, printed by permission of Linda Kutner, RN, BSN, IBCLC.

ing. Then, if he does bring up an air bubble there is less chance of bringing up milk with it. Because milk allergy and nicotine can cause spitting, the mother may want to make some adjustments in her lifestyle and diet (Luck, 1987). Her baby will benefit if she decreases cigarette use, or better yet, stops completely. She can burp her baby more often during a feed to bring up air bubbles and may even want to burp him before a feed for any tiny bubbles that have coalesced into one big enough to come up. More frequent feeds may help, as may limiting the baby to one breast at a feed to avoid overfullness.

▼ Projectile Vomiting

Spitting can be distinguished from vomiting in terms of the force with which it is expelled. The baby may dribble milk out with every burp, or he may expel it with some force. A violent expulsion of milk, one that travels 5 to 10 feet, is considered to be projectile vomiting and may require a physician's attention.

If a baby violently expels the contents of his stomach more than once or twice a day, it may indicate a serious medical condition. If he suddenly begins vomiting when he is several weeks old, or if the vomiting gets progressively worse with a decreasing number of wet diapers, he may have **pyloric stenosis**. This is a condition in which the outflow valve of the stomach will not open satisfactorily to permit the contents of the stomach to pass through. It seems to be most common in firstborn white male infants. Such a sudden onset of vomiting can also indicate an obstruction of the intestines or a strangulated hernia. All of these conditions require careful medical observation and may result in surgery.

▼ Gastroesophageal Reflux

Some infants spit every time they are fed or burped, and others seem to spit all the time. This spitting is caused by gastroesophageal reflux (GER). GER is a backflow of the contents of the stomach into the esophagus. It is often the result of failure of the lower esophageal sphincter to close. Gastric juices are acidic and produce burning pain in the esophagus. Infants with reflux may spit several times after a feed, whereas some will spit even during the feed. The constant regurgitation of milk into the esophagus can cause severe irritation and pain for the infant.

Some infants with GER learn to limit their intake, having made the association between a full stomach and the pain that may accompany the reflux. Because of the frequent spitting and the limited amount of intake, these infants may have poor weight gain. Regurgitating human milk is not as irritating as it is with formula. Because human milk is digested more quickly than infant formulas, more milk can be absorbed in the same amount of time. Infants who are breastfed also have a lower pH (measure of the acid level) in their stomach. For these reasons, it is not appropriate to switch a breastfed infant to formula as a treatment for GER.

Infants who experience GER need to be fed in an upright position so that gravity will help the milk stay down. They also benefit from frequent feeds and nursing from only one breast at a feed provided that the mother has adequate milk production. Both of these suggestions will help limit the amount of milk the infant takes in at a feed, and allows him to digest and retain more of the milk.

TABLE 11.2 (CONTINUED)
Intake and Output Patterns of Nine Breastfed Newborns in Hospital

Total Stools 1st 24 Hours	Total Voids 1st 24 Hours	Weight 2nd 24 Hours	Total Feeds 2nd 24 Hours	Total Stools 2nd 24 Hours	Total Voids 2nd 24 Hours	Weight 3rd 24 Hours	
7	1	7 lb 10 oz	Discharged at 36 hours				
5	2	7 lb 1 oz	7	0	2	Discharged	
3	4	8 lb 11 oz	5	4	6	Discharged	
8	3	8 lb 6 oz	8	5	5	Discharged	
3	7	8 lb 12 oz	Discharged				
4	5	7 lb 10 oz	8	3	7	Discharged	
6	7	6 lb 1 oz	10	6	3	5 lb 13 oz	Discharged
5	2	7 lb 3 oz	5	0	3	7 lb 11 oz	Discharged
4	1	8 lb 5 oz	9	3	3	8 lb 2 oz	Discharged

One family physician distinguishes between severe reflux—that requires medical attention and the kind that is merely a laundry nuisance. With the laundry type reflux, the mother can work with her positioning and milk production. If the infant has more severe reflux then the physician needs to be more involved in the infant's care. At times this problem is severe enough that the pediatrician needs to prescribe medications for the infant. Some of these medications decrease the acid level in the infant's stomach; others encourage the infant's stomach to pass the mother's milk along more quickly into the infant's intestines. In the past, physicians frequently requested that the mother mix her milk with cereal to see if the thicker fluid would stay down better. This treatment has not been shown to have a positive impact on this condition and is not commonly used today.

▼ Elimination

Infant elimination patterns are significant indicators of the infant's intake—what goes in, has to come out! In order to assess the baby's intake clearly, new parents may be asked to keep a diary of feeds, voids, and stools for the first several days after birth. This also helps them begin to understand patterns in their new baby's behavior. There is wide variability in stooling and voiding among infants in the early days, especially when there are differences in breastfeeding management.

Tables 11.1 (page 198) and 11.2 (pages 198–199) show patterns for nine breastfed infants in a North Carolina suburban hospital. As these tables indicate, infants varied as to when they went to the breast for the first time, the number of feedings they received in a 24-hour period and the frequency with which they stooled and voided. Interestingly, although the number of stools decreased from day one to day two, the number of voids increased.

Current recommendations are based on clinical observation and bits of information gleaned from unrelated research. The problem with such observations and studies is that often they are based on infants who have had birth and postpartum interventions that do not allow for exclusive, uninterrupted breastfeeding in the early days of life. Recording intake and output patterns of infants in your practice may shed some light on the relationship of these patterns related to breastfeeding management. Table 11.3 illustrates one method for recording this.

Voiding

Urine should be in the range of pale yellow to clear in color. In the first week of life, the baby should have an increasing number of voids each day. By the time he is 6 days old, he should be voiding at least six times in 24 hours. Pink (copper or brick dust) stains that appear with urination generally are not significant in the first 1

to 3 days of the newborn period. However, assessment of the baby's hydration status is warranted, particularly if the stains appear after this time.

Stools

A breastfed baby's stools differ greatly from those of a formula-fed baby. The newborn's first stools are a black, tarry meconium that should be passed within the first 24 to 36 hours. Transitional stools are greenish black to greenish brown, as the meconium gives way to brown and then to golden or mustard yellow color at about 48 to 72 hours of age. The texture may range from watery, to seedy yellow, to a toothpaste consistency. There is virtually no odor to the stools.

Infants in the first month of life should have at least four or more soft yellow runny stools a day. Less than four stools in a 24-hour period may indicate insufficient caloric intake. Such an infant will need to be weighed, examined, and monitored for adequate intake. You can teach parents to observe their baby's stooling patterns. Every baby's digestive system is different, and each one will determine his own pattern for expelling waste.

Babies' bowel habits change with age, and exclusively breastfed infants will frequently decrease the number of stools they have each day. A mother may find that after 1 month of age, her baby will begin going for longer periods between bowel movements. In older infants, one breastfed baby may have several stools every day and another may have a stool only once every 3 or 4 days. Both patterns are perfectly acceptable. The characteristics of healthy breastfed stools are described in Table 11.4, along with variations and their possible causes.

Constipation

Constipation is rare in breastfed infants. As long as the infant's stool is soft, he is not constipated. Neither lack of a daily bowel movement nor straining at stooling indicate constipation. These are normal aspects of toileting. Constipation is diagnosed by the consistency of the infants's stools, not by the frequency. Constipated stools are molded and firm to the touch like pellets or marbles. In young infants, more frequent nursings will solve most constipation problems. Iron supplements have been noted to contribute to an infant's constipation and may need to be discontinued for a few days until the infant's system returns to normal.

Constipation sometimes occurs when solid foods are added to the older infant's diet. If the mother is giving large amounts of cereal, she can stop or decrease the cereal for several days until normal stooling is re-established. She can then reintroduce the cereal in smaller amounts less frequently. She might also offer the infant more fruits and vegetables. If the baby is old enough, he can be given yogurt, oatmeal, or prune juice. The mother

TABLE 11.3

My Breastfeeding Record for the First Week

Use this record when you breastfeed and when your baby needs a diaper change during the first week. This will help you keep track of how well your baby is breastfeeding. Look at the sample.

1. Circle the hour closest to when your baby starts each breastfeeding.

2. Circle the W when your baby has a wet diaper.

3. Circle BM when your baby has a bowel movement.

It is OK for your baby to have more wet diapers or more bowel movements than the goal. Call your breastfeeding helper if your baby has less than the goal on the record.

Birth Date: _____ / _____ / _____   Time: _____ AM   PM

Birth Weight _____   Discharge Weight _____

Sample for Day One		GOAL
		(at least)
12 1 2 3 4 ⑤ 6 ⑦ 8 9 10 ⑪ noon ① 2 3 4 5 ⑥ ⑦ 8 9 ⑩ 11		6 to 8 or more
Wet Diaper	Ⓦ	1
Black tarry bowel movement	ⒷⓂ Ⓑⓜ	1

On the first day this baby fed 7 times, wet one diaper, and had two bowel movements.

Day One		GOAL
		(at least)
12 1 2 3 4 5 6 7 8 9 10 11 noon 1 2 3 4 5 6 7 8 9 10 11		6 to 8 or more
Wet Diaper	W	1
Black tarry bowel movement	BM	1

Day Two		GOAL
		(at least)
12 1 2 3 4 5 6 7 8 9 10 11 noon 1 2 3 4 5 6 7 8 9 10 11		6 to 8 or more
Wet Diaper	W W	2
Brown tarry bowel movement	BM BM	2

Day Three		GOAL
		(at least)
12 1 2 3 4 5 6 7 8 9 10 11 noon 1 2 3 4 5 6 7 8 9 10 11		8 or more
Wet diapers	W W W	3
Green bowel movement	BM BM	2

Day Four		GOAL
		(at least)
12 1 2 3 4 5 6 7 8 9 10 11 noon 1 2 3 4 5 6 7 8 9 10 11		8 or more
Wet diapers	W W W W	4
Yellow bowel movement	BM BM BM	3

TABLE 11.3 (CONTINUED)		
My Breastfeeding Record for the First Week		

Day Five		GOAL
		(at least)
12 1 2 3 4 5 6 7 8 9 10 11 noon 1 2 3 4 5 6 7 8 9 10 11		8 or more
Wet diapers	W W W W W	5
Yellow bowel movement	BM BM BM	3

Day Six		GOAL
		(at least)
12 1 2 3 4 5 6 7 8 9 10 11 noon 1 2 3 4 5 6 7 8 9 10 11		8 or more
Wet diapers	W W W W W W	6
Yellow bowel movement	BM BM BM BM	4

Day Seven		GOAL
		(at least)
12 1 2 3 4 5 6 7 8 9 10 11 noon 1 2 3 4 5 6 7 8 9 10 11		8 or more
Wet diapers	W W W W W W	6 or more
Yellow bowel movement	BM BM BM BM	4 or more

_____ Baby's weight at 1 week

Questions to ask when baby is 1 week old

If you can answer "yes" to each of these questions when your baby is one week old, then you know breastfeeding is going well. If you answer "no" to any of these questions, call your baby's doctor or a breastfeeding helper. Getting help early is best for enjoyable breastfeeding.

1. Is breastfeeding going well?

2. Does your baby breastfeed at least eight times each 24 hours?

3. Does your baby have at least six very wet diapers each day?

4. Does your baby have at least 4 large yellow bowel movements each day?

5. Is your baby getting only your milk? (no formula or water)

6. Do you let your baby finish the first breast before you offer the other side?

7. Is your baby happy or sleepy after breastfeeding? (not in need of a pacifier)

8. Are your breasts and nipples comfortable?

You may copy this paper written by Kay Hoover, M Ed, IBCLC, Lactation Consultant.

1101 Market Street, 9th Floor, Philadelphia, PA 19107

Phone 215-685-5225 or 215-685-5282 FAX 215-685-5257

Name and telephone number of a breastfeeding helper

Printed by permission of Kay Hoover (9/98).
Neifert M: Early assessment of the breastfeeding infant. *Contemporary Pediatrics* 13(10):142–165; 1996.

TABLE 11.4
Stool Patterns of a Breastfed Baby

Characteristics	Normal Stool	Variations	Possible Causes
Color	A newborn's stool is black, brown, or green in the first 3 days. This is meconium. Later, color ranges from brown or green to mustard yellow	Unexplained color changes Black, brown, or red spots	Mother's or baby's diet Mother's cracked nipples (possible bleeding—there is no harm to the baby). Bleeding from baby's rectum. If no known cause, the mother should consult the physician
Consistency	Ranges from a toothpaste-like texture to a liquid with curds	Very watery	Foods in diet other than mother's milk, antibiotics, or illness
		Hard pellets	Foods in diet other than mother's milk, insufficient fluids, or baby tense or ill
		Mucous	Newborn mucus, cold, congestion, or allergy to mother's or baby's diet
		Fibrous	Bananas and cereal present in the baby's diet
Odor	Very little, not unpleasant	Unpleasant	New foods in addition to mother's milk, antibiotics, or illness
Frequency	Ranges from one with every feed to four a day under one month of age. Decrease in frequency after the first month of life	Sudden change in frequency Watch carefully and look for other symptoms	Foods, maturity, or illness
Volume	Varies with frequency. More frequent stools mean less volume per diaper	Any sudden change. Watch carefully and be alert to other symptoms	Foods, maturity, or illness
Ease of Expulsion	Easy and semicontrolled with some straining by the baby	Flows out continually	Foods other than mother's milk, illness, or antibiotics
		Very difficult with extreme straining	Foods other than mother's milk or insufficient fluids

should not treat her infant with suppositories unless the physician prescribes them.

Diarrhea

Teach mothers to distinguish between diarrhea and the typically loose stool of a breastfed baby. A mother who had been supplementing with formula and has returned to exclusive breastfeeding may mistakenly believe her baby has diarrhea because of the typically loose consistency of the exclusively breastfed baby's stool. A mother whose other children were not breastfed might also need to understand this distinction.

In the case of diarrhea, the stool is much looser than normal, is very watery, and may be foul smelling. It may indicate the beginning of an illness, a food allergy, or a reaction to antibiotics taken by either the mother or the baby. If diarrhea is suspected, advise the mother to continue breastfeeding. Diarrhea removes valuable intestinal bacteria that help in the digestion of food, and such bacteria can be built back up with human milk. If the infant's diarrhea does not improve quickly, or if the infant appears sick or dehydrated, the mother should contact her infant's physician immediately.

Infrequent Stooling

When an infant in the first month of life is not stooling appropriately, a full feeding assessment must be performed. Infrequent stooling in the first month of life is almost always due to insufficient intake of milk. A baby who is voiding but not stooling or gaining weight may not be receiving enough high fat hindmilk. Stooling frequency will correct itself with additional feeds or making sure the infant receives more hind milk at a feed.

If it is established that the mother has good milk production, and the infant is gaining at least 1 oz/day and has established a good pattern of weight gain, then **Hirschsprung's disease** may be the cause of infrequent stooling. In Hirschsprung's disease a part of the infant's intestines lacks proper nerve innervation and the stool is not passed easily beyond that point. These infants frequently have large bloated abdomens from the collection of stool and gas. Breastfed infants with this condition may escape detection until solid foods are added to their diet and their stools become more bulky and less liquid. Although this is a rare condition, any exclusively breastfed infant who is gaining nicely but not stooling frequently needs to be watched carefully.

▼ INFANT COMMUNICATION

A 1994 study in the Netherlands revealed that infants have more positive social behavior when their mothers are given special training in responding sensitively to infant signals. At 12 months of age, the infants demonstrated more secure attachments (Vanden Boom, 1994). In the previous year, Graham (1993) reported that parents who were better at recognizing cues were more empathetic when their infants were 3 months old. You can play an important role in teaching parents to recognize infant signals and praising them when they respond to their babies' cues.

▼ Approach and Avoidance Behaviors

An infant will exhibit specific behavior that indicates a willingness to be approached. Approach behavior is integrated, stable, balanced, exploratory, and self-regulated. These signals are characteristic of the more mature infant (Fig. 11.6). Conversely, infants display avoidance behavior, which indicates a desire to withdraw (Fig. 11.7 and Fig. 11.8). Recognizing these behaviors will help parents know how to respond to their baby. Infant approach and avoidance behaviors are described in Tables 11.5 and 11.6 respectively.

▼ Feeding Cues and Stages of Alertness

Many of the infant approach behaviors signal an interest in feeding. Teaching feeding cues to parents will help them know when their baby is ready to be put to breast. If parents wait until their baby cries, he will already be exhibiting the final sign of hunger. The baby may demonstrate feeding cues when he is hungry, when he is thirsty, or when he needs to be comforted at the breast. He will give cues the same way regardless of the reason. His interest in feeding is influenced by his level of alert-

FIGURE 11.6 An infant exhibiting approach behavior

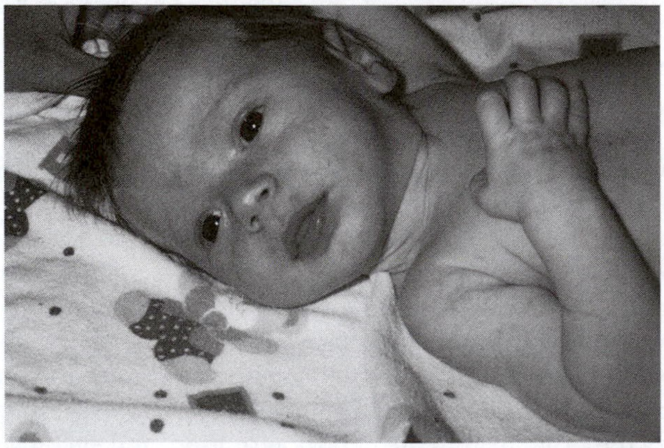

Printed by permission of Linda Kutner.

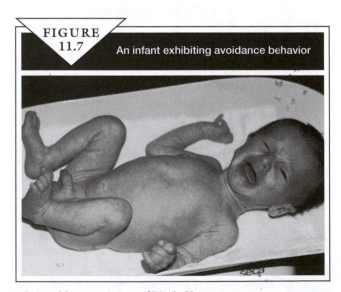

FIGURE 11.7 An infant exhibiting avoidance behavior

Printed by permission of Linda Kutner.

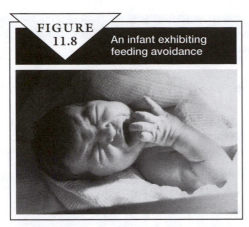

FIGURE 11.8 An infant exhibiting feeding avoidance

Printed by permission of Carole Peterson.

ness, as described in Table 11.7. Watching for feeding cues during a breastfeeding assessment is important. This will help you teach the mother what to look for as well.

Knowing When to Attempt a Feed

Feeding cues may be evident during the light sleep, drowsy, and quiet alert states. The baby will begin to wriggle his body, and his closed eyes will exhibit rapid eye movement (REM). He will pass one or both of his hands over his head and will bring his hand to his mouth (Fig. 11.9). He will make sucking motions, and if his cheek or mouth is touched at this stage, he will begin to root. Soon, more vigorous sucking begins. Finally, the baby settles back into a less active state.

TABLE 11.5

Infant Approach Behaviors

Behavior	Description
Tongue extension	The infant's tongue either is extended toward a stimulus or it repeatedly extends and relaxes.
Hand on face	The infant's hand or hands are placed onto his face or over his ears, and are maintained there for a brief period.
Sounds	The infant emits undifferentiated sounds. At times, it may sound like a whimper.
Hand clasp	The infant grasps his own hands or clutches his hands to his own body. His hands each may be closed and touch each other.
Foot clasp	The infant positions his feet against each other, foot sole to foot sole. Or he folds his legs in a crossed position with his feet grasping his legs or resting on them.
Finger fold	The infant interweaves one or more fingers of each hand.
Tuck	The infant curls or turns his trunk or shoulders, pulls up his legs, and tucks his arms. He uses the examiner's hands or body to attain tuck flexion.
Body movement	The infant adjusts his body, his extremities, or his head into a more flexed position. He may turn to the side or attempt to attain a tonic neck response.
Hand to mouth	The infant attempts to bring his hand or fingers to his mouth. He does not have to be successful.
Grasping	The infant makes grasping movements with his hands. He may grasp either toward his own face or body, in midair, toward the examiner's hands or body, or toward the side of the bassinet.
Leg and foot brace	The infant extends his legs and/or feet toward an object in order to stabilize himself. He may push against the examiner's body or hands, the surface he is on, or the sides of the bassinet. Once touching, he may flex his legs or he may restart the bracing.
Mouthing	The infant makes mouthing movements with his lips or jaws.
Suck search	The infant extends his lips forward or opens his mouth in a searching fashion, usually moving his head at the same time.
Sucking	The infant sucks on his own hands or fingers, clothing, the examiner's fingers, a pacifier, or other object that he has either obtained himself or that the examiner has inserted into his mouth.
Hand holding	The infant holds onto the examiner's hand or finger with his own hands. He may have placed them there himself, or the examiner may have positioned them there. The infant then actively holds on.
Ooh face	The infant rounds his mouth and purses his lips or extends them in an ooh configuration. This may be with his eyes open or closed.
Locking visually and/or auditorily	The infant locks onto the examiner's face or an object or sight in the environment. He may lock on above or to the side of the examiner's face and maintains his gaze in one direction for observable periods. The sound component of an environmental stimulus may contribute to his locking.

The behaviors described are adapted and printed by permission of Sarah Coulter Danner.

TABLE 11.6

Infant Withdrawal or Avoidance Behaviors

Behavior	Description
Spit up	The infant spits up, with more than a passive drool. However, the amount of vomit may be quite minimal.
Gag	The infant appears to choke momentarily or to gulp or gag. Swallowing and respiration patterns are not synchronized. This is often accompanied by at least mild mouth opening.
Hiccough	The infant hiccoughs.
Bowel movement grunting or straining	The infant's face and body display the straining often associated with bowel movements. He emits the grunting sounds often associated with bowel movements.
Grimace, lip retraction	The infant's lips retract noticeably. His face is distorted in a retracting direction.
Trunkal arching	The infant arches his trunk away from the bed or the mother's body.
Finger splay	The infant's hands open strongly, and the fingers are extended and separated from each other.
Airplane	The infant's arms either are fully extended out to the side at approximately shoulder level or the upper and lower arm are at an angle to each other and are extended out at the shoulder.
Salute	The infant's arms are fully extended into midair, either singly or simultaneously.
Sitting on air	The infant's legs are extended into midair, either singly or simultaneously. This may occur when the infant is lying flat on his back or upright.
Sneezing, yawning, sighing, or coughing	The infant sneezes, yawns, sighs, or coughs.
Averting	The infant actively averts his eyes. He may momentarily close them.
Frowning	The infant knits his brows or darkens his eyes by contracting his muscles.
Startle	The infant's limbs jerk once, occasionally followed briefly by a slight amount of jitteriness and possibly crying.

The behaviors described are adapted and printed by permission of Sarah Coulter Danner.

TABLE 11.7

The Six Infant States

Infant State	Description
Deep sleep	Characterized by limp extremities, a placid face, quiet breathing, no body movement, and no rapid eye movement (REM). The baby lies very still, with an occasional twitch or sucking movement. He cannot easily be aroused.
Light or active sleep	Resistance in the extremities when moved, mouthing or sucking motions, body movement, and facial grimaces. The baby is awakened more easily and is likely to remain awake if disturbed. Most of the baby's sleep is spent in this state, with less regular breathing and rapid eye movement (his eyes flutter beneath the eyelids). Although he may stir and move about, he can return to sleep if left undisturbed.
Drowsy	The baby is aroused easily and may drift back to sleep. His eyes may open and close intermittently, and he may murmur, whisper, yawn, and stretch.
Quiet alert	The baby looks around and interacts with others. This is an excellent time to breastfeed. The baby is extremely responsive. His body is still and watchful, his eyes are bright, and his breathing is even and regular.
Active alert	The baby moves his extremities and plays. He is even more attentive, being wide-eyed, with rapid and irregular breathing. He may become fussy and is more sensitive to the discomfort of a wet diaper or excessive stimulation.
Crying	The baby is agitated and needs comforting.

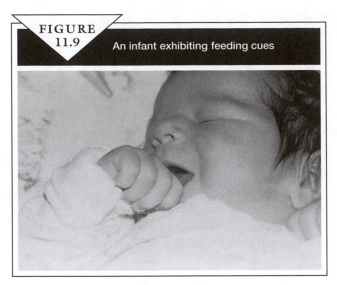

FIGURE 11.9

An infant exhibiting feeding cues

Printed by permission of Kay Hoover.

The baby may do this several times in the span of 20 to 30 minutes. If his signals remain unheeded, he may become very frustrated and cry. At the other extreme, he may become exhausted and fall back asleep without having received any nourishment. The missed feeding opportunity can have consequences for the next feed. This is a common occurrence in preterm or compromised infants and when infants are left in a hospital nursery, fed by the clock, or ignored in an attempt to train him when to feed.

When a newborn begins to cry, he can easily become disorganized and it may take several minutes for him to settle enough to breastfeed. Or he may be unable to breastfeed at all until he has slept again for awhile. In either case, the mother has missed an opportunity for feeding. If a baby needs to be awakened for a feed, advise the mother to wait until he is in a light sleep or a drowsy state. Most babies will move from deep to light sleep in approximately 20- to 30-minute cycles.

INFANT BEHAVIOR PATTERNS

The first few weeks of a baby's life is a series of adjustments and readjustments for everyone. For parents, it is a period when love, patience, and understanding for their infant is most important. In the beginning, the baby is not aware that anything exists outside himself. He believes that everything, including nourishment and comfort, comes from within himself. Because her baby totally relies on her to meet all his needs, a mother may spend nearly all of her time and energies during the first month caring for her baby. At times, she may feel physically drained and emotionally frustrated by his helplessness, while at the same time enjoying the closeness and warmth of their growing loving relationship.

A baby's pattern of sleeping and eating, as well as his disposition, can affect his nourishment. First-time mothers sometimes become concerned about their babies' dispositions, whether they are easygoing and undemanding, or active and fussy. It helps for these mothers to know that babies experience a variety of behavior patterns. Although their baby's pattern may be different from the average, it is still perfectly normal and manageable.

A mother may worry that she is causing her baby to act in a certain manner, or she may overreact to some perceived behavior. However, studies show that an infant's temperament is inborn. Your specific advice to a mother concerning breastfeeding may depend on the type of baby she has. Understanding the various behavior patterns, disposition, and sleeping and eating patterns will help you offer appropriate suggestions.

Average Baby

The average newborn who is exclusively breastfed will nurse anywhere between 6 and 14 times in 24 hours. He sleeps from 12 to 20 hours a day, with one or two longer periods of sleep balanced by one or two fussy periods. Usually responsive when handled, he is generally quiet, alert, and listening when is awake. He soon may learn to soothe himself by sucking on his fist or displaying some other type of comfort measure.

Easy Baby

The breastfeeding pattern of an easy baby is the same as that of an average baby. He will, however, have longer sleep periods and will be less demanding with relatively no fussiness. The mother may need to make a conscious effort to give her baby the tactile stimulation and attention he needs for his emotional growth and physical development. Her undemanding baby may allow her more free time, and she will want to take care not to overexert herself physically. She can make good use of her free time by devoting some of it to her baby, even though he does not make many bids for attention.

Placid Baby

A placid baby may request as few as four to six feeds a day. The mother will need to monitor him to guard against his becoming undernourished. Because he is sleeping as much as 18 to 20 hours a day, he is usually quietly alert and tranquil when awake. Although he makes few demands for attention, the infrequent feeds do not indicate a lack of hunger. He may wake, feel hungry and need to be fed. But he will not cry or demonstrate specific feeding cues to let his mother know he is awake and hungry. Rather, he soon falls back asleep until he awakes again and repeats the same pattern. The result can be an undernourished baby.

A lack of attention and stimuli can result in the placid baby being poorly nourished emotionally as well. Unlike the easy baby, this baby's needs for nourishment are not being met because he does not know how to give the necessary cues to his mother. With such vital physical and emotional needs going unfulfilled, he may become withdrawn and lethargic. Mothers often describe a placid baby as, "such a good baby who doesn't cry and sleeps through the night." You can discreetly ask the mother of a "good" baby about his breastfeeding pattern. These babies are typically slow weight gainers.

The mother of a placid baby must take care to meet his needs without receiving many cues from him. She can place a noise device in his crib, such as a rattle, bell, or squeaky toy, which will be triggered when he awakes and moves about. The mother can set an alarm clock for herself and check on her baby every two to three hours. When she finds him awake, she can pick him up, stimulate him and encourage him to nurse. Any pacifying techniques such as pacifiers, cradles, or swings should be avoided. If her baby sucks his thumb, she can encourage him to satisfy his sucking needs on the breast instead of his thumb.

▼ Active and Fussy Baby

An active, fussy baby may nurse more frequently than the average baby, perhaps because of a greater need to calm or comfort himself. He may seem insatiable at the breast and impatient for the milk to let down. He will sleep fewer hours than average and, when awake, will be active and frequently unable to calm himself. He may have several periods during the day when he cries and cannot easily be quieted. He may overreact to freedom and stimulation, and will need gentle, slow, and soothing movements. He may also find comfort in being kept warm and **swaddled**, and by being held closely and frequently by his caretakers.

An active, fussy baby may respond well to being allowed to nurse, doze, and play at the breast for generous periods of time. His greater need to use the breast for calming and comforting, combined with more frequent feeds, may cause him to spit up often from being overly full. The mother might try limiting him to one breast at a feed, so that he can nurse at his leisure on an empty breast and not take in more milk than he can handle. Although he will exhibit no true colicky symptoms, he may have a greater need to be burped than the average baby. This may be due to his overeagerness at

feeds, causing him to swallow more air. Some of these babies do well when they are worn in a sling.

▼ INFANT GROWTH

When assessing infant growth, it is important to note the infant's specific weight gain since his last weight check. Consider also the overall pattern of gain since the lowest weight he experienced below his birth weight. His growth in length and head circumference are also an issue. Other signs of adequate intake must be observed in relation to weight gain as well. These include alertness, skin turgor, moist mucous membranes, and adequate output.

▼ Caloric Intake

There is ample evidence that infants are able to control their own intakes of food, provided that no arbitrary scheduling or limits on feeding duration are imposed. Giving breastfed babies water can also affect their caloric intake. Sterile water has no calories, and sugar water (D_5W) has 6 kcal/oz. Colostrum has 18 kcal/oz. Therefore, for every ounce of sugar water the baby takes in, his caloric intake is reduced by two-thirds. These calories are also needed to prevent reabsorption of bilirubin from meconium.

There is as much individual variability among infants as among the adult population. This was studied by Dewey (1991), who advises that lower caloric intake among breastfed infants probably results from individual differences in their ability to self-regulate. These lower caloric (energy) intakes by breastfed infants explain their lower percent body fat beginning at 5 months (Dewey, 1993a).

In a 1993 study, Heinig found that breastfed infants' energy intake was lower throughout the first 12 months. According to Whitehead (1995), energy needs per day decrease as the baby gets older. At birth, the infant needs 115 kcal/kg/day. At 1 month, he needs 110; at 2 months, 105; at 3 months, 100; and at four months, 95. Energy needs drop to 82 kcal/kg by 6 months and then rise slightly. Garza (1990) additionally notes that breastfed infants have lower sleeping metabolic rates, rectal temperature, and heart rates, which may account for the differences in energy intake and expenditure. The gain in lean body mass has also been shown to be greater in breastfed infants (Heinig, 1993). Dewey (1993b) cites a need for new growth charts that reflect typical weight gain for breastfeeding infants. Present growth charts are based on infants who are fed artificial baby milk. These charts do not reflect growth patterns of breastfed infants.

TABLE 11.8	
Baby's Weight Gain	
Baby's Age	**Baby's Weight**
First month	5–10 oz/week
1–3 months	5–8 oz/week
3–6 months	2.5–4.5 oz/week
6–12 months	1–3 oz/week

Source: Dewey, 1993b

Weight Gain

Initially after birth, the baby may lose up to 7 percent of his birth weight due to loss of fluids and passage of me-co-nium. If the mother receives excessive intravenous fluids there may be a fluid shift to the infant, which artificially increases the baby's birth weight. These infants typically void large amounts of urine in the first 24 hours of life and may lose more weight than the average infant. Additionally, the exposure to medications during labor may depress the baby's central nervous system. This can lead to less frequent feeds in the first days of life.

A weight loss of more than 7 percent indicates the need for evaluation and perhaps assistance with breastfeeding. By the end of the first week, weight loss is stabilized and by 10 to 14 days birth weight should be regained. Infants who are not back to birth weight by this time need to be evaluated. Table 11.8 presents a typical weight gain pattern for a breastfeeding baby. It is important to recognize that this pattern may vary from one baby to the next.

SLEEPING PATTERNS

Although the specific amount of sleep each baby needs varies, all babies require a great amount of sleep. Although a few babies sleep as few as 8 hours in 24-hour period, some sleep as many as 20 hours. Understanding her baby's typical sleep patterns will help a mother adapt to his needs. There are many factors that can cause individual variations among babies' sleep patterns. The factors may be developmental, environmental, or nutritional. Overtiredness or overstimulation can cause fretfulness before and during sleep. Sounds, lights, the temperature of the room and bedding, and low humidity, which causes difficulty in breathing, can interfere with sleep.

Babies may wake at night for nursing and physical contact even if they were held a lot and nursed frequently during the day. Anna Freud, in *Psychoanalysis and Education* (1954), has commented on the close in-

terrelation between sleep and skin contact. She states that "falling asleep is more difficult for the infant who is kept strictly separated from the mother's body warmth". Ashley Montagu (1972) also believes that children who have been separated briefly from their mothers may suffer disturbed sleep. See Chapter 15 for a discussion of developmental variables.

Encouraging Baby to Sleep

Many parents voice concerns about their babies' sleep habits. You can help a mother determine whether or not she has realistic expectations. Perhaps she can keep a written record for several days of her baby's sleep patterns over a 24-hour period, including even 5 minute naps. Gaining a better understanding of her baby's behavior may help her relax and not allow sleep to be such an important goal for her baby. If she finds that her baby's sleep habits are robbing her of her own sleep, she could make it a practice to sleep when her baby does, taking a number of daytime naps. She can go to bed early in the evening and take her baby to bed with her. During the night, the baby's father can bring the baby to bed for feeds, allowing her to stay in bed.

Establishing a bedtime ritual can be enjoyable for both parents and baby. A routine will help teach the baby to go to sleep easily at an established time every night. Quiet, soothing activities directly before bedtime such as a bath, story, rocking, and nursing will be effective in preparing the baby for sleep. His room should be dark and his bed could be warmed with a heating pad or hot water bottle before putting him in it. Flannel sheets may also help keep him from being awakened by the initial coolness of cotton sheets.

If a baby is sleeping for longer periods during the day, the parents may want to condition him gradually to reverse his schedule so that his longer sleep periods occur at night. The mother can wake her baby every 2 to 3 hours during the day to discourage him from sleeping for longer periods. This will allow her to nurse him more frequently and will let him know that undisturbed sleep is meant for nighttime, not daytime.

Breastfeeding Issues with Sleep

An older baby who is well nourished will be able to sleep for longer periods at night. Therefore, the mother will want to nurse her baby during the day as frequently as he should for his age. If the baby still seems to have trouble sleeping, perhaps the mother is consuming too much caffeine, which is being passed to the baby through her milk. Nursing him directly before bedtime will help soothe him and will give him a full stomach. If she nurses him while lying down in the middle of the bed, she can leave him there when he falls asleep. She can later move him to his crib when he is in a deeper sleep, or leave him in her bed until morning or until after the next feed.

When the baby wakes in the middle of the night to nurse, the mother will want to stimulate him as little as possible. Placing a night light in the baby's room will avoid the need to turn on a bright light, and will maintain a dark atmosphere. If the baby's diaper needs to be changed, it can be done before he is put to the second breast. He then will be able to nurse on the second breast and fall back to sleep without being disturbed for a diaper change. The baby and mother need to be kept warm so they can both return to sleep more easily.

▼ Cosleeping

In many non-Western cultures, and among many subgroups within Western cultures, an infant stays with his mother continually, both day and night. While sleeping in his parents' bed (referred to as cosleeping), the infant is comforted by the warmth and familiar smell of his mother and can nuzzle at her breast and nurse whenever he wishes. The mother is not required to get out of bed to nurse her hungry infant, and she is then able to get the sleep she needs.

McKenna (1994) found that cosleeping infants arouse more often and in synchrony with their mothers than do separate sleepers. This suggests that cosleeping may reduce the risk of sudden infant death syndrome (SIDS) (Stuart-Macadam, 1995). The more frequent arousal also promotes nighttime breastfeeding. Mothers who cosleep with their babies nurse them three times more frequently than do those whose babies sleep in a

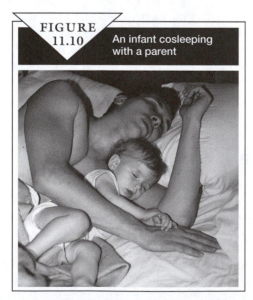

FIGURE 11.10   An infant cosleeping with a parent

Printed by permission of Debbie Shinskie.

separate room (McKenna, 1997). Contrary to popular thinking, research shows that routinely bedsharing and breastfeeding mothers and infants receive more total sleep than do routine solitary sleeping and breastfeeding mothers. Moreover, the routine bedsharers evaluate their sleep more positively than do the solitary sleeping and breast feeding mothers (Mosko, 1997).

Cosleeping is characteristic of middle class life in America. It is becoming much more popular, and the numbers are growing. A family bed, shared by mother, father, and baby, may be an effective alternative for parents whose baby has difficulty falling asleep or who falls asleep in their arms and cries out when placed in his bed (Fig. 11.10). It will also be helpful with a baby who wakes frequently during the night. Parents may also wish to use a crib that attaches to their bed. See the discussion of attachment parenting in Chapter 17.

Some parents are uncomfortable with cosleeping, fearing that it is emotionally unhealthy for an infant to share the same bed as his parents or that it may be difficult to break the habit after it has been established. Some fear the mother may harm her baby by inadvertently rolling over onto him while she is asleep. Most mothers, however, instinctively recognize their babies' presence and respond accordingly. The baby would most likely cry out and awaken the mother if she were to roll too close to him. Mothers who are ill or under the influence of medications, alcohol, or recreational drugs may not be as responsive to the baby's presence. Also it is not advisable to cosleep in a water bed.

▼ Sudden Infant Death Syndrome

It was noted earlier that cosleeping may reduce the risk of SIDS. In SIDS, a seemingly healthy infant is found lifeless in bed. Most SIDS deaths occur between the ages of 2 and 6 months. The occurrence peaks at about 10 weeks of age. It has been suggested that a baby not being breastfed may place him at greater risk for SIDS. This is presumably because of the immunologic protection from human milk that he does not receive. It also may be related to differences in mothering styles between mothers who breastfeed and those who bottle feed (Bernshaw, 1991).

The position in which the baby is placed for sleep is a major factor in the risk of SIDS. Placing the baby in a **supine** position (on his back), rather than in a prone position (on his stomach) reduces the incidence of SIDS substantially (Guntheroth, 1992; Irgens, 1995). Breastfed babies are almost exclusively found to sleep next to their mothers in the safer supine position. Breastfeeding mothers almost always put their babies on the back to facilitate reaching the breast.

Bedsharing low income mothers have an increased risk for SIDS because many of these women smoke in conjunction with bedsharing, put the baby prone, and fail to breastfeed. Sleeping prone and maternal smoking are two of the most significant risk factors for SIDS—quite independent of bedsharing—and all three factors together increases the risks even further (Gilbert, 1995). Another risk factor is the baby's inhalation of passive smoke (Klonoff-Cohen, 1995; Malloy, 1992). This factor has counseling implications for parents who smoke around their baby, and parents need to be educated about the dangers to their baby.

▼

CRYING AND COLIC

The perception of a baby is one of smiles, cooing, and snuggling. Parents never expect to have a crying, fussy baby. They often feel that infant crying is a reflection on their ability to parent. People stare at the parents of a crying baby, and the parents may feel out of control. During pregnancy, the mother was in control and was the center of attention. Now it seems that the baby has all the attention and the control. Mothers are vulnerable to the negative reaction from their colicky baby. Many times the problem lies in the parents expectation of what parenting will be like.

Sears (1985) reassures parents that "Your baby fusses because of her own temperament and not because of your parenting abilities." You can help parents focus on positive elements, i.e., "You have a high-need baby . . . your baby is fortunate to have parents who are so tuned into his needs." Several combinations of temperament that can affect a baby's disposition are described in Table 11.9.

TABLE 11.9

Influences on Baby's Disposition

Baby's Disposition	Mother's Disposition	Probable Outcome
Easy baby	Responsive mother	This is a predictable and cuddly baby whose mother is in tune with him. The mother feels good about her parenting based on the positive interactions with her baby.
Easy baby	Restrained mother	This baby is not very demanding, and such behavior may lead the mother to feel somewhat unnecessary. The mother initially may not develop comfort skills, believing they are unnecessary. She may divert her energies elsewhere, and her baby may, in time, exhibit more fussy behavior.
High-need baby with good attachment-promoting behaviors	Responsive mother	The mother cannot ignore the needs of her baby and responds to him. She is rewarded with occasional satisfied responses from her baby. She will continue to explore alternative responses until she finds one that reaches her baby. Because of his mother's responsiveness, the baby will also fine-tune his attachment-promoting skills, resulting in a parent-child relationship of mutual sensitivity.
High-need baby with poor attachment-promoting skills	Responsive mother	This type of baby often is referred to as slow to warm up. He shows little or no effort to respond to or be comforted by his mother's efforts. The mother's nurturing responses are fine tuned by her baby's responses. When the baby's responsiveness is lacking, this may seriously jeopardize the mother-baby relationship. In some situations, it is helpful for the mother to seek assistance from a professional who is trained in interaction counseling.
High-need baby	Restrained mother	This situation places the mother-baby relationship at risk. Often, the mother has been advised to let the baby cry it out or to not spoil him. Continued lack of response to his needs will lead this baby to one of two outcomes. He will intensify his high-need behaviors, or he will give up. The baby who gives up essentially shuts down his communication and withdraws into himself. He is prone to attach to objects rather than persons.

From Sears W. *The Fussy Baby*. Franklin Park, IL: La Leche League International; 1985.

▼ Crying

All parents face a common dilemma. Should they pick up their crying infant or leave him for a while and let him cry it out? Salk states that "a baby repeatedly left to cry alone ultimately learns to give up and tune out the world" (Sobel, 1981). Infant crying is not merely a distress signal. It is a powerful communicator used by the baby in order to interact with his environment. In a cause-and-effect relationship, the infant learns that he has the ability to make things happen through crying. By crying and eliciting his parents' response, he learns that his needs will be met. He forms a greater attachment to his parents, develops trust more readily, and cries less.

Mothers may perceive infant fussiness as dissatisfaction with breastfeeding and may conclude that supplementing with infant formula or cereal will provide a solution. Parents tend to perceive the level and amount of crying as greater than it actually is. It is important that parents understand that crying is a baby's method of communicating with his world. It is meant to get attention. The decibel level of a baby's cry is actually higher than street noise and 20 decibels louder than normal speech. A study by Ann M. Frodi at the University of Rochester reveals a different crying pattern for a premature infant than for a full-term infant (Sobel, 1981). The premature infant has a different rhythm, pause, and inhalation-exhalation pattern. His cry is a full octave higher, signaling a greater urgency. In response to a baby's cry, the mother's heart beats louder, her blood pressure increases, and the temperature in her breasts increases (Fig. 11.11). Crying is basically a disturbing and aggravating noise. Perhaps, it is nature's design to ensure that the newborn infant receives the attention that he needs.

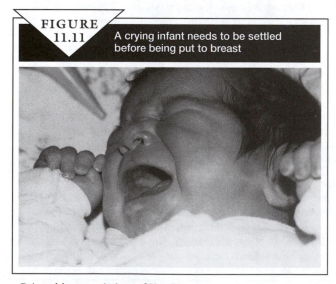

FIGURE 11.11 A crying infant needs to be settled before being put to breast

Printed by permission of Kay Hoover.

The Effect of Crying on the Infant

William Sears (1993) suggests that "crying is good for the lungs like bleeding is good for the veins". Babies who have been crying have difficulty breastfeeding. They are often unable to organize themselves and their behavior for a period of time after the crying spell. When an infant cries or startles during the first 4 to 5 days of life, there is an increase in blood pressure, which, in turn, increases intracranial pressure. Poorly oxygenated blood flows back into the systematic circulation rather than into the lungs. When large fluctuations in blood flow occur, cerebral blood volume increases and cerebral oxygenation decreases. A fluctuating pattern of cerebral blood flow is associated with intracranial hemorrhage (Anderson, 1989).

Crying in the newborn obstructs venous return in the inferior vena cava and re-establishes fetal circulation to the heart. Further, it increases alveolar distention within the lungs where it is not needed and may, in the extreme, lead to a **pneumothorax** (collection of air or gas in the chest causing the lung to collapse) (Dinwiddie, 1977, 1979). Metabolically, crying leads to increased glucose expenditure. In the immediate postpartum period, this may result in hypoglycemia. Crying also increases gastric distention and may result in a very discontented baby due to gas pain.

▼ Identifying the Cause of Crying

Although some babies may cry periodically as a way of releasing tension, a baby's cry usually indicates some form of physical discomfort. As parents become accustomed to their baby, they will learn to distinguish among different types of cries. An infant's cry may indicate hunger, physical discomfort, or a reaction to his environment. Too often, a mother assumes immediately that hunger is the cause and may blame low milk production or poor quality milk for her baby's fussy disposition. You can encourage mothers to investigate other causes for crying, especially if the baby has nursed recently and does not appear to be hungry. As parents become better acquainted with their baby's own particular communication, they will learn to distinguish the cause for his crying.

Crying from Hunger

In the early weeks of breastfeeding, it is common for the baby to require frequent feeds and to sleep for short, frequent periods of time. The mother's usual response to her crying infant is to question whether or not he is hungry. As she becomes tuned into his pattern of sleeping and waking, she will learn to recognize a hunger cry. She will want to consider the length of time since the last feeding, how well he nursed at the previous feed, his general disposition, and whether he can easily be soothed.

A breastfed baby usually cries from hunger about 1½ to 2 hours or more after a feed. A hunger cry is more prevalent in the evening hours when the mother's milk production is lowest. Thus, cluster feeding is common in the early evening. Mothers who respond to hunger cries by nursing their babies will most likely find a more contented baby. The baby will cry less frequently than one whose mother maintains a strict feeding schedule regardless of her baby's cries. Dunn (1977) states that, "mothers in a study who were willing to feed their newborn babies when they cried were more likely to be successful breastfeeders later." You can teach mothers to recognize hunger cues so that they feed on cue rather than waiting until the baby cries.

Crying from Body Discomfort

Wet or soiled diapers themselves are not sufficient to cause crying. However, when the diaper leads to cooling, the drop in temperature is a potential cause of discomfort. Cooling may actually make the baby more responsive to stimulation and more likely to cry for other reasons. Babies may also cry from too much heat. First-time mothers tend to overdress a new baby even on the hottest summer day, fearing he may become chilled. Assure parents that, in warm weather and cold weather alike, babies can be dressed in the same type of clothing that an adult would wear.

Even when temperature is controlled, babies are likely to cry when they are undressed, having lost the warm secure feeling of clothing and blankets. A baby who is especially sensitive to this may need to be swaddled in order for cloth to contact all parts of his body, including his arms and legs. The texture of the cloth that touches his body is also important. Plastic or rubber is more irritating than soft toweling or blanketing. Other skin irritations such as heat rash or diaper rash can also be a cause of a baby's cries. In addition to comfortable body temperature, swaddling, and avoidance of skin irritants, a baby may find comfort in close skin-to-skin contact with his parents. You might suggest to the mother that she take her baby into the bathtub with her or lie in bed with him.

A baby may cry from an internal discomfort such as gas or overfullness. If the mother finds her baby is constantly fussy during feeds, and she is confident that breastfeeding management is not the cause, she may need to burp him more often to help him bring up a bubble of air. Gas in the intestines can also cause discomfort. The mother can help her baby pass his gas by using the techniques for comforting a colicky baby described later in this chapter. Some babies take in more milk than they are able to handle. Such overfullness causes pressure, which, in turn, can produce discomfort. Limiting feeds to one breast may help in these instances.

External Stimuli That Cause Crying

Some babies react unhappily to sensations such as movement, touch, smell, light, noise, and excessive handling. Anything that happens suddenly can cause a baby to startle and cry. On the other hand, a background of constant rhythmic stimulation can be an effective source of comfort to a crying baby. When parents have tended to the physical needs of their baby and he continues to cry, they will want to look for an external cause for the crying.

Swaddling and being held by a parent are the most effective sources of comfort to a newborn. Swaddling provides a baby with constant touch stimulation, which reduces the amount of movement he can make and thus the amount of stimulation he experiences from his own movements. Confining his arms and legs will prevent him from startling himself and provide him with a feeling of warmth and security. Although this may increase the time a baby sleeps and decrease time spent crying, it does not necessarily do so at the expense of time spent quietly awake. Another comforting technique very similar to swaddling is "wearing" the baby in a sling (Fig. 11.12). This provides him with the secure feeling of swaddling, with the added benefit of closeness to the person who "wears" him.

Some babies do not like to be swaddled. They will cry or squirm frantically if they are wrapped too tightly or held too snuggly against the parent. Such a baby may

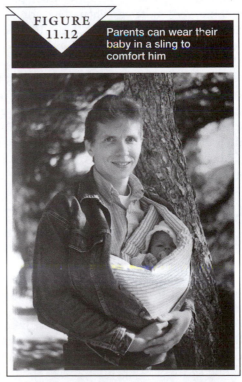

FIGURE 11.12 Parents can wear their baby in a sling to comfort him

Printed by permission of Debbie Shinskie.

push away from the breast when held too closely. He may need to be nursed in such a way that he has no constraints on his movements. For a young baby this could be done with the mother lying on her side to nurse. She can either lightly support the baby from behind or put a pillow behind him for support. She could also lean above a reclining baby and put him to breast.

Through touch, a baby gets important information about the world around him. If a mother's touch is tentative and light, she is likely to find that she has an irritable baby who cries frequently. With a good firm touch, a mother communicates to her baby that she is confident and that he can relax and trust in her. Gently stroking an infant's body during a feed—called **grooming**—increases the mother's prolactin level. Such quiet gentle touching does not usually interfere with feeds. However, if a mother distracts her baby during a feed by poking or jiggling him she may make it difficult for him to relax and he may react by crying.

Unfamiliar or unpleasant smells may be disquieting to a baby, as are bright lights and loud or sudden noises. This often accounts for the initial fussiness when the baby makes the transition from hospital to home. Constant, soft, soothing noise can prove to be an effective comfort measure. Steady movement from being rocked will be comforting, as will the motion of a car ride.

Overhandling by well-meaning adults can cause a baby to cry in an attempt to tell them to "Please leave me alone!" Babies at times may prefer to lie quietly in their cribs and may react unhappily when picked up. Some become very agitated when they are tired and might need to cry themselves to sleep. If the parents have ruled out hunger or discomfort and if the baby indicates that he does not want to be held, they may try to let him cry for 5 or 10 minutes. For some young babies, this is the only way they can fall asleep. Parents need to be encouraged to focus on the cues their baby gives in response to their parenting approach. If their baby is responding positively to a technique, it can be encouraged. If their baby exhibits withdrawal or avoidance behaviors, they will want to try a new approach.

▼ ### Distinguishing Crying from Colic

Much of the fussiness that practitioners see and parents describe is actually colic-like behavior and not true colic. The accepted research definition of colic is "unconsolable crying for which no physical cause can be found, which lasts more than three hours a day, occurs at least three days a week and continues for at least three weeks; spasmodic contractions of smooth muscle, causing pain and discomfort" (Wessel, 1954). This is quite different from the one or two fussy periods a day experienced by most infants. Barr (1992) found evidence for a definable

syndrome of colic, and identified duration as more important than frequency in defining it.

A colicky baby exhibits unexplained fussiness, fretfulness, and irritability. He appears to suffer from severe discomfort most of the time. His cries are piercing and explosive attacks, and a rumbling sound may be audible in the baby's gut. Excessive **flatulence** (gas) and apparent abdominal pain may cause the baby to draw his legs up sharply into his abdomen. His fists may be clenched and he may appear intense, energetic, excitable, and easily startled. He may grimace, stiffen, and twist his body, and may awaken easily and frequently. Continuous crying may cause the infant to swallow air and further aggravate the discomfort.

Colic derives from the Greek word *kolikos*, an adjective derived from Kolon, meaning large colon. It is estimated that as many as 16 to 30 percent of all infants experience colic-like symptoms, and in the majority of infants, these symptoms subside by 16 weeks of age (Pinyerd, 1992). There seems to be no distinction between bottle-feeding and breastfeeding infants. Colic does seem to be more common when solid foods are started in infants younger than 3 months of age.

Causes of Colic

The exact cause of colic has not been determined medically. Not everyone is in agreement about the incidence of colic. Some theories relate colic to stress and tension in the mother and child, both during pregnancy and lactation. Others believe the cause to be an immature digestive and intestinal system or allergies. A Danish study reported that pregnancies with **hyperemesis** (pregnancy marked by long-term vomiting, weight loss, and fluid and electrolyte imbalance), pelvic pain, and distress were more often related to infants with colic. A similar relationship was found for second-born infants and those with a family history of colic (Hogsdall, 1991). Possible causes of colic are explored in the following sections.

Immature Gastrointestinal and/or Neurologic Systems

Compared with other young mammals, a human baby is born in an extremely immature state. He is essentially neurologically incomplete. At 1 month, the infant's stomach capacity is one-tenth the size of an adult stomach. He has only 4 percent of the gastric glands that secret digestive enzymes. The muscle layers surrounding the stomach and intestines are thin and weak, and his intestines lack the ridges and hairlike filaments that help process food.

Colicky infants have been found to transmit more macromolecules across the **epithelium** (lining) of the gut than those without colic symptoms (Lothe, 1990a). **Peristalsis** (wavelike rhythmic contraction of smooth muscle) can be irregular, faint, forceful, or spasmodic.

Additionally, lack of muscle tone can cause food to move up out of the stomach as well as down into the intestines. The colons of colicky infants contract violently during feeds (Jorup, 1952). Whereas the colon in normal infants takes several hours to empty, with some colicky infants, the colon may empty in less than 1 minute.

Hormones

At birth, babies have high levels of progesterone, which helps relax the muscles of the intestines. The level drops after 1 to 2 weeks and may account for the increase in colic symptoms at that time. Infants with colic-like behavior have been found to have high levels of motilin from the first day of life. Motilin is a digestive hormone that stimulates muscle contractions. Human milk has high levels of many enzymes that are necessary for digestion and thus may aid in reducing the intensity of colic in some infants.

Intrauterine and Birth-Related Problems

Increased crying is seen in infants who were born prematurely, who were **small for gestational age (SGA)**, or who experienced birth trauma or **anoxia** (lack of oxygen). There are also reports of increased excitability and fussiness seen in infants whose mothers were **hypertensive** (had high blood pressure). Two separate studies conducted in 1981 suggested a correlation between colicky babies and mothers who received epidural anesthesia (Murray, 1981; Thomas, 1981). By the fifth day of life, these babies cried more and, at 1 month, were less adaptable, more intense, and difficult to manage. The tincture of time is the most effective course for colic-like behavior caused by birth interventions. Some parents seek help from a chiropractor or craniosacral therapist.

Prenatal Intake of Street Drugs

Prenatal abuse of heroin, marijuana, barbiturates, or cocaine can result in colic-like behavior in the infant. Infants born of an abuser often exhibit signs of nervous system instabilities. Symptoms may not appear until a week or more after birth. Symptoms include excitability; trembling; restlessness; ravenous appetite; jitteriness; hyperactivity, shrill scream; feeding problems; and either hypertonia or hypotonia.

Smoking Parent

A clear correlation is seen between infant fussiness and parental intake of nicotine. The infants of smokers are more irritable and agitated. A 1984 study reported that 91 percent of infants with two smoking parents were fussy, whereas 57 percent were fussy if only the mother smoked (Said, 1984). Only about 20 percent of women who smoke will initiate breastfeeding. In one study, 40 percent of infants who were breastfed and whose mothers smoked had colic. Of infants who were breastfed and whose mothers did not smoke, 26 percent had colic-like symptoms (Matheson, 1989).

The levels of the peptide somatostatin are higher in smoking mothers. This peptide inhibits the release of prolactin, which can lead to a decrease in maternal milk production and cause even more infant crying and fussing. Smoking 15 or more cigarettes per day significantly lowers **basal** prolactin levels (Anderson, 1982). Advise the mother to stop or decrease the amount of cigarettes she smokes. Discuss with both parents the need to refrain from smoking in the same room or car as the baby. The mother may need help maintaining adequate milk production.

Food Sensitivity

A typical symptom of an infant who is reacting to something in his mother's diet is an infant who is calm at the start of a feed and then begins to pull off the breast, stiffens his body, cries, and then reattaches. He may repeat this many times during the feed, and symptoms can be continuous or start after a feed. Other signs of food sensitivity are

- A stuffy or drippy nose without any other sign of having a cold.
- An itchy nose.
- A red, scaly, oily rash on the forehead or eyebrows, in the hair, or behind the ears.
- Eczema.
- A red rectal ring.
- Fretful sleeping or persistent sleeplessness.
- Frequent spitting up or vomiting.
- Diarrhea or green stools, perhaps with blood in them.
- Wheezing.
- Typical colic symptoms and behaviors.

▼ Cow and Soy Milk Intolerances

Cow's milk protein is a common cause of allergy in infants. In one study, the mean level of bovine immunoglobulin G (IgG) in colicky babies mothers' milks was higher than levels for noncolicky babies. Almost all mammal milks contained some IgG (Clyne, 1991). In this study, bovine IgG levels were found to be at least 0.42 μg/ml. Levels were lower than 0.32 μg/ml in mother's milk whose infants did not have colic. The range in human milk was from 0.1 to 8.5 μg/ml. In cow's milk formulas the range is 0.6 to 128 μg/ml. The highest levels were found in the powdered form and the lowest levels were found in the concentrate. Levels can be so high, or the **half-life** of bovine IgG is so long, that trials of 2 to 7 days on a diet free of cow's milk may not be long enough to see results. A 14-day trial may be needed. No bovine IgG is found in soy or hydrolysate formulas. It is estimated that 30 percent of colic-like behavior in breastfed infants is due to cow's milk protein intolerances.

A mother who suspects that her baby is intolerant to cow's milk can try eliminating dairy foods from her diet for 2 weeks. If cow's milk was the cause of her infant's colic-like behavior, she may see some improvement in 48 hours. For others, it may take several days. The mother can gradually reintroduce dairy slowly into her diet after 2 weeks of a dairy-free diet. She can start with hard cheeses or yogurt the first week, add soft cheeses the second week, butter and ice cream the third week, and cow's milk in small quantities the fourth week. Any time the infant becomes fussy or other symptoms return, the mother can once again reduce her intake of dairy products.

▼ Mother's and Infant's Diets

Removal of possible sources of intolerance may provide relief to the colicky baby. The mother of a colicky baby would be well advised to feed her baby nothing but her own milk. Vitamins, fluoride, and iron supplements may even be a source of discomfort. Infants who receive antibiotics may be at a greater risk for developing food allergies. Antibiotics are linked to **leaky gut syndrome**, a condition in which the intestinal lining becomes inflamed, and then thin and porous. Proteins that are incompletely digested may then cross from the intestines into the bloodstream. **Leukocytes** attack such proteins and lead to an antigen-antibody reaction, which manifests itself as an allergic reaction with subsequent exposure to that protein.

The mother also may want to monitor her own food intake, because some of what she consumes may pass through her milk to her baby. Medications, vitamin supplements, caffeine, high-protein foods, milk, wheat, chocolate, eggs, and nuts are all potential sources of discomfort to the intolerant baby. Because many colicky babies become food-intolerant children, there may be some validity to the theory of allergy as a cause of colic-like behavior.

▼ Lactose Overload

Colic-like symptoms can occur when an infant consumes too much lactose and not enough fat. This results in the lactose fermenting in the baby's gut, which leads to gasiness and fussiness. Lactose overload can be caused by an overactive letdown, overabundant milk production, or insufficient hindmilk intake. Woolridge (1988) contends that colic-like symptoms can result from mismanagement of breastfeeding. When limits are placed on a baby's time at the breast, he may be removed from one breast before letdown has occurred or before he has been able to obtain the amount of hindmilk he needs. This results in the baby ingesting a large quantity of foremilk. He is then placed on the other breast and fills up on foremilk again.

In addition to typical colic-like symptoms, the infant may have stools which are green, frothy, loose, and frequent. He may have poor weight gain, a bloated abdomen, and a great deal of gas. Lactose overload can be a temporary problem when either the mother or the infant have been on prolonged antibiotic therapy. To avoid lactose overload, it is important that the baby be allowed to feed from the first breast until he has received the fatty hindmilk. Some babies may need to nurse repeatedly on the same breast before being put to the other breast. If the mother has overabundant milk production, she may try nursing on one breast for several feeds before switching. Although some physicians prescribe simethicone (Mylicon) drops for colic due to gas, these aids have not proved to be effective.

Treatment of Colic-Like Symptoms

One theory holds that colic indicates an overreactive nervous system. This causes the infant to become tense easily and to react with discomfort to most stimuli, including parental handling. For this reason the infant often appears to reject his mother by crying and pushing her away when he is picked up. The mother needs to learn that these reactions by the infant are not caused by his dislike of her but that her baby needs to be soothed (Vatanen-Dahlin, 1977).

Vatanen-Dahlin suggests that massage is the most effective way to soothe an infant with colic-like symptoms. She recommends that the mother hold the naked baby on her lap with his head on her knees. She gently massages his stomach, shoulders, head, hands, and feet, and then turns him over to massage his back. Then she holds her baby against her shoulder and soothes him until he is calm. Most times, the infant will cry throughout the massage, for perhaps 10 to 15 minutes, and will usually be calm by the end. Vatanen-Dahlin believes that if this procedure is continued regularly, the colic-like symptoms may disappear within 1 or 2 weeks rather than the usual 3 to 6 months.

Tincture of time seems to be the actual cure for colic-like behavior (Parkin, 1993). Parkin found in a randomized controlled trial that none of three interventions was better than the other in the management of persistent crying. Even when an intervention temporarily stops the crying, it cannot be assumed that the cause has been identified (Pinyerd, 1992). Some interventions that parents may wish to try are identified in Figure 11.13. If all measures used to comfort the baby fail, the

FIGURE 11.13   Measures for comforting a colicky baby

◆ **Holding techniques**

"Wear" the baby around the house in a cloth baby sling, walking and dancing in a soothing manner.
Hold the baby upright against the parent's shoulder near the neck.
Place the baby on his stomach across the parent's lap or knees.
Carry the baby against the parent's hip.
Lay the baby face down on the parent's chest.
Lay the baby face down on the inside of the parent's forearm with the baby's head held in the crook of the parent's hand. The pressure on the stomach feels good and the parent can use the free hand to pat and rub the baby's back.
Pick up the baby as soon as he starts to fuss. This will decrease the length of time he is fussy and prevent it from escalating.

◆ **Sounds and motion**

Provide a steady noise from a vacuum, clothes dryer, music, humming, or tapes of the mother's heartbeat.
Play a recording of the baby's own cry.
Parents speak closely and softly in whispers.
Baby look at the mother's and father's face.
Provide an unexpected distraction to startle the baby to cease crying.
Take the baby for a car ride to provide soothing, rhythmic motion.
Bounce, swing, rock and walk in slow, rhythmical movements.

◆ **Security and warmth**

Place the baby in a warm bath.
Check for any rashes which could indicate reaction to the fiber or detergent in clothing or blankets.
Swaddle the baby to provide closeness and security, or unswaddle him if the blanket seems too constricting.
Check the diaper for dampness and keep the baby warm with sweaters or blankets.
Place a warmed hot water bottle against the baby's stomach area to help him release tension and thereby encourage the passing of gas.
Fold his legs up to his stomach in a bicycle motion to help him eliminate gas.

parents may want to consult their baby's physician to rule out illness.

Supporting the Parents of a Baby with Colic-Like Symptoms

When a baby experiences colic-like symptoms, parental stress and concern increase. Colic is severe enough to some parents that they visit the hospital emergency room (Nacey, 1993). Beebe (1993) reported that 10 to 30 percent of infants cry for 3 hours or more a day in the first 3 months, and stress was higher for the mothers of these babies. Parents will need support, frequent contact, and reassurance. Depending on their reading level and desire, you can suggest appropriate reading material. *The Fussy Baby* and *The Baby Book*, both by Sears (1992, 1993); *Curing Infant Colic* by Taubman (1990); and *Crying Baby, Sleepless Nights* by Jones (1992) are all helpful sources.

The mother of a colicky baby may experience feelings of frustration and guilt for resenting her fussy baby. She may believe that her baby is rejecting her. Physical exhaustion is common from constantly trying to soothe and comfort a crying baby. Because a baby's disposition can be affected by his mother's emotional state when she is holding him, the mother may find that her baby is comforted immediately when another person picks him up. This may further add to her feelings of guilt and may make the

mother feel that she is the cause of her baby's colic-like behavior. The mother will need a great deal of emotional support and frequent close contact with a support person. Because tension can aggravate the baby's condition, she will need an avenue for venting her anger and frustration, and will benefit from having a listening ear that is receptive, caring, and reassuring. Parents may also need to take a break and spend some time away from the baby when necessary in order to keep their perspective.

▼

SUMMARY

Infant assessment is a significant part of your role with breastfeeding mothers. Recognizing deviations from normal in the infant's posture, skin, head, and reflexes will provide important clues to his condition. An assessment of the infant's oral cavity and patterns of voiding and stooling will assist you in determining any need for changes in approach. Teaching parents how to recognize and interpret infant signals will help them become attuned to their baby's needs. Understanding typical patterns of behavior, growth, sleeping, crying, and digestion will be a source of comfort to parents as they learn to interpret their own baby's patterns.

▼
REFERENCES

Anderson AN et al. Suppressed prolactin but normal neuro-physin levels in cigarette smoking breastfeeding women. *Clin Endocrinol* 17:363; 1982.

Barr R et al. The crying of infants with colic: A controlled empirical description. *Pediatrics* 90:14–21; 1992.

Beebe S et al. Association of reported infant crying and maternal parenting stress. *Clin Pediatr* 32:15–19; 1993.

Bernshaw NJ. Does breastfeeding protect against sudden infant death syndrome? *J Hum Lact* 7:73–79; 1991.

Clyne P and Kulczycki A. Human breast milk contains bovine IgG. Relationship to infant colic? *Pediatrics* 87:439–444; 1991.

Dewey K et al. Adequacy of energy intake among breast-fed infants in the DARLING study: Relationships to growth velocity, morbidity, and activity levels. *J Pediatr* 119:538–547; 1991.

Dewey K et al. Breast-fed infants are leaner than formula-fed infants at 1 year of age: the DARLING study. *Am J Clin Nutr* 57:140–145; 1993a.

Dewey K et al. Growth of breast-fed and formula-fed infants from 0 to 18 months: The DARLING study. *Pediatrics* 89: 1035–1041; 1993b.

Dinwiddie R et al. Transient hypoxemia in the crying neonate recovering from respiratory distress syndrome. *Pediatr Res* 10: 460; 1976.

Dinwiddie R et al. Cardiopulmonary changes in the crying neonate. *Pediatr Res* 13:900–903; 1979.

Dunn J. *Distress and Comfort*. Boston: Harvard University Press, pp. 8–23; 1977.

Freud A. The psychoanalytical study of the child. *Psychoanalysis and Education* 9:12; 1954.

Garza C and Butte N. Energy intakes of human milk-fed infants during the first year. *J Pediatr* 117(Suppl):S124–S131; 1990.

Gilbert RE. Bottle feeding and the sudden infant death syndrome. *Br Med J* 310:88–90; 1995.

Graham M. Parental sensitivity to infant cues: Similarities and differences between mothers and fathers. *J Pediatr Nurs* 8:376–384; 1993.

Heinig M et al. Energy and protein intakes of breast-fed and formula-fed infants during the first year of life and their association with growth velocity: The DARLING study. *Am J Clin Nutr* 58:152–161; 1993.

Hogsdall C et al. The significance of pregnancy, delivery and postpartum factors for the development of infantile colic. *J Perinat Med* 19:251–257; 1991.

Jones S. *Crying Baby, Sleepless Nights*. Boston: Harvard Common Press; 1992.

Klonoff-Cohen HS et al. The effect of passive smoking and tobacco exposure through breast milk on sudden infant death syndrome. *JAMA* 273:795–798; 1995.

Kramer LI. Advancement of dermal icterus in the jaundiced newborn. *Am J Dis Child* 118:454–458; 1969.

Lothe L et al. Macromolecular absorption in infants with infantile colic. *Acta Paediatr Scand* 70:417–521; 1990a.

Luck W and Nau H. Nicotine and cotinine concentration in the milk of smoking mothers: Influence of cigarette consumption and diurnal variation. *Eur J Pediatr* 146:21–26; 1987.

MacArthur C. More evidence against the routine use of epidurals. *Births* 21:3; 1994.

Malloy M et al. Sudden infant death syndrome and maternal smoking. *Am J Public Health* 82:1380–1382; 1992.

Matheson I and Rivrud GN. "The effect of smoking on lactation and infantile colic. *JAMA* 261:42; 1989.

McKenna J et al. Bedsharing promotes breastfeeding. *Pediatrics* 100:214–219; 1997.

McKenna J and Mosko S. Sleep and arousal, synchrony and independence among mothers and infants sleeping apart and together (same bed): An experiment in evolutionary medicine. *Acta Paeidatr Suppl* 397:94–102; 1994.

Montagu A. *Touching: The Human Significance of the Skin*. New York: Harper & Row; 1972.

Mosko S et al. Maternal sleep and arousals during bedsharing with infants. *Sleep* 201(2):142–150; 1997.

Murray AD et al. Effects of epidural anesthesia on newborns and their mothers. *Child Dev* 52:71–82; 1981.

Nacey K. Infant colic. *J Emerg Nurs* 19:65–66; 1993.

Parkin P et al. Randomized controlled trial of three interventions in the management of persistent crying of infancy. *Pediatrics* 92:197–201; 1993.

Pinyerd B. Strategies for consoling the infant with colic: Fact or fiction. *J Pediatr Nurs* 7:403–411; 1992.

Said G et al. Infantile colic and parental smoking. *Br Med J* 289:660; 1984.

Sears W and Sears M. *The Baby Book: Everything You Need to Know About Your Baby—From Birth to Age Two*. Boston: Little, Brown and Company; 1993.

Sears W. *Keys to Calming the Fussy Baby*. New York: Barrons; 1991.

Sears W. *The Fussy Baby*. New York: Penguin Group; 1985.

Sobel D. Don't let baby just keep crying, inattention now may cause real problems later (quoting Dr. Lee Salk). *Philadelphia Bulletin*, pp. D1–2; November 8, 1981.

Stuart-Macadam P and Dettwyler K (eds). *Breastfeeding: Biocultural Perspectives*. New York: Aldine de Gruyter; 1995.

Taubman B. *Curing Infant Colic*. New York: Bantam Books; 1990.

Vanden Boom D. The influence of temperament and mothering on attachment and exploration: An experimental manipulation of sensitive responsiveness among lower-class mothers with irritable infants. *Child Dev* 65:1457–1477; 1994.

Vatanen-Dahlin I. Presentation at ASPO Western Regional Conference. San Francisco; 1977.

Volpe J. *Neurology of the Newborn*, 3rd ed. Philadelphia: W.B. Saunders; pp. 769–792; 1995.

Wessel M et al. Paroxysmal fussing in infancy, sometimes called "colic". *Pediatrics* 114:421–434; 1954.

Whitehead RG. For how long is exclusive breastfeeding adequate to satisfy the dietary energy needs of the average young baby? *Pediat Res* 37(2): 239–243; 1995.

Woolridge M. Colic, "overfeeding", and symptoms of lactose malabsorption in the breast-fed baby: A possible artifact of feed management? *Lancet* 2:382–384; 1988.

BIBLIOGRAPHY

American Academy of Pediatrics (Work Group). Infant feeding practices and their possible relationship to the etiology of diabetes mellitus. *Pediatrics* 94:752–754; 1994.

Anderson G. Risk in mother-infant separation postbirth. *Image* 21:196–199; 1989.

Barr RG et al. Nursing interval and maternal responsivity: Effect on early infant crying. *Pediatrics* 81:529–536; 1988.

Behraman R and Victor V. *Nelson Textbook of Pediatrics*, 13th ed. Philadelphia: W.B. Saunders Company; 1987.

Crook W. *Allergies: How It Affects You and Your Child*. Jackson, TN: Professional Books; 1984.

Crook W. *Yeasts and How They Can Make You Sick*. Jackson, TN: Professional Books; 1991.

Fanaroff A and Martin R. *Behrman's Neonatal-perinatal Medicine: Diseases of the Fetus and Infant*, 3rd ed. St. Louis: C.V. Mosby Company; 1983.

Guntheroth WG and PS Spiers. Sleeping prone and the risk of sudden infant death syndrome. *JAMA* 267:2359–62; 1992.

Gurry D. Infantile colic. *Aust Fam Phys* 23:337–346; 1994.

Irgens LM et al. Sleeping position and sudden infant death syndrome in Norway 1967–91. *Arch Dis Child* 72:478–82; 1995.

Lothe L et al. Motilin and infantile colic: A prospective study. *Acta Pediatr Scand* 79(2):410–416; 1990b.

Matheny R et al. Control of intake by human-milk-fed infants: Relationships between feeding size and interval. *Dev Psychobiol* 23:511–518; 1990.

Minchin M. *Food For Thought*. Sydney, Australia: Unwin Paperbacks; 1986.

Mohrbacher N and Stock J. *The Breastfeeding Answer Book*. Franklin Park, IL: La Leche League International; 1991.

Neville M and Neifert M. *Lactation Physiology, Nutrition, and Breastfeeding*. New York: Plenum Press; 1983.

Rapp D. *Is This Your Child?* New York: William Morrow and Company, Inc.; 1991.

Riordan J and Auerbach K. *Breastfeeding and Human Lactation*. Boston: Jones and Bartlett Publishers; 1993.

Taubman B. "Parental counseling compared with elimination of cow's milk or soy milk protein for the treatment of infant colic syndrome: A randomized trial. *Pediatrics* 81:756–761; 1988.

Weissbluth M. *Crybabies: Coping With Colic—What to Do When Your Baby Won't Stop Crying!* New York: Berkley Books; 1985.

12

GETTING BREASTFEEDING STARTED

Breastfeeding can be mastered by virtually every mother and baby. Breastfeeding is a combination of instincts and learned skills for both mother and baby, and it may take a while for breastfeeding to become familiar to them. Mothers have the desire to snuggle and cuddle with their newborns. Often they hold their babies in positions that are very close to actual breastfeeding during nonfeeding times. Being a novice at breastfeeding, the baby may have difficulty in his initial attempts or he may be a natural pro. Both mother and baby will learn the art of breastfeeding with time, patience, and gentle guidance as they learn to coordinate their natural behaviors with one another as individuals.

GETTING READY TO NURSE

Mothers typically look forward to their first breastfeeding session with anticipation and excitement. Ideally, a mother will nurse her baby directly after birth on the same bed in which she delivered him. The earlier she begins to breastfeed, the earlier her baby will receive colostrum and the sooner he will begin stooling. This early suckling will also begin milk production earlier than that of a woman whose first breastfeed has been delayed. In some birth facilities the newborn may be taken to a nursery and observed for a short period of time. Parents should question the need for this separation.

Delays in initiating breastfeeding can contribute to engorgement and low milk production (DeCarvalho, 1983; Newton 1961). There is also evidence that a delay may affect the duration of breastfeeding. "A study was done . . . with two groups of mothers who had expressed a desire to breastfeed. One group was given their babies to suckle shortly after birth. The other group did not have contact with their babies until sixteen hours later. No mother in either group had to stop breastfeeding for physical reasons. Two months later, the mothers who had had their infants to suckle right after birth were all still breastfeeding. In the other group, five out of six had stopped" (MacFarlane, 1997).

ESTABLISHING A BREASTFEEDING ROUTINE

Some mothers, when breastfeeding a baby for the first time, feel an initial awkwardness in trying to achieve a comfortable position while the baby is settling onto the breast. Assure mothers that this feeling of awkwardness is common and to be expected. Breastfeeding is a new venture for the mother, and she needs time to learn it. These first sessions are ideal practice times for both the mother and her baby as they both learn how to approach a feed.

By establishing a regular routine for every feed, the mother will develop self-confidence, increase the ease with which she breastfeeds, and ensure effective breastfeeding management. Before settling down for a feed, the mother can attend to her physical needs, using the bathroom, washing her hands, and gathering whatever she will need during the feed. She may want pillows to help position herself and her baby, a beverage, a cloth for burping her baby, reading material, breast pads, diapers, wipes, and a change of clothes for her baby. After she is home from the hospital, the mother may wish to gather a basket of such items that she will want during a feed. This can be carried anywhere in her house for feeds throughout the day. She may also want to turn off the telephone so that she and her baby will be undisturbed.

ENCOURAGING BABY-LED FEEDS

Newborns have an amazing ability to tell their parents when they need to eat and when they are finished with a feed. The feeding cues described in Chapter 11 show the mother when her baby is ready for a feed. The baby is equally able to let her know when he has fed long enough and wishes to end the feed.

In contrast to older literature regarding the duration of feeds, babies have the ability to self-regulate their feeds to meet their individual needs for optimal growth (Woolridge, 1990). Encourage mothers to allow the baby to begin the feed on the appropriate side (the one that received the least stimulation at the previous feeding) and allow him to continue nursing on that breast until he removes himself. If it has been only a short time and he unlatches for burping or discomfort, the mother may address the cause and resume nursing on that breast again. If he has been on one breast for some time, the mother may watch for further feeding cues and then switch him to the other breast. Using both breasts at a feed is unnecessary unless the baby wishes to do so.

Each baby is an individual who will pace himself in a way that is not like every other baby. Confusing a mother and baby with times for feeding length will lead to frustration for both. No adult eats a meal in exactly the same amount of time as all other adults. Nor do adults enjoy having their meals regulated by a clock. The same is true with babies. Imposing time restrictions will alter a baby's natural regulation of his intake of foremilk and hindmilk. Woolridge (1988) found that switching breasts overrides a baby's natural ability to self-regulate his feeds. Such overriding of a baby's freedom can set up negative reactions and behaviors in the newborn that may lead to breast refusal.

Woolridge also notes that interference with the intake of foremilk and hindmilk may lead to colic-like symptoms in babies, as discussed in Chapter 11. Limiting a baby's time on one breast in order that he will nurse on the other breast results in less hindmilk intake in the overall feed. The increased foremilk intake, coupled with less hindmilk, results in lactose dumping into the small intestine. This overload in the small intestine causes fermentation, which results in increased gas and gut **motility** in the gastrointestinal tract. Ultimately, this situation may lead to a very uncomfortable, fussy baby.

Imposing time-related rules for breastfeeding is a frustration for a new mother that is an unnecessary burden on her during a time meant for becoming acquainted with her new baby. Such restrictions on feeds can lead to frustration and physical symptoms in the baby. Mothers need to be encouraged to watch their babies, not the clock. Their babies cannot tell time. They only know that they are unhappy when they are hungry and content when they are full.

POSITIONING FOR FEEDING

When a mother learns how to recognize when her baby wants to feed, she is able to let her baby lead the way. Help mothers learn how to observe their baby's feeding readiness. A baby who is often placed in a position for feeding at times when he is not ready to feed can become frustrated and wary of the whole process. Only the baby knows when it is time to nurse, and he will exhibit a progression of signs that indicate a desire to feed. See Chapter 11 for a description of infant feeding cues.

The manner in which the mother brings her infant to breast forms the foundation for the entire breastfeeding experience. When discussing positioning, it is convenient to consider four zones within which the mother and baby interact. These zones include the mother's body, the mother's breast, the infant's body, and the infant's mouth (Kutner, 1996). A mother must be in a comfortable position to support her baby during a feed, and the baby's position needs to enable him to latch onto the breast and keep it in his mouth. The mother is easiest to work with, because she can respond to verbal communication. The infant can usually be positioned easily. Even when the infant has idiosyncrasies in his position or his relaxed body is controlled by gravity, he can be positioned to accommodate breastfeeding. In most cases, the infant's mouth will work correctly if the mother's and baby's body positions do not interfere (Minchin, 1989).

The Mother's Body: Zone One

The mother needs to be positioned comfortably, with her back and arms supported by pillows where necessary (Fig. 12.1). A mother who delivers by cesarean birth may want to place a pillow on her lap to protect her abdominal incision. Alternatively, she may choose to position the baby at her side. Pillows are also helpful when placed under the baby to raise him to a level near the breast. This position is especially helpful for a woman who delivered by cesarean because it protects her abdomen.

When the mother is positioned well, her posture will be relaxed, with her shoulders resting comfortably against the back support. If she is sitting, her feet will rest comfortably on the floor or a footstool, so that her knees are

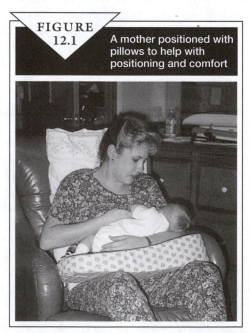

FIGURE 12.1 A mother positioned with pillows to help with positioning and comfort

Printed by permission of Linda Kutner.

higher than her hips. This encourages the infant to remain close to the mother's chest rather than away from her. Placing her knees higher than her hips also helps prevent the mother from leaning over her infant to breastfeed.

Typical postpartum pains and discomforts need to be addressed, particularly perineal and incision areas. Positioning should place the least stress on any sore areas. If the mother is in pain, you may see her toes curled, facial grimacing, or hunched shoulders. She may also become uncomfortable if she remains in the same position for a long time. When the mother is positioned comfortably, she is ready to bring her baby to breast.

▼ The Mother's Breast: Zone Two

For the first few weeks, it is often helpful for the mother to support her breast during feeds. The weight of the breast may cause it to be pulled slightly from the infant's mouth, causing the infant to nipple suck rather than breastfeed. The preferred method of supporting the breast is a technique referred to as the **C-hold.** The mother cups her free hand to form the letter C, with her thumb on top and her fingers curved below the breast, well behind the areola, as in Figure 12.2. She can then gently guide her baby to the breast so that the nipple is centered in his mouth. Some infants latch on better when the nipple is angled up toward the hard palate. This helps trigger the infant's suck and encourages him to take in more of the areola below the nipple. After the mother and baby have mastered the technique and the baby is older, it will not be necessary for the mother to support her breast. In the early weeks, however, some sort of support will be helpful in preventing nipple soreness and encouraging positive milk transfer.

In past years, women were advised to use a scissor hold, in which the breast is held between the first two

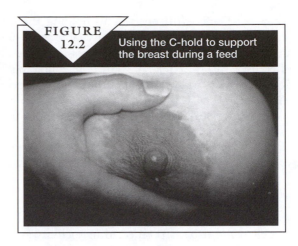

FIGURE 12.2 Using the C-hold to support the breast during a feed

fingers of the mother's free hand. Some texts still illustrate this hold. Such a technique can place pressure on the milk ducts and cause plugged ducts. If the fingers are placed too close to the nipple, the infant may be unable to take sufficient breast tissue into his mouth. This can result in nipple soreness for the mother and inadequate milk intake for the infant. Mothers should be discouraged from using the scissor hold unless they are able to spread their fingers wide enough so that they do not interfere with latch or milk flow.

A slight variation of the C-hold can be used with premature infants and other babies who have weak muscle development and find it difficult to hold the jaw steady while they suck. This position, the **Dancer hand position**, begins in the C-hold position. The mother then brings her hand forward so that her breast is supported with the first three fingers. The infant's chin is supported by the area of her hand between her thumb and index finger (Fig. 12.3). The mother bends her index finger slightly so that it gently holds the baby's

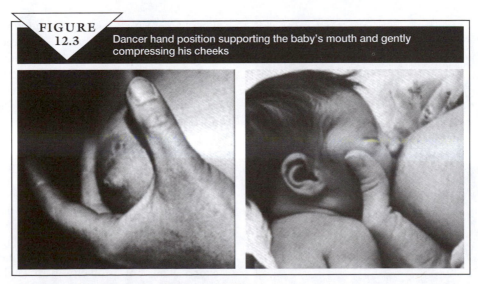

FIGURE 12.3 Dancer hand position supporting the baby's mouth and gently compressing his cheeks

Courtesy of Childbirth Graphics Ltd., 1985.

cheek on one side, with her thumb holding the other cheek. This hold helps decrease the available space in the infant's mouth and increase negative pressure. When the mother uses steady, equal pressure while holding her baby's cheeks, she will avoid interfering with the rooting reflex. As muscle tone begins to improve, the thumb can be placed back on top of the breast, and the index finger can support the baby's chin.

The Baby's Body: Zone Three

Improper positioning of the baby at the breast is the major cause of nipple soreness. Breastfeeding should not hurt! When the baby is positioned in such a way as to avoid pulling on the nipple, the mother will not experience pain. That's not to say that mothers will not be surprised by the sensation of the first latch, as evidenced in Figure 12.4. Properly positioned, the baby will be well supported and cuddled around the mother. He is held chest to chest with the mother, level with her breast. His ear, shoulder, and hip are all aligned, and his body is flexed. The baby's cheeks are both the same distance from the breast, and he is held closely enough so that the tip of his nose and his chin both indent the breast. If his breathing becomes obstructed by the mother's breast, his lower body can be pulled in toward her body. This will angle his head slightly away from the breast and allow him to breathe freely.

The Baby's Mouth: Zone Four

With her baby positioned as described in zone three, the mother is ready to begin the feeding session. If her baby turns his head away from the breast, she can entice him to turn back toward the breast and open his mouth by stimulating his rooting reflex. Either gently stroking his

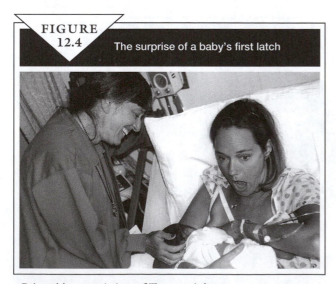

FIGURE
12.4
The surprise of a baby's first latch

Printed by permission of Tammy Arbeter.

cheek with her nipple or tickling his lower lip with it will provide the signal for him to open his mouth. The mother will want her baby's mouth to be opened wide and positioned slightly below the center of the breast. This will result in his lower lip covering more of the areola than his upper lip. His tongue will extend over his lower gum (alveolar ridge), many times far enough to extend out to the lower lip.

Rooting Reflex

When eliciting the rooting reflex, the mother will want to take care not to touch any other part of her baby's face because he will instinctively root toward the source of the stimulation and may become confused and frustrated. A 1993 study by Widstrom looked at the placement of the infant's tongue during rooting and prior to the first suckle. The infants were between 1 and 2 hours old. When they showed an interest in feeding, the mother elicited the rooting reflex by touching the cheek with her nipple. In 10 of the 11 infants, as the infant turned his head toward the stimulus, his mouth opened wide and the tongue extended out of the mouth. Licking movements preceded the rooting when the infant was in an alert state.

A baby who is crying will place his tongue up toward the palate. If forced to the breast (even with gentle force), the infant may remember the forced situation and defend itself by placing his tongue in the palate at subsequent feeds. This may also occur when a baby who is not hungry is forced to the breast. Forcing the baby to the breast can disturb the rooting-tongue-reflex system. Figure 12.5 illustrates the process of the baby latching on for a feed. The subject of latch-on is discussed in greater detail in Chapter 13.

USING A VARIETY OF BREASTFEEDING POSITIONS

There are a variety of positions in which the mother can hold her baby at the breast. The most common positions are the cradle hold, clutch hold, cross cradle hold, and lying down. Posture feeding and some other unique variations are also useful in particular circumstances. The following breastfeeding positions describe a mother nursing her baby at her right breast.

Cradle Hold

The cradle hold is the traditional sitting position whereby the mother sits with her baby's body across her abdomen. She places his head in the crook of her right arm and supports his body with her right hand (Fig. 12.6). This position is not a good one to use if the mother and baby are experiencing any problems with latch or milk transfer. When using this hold, the mother has limited control

FIGURE 12.5 The process of latch-on

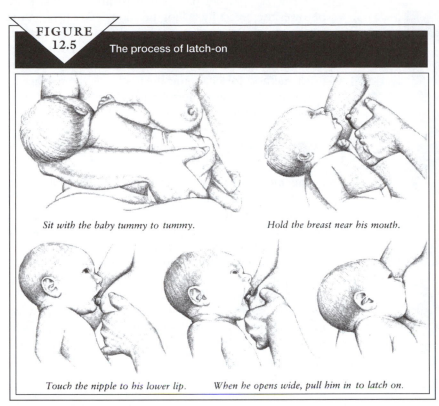

Sit with the baby tummy to tummy.   *Hold the breast near his mouth.*

Touch the nipple to his lower lip.   *When he opens wide, pull him in to latch on.*

Source: Huggins K. *The Nursing Mother's Companion,* The Harvard Common Press, 1986.

FIGURE 12.6 Cradle hold nursing position

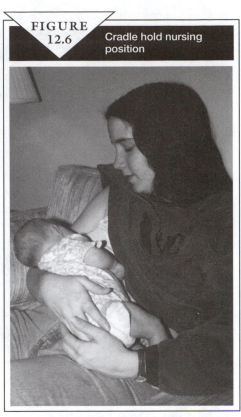

Used by permission of Debbie Shinskie.

over the movement of her baby's head. Thus, she cannot assist or guide him to a better latch.

Clutch (Football) Hold

In the clutch hold, the mother holds her baby under her arm much in the same way she clutches a purse to her side or as a football player holds the ball while running. She places her baby with his body along her side and his feet toward her back. Pillows will be needed to support the baby and the mother's arm. Holding the baby's head in her right hand, she supports his body with her right forearm and raises his head to breast level (Fig. 12.7). Such positioning is especially effective for nursing a premature baby, who fits snugly under the mother's arm. It is also useful for full-term infants who have difficulty latching on. The mother is able to hold her baby's entire body on her arm and can control his body movements better. The clutch hold could be helpful in tricking a baby into nursing on a breast that he refuses in the traditional sitting position. It is also useful for nursing twins.

Dominant Hand Position

The dominant hand position combines the clutch hold and cradle hold, with the mother holding her baby with her dominant hand. Some refer to this position as the

FIGURE 12.7 Clutch (football) hold nursing position

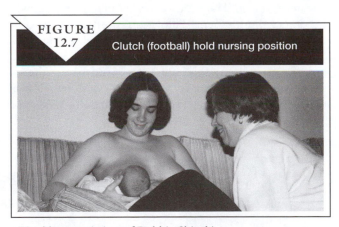

Used by permission of Debbie Shinskie.

cross cradle hold. However, the cross cradle hold can be used with both the dominant and less dominant hand. In the dominant hand position, the right-handed mother holds the baby's head in her right hand and supports his body with her forearm. She then moves her arm with the baby across her body to the opposite breast (Fig. 12.8). This makes it possible to begin the feed at one breast in the clutch hold and end it with the cross cradle hold on the opposite breast without repositioning her hold on the baby. The cross cradle hold is especially helpful in early feeds, because it enables the mother to control her baby's movements. Feeds are easier to manage, and the mother's self-confidence increases.

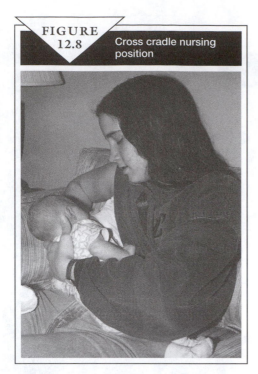

FIGURE 12.8   Cross cradle nursing position

Used by permission of Debbie Shinskie.

Lying Down Position

When the mother nurses while lying down, it helps her get needed rest. The mother lies on her right side, with her knees slightly bent. Pillows are positioned for comfort under her head and upper leg, and behind her back. She can position her right arm under her head, using her left arm to support the baby's head and back. Alternatively, she can place her right arm under the baby's head or along the back of his body, using that arm to support

him. She can put her baby to breast first and then raise or lower the breast by rolling her body. To nurse on the left breast, she can roll toward the baby so that her left breast is level with his mouth. She may need to rearrange the pillows to provide necessary support. Another method for changing breasts is for the mother to hug her baby against her chest and roll together with him to the opposite side (Fig. 12.9).

Posture Feeding

If the mother has an overabundant milk supply that causes excessive amounts of milk to gush into her baby's mouth, posture feeding may be useful. Posture feeding is a term that was popularized in Australia, where women tend to have copious milk production. In this position, the baby is positioned above the breast and has better control over milk flow [Nursing Mothers Association of Australia (NMAA), 1995]. The mother lies flat on her back with her baby lying tummy to tummy on top of her (Fig. 12.10). To get into this position easily, the mother can begin in a sitting position, put her baby to breast, and then lie down. She may need to support his forehead with the heal of her hand to help him hold his head up and away from the breast.

Posture feeding may be needed only at times of the day when milk is most plentiful, as in the early morning. It is also used for babies who bite or retract their tongue. This position encourages the jaw to fall forward by gravity. Posture feeding should be used judiciously, however. Because gravity does not aid milk flow, there is a danger of incomplete milk removal if this position is used too often. Also, the infant can become accustomed to nursing in this position and refuse to nurse in any other position.

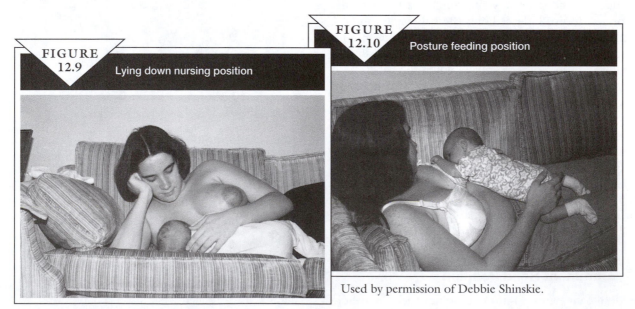

FIGURE 12.9   Lying down nursing position

Used by permission of Debbie Shinskie.

FIGURE 12.10   Posture feeding position

Used by permission of Debbie Shinskie.

Other Creative Breastfeeding Positions

Women who have experienced difficulties in using traditional nursing positions have devised some unusual positions to meet their needs. A sore spot on the nipple can be aggravated by conventional nursing positions, or a plugged duct may not be cleared by using such positions. The mother may then want to try a special position to alleviate her problem. In one variation, she can place her baby on the bed, as in Figure 12.11, and lean over him on her hands and knees. She can then position the breast in his mouth by rotating his body. To avoid back strain, she may wish to raise the baby by placing pillows or blankets under him. This position is useful for babies who are in traction or following surgery. As an alternative, the mother can lie on her back and place the baby on his stomach with his feet over her shoulder, as in Figure 12.12. There are doubtless other unique variations devised by mothers. There is no one correct position for nursing. As long as the baby is held with his head positioned appropriately at the breast, mothers can continue to be creative in their approach.

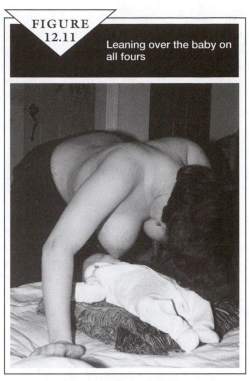

FIGURE 12.11 Leaning over the baby on all fours

Printed by permission of Debbie Shinskie.

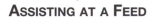

ASSISTING AT A FEED

During the early postpartum weeks, the most important adjustment for parents is becoming acquainted with their baby. New roles are being explored, and the mother's physical recovery is taking place. Parents learn to become sensitive to their baby's physical needs, his disposition and his behavior at the breast. He may prefer quiet at one time and stimulation at another time. During these early weeks, parents learn the many things that make their own baby unique.

Acquainting parents with typical infant patterns will help them adapt their routines to meet the needs of their baby. Learning these patterns of behavior may be challenging in the early days. Help parents understand

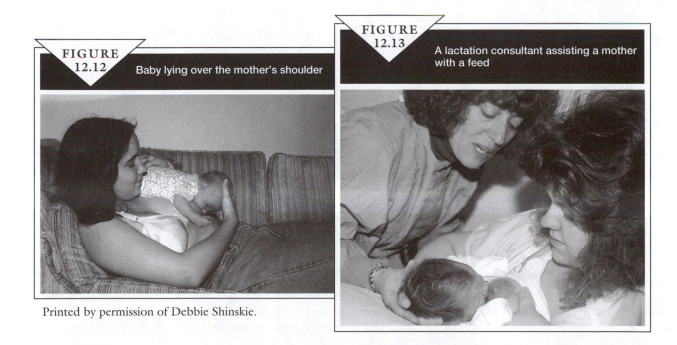

FIGURE 12.12 Baby lying over the mother's shoulder

Printed by permission of Debbie Shinskie.

FIGURE 12.13 A lactation consultant assisting a mother with a feed

that it will become more natural and instinctual with time. Let them know, too, that it may be learned more slowly with babies who demonstrate ambiguous signals than it is with those whose signals are more clear. You can explore with the mother ways to modify her baby's patterns, when necessary, to help her adapt to her baby's nuances. Being available to assist her at early feeds will help to build her confidence and put them on the road to long-term enjoyment (Figure 12.13).

▼ Observing the Feed

After the baby is latched on, this is an ideal opportunity for you to sit back and watch the mother and baby. Observe the mother's posture. Note whether she is comfortable and has her back supported. Watch how she holds the baby, and how she holds her breast for the feed. Note the position of the baby at the breast as he is being held, the position of his mouth, the placement of his tongue, and the position of his head and hands. He should appear comfortable, with his body in good alignment. His lips should be flanged out, and his cheeks should be smooth and each an equal distance from the breast.

The baby should settle into long, deep sucks, with one suck per second. You should be able to hear swallowing with the absence of clicking sounds. Listen for a suck-swallow-breathe pattern. When a large quantity of milk is flowing a baby suckles about once per second. He suckles about twice per second when there is little milk flow. This may signal the time between milk ejection reflexes or the end of the feed on that breast. If this latter pattern is observed throughout an entire feed, it may indicate that the baby is not attached well or that there is little milk available.

▼ Assisting the Reluctant Nurser

In the early days of breastfeeding, when a baby seems reluctant to breastfeed, it is frequently caused by something unrelated to feeding. The mother and baby may simply need time to learn how to respond to one another. Observe the mother and baby at a feed to consider what is happening. Learn from the mother and baby, and trust that they will work it out. Do not be in a hurry to do or say anything until you have determined that they need help. If the baby's reluctance continues for several hours or days, the mother will need to use a breast pump to maintain milk production and prevent engorgement.

It is not unusual in the early days of breastfeeding for the baby to seem unresponsive to the mother's attempts to breastfeed. He may be sleepy or medicated from the delivery or from the mother's pain medication during her postpartum recovery. He simply may not be hungry at the time a feed is attempted. Often he can be encouraged to nurse by expressing milk onto his lips so that he will take the breast into his mouth. There also may be times during the early days that a baby will not be ready to breastfeed when the mother wants or needs to nurse. When this occurs, the mother can stimulate the baby to nurse through the use of one or more of the rousing techniques listed in the following section. These techniques can be used both before and during a feed to stimulate a baby who has fallen asleep before completing the feed. If the mother notices that her baby develops a pattern of being reluctant to nurse at a particular time of day, she may consider whether he really needs to be fed at that time. Watching her baby for feeding cues will help her determine the times when he is most receptive for feeding.

The Baby Who Is Sleepy

There may be times when a mother needs to wake her baby in order to feed him. This often happens in the early days when the baby may still be sleepy from labor medications or simply due to his immature system. Because the mother needs to nurse frequently enough to establish milk production, it may be necessary to wake her baby at times to establish a pattern of good feeds. Most newborns prefer to sleep for longer periods during the day and nurse more at night. Waking these babies periodically during the day will help turn the schedule around and encourage longer sleep periods at night. Parents will need to be patient because it may take several weeks to reverse the baby's schedule.

Possible Causes of the Baby's Sleepiness

You can help the mother explore possible causes for her baby's sleepiness. The cause may be

◆ Medications during labor.

◆ Traumatic birth, caused by long labor or long second stage labor.

◆ Usual sleepy period.

◆ Delayed first feed.

◆ Overlooked feeding cues.

◆ Sensory overload, as in a loud nursery.

◆ Crying related to interventions, particularly circumcision.

◆ Jaundice.

◆ Schedule imposed on feeds.

◆ Cesarean delivery.

◆ Hypothermia.

Plan of Care for a Sleepy Baby

After exploring causes of the baby's sleepiness, you and the mother can determine a plan of care. In the hospital, you can encourage 24-hour rooming in, along with skin-to-skin contact. Help parents learn to distinguish between deep sleep and light sleep, and teach feeding cues to the parents so they learn how to respond to their baby. The mother can attempt to put her baby to breast every half hour to hour, when he shows signs of a light sleep state.

Until feedings are established, advise the mother to pump or hand express her milk to feed by cup to her baby. Using a cup will avoid the potential for the nipple preference that would result if a bottle were used. If her own milk or donor milk are not available, she will need to feed the baby artificial baby milk. It is important that the mother monitor her baby's output and watch for symptoms of dehydration or hypoglycemia (Maccagno-Smith, 1993).

Rousing Techniques

There are a number of rousing techniques parents can try when attempting to interest their baby in feeding. Such attempts should be made in conjunction with the baby demonstrating feeding cues. Attempting to feed a baby who is in a deep sleep is futile. The first step, on picking him up, is to loosen his blankets to expose him to the air. Because he will likely be in need of a diaper change anyway, this can be the next step. Skin-to-skin contact often facilitates an interest in nursing. Therefore, the mother can unclothe her baby and cuddle him upright between her bare breasts. If he is still not awakened, the mother can unclothe him, hold him in an upright position, and talk to him. Dimming the lights will encourage the baby to open his eyes. If he does not waken, the mother can allow him to sleep for another ½ to 1 hour and then try again.

Techniques used to rouse a baby. Rousing techniques include the following techniques:

- Talk to the baby and try to make eye contact.
- Loosen or remove blankets.
- Hold the baby upright in a sitting or standing position.
- Partially or fully undress the baby.
- Change the baby's diaper.
- Stimulate the baby through increased skin contact, such as massage or gently rubbing his hands and feet.
- Stimulate the baby's rooting reflex.
- Stimulate the baby's sense of smell by bringing him close to the breast so that he can detect the scent of the mother's skin.
- Stimulate the baby's sense of taste by expressing milk onto the nipple or into his mouth.
- Wipe the baby's forehead and cheeks with a cool moist cloth.

- Manipulate the baby's arms and legs by playing pat-a-cake, doing baby exercises, and so on.
- Give the baby a bath or, better yet, take a bath with the baby to provide increased skin-to-skin contact.
- If the baby takes the breast but does not maintain a rhythmic suck-swallow-pause pattern, try stroking under his chin from front to back. Also, compress the breast, as with manual expression.

The Baby Who Cries and Resists Going to Breast

At times, a baby may seem to resist being put to breast. When moved toward the breast, instead of starting to suckle, the baby cries loudly. The longer the mother tries, the more the baby cries and fights against being brought to breast. Some babies seem to be more fussy and irritable during the first month of life. These babies may cry frequently, and require continuous attention during their waking hours. They are easily stimulated and excited, and may be especially sensitive to being handled, or frightened by their own flailing arms and legs. Swaddling the baby to restrict startling and movement may help.

Nursing itself can have a calming effect on a fussy baby. The baby first may need to be soothed before being put to breast. A crying baby will have difficulty coordinating breathing and swallowing, and may choke or swallow air. Similarly, a baby who is overly hungry may choke and gag due to his overeagerness to nurse. The mother can prevent these problems from occurring by carefully observing her baby and beginning the feed before he becomes too upset or overly hungry. The mother may not always be able to anticipate hunger or fussiness, however, and will benefit from suggestions for calming a fussy baby. She can try these suggestions before and during the feed, as well as at other times during the day.

Sometimes when a sensitive baby becomes upset, the mother will become tense and frustrated by his behavior. The baby may pick up on this tension, causing him to cry and scream even more. When this happens, the mother needs to break the cycle by changing her behavior in some way. She can leave the room for several minutes, and use relaxation and breathing techniques to calm herself. She can get relief away from the baby for longer periods by enlisting the help of the father, other relative, or friend to care for the baby. Talking with you or someone close to her about her feelings of anger, frustration, and inadequacy will help relieve her tension. She may also benefit from a walk outdoors or a trip to a shopping mall or grocery store.

The mother can improve her outlook by keeping her body in good condition and eating nutritious foods. Advise her to plan easy meals and snacks that include sufficient protein to ensure a feeling of well-being, and adequate B vitamins for calm nerves. She will want to rest whenever possible, nursing while lying down and enlisting the help of others to care for the baby while she naps. See Chapter 11 for further discussion on crying and care of the fussy or colicky baby.

Possible Causes of Fussiness

You can problem solve with the mother to find out what is causing her baby to be fussy. Some possible reasons are

◆ The baby has been handled too much by caregivers.

◆ The baby is in pain or has experienced pain.

◆ The mother received medication during labor that was transmitted to the baby.

◆ The baby has discomfort from forceps, vacuum extraction, internal monitor lead, or cephalhematoma.

◆ The baby experiences oral aversion as a result of deep suctioning.

◆ The baby is irritable.

◆ The baby was given artificial nipples or pacifiers, which have resulted in nipple preference.

◆ The mother's lack of confidence causes her to hold her baby tentatively.

◆ The baby needs to be swaddled to provide boundaries, or needs to be soothed by being cuddled skin to skin with the parent.

◆ The baby has shut down from too much intervention, such as someone attempting to push the baby on the breast.

◆ The mother and infant have been separated, resulting in missed feeding cues.

Plan of Care for a Fussy Baby

You can help the mother by encouraging her to hold her baby calmly and to cuddle him skin to skin at the breast. Limit attempts to attach him to no more than a few minutes at a time. If he starts to cry or fight the breast, stop and try again about 15 minutes later, after the baby is calmed. Avoid placing pressure on a potentially painful site or holding the baby in a feeding position when administering medical treatment. As with a sleepy baby, until feeds have become established, it is important for the mother to express or pump her milk and feed it to the baby in a cup. No bottles or pacifiers should be used. The baby's physician may prescribe medication to calm the baby. Encourage the mother to ask questions about its possible side effects.

Calming Techniques

◆ Limit invasive procedures to minimize crying.

◆ Provide skin-to-skin contact.

◆ Cuddle without pushing the baby to breastfeed.

◆ Work with the baby in short cycles.

◆ Be sensitive to and respect the baby's cues.

◆ Build the mother's confidence.

◆ Use slow, calm, deliberate movements in caring for the baby.

◆ Cuddle, hold, and walk with the baby.

◆ Talk or sing to the baby in a soft voice.

◆ Swaddle the baby.

◆ Nurse in a dark, quiet room.

◆ Rock in a rocking chair to relax both the mother and baby.

◆ Burp the baby often (unless burping seems to upset him). Burp before switching to the other breast at a feed. After the feed, take as long as a half-hour to burp, if necessary.

◆ Carry the baby in a position that puts gentle and firm pressure on his abdomen, for example, on the mother's hip or shoulder.

◆ Play music, create a monotonous noise by running a vacuum cleaner or dishwasher, or play a tape recording of such sounds.

◆ Change the baby's diaper when it becomes damp or soiled.

◆ Mother and baby sleep or nap together so the baby is comforted by her body warmth and heartbeat.

◆ Massage the baby for 10 to 15 minutes (the baby may fuss during the massage, and will become quiet afterward).

◆ Use a sling to carry the baby close to the mother's body.

◆ Use a baby swing for times when individual attention is not possible.

◆ If the baby is full term and has established good temperature control, remove his clothes and expose him to the air for limited amounts of time.

◆ Lie the baby on his stomach on the mother's lap while she gently bounces her knees or moves them back and forth.

◆ Have the mother and baby take a bath together.

◆ Provide monotonous movement by giving a carriage or car ride.

◆ Remove allergens from the mother's diet.

Ending the Feed

When the baby is allowed to determine the length of a feed, his mouth will gently release the breast when he is finished (Fig. 12.14). If the mother needs to remove her baby from the breast before this occurs (i.e., to achieve a

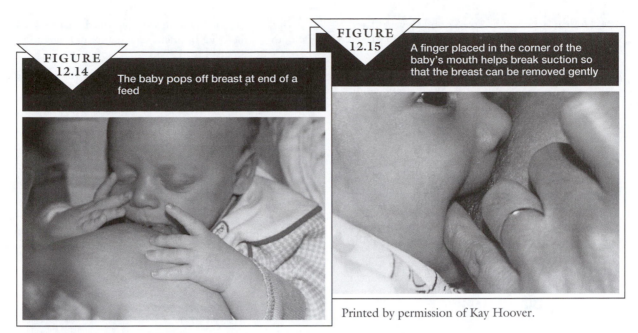

FIGURE 12.14 The baby pops off breast at end of a feed

FIGURE 12.15 A finger placed in the corner of the baby's mouth helps break suction so that the breast can be removed gently

Printed by permission of Kay Hoover.

Printed by permission of Kay Hoover.

better latch), she can break the suction by inserting her finger gently into the corner of his mouth between his gums (Fig. 12.15). Also, she can press a finger against her breast near the corner of the baby's mouth. Her breast should then slip easily out of his mouth.

There should be no chewing or tugging on the end of the nipple. If the mother notices her baby chewing on her nipple toward the end of a feed, to the extent that it causes discomfort, she may need to use this method to end the feed. When the mother's finger touches the infant's lips to begin breaking suction, the infant will automatically begin to suck faster. This is a reflex to having his lip touched while at the breast. The mother can continue her efforts to remove her baby from the breast.

Generally, however, advise the mother to continue the feed until the baby releases the breast spontaneously. She can put him to breast on the other side after he has finished the first breast and continue to nurse at both breasts, one after the other, for as long as the baby wants to continue to breastfeed. There is always milk in the breast. Unless the mother feels pain or discomfort, encourage her to allow her baby to stay at the breast when he is still suckling and swallowing.

breastfeeding. Establishing a routine for feeds will help the mother become comfortable with the process. Teach mothers how to recognize feeding cues and to trust in their own instincts in nurturing their babies. Ensure that mothers have a sound basis for breastfeeding management. Teach them the principles of positioning and attachment, and make it a goal to observe every mother and baby at a breastfeed to assess technique and offer any necessary assistance. Be available to assist with babies who have difficulty latching on, and provide support for mothers whose babies are sleepy or fussy, offering suggestions for rousing or calming the baby. The time spent by caregivers assisting mothers in these early feeds will determine the course of the mother's long-term breastfeeding.

REFERENCES

DeCarvalho M. Effects of frequent breastfeeding on early milk production and infant weight gain. *Pediatrics* 72:307–311; 1983.

Kutner L. *Lactation Management Course.* Chalfont, PA: Breastfeeding Support Consultants Center for Lactation Education; 1996.

Maccagno-Smith R and Young M. Breastfeeding the sleepy infant. *Can Nurse* 89:20–22; 1993.

Minchin M. Positioning for breastfeeding. *Birth* 16:67–73; 1989.

SUMMARY

Learning to recognize their baby's instincts, reflexes, and responses will guide parents in meeting their baby's needs. The mother's early days with her baby are important in the establishment of a strong foundation for

Newton M. Human lactation. In Kon SK and Cowie AT (eds): *Milk: The Mammary Gland and Its Secretion*, Vol. 1. New York: Academic Press, Inc.; 1961.

Nursing Mothers Association of Australia (NMAA). *Too Much, Coping with an Over-Abundant Milk Supply*. Nunawading; 1995.

Widstrom AM et al. The position of the tongue during rooting reflexes elicited in newborn infants before the first suckle. *Acta Paediatr* 82:281–283; 1993.

Woolridge MW and Fisher C. Colic, overfeeding, and symptoms of lactose malabsorption in the breastfed baby: A possible artifact of feed management. *Lancet* 2:382–384; 1988.

Woolridge MW et al. Do changes in pattern of breast usage alter the baby's nutrient intake? *Lancet* 336:395–397; 1990.

------------------------------▼------------------------------

BIBLIOGRAPHY

Danner SC and Cerutti ER. *Nursing Your Premature Baby*. Waco, TX: Childbirth Graphics, Ltd.; 1984.

Dewey K. Growth patterns of breastfed infants and the current status of growth charts for infants. *J Hum Lact* 14:89–92; 1998.

Fleming P. *Reducing the Risk of SIDS. Where Should Babies Sleep? Alone or with Parents*. Conference Proceedings: Breastfeeding '99: The Vital Gift. Atlanta, GA; March, 1999.

Levindon P et al. Randomised controlled trial of sucrose by mouth for the relief of infant crying after immunisation. *Arch Dis Child* 78:453–456; 1998.

Lucassen P et al. Effectiveness of treatments for infantile colic: Systematic review. *Br Med J* 316:1563–1569; 1998.

MacFarlane A. *The Psychology of Childbirth*. Boston, MA: Harvard University Press, pp. 100–101; 1997.

Matthews MK. Mothers' satisfaction with their neonates' breastfeeding behaviors. *JOGNN* 20(1):49–55; 1991.

Renfrew M. Positioning baby at the breast: More than a visual skill. *J Hum Lact* 5(1):13–15; 1989.

Skadberg B et al. Abandoning prone sleeping: Effect on the risk of sudden infant death syndrome. *J Pediatr* 132:340–343; 1998.

Titus K. When the full term newborn will not nurse. *J Hum Lact* 4(1):12–14; 1989.

Walker M. Functional assessment of infant breastfeeding patterns. *Birth* 16(3):140–47; 1989.

Wolke D et al. An epidemiologic longitudinal study of sleeping problems and feeding experience of preterms and term children in southern Finland: Comparison with a southern German population sample. *J Pediatr* 133:224–231; 1998.

CHAPTER

13

INFANT ATTACHMENT AND SUCKING

Contributing Authors: Linda Kutner and Jan Barger

Although there may be an occasional baby who needs assistance in initiating effective suckling, the vast majority of babies need no help. Health care professionals need a sound understanding of sucking as described in this chapter. This understanding will help in evaluating the appropriateness of any intervention. Armed with this fundamental understanding, the helper then needs to step back and take a noninterventive approach. There is a great deal of biologic variability among women and babies. Caregivers need to trust in the innate abilities, reflexes, and intuitive instincts of both the mother and baby. Always remain aware of the fact that you must have a good reason for putting anything in the baby's mouth other than the breast. The baby's sucking and suckling are explored in this chapter, in order to form a basis for discussing the relationship between suckling, attachment, and milk transfer.

SUCKING AND SUCKLING

Sucking is a means of comfort and nourishment to a baby. In addition to being pleasurable both physically and emotionally, the sucking associated with nursing stimulates saliva, which contains enzymes that help predigest food before the stomach enzymes begin to work on it. Further down in the gut, sucking stimulates gastrointestinal secretions, hormones, and motility. The release of certain hormones in the gut also promote satiety and sleepiness in the baby.

Sucking can have a calming effect on the baby and helps him pass gas and move his bowels. It serves the mother by activating prolactin release, thus stimulating her milk production and feelings of yearning for her baby. As sucking continues, oxytocin—which also causes cuddly and warm feelings in the mother—is released. This causes her milk to let down and helps her uterus to return to its prepregnant size.

It is understandable that sucking needs vary from one baby to another. Many babies are born with red marks or blisters on their hands or wrists, an indication that they were sucking in utero. Thumbs, fingers, and hands are used by many babies as a means of soothing and calming themselves. The need for sucking is usually greater in the first 3 months than at any other time. Encourage mothers to be sensitive to this important aspect of their babies' health. Satisfying a baby's sucking needs will enhance his emotional well-being and growth.

The Infant's Sucking Pattern

A breastfeeding baby sucks in a rhythm that corresponds inversely to the amount of milk that is available. High rates of milk flow result in slower sucking rates of about one suck per second. As the milk is removed, sucking rates increase until they reach about two sucks per second, when milk removal is minimal (Bowen-Jones, 1984; Mathew, 1989). These rates of sucking are termed nutritive and non-nutritive, respectively, and comprise two distinctly different patterns. Another distinction is made between sucking and suckling. Sucking describes the act of the baby drawing the breast into his mouth and maintaining negative pressure to keep it there. To receive milk, he then actively suckles the milk out with a peristaltic action of his tongue.

Suckling and feeding develop in a predictable and organized way after birth (Widstrom, 1987). Several investigators have found that nutritive sucking is adversely affected by central nervous system depressant drugs given to the mother in labor (Crowell, 1994; Matthews, 1989; Righard, 1990). Letting the baby cry can also compromise his innate sucking behavior and result in a disorganized suck (Anderson, 1989).

Changes in sucking rate during breastfeeding are gradual (Bowen-Jones, 1982). At the breast, the cycle begins with rapid suckling until letdown occurs. As the baby swallows, his sucking pace slows. He returns to more rapid suckling for stimulation and then slower sucking as milk is released. This pattern continues until the decreased milk reserve results in a faster non-nutritive sucking. When the baby switches to the other breast, he resumes the same pattern. Studies reveal that the full-term **neonate** younger than 24 hours old showed less rhythmic sucking than the older term infant. This could bolster the evidence that normal sucking is partly a learned behavior (Medoff-Cooper, 1989).

Additionally, it has been found that babies who exhibit short suckling bursts and shorter overall suckling times have more feeding difficulties at 6 weeks of age than those who have longer, continuous bursts of suckling and spend more of their time suckling (Ramsay, 1996). For this reason, it is important that you thoroughly assess the baby's early sucking pattern and work with the mother to help her baby continue at feeds rather than stop after short efforts.

In the first 2 or 3 days, the baby exhibits several short, fast bursts of suckling per swallow. This pattern is an indication that volume of colostrum is relatively small. After around the third or fourth day, a regular feeding rhythm becomes established. It is no coincidence that this timing correlates with the point at which the mother's milk progresses from the colostral phase to transitional milk with increased volume. At around 4 to 5 days, the full-term infant swallows with every suck, which indicates milk flow following letdown.

▼ **Physiology of Suckling**

In suckling, the baby uses his tongue to draw the nipple and areola into his mouth to form a cone-shaped extension of the breast that conforms to the shape of the baby's mouth (Fig. 13.1). It is important to recognize that when sufficient breast tissue is drawn into his mouth, the baby's tongue is free from frictional movement against the breast. There is no in-and-out movement—only a one-way exchange of milk from the breast to the baby. The baby's tongue ripples in a rhythmic, wavelike motion from the front of the mouth toward the back.

The areola and nipple are pressed upward progressively against the upper gum, the hard palate, and the soft palate at the back of the mouth. This action, along with the alternate compression and release of the gums, moves the milk through the lactiferous sinuses and out of the nipple. When the baby's jaw drops, it creates negative pressure, which allows the milk to move from the nipple to the baby's mouth.

A 1994 article by Yokoyama documents the pulsatile manner in which oxytocin is released by suckling and the increase in prolactin level as a result of suckling. Another study conducted during that year revealed how quickly the newborn is capable of adjusting his sucking rate. Although the study involved bottle-feeding babies, the authors believe it can be applied to the breastfeeding baby's ability to cope with letdown (Al-Sayed, 1994).

A 1989 study demonstrated that bottle feeders breathe less often than breastfeeders, with two of the 15 bottle feeders experiencing decreased heart rates. The number of sucks per minute was also higher in breastfeeders (Mathew, 1989). Because swallowing cannot occur simultaneously with breathing and because a pattern of more sucks per minute is associated with fewer swallows, higher sucking frequency correlates with more breaths and higher oxygen saturations. Babies pause between bursts of suckling and are able to regulate their breathing. Suckling develops on a continuum with fewer sucks per burst and longer pauses in preterm infants.

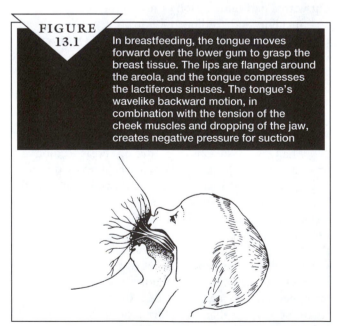

FIGURE 13.1 In breastfeeding, the tongue moves forward over the lower gum to grasp the breast tissue. The lips are flanged around the areola, and the tongue compresses the lactiferous sinuses. The tongue's wavelike backward motion, in combination with the tension of the cheek muscles and dropping of the jaw, creates negative pressure for suction

Source: King FS. *Helping Mothers to Breastfeed*, Revised Edition, p. 14. Nairobi, Kenya: AMREF. Reprinted with permission.

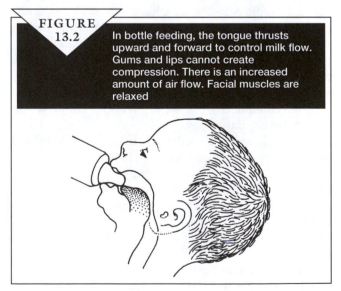

FIGURE 13.2 In bottle feeding, the tongue thrusts upward and forward to control milk flow. Gums and lips cannot create compression. There is an increased amount of air flow. Facial muscles are relaxed

Illustration by Marcia Smith.

Suckling at the Breast Versus Sucking on a Bottle

The suckling mechanism for a breastfeeding infant involves his entire mouth—his lips, gums, tongue, cheeks, and his hard and **soft palate;** the soft breast molds to the baby's mouth. A breastfeeding infant actively suckles the breast in order to receive milk. It is quite different from the sucking motion that is used for extracting milk from a bottle (Fig 13.2). In bottle feeding, the baby draws the nipple into his mouth and he must alter his mouth to accommodate the shape of the artificial nipple. He must generate suction pressure so that the milk flows freely from the bottle. This is a very different action from the peristaltic tongue motion used by the breastfeeding baby. The use of an artificial nipple may alter proper development of swallowing, alignment of the teeth, and the shaping of the hard palate (Palmer, 1999). Additionally, artificial nipples weaken the baby's suck. They reduce the strength of the **masseter muscle** and increase the strength of the **orbicularis oris muscles**. This causes the facial muscles to develop in the exact opposite pattern from which they were intended (Legovic, 1991).

In 1994, Meier emphasized the difference in sucking between breastfeeders and bottle feeders. What may appear to be dysfunctional on a bottle, that is, wide jaw excursions, is not dysfunctional in breastfeeding. Wide jaw excursions are indicative of nutritive suckling in a breastfeeding baby. This supports the argument against the idea that preterm infants must "prove" themselves on a bottle before they are allowed to go to breast. Further, high flow rates from artificial nipples cause preterm infants to swallow continuously, thus limiting their chances to breathe.

Because of the very different way in which babies suck on a bottle and the breast, alternating between the two can create problems. This is especially true in the early weeks when the baby is mastering his technique. Artificial teats—both bottle nipples and pacifiers—can cause the baby to develop a preference for this teat over the breast. Milk flows more readily and quickly from a bottle nipple. When he returns to the breast, he must suckle actively to receive milk. It is for this reason that breastfeeding babies should be given no artificial nipple.

LATCHING THE BABY ON

Now, with a firm understanding of the baby's suckling, we can address the relationship of suckling to the manner in which the baby is attached at the breast. The moment of contact of the baby's mouth on the mother's breast is referred to as *latching on* or *attachment*. A good latch enables the infant to take a large amount of breast tissue into his mouth. He needs to get as much of the areola as possible into his mouth so that his lips are positioned behind the lactiferous sinuses and can strip milk from them. With this accomplished, the baby is then able to suckle and obtain milk. Removal of milk, in turn, relieves milk pressure in the breast so that milk production is maintained. This process should occur without causing the mother any discomfort, pain, or trauma.

When a baby is latched on well, the mother will be able to observe audible swallows or long, drawing, nutritive, high flow sucks. In the first 24 to 48 hours, the swallows often sound like little puffs of air after three to four high-flow, nutritive sucks. The mother may report a tugging or pulling sensation with a good latch. However, she should be free of pain, both during and after the feed. If she experiences pain, she needs to adjust her baby's position. Figures 13.3 and 13.4 show the differences between a baby who has a good latch and one who does not.

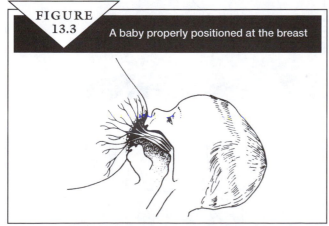

FIGURE 13.3 A baby properly positioned at the breast

Source: King FS. *Helping Mothers to Breastfeed,* Revised Edition, p. 14. Nairobi, Kenya: AMREF. Reprinted with permission.

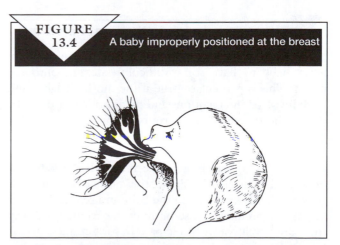

FIGURE 13.4 A baby improperly positioned at the breast

Source: King FS. *Helping Mothers to Breastfeed,* Revised Edition, p. 14. Nairobi, Kenya: AMREF. Reprinted with permission.

Principles of a Good Latch

In order to achieve a good latch, the baby needs to be in a receptive state in which he can settle and organize. He will turn his head toward the mother's breast and open his mouth wide. The proper position for optimal suckling is for the breast to be slightly above the center of the baby's open mouth. His lips are **flanged** out and open wide at an angle of at least 140 degrees. His bottom lip will cover most of the areola and his top lip will cover somewhat less of the areola. This ensures more adequate compression of the lactiferous sinuses, which lie deeper in the breast.

If the baby does not take enough breast tissue into his mouth, he will have difficulty extracting milk and will compensate by increasing suction and compressing his lips to hold the nipple securely. This could result in nipple soreness. A 1992 case study reported by Morton demonstrated how a change in positioning improved suckling. The protractility of the mother's nipple and flexibility of the breast tissue are important to the infant's ability to latch on effectively. If the breast tissue is not drawn into the baby's mouth back to the soft palate, he may have difficulty with feeds and fail to gain weight.

The baby's tongue will be positioned under the breast and will extend outward far enough to cover the alveolar ridge (bottom gum line). With his mouth open wide and his lips flanged, he will take in a large mouthful of breast tissue, forming a trough with his tongue, and drawing the nipple into the center of his mouth or tongue. He will position his jaws behind the lactiferous sinuses and compress them rhythmically, continuing to hold the breast in his mouth as he establishes a pattern of repeated bursts of suck/swallow/pause ... suck/swallow/pause. In order for this to be considered a good latch, all of this must be done without the mother experiencing any discomfort (Kutner, 1996).

The Baby's Latch in the First Few Days

In the early days of breastfeeding, it is not uncommon for a baby to have some difficulty latching onto the breast. This is particularly true if the mother's labor and birth involved interventions and medications. If the baby misses the nipple when he roots toward it, the mother can wait a few seconds and stroke his cheek again. If his rooting reflex appears to be weak, she can express milk onto his lips to lead him to the breast. If the baby still does not latch onto the nipple, the mother can withdraw her breast, relax, reposition the baby and repeat the rooting reflex stimulation. Establishing this routine will help the baby develop a workable pattern for getting onto the breast. Encourage the mother to think of her early days

of breastfeeding as a learning period and not to become discouraged if she and her baby experience some difficulties in getting started. It is all part of the process!

THE TRANSFER OF MILK TO THE BABY

Before addressing possible problems with suckling and attachment, it is helpful to first understand how milk is transferred from the mother to her baby, and how interaction between them can affect that transfer. The two essential elements for efficient milk transfer are a functioning letdown in the breast and appropriate suckling by the infant. It is important that everyone involved in the mother's and baby's care understand that milk transfer is an interaction between the mother and her baby, and they each exert influence over one another. The manner in which the baby's mouth physically meets and then stimulates the breast is crucial to effective milk transfer (Woolridge, 1986). The mother's physical comfort, as well as her confidence in her ability to nurture and nourish her infant, is communicated to her baby in the way she holds him. Both of these factors can affect her letdown reflex.

As depicted in Figure 13.5, the mother's breast completely fills the baby's oral cavity. Milk is transferred from the breast to the baby when suckling causes a **bolus** of food to be delivered to the **pharynx**. A peri-

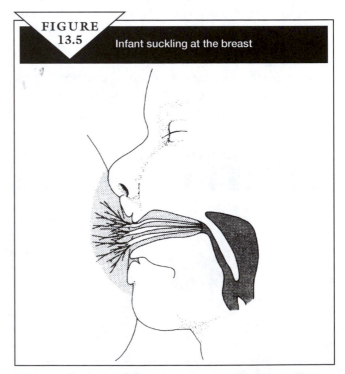

FIGURE 13.5 Infant suckling at the breast

Source: Woolridge MW. The anatomy of infant sucking. *Midwifery* 2:164–171; 1986. Reprinted with permission.

staltic wave of contraction in the tongue muscle progresses backward along the teat from an anterior to posterior direction. The baby needs a large mouthful of breast in order to remove milk effectively. In order for the baby to take a large enough amount of breast tissue into his mouth, he must be held close to and facing the mother's breast. Suckling occurs in a continuous cycle of suck/swallow/breathe (Mathew, 1989). This occurs all within about 1 second per cycle. With the mother's nipple, areola, and breast tissue forming a teat within the baby's mouth, the baby's tongue cups along the sides of the teat and forms a trough. A wave of compression then moves along the tongue to push the milk toward the back of the mouth, and the baby swallows when the back of his mouth fills with milk.

Table 13.1 describes this action in detail. The infant draws the breast into his mouth and forms a teat of the breast and nipple that conforms to his mouth. During this formation, the baby's tongue cups along the sides of the teat, and it covers the alveolar ridge throughout the suckling cycle. The combination of positive pressure in the alveoli, created by the letdown reflex, and suction caused by the jaw lowering causes milk to enter the teat. The end of the nipple is drawn back to the soft palate. Next, the front tip of the tongue wells up, and the lower jaw raises to compress the breast, thus pinching off milk

---

TABLE 13.1

The Process of Milk Transfer

Step	Description
1 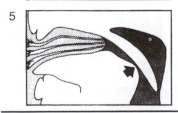	The baby takes breast tissue into his mouth and forms a teat from the mother's nipple, areola, and breast tissue. It is important to note that the teat formed by the breast and nipple fills the baby's mouth, leaving no room for movement of the breast within the mouth. As he draws the teat far into his mouth, his tongue cups around the teat to form a trough for the milk. The baby's tongue stays cupped along the sides of the breast and nipple teat, and covers the alveolar ridge throughout the suckling cycle.
2 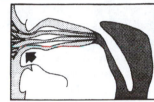	The suck cycle begins. The end of the nipple is drawn back to the soft palate by a combination of suction and compression. When it is fully extended, the nipple is approximately three times as long as it is at rest. This suggests that the baby cannot traumatize the breast tissue if he has a good mouthful of breast. It is compressed for only a fraction of a second and will not look flattened or compressed when the feed ends if the baby was attached correctly. When the nipple touches the soft palate at the back of the oral cavity, it elicits the baby's suck reflex. The baby then raises his lower jaw to pinch off milk that collects in the lactiferous sinuses. At the same time, the anterior tip of his tongue begins to push upward against the breast tissue.
3 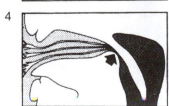	The baby strips milk from the lactiferous sinuses. A peristaltic wave of compression moves along the underside of the teat. The baby's tongue pushes against his hard palate, thus compressing the sinuses. A bolus of milk is then squeezed from the teat. Note that when the sinuses are compressed, milk flows from the breast. The baby does not get milk from the breast by suction.
4 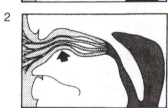	The wave of compression continues to the back of the tongue, which pushes against the soft palate and rises to seal the nasal cavity. The trachea and vocal chords are closed off by the **epiglottis**, and milk is propelled into the esophagus. This, in turn, initiates the baby's swallow reflex.
5 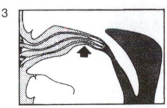	The compression ends at the posterior base of the tongue. The back of the tongue depresses, which creates negative pressure. The breast is then drawn back into the baby's mouth to begin another cycle.

Source: Woolridge MW. The anatomy of infant sucking. *Midwifery* 2:164–171; 1986. Reprinted with permission.

in the lactiferous sinuses. A peristaltic wave of compression moves along the tongue toward the back of the mouth. The tongue continues in its action, pushing against the hard palate, compressing the lactiferous sinuses, and making milk flow.

As the peristalsis moves to the back of the mouth, the tongue pushes against the soft palate. Through the rolling motion of the tongue, the milk is brought out of the nipple to fill the back of the baby's mouth, causing the baby to swallow. To complete the cycle, the back of the tongue depresses to create negative pressure. This retains the breast in the baby's mouth and refills the lactiferous sinuses. Thus, the amount of breast tissue that is taken into the baby's mouth will determine how easily the milk is nursed out. Watching the baby's sucking action and jaw movement in relation to the frequency of swallowing can give clues to the amount of milk that is being transferred to the baby.

Signs of Good Milk Transfer

After observing that the baby is latched on effectively, you can evaluate the transfer of milk from the mother to her baby. Signs to watch for include

- The baby moves from short rapid sucks to slow deep sucks early in the feed.

- The mother notices signs of the milk ejection reflex.

- No dimpling or puckering of the baby's cheeks is noted.

- Breast tissue does not slide in and out of the infant's mouth when the baby sucks or pauses.

- No smacking or clicking sounds are noted with sucking.

- Swallowing is noted after every one to four sucks.

- The baby is able to maintain his latch throughout the feed.

- The mother's breast softens as the feed progresses (noted after Stage II lactogenesis).

- The baby spontaneously unlatches and is satiated.

- The mother's nipple is not blanched or compressed when the baby unlatches.

- The baby is content between most feeds.

- The baby's voiding and stooling are appropriate for his age.

We now have a clear picture of the manner in which a baby attaches to the breast, and how he obtains milk through an intricate suckling action. The vast majority of babies will accomplish this feat remarkably well when the mother uses sound breastfeeding management. There are some babies, however, who may have difficulty and require assistance.

▼

PROBLEMS GETTING THE BABY LATCHED ONTO THE BREAST

It is not uncommon for a baby to have some difficulty latching onto the breast in the early attempts. Help mothers approach early feeds in a calm manner and with a sense of humor. This will decrease potential frustration in both the mother and the baby. When there are difficulties, encourage mother's to keep the attempts to breastfeed very short. Depending on the baby's tolerance, the mother may be able to work with him for as long as 10 minutes. As soon as the baby cries or pushes away or demonstrates other withdrawal or avoidance behaviors such as hiccoughs, coughing, gagging, or sneezes, she can stop that attempt, calm the baby, and try again. She may also try feeding on the other breast or hold her baby in a different position.

If the baby rejects the breast after three such attempts, advise that she stop all efforts for that feed. Simply snuggling skin to skin with her baby in a relaxed manner may be the best approach at this point. The mother can watch for the return of approach behaviors such as tongue extension, bringing the hand to the mouth, or rooting. She can then gently bring him to breast again. The mother will need to express milk from her breasts to maintain milk production if the infant continually refuses to nurse. Until an effective latch is achieved, the baby can be given expressed milk with a cup. Occasionally, latch problems are due to oral intrusion such as vigorous oral suctioning or unnecessary digital exams. Care should be taken that the first thing introduced into a baby's mouth is the breast, and that he is put to breast in a gentle manner. The information in Table 13.2 will help you explore the possible causes for problems with latch-on and then to determine appropriate management.

Possible Signs of a Poor Latch

- The baby is unable to stay on the breast for more than several sucks.

- Pain is reported by the mother during or after feeds.

- Dimpling or puckering of the baby's cheeks is noted.

- The breast slides in and out of the baby's mouth throughout sucking.

- Clicking or smacking noises are heard when the baby suckles.

- Little or no swallowing is noted during a feed.

- The baby is discontented during or after feeds.

- The mother's nipple appears flattened, creased, or blanched after the baby unlatches.

TABLE 13.2	
The Baby Who Cannot Get Attached	
Cause	**Suggestions for Management**
The baby is being held in a position that requires him to twist his neck in order to breastfeed.	Help the mother hold her baby close, directly facing and slightly lower than the center of the breast.
The baby does not open his mouth large enough.	Tease the baby with the nipple, by gently touching his lower lip, until he opens his mouth wide before attaching.
The baby has been given an artificial nipple and has a sucking preference. He may thrust or hump his tongue when he tries to attach and suckle.	Give no artificial nipples to the baby; allow him only to suckle at the breast. If supplementation is necessary, use a small cup or a tube at the breast.
The mother's nipples are flat because of engorgement.	Be sure the mother's breasts do not become too full because of limited feeds. If the breasts are engorged, express milk to help the nipple protrude and soften the areola.
The mother's nipples are inverted to the point that the baby cannot get attached.	Draw out an inverted nipple with mild suction before the feed, using an inverted syringe or pump. Note that most inverted nipples do not interfere with breastfeeding. Babies attach to the breast, not to the nipple.

- Little or no breast changes occur from the beginning to the end of a feed after Stage II lactogenesis.
- The baby has inadequate voiding or stooling, or both.

Feeding Adjustments to Improve Latch-On

When an infant continues to have difficulty with latch-on, the mother will need to explore alternative ways to manage feeds. Suggest that she provide lots of skin-to-skin contact without attempting to put the baby to breast. She can lie on her back, with the baby between her breasts, just as she would immediately after birth. If the baby begins to root around for the breast, she can help guide him to the breast, making sure to not push him on.

The mother may have more success getting her baby attached if she holds him in a position where her dominant hand is in control. A right-handed mother would use the clutch hold on the right breast or cross cradle with the left hand supporting the left breast. This is reversed for a left-handed mother. Such positions will give the mother some control over the baby's head movement and help her hug the baby to the breast quickly as soon as his mouth is opened wide enough.

If her baby tends to approach the breast without opening his mouth, the parents can encourage him to open his mouth wider. When the baby is content, awake, and happy, mom or dad can tickle his lower lip with a finger, talking to him all the time, saying slowly "o. .p. .e. .n. .w. .i. .d. .e." When he responds, they can put the finger into his mouth, pad side up, to suck on as a reward. Dipping the finger into the mother's expressed colostrum or milk, or sweetened water will be an added incentive. Also, babies often imitate facial expressions. Parents can demonstrate a wide mouth by opening their mouths wide so that the baby will mirror the action.

The Baby Who Cannot Stay Attached

Some babies may achieve a good latch initially and then will form a pattern of popping on and off the breast during a feed. The baby attaches and begins to feed, and then after a short time, falls away from the breast and cries or chokes. This happens several times during a breastfeed. Table 13.3 will help you explore the causes and then determine the appropriate course of management.

Consequences of a Poor Latch

A mother whose baby is not latched on effectively will very likely experience nipple soreness. An incorrect latch, in fact, is the primary cause of nipple soreness. In turn, the pain—or anticipation of pain—when the mother latches her baby on may inhibit her milk ejection reflex and prevent any milk from reaching her baby. Because a poorly latched baby is unable to remove milk from the mother's breasts adequately, the mother is at risk for engorgement, plugged ducts, and mastitis. Her milk production will also be seriously compromised, and lactation

T A B L E 13.3	
The Baby Who Cannot Stay Attached	
Cause	**Suggestions for Management**
The baby must reach or twist his neck to keep the breast in his mouth.	Be sure the mother is holding her baby close, directly facing and slightly lower than the breast, with his nose and chin touching the breast and the baby's ear, shoulder, and hip in alignment.
The baby is unable to breathe when he is at the breast.	Avoid flexing the baby's head forward in such a way that his nose is pushed against the breast. His head needs to be slightly extended so that his chin and nose are just touching the breast. Pull his bottom in more, and his head will angle out.
The mother is moving either her breast or her baby, or not supporting the baby enough so that the breast falls away.	Hold the baby in a side-sitting position with his head cradled in the mother's hand for greater head control (avoiding pushing at the back of his head). Help the mother identify a good attachment and focus on what it feels like in order that she can recognize the baby's gradual slipping off the breast. Put pillows or blankets under her arm so a fatigued arm muscle will not let the baby slip. Help her check during the feed for good attachment and learn trauma-free unlatching and relatching so that both she and the baby develop the habits of a wide-open, mouth-full attachment. If you can see the problem and the mother cannot, she will continue doing the wrong thing.
The mother's milk is flowing too forcefully.	Be sure the mother's breasts do not become too full because of limited feeds. If the breasts are engorged, expressing milk will help the nipple to protrude. Suggest that the mother express milk before a feed so that the flow is less forceful. Allow the baby to feed on only one breast per feed, with no time limitations, until the initial oversupply has diminished. The mother may need to express milk from the other breast for comfort. If she has an overabundance of milk, she may want to nurse the baby on the same side two or three times before changing to the other breast.

failure is likely to result in the absence of any intervention. It is important that the mother pump or express her milk if the baby is not latching on and breastfeeding effectively.

Consequences of a poor latch are inevitable for the baby as well. Because of the mother's decreased milk ejection reflex, the baby receives primarily foremilk. This results in increased hunger, increased fussiness, and perhaps colic-like symptoms. His urine and stool output may be low, and he may develop jaundice. The baby will be unable to obtain the high-fat hindmilk, resulting in failure to gain weight or even in weight loss. To preserve the baby's health, infant formula supplements may need to be initiated. This could mark the beginning of the end to breastfeeding, unless the plan of care includes suggestions on ways to increase the mother's milk production. Making adjustments in the baby's latch can prevent the situation from progressing to this point.

Physical Pathologies That Can Affect Attachment

In some cases, difficulty with latch may be a result of the mother having breast or nipple abnormalities. It could also be caused by acute or chronic physical conditions such as low back pain, carpal tunnel syndrome, or pain related to delivery, particularly perineal pain. Difficulty could also be a result of the infant having a cleft lip or palate, neurologic or orthopedic problems, Down syndrome, a fractured clavicle, ankyloglossia (tight frenulum), or a high palate. If comfort measures have not resulted in improvement, you may want to explore these factors as possible causes for the baby's difficulty with attachment.

Some babies also engage in rapid side-to-side head movements, making it impossible to achieve a good latch. You can use a dropper of the mothers milk or water to touch the midline of the baby's upper lip. When the baby stops his head movement, you can lead him to the breast. Then place a couple of drops of fluid on his tongue as he opens his mouth. You can also do this with tubing and a syringe.

The Use of Feeding Devices to Help with Attachment

If the mother is getting frustrated to the point of weaning, you might suggest that she feed her baby her expressed milk using an alternative feeding method, as discussed in Chapter 19. She can also continue to put the baby to breast at each feed. If the baby will tolerate a nipple shield, she may consider this as a last resort. The mother will need to continue to express milk from her breasts to maintain milk production until the baby is weaned from the shield. It is important to remain flexible in your approach with mothers. Do only what a particular mother can tolerate. This may require more alternatives in some cases than in others.

Be careful about using a syringe with a plunger to feed babies. This removes control from the baby and places it in the hands of the mother or caregiver. Some practitioners have recommended using periodontal syringes for finger feeding or for supplementing at the breast. However, the syringe is sharp and potentially could be harmful to the baby. If the baby were to move suddenly, he could be poked or scratched. For all of these reasons, use of a syringe in an infant's mouth is not recommended. See the discussion of feeding alternatives in Chapter 19.

BABIES WHO HAVE DIFFICULTY SUCKLING

Most feeding difficulties are caused by improper or incorrect attachment or faulty positioning of the baby at the breast. In many cases, patience, practice, and proper positioning of the baby's body, and of his mouth on the breast, will alleviate these suckling difficulties. Righard and Alade demonstrated the importance of correcting early sucking problems. Their 1992 study revealed that uncorrected babies stopped nursing sooner. Hence, there is danger in suggesting that the "baby will figure it out when the milk comes in". Another 1992 report revealed that after correcting positioning, the baby's suckling improved (Morton, 1992).

A thorough assessment of both the mother and baby will help determine if the problem is one of attachment or if the baby truly does have a dysfunctional suck. There are numerous factors that can potentially cause attachment or sucking difficulties. Most of them are relatively short lived, and are resolved by time and by making sure the baby receives sufficient calories. A baby may have a weak or dysfunctional suck because he is actually weak from insufficient nourishment. Many times, a baby's suckling can be improved by getting more calories into him. **Intubation** is another factor to consider when evaluating an infant's suck, especially with preterm infants. A 1993 study showed that it took intubated babies longer to develop a normal nutritive suck. Both breastfeeders and bottle feeders were included in this study, and they were not analyzed separately (Bier, 1993).

The Baby Who Attaches and Is Not Suckling Nutritively

An occasional baby may achieve a good latch and yet makes no effort to establish a nutritive suck. It is possible that he is sleepy and not hungry at that moment. For these babies, you need to determine whether they are receiving any artificial feeds of water or infant formula, or are using a pacifier. These are fairly simple factors to correct once the baby is back exclusively at the breast.

Some babies, however, will have difficulty initially mastering the physical process of suckling. Suckling can be disorganized due to illness, prematurity, drugs given to the infant or mother, or a delay in the first breastfeed after birth. Suckling ability may also be affected by neuromotor dysfunction, variations in oral anatomy, and nipple preference due to the introduction of an artificial nipple. Table 13.4 presents a summary of the causes of a baby having difficulty suckling and suggests possible actions the mother can take to overcome these problems. It is clear in reviewing these causes that a careful assessment is an integral part of determining the appropriate course of action.

DEVELOPING A PLAN OF CARE

It is important that the plan of care be based on the assessed problem and not on an assumption of dysfunctional suck. The goal is to resolve the cause of the problem, not just the symptoms (i.e., resolve why the baby has poor weight gain, not just give formula). Take the mother's situation and emotional state into account, and include her in the planning. Be cautious not to overwhelm the mother with too many things to do. Consider the long-term consequences of your plan of care as well. Will using a bottle cause a nipple preference? Might a nipple shield lower the mother's milk production? Will feeding become a chore for the mother and a difficult procedure for the baby? You need to develop a plan that the mother is likely to follow.

Keep in mind that most breastfeeding problems are related to incorrect attachment at the breast, not to dysfunctional sucking. There is a difference between a disorganized suck and a dysfunctional suck. Babies may exhibit an uncoordinated suck in the first few days of life as a result of sucking habits in utero, birth interventions, or early artificial nipple feeds. In some cases, the cause is unexplained. Most uncoordinated sucking is resolved with the passage of time and with increasing the baby's caloric intake. The initiation of any intervention in the hospital for the healthy term infant is rarely indicated. Putting your finger into the baby's mouth should be done only in

TABLE 13.4
Issues That May Cause Problems With Latch-On or Suckling

Cause	Suggestions for Management
Medication received by the mother during labor	Encourage childbirth educators to focus on labor support issues. Encourage labor and delivery staff to focus on nonpharmacologic comfort measures for labor.
Forceps delivery or vacuum extraction	Watch positioning of the infant to avoid pressure on the infant's head.
Post birth interventions such as deep laryngeal suctioning or circumcision	Avoid putting the baby to breast immediately following deep suctioning or other oral insult until the baby demonstrates readiness. Avoid circumcision until the baby has fed well at the breast at least 3 times.
Prolonged crying, especially due to interventions	Prevent prolonged crying by helping the mother with her baby. Comfort the baby before putting him to breast. Teach the mother and staff the importance of feeding on cue rather than when the infant cries. Keep the mother and baby together rather than having the baby in the nursery.
Baby has a fractured clavicle or **cephalhematoma**	Position the baby in a manner that prevents pressure on the affected area.
Mother has tight, taut breast tissue with flat or inverted nipples	Massage breast before the feed. Use a hold that enables the mother to maintain control over her baby's head movement (clutch hold or cross cradle hold). Use an inverted syringe to form the nipple (see Chapter 19). The mother may need to use a nipple shield (see Chapter 19).
Incorrect positioning at the breast	Correct any positioning problems. Make sure both mother and baby are comfortable.
Mom's lack of confidence in handling baby and putting baby to breast	Give encouragement to the mother and help her see that she and her baby will become more comfortable with one another with practice and time. Show the mother how to handle her baby and put him to breast. Avoid doing it for her.
High-arched or bubble palate	Use the clutch hold. Take the infant off the breast after 30–60 seconds and reattach. The second latch helps draw more tissue farther back into the infant's mouth.
Short or tight frenulum	Contact the pediatrician, dentist, oral surgeon, or ear-nose-throat specialist for evaluation and possible clipping of the frenulum.
Cleft lip	The lip usually molds around the breast to form suction. If this is not the case, the mother can cover the cleft area with her breast or finger. Massage the breasts before and during the feed.
Cleft palate	Nurse in a semiupright position. Hold the breast in the baby's mouth during feeds. Interrupt feeding as necessary to allow the baby to burp or breathe. If the baby cannot obtain sufficient milk through suckling, express and feed milk in a tube feeding device or cup. An **obturator** (a feeding plate placed over the cleft) may be helpful. The mother will need a referral to a cleft palate team if one is available in your area.
Hypoglycemia in the infant	Feed the baby. Give expressed colostrum via cup or spoon. Use an artificial baby milk if expressed mother's milk is not sufficient for the baby's needs. Make sure that the infant is fed at regular intervals. Wake him to feed if necessary.
Hypotonia or hypertonia in the infant	Positioning is the key. Some hypertonic babies may need to find their own position of comfort. A hypotonic baby will need to be supported well. The mother may need to use a tube-feeding device if the infant does not feed well. Decrease external stimulation for the hypertonic infant. Use rousing techniques for the hypotonic infant, starting with infant massage. Use gentle massage to calm the hypertonic infant. Short, very frequent feeds (every 1½ to 2 hours) will be more effective than longer feeds at longer intervals. Condition the baby by establishing a routine for getting on the breast, especially if the baby's rooting reflex is not well developed. Supplement with expressed milk in a cup or bottle after nursing if the infant is unable to obtain enough through use of a tube-feeding device at the breast. Express milk, and supplement the baby until the condition improves.

TABLE 13.4 (CONTINUED)	
Issues That May Cause Problems With Latch-On or Suckling	
Cause	**Suggestions for Management**
Baby engages in tongue sucking or tongue thrust	A baby who consistently sucks his tongue has been doing so in utero for months. Have the baby learn to suck progressively on mom's small finger, middle finger and then thumb to gradually increase the baby's comfort level with larger sizes of objects in his mouth. Use finger feeding until the infant can latch on.
Baby has received bottles and prefers an artificial nipple	Because babies suck differently on an artificial nipple than they do on the breast, it is important to avoid using a rubber/silicone teat as much as possible. The long, firm object stimulates his palate and initiates a suck almost immediately. He does not have to draw it into his mouth. Any kind of sucking stimulus on the bottle teat will cause fluid to flow into his mouth; hence, he will be unable to suck non-nutritively on the bottle as he can on the breast. He will have to hump his tongue at the front of the teat to control milk flow. When the breast is drawn into the baby's mouth, it conforms to the shape of his mouth, whereas the bottle teat not only does not fill the baby's mouth but he must alter his mouth shape to work with the artificial nipple. Discontinue the bottle and supplement with a cup, spoon, or medicine dropper.
Baby has a stuffy nose due to a cold or allergies	Nurse the baby in an upright position. Saline nose drops or a drop of the mother's milk in the baby's nostrils helps clear a stuffy nose. Using a bulb syringe to clear the nose may irritate the delicate mucous membranes and cause swelling.
Mother is taking medication that affects the baby through her milk	Ask the physician about switching to a drug that will have less effect on the baby. Alter feeding times and drug administration so that the baby nurses when the amount of drug in the mother's milk is lowest. If possible, delay drug use until the baby is older. If reactions are serious (i.e., extreme colic-like behavior or lethargy) and the drug cannot be discontinued, do not breastfeed.

special circumstances and should be done very carefully by a trained person. The baby's oral cavity is extremely sensitive, with many complex innervations. Too much inappropriate manipulation can result in an aversion to anything going into his mouth, including the breast.

Barger (1998) identifies five levels of intervention for infants who have difficulty suckling. When assistance is indicated, the caregiver should start with the least complex method and progress to the highest degree of intervention only when indicated. Whenever possible, follow a course that places the baby in control of the feeding rather than special devices or techniques. Refer to Chapter 19 for further details on the techniques described.

▼ Noninterventive Techniques

First, you will need to determine the probable cause of the suckling difficulty and consider whether the situation is one that will improve with time. If poor positioning is the cause, help the mother correct the positioning. Then wait for the "golden moment," the time before crying begins when the baby is rooting, hungry, and opens his mouth wide. The mother can express colostrum onto her nipple to entice the baby. Alternatively, she may drip some glucose water on the nipple to stimu-

late sucking. The sweeter the solution, the faster the baby will suck.

▼ Minimal Level of Intervention

You or the parent can place an index finger in the baby's mouth to pacify him or to initiate rhythmic sucking. Using a supplemental feeding device at the breast will help get calories into the baby and stimulate sucking at the same time. Either expressed mother's milk or formula can be given through the device, depending on the availability of mother's milk. Keep in mind that if the baby is not latching on to the breast, a feeding tube at the breast will not be helpful. However, a feeding tube is helpful for a baby who attaches and does not suckle adequately.

▼ Low-Level Intervention

You can insert your index finger into the baby's mouth to evaluate his oral cavity and his suck. Please note that it is not necessary to assess infant oral structure routinely other than visually. Oral examination is an invasion of the baby's mouth and should be done only if a problem is suspected. If a short frenulum is causing difficulty, you can help the mother find someone to clip the frenulum.

A baby who is not feeding effectively will need to receive nourishment by either a cup or finger feeding. These techniques are also considered to be low-level interventions.

▼ Moderate-Level Intervention

If other measures have been unsuccessful, you can place your index finger in the baby's mouth, with the pad side up, to organize his sucking. Slight pressure is placed on the midline of the tongue, and the finger is pulled out slowly to encourage the baby to suck it back in. Verbal reinforcement is given when the baby sucks correctly. Notice that in the minimal level and low level interventions, the baby was in control. This intervention involves more control by the caregiver through manipulation of the finger in the baby's mouth. It should be performed only after other measures have failed to elicit effective suckling.

▼ High-Level Intervention

The highest degree of intervention is suck training. This degree of intervention is beyond the scope of most nurses and lactation consultants. If there is a need for suck training, there are often other neurologic problems (such as cerebral palsy) and the suck is often the first area in which the problem presents. This technique involves placing the index finger in the baby's mouth to stimulate certain portions of his oral anatomy in order to train him to suck. A baby who needs suck training must be referred to a professional who is trained and skilled in this field, such as a physical or speech therapist with further specialization as a neurodevelopmental therapist. You will need to work in concert with the baby's physician and other specialists. A referral to an organization that assists the neurologically impaired child and his family may be necessary. It is important to recognize that the incidence of a need for suck training is extremely rare.

▼ SUMMARY

An awareness of the mechanics of infant sucking will help caregivers understand the transfer of milk from the breast to the baby. The manner in which a baby suckles the breast, his sucking needs, and the pattern he establishes will impact this transfer. Although a small number of infants may have difficulty suckling, most causes of attachment or suckling difficulties can be reversed without direct intervention by the caregiver (Table 13.5). When it becomes necessary to intervene, the least invasive

---

TABLE 13.5

Chapter Summary—Teaching Points for Helping Mothers Get Started With Breastfeeding

Helping mothers with breastfeeding

◆ Have the baby breastfeed within the first hour after birth.

◆ Keep babies and mothers together from birth.

◆ Offer help with breastfeeding within 6 hours of delivery.

◆ Help mothers learn how to respond to their babies' needs.

◆ If the baby seems too sleepy to feed, wait half an hour and try again.

◆ Place no restrictions on the frequency or length of feeds.

◆ If there is pain during breastfeeds, check the baby's latch.

◆ Teach mothers to let their babies come off the breast of their own accord.

What to look for when observing a breastfeed

◆ Signs that the baby is attached for effective suckling.

◆ Signs that the baby is suckling and that milk is flowing.

◆ Signs that the mother may need help.

Signs of good attachment

◆ The baby's mouth is open wide.

◆ The baby's chin is touching the breast.

◆ The baby's lower lip is curled outward.

◆ The baby suckles, pauses, and sucks again—in slow, deep sucks.

◆ The mother hears the baby swallowing.

Signs of poor attachment

◆ The nipple looks flattened or striped as it leaves the baby's mouth at the end of the feed.

◆ The mother experiences nipple soreness during and after feeds.

◆ The mother's breasts are engorged.

◆ There is inefficient removal of milk from the breast.

Factors in helping mothers with attachment

◆ Getting herself and her baby comfortable and ready for a feed.

◆ Holding the baby so that he can attach effectively.

◆ Attaching the baby to the breast.

◆ Keeping the baby attached during the feed.

◆ Ending a breastfeed.

method should be used. Refrain from high level interventions until other alternatives have been exhausted. The vast majority of suckling difficulties will be resolved by time and by making sure the baby is receiving sufficient calories.

▼

REFERENCES

Al-Sayed L et al. Ventilatory sparing strategies and swallowing pattern during bottle feeding in human infants. *J Appl Physiol* 77:78–83; 1994.

Anderson G. Risk in mother-infant separation postbirth. *Image Journal of Nursing Scholarship* 21:196–199; 1989.

Barger J. *Lactation Management Course*. Breastfeeding Support Consultants Center for Lactation Education, Chalfont, PA.; 1998.

Bier J et al. The oral motor development of low-birth-weight infants who underwent orotracheal intubation during the neonatal period. *Am J Dis Child* 147:858–862; 1993.

Bowen-Jones A et al. Milk flow and sucking rates during breast-feeding. *Devel Med Child Neurol* 24:626–633; 1982.

Lactation Management Course, Breastfeeding Support Consultants, Chalfont, PA.

Legovic M and Ostric L. The effects of feeding methods on the growth of the jaws in infants. *J Dent Children* 58(3):253–255; 1991.

Mathew O and Bhatia J. Sucking and breathing patterns during breast- and bottle-feeding in term neonates. *Am J Dis Child* 143:588–592; 1989.

Matthews MK. The relationship between maternal labor analgesia and delay in the initiation of breastfeeding in healthy neonates in the early neonatal period. *Midwifery* 5:3–10; 1989.

Medoff-Cooper B et al. Neonatal sucking as a clinical assessment tool: Preliminary findings. *Nurs Res* 38:161–165; 1989.

Meier P. Transitional suck patterns in premature infants. *J Perinat Neonat Nurs* 80:vii–viii; 1994.

Morton J. Ineffective suckling: A possible consequence of obstructive positioning. *J Hum Lact* 8:83–85; 1992.

Palmer B. Breastfeeding: Reducing the risk for obstructive sleep apnea. *Breastfeeding Abstracts* 18(3):19–20, 1999.

Ramsay M and Gisel E. Neonatal sucking and maternal feeding practices. *Dev Med Child Neurol* 38:34–47; 1996.

Righard L and Alade M. Sucking technique and its effect on success of breastfeeding. *Birth* 19:185–189; 1992.

Righard L and Alade M. "Effect of delivery room routines on success of first breastfeed." *Lancet* 336:1105–1107; 1990.

Widstrom AM. Gastric suction in healthy newborn infants. *Acta Pediatr Scand* 76:566–572; 1987.

Woolridge M. Anatomy of infant suckling. *Midwifery* 2:164–171; 1986.

Yokoyama U et al. Releases of oxytocin and prolactin during breast massage and suckling in puerperal women. *Eur J. Obstet Gynecol Reprod Biol* 53:17–20; 1994.

▼

BIBLIOGRAPHY

Ardran GM and Kemp FH. A cineradiographic study of breast-feeding. *Br J Radiol* 31:156–162; 1958.

Auerbach KG and Eggert LD. The importance of infant suckling patterns when the breastfed baby fails to thrive. *J Trop Pediatr* 33:156–157; 1987.

Crowell MK et al. Relationship between obstetric analgesia and time of effective breastfeed. *J Nurse Midwifery* 39(3): 150–56; 1994.

Kutner L. *Lactation Management Course*. Breastfeeding Support Consultants Center for Lactation Education, Chalfont PA.; 1996.

Maher S. An overview of solutions to breastfeeding and sucking problems. La Leche League, International, No. 67; 1988.

Matthews MK. Developing an instrument to assess infant breastfeeding behaviour in the early neonatal period. *Midwifery* 4:154–165; 1988.

Morris SE. *Overview of the anatomy and physiology of the oral pharyngeal mechanism*. In Palmer MM (ed). The normal acquisition of oral feeding skills: Implication for assessment and treatment. New York, Therapeutic Media; pp. 19–32; 1982.

Narayanan I et al. Sucking on the 'emptied' breast; Non-nutritive sucking with a difference. *Arch Dis Child* 66(2): 241–244; 1991.

Neville M. Milk production by the mammary cell. In *Proceedings of the Invitational Asian Regional Lactation Management Workshop and Related Events*. Bali, Indonesia; June 29–July 9; 1988; pp. 278–291.

Prieto C et al. Sucking pressure and its relationship to milk transfer during breastfeeding in humans. *J Reprod Fertil* 108:69–94; 1996.

Smith WL et al. Physiology of sucking in the normal term infant using real time ultrasound, *Radiology,* 156:379–381; 1985.

Stevenson RD and Allaire JH. The development of normal feeding and swallowing. *Pediatr Clin N Am* 38(6): 1439–1453; 1991.

Weber F et al. An ultrasonographic study of the organization of sucking and swallowing by newborn infants. *Dev Med Child Neurol* 28:19–24; 1986.

14

BREASTFEEDING ISSUES IN THE EARLY WEEKS

The early weeks with a new baby are a time of great adjustment for families. Some mothers seem to sail through this time with little difficulty. Others encounter situations that require extra assistance. Providing anticipatory guidance at key times will help the mother manage difficulties with minimal disruption. During the early weeks of breastfeeding, the mother will be establishing milk production and refining her management of feeds. She will benefit from your guidance and support as she learns how to respond to the needs of her baby. Your assistance at this critical time can also help her avoid problems with sore nipples, engorgement, plugged ducts, and mastitis. These issues are explored in this chapter.

CONFIDENCE AND COMMITMENT TO CONTINUE BREASTFEEDING

Why do some women breastfeed for months and years, whereas others limit their breastfeeding experience to a few days or weeks? In the industrialized world, there is a clear perception that breastfeeding is best *but* that alternatives are acceptable. Generally, mothers who breastfeed are doing so out of choice, not because of a perceived necessity or tradition. This has a significant impact on duration. When an alternative exists and it is deemed acceptable, confidence and commitment may wane in the absence of support and encouragement.

Bottorff (1990) looked at a woman's continuing to breastfeed beyond the early days. She noted that it may be influenced by the baby's responsiveness, as well as the mother's own satisfaction, and the compatibility of breastfeeding with her lifestyle. She also identified the key role a mother's persistence and commitment play in the decision. There is a difference between a woman saying, "I will *try* to breastfeed," and one who says, "I *will* breastfeed." When a woman decides to breastfeed, the capacity to breastfeed opens up and the mother is able to do so despite any difficulties that may arise. Breastfeeding is a journey into the unknown—the unpredictable. It involves ongoing learning and takes courage.

Bottorff notes the importance of support and help with breastfeeding to the new mother. She speculates that part of a mother's persistence is recognizing the need for help and then finding that help.

Lindenberg (1990) found that early contact and feeding contribute to how long a woman breastfeeds. Leff (1994) further identified areas that are important in evaluating the overall breastfeeding experience. Mothers reported that seeing their babies grow, gain weight, rarely become ill, settle with breastfeeding, and fall asleep during or after breastfeeding increased their likelihood to view breastfeeding as successful. There was increased satisfaction when breastfeeding was comfortable and when any painful phases were short lived. Breastfeeding was identified by the mothers as an important part of the maternal role. They spoke of a harmonized relationship between themselves and their babies that made breastfeeding feel successful. In other words, breastfeeding was working for both the mothers and their babies.

Women in the Leff study rated their breastfeeding success relatively low if the baby was perceived as not being satisfied. If the baby was satisfied, high levels of success also depended on maternal enjoyment, attainment of the desired maternal role, and lifestyle compatibility. The baby's satisfaction is not totally the mother's responsibility. His sucking competence, alertness, stamina, and abilities to self-regulate and to respond to soothing also influence his own satisfaction. Lothian (1995) asserts that it takes time for mothers to find ways to work with the individual characteristics of their babies.

Your role in encouraging the continuation of breastfeeding involves recognizing both the mother's and baby's needs, and assisting them in balancing the breastfeeding relationship. Boosting a mother's confidence empowers her to continue with breastfeeding. Her confidence will soar when you point out positive things about her baby—"He is growing so fast," "He looks so healthy."—and her own abilities—"You're such a good mom," "You pick up on your baby's cues really well." Help the mother recognize her baby's language and cues, and encourage her responsiveness to them.

Also, assure the mother that she knows her baby better than anyone else possibly could. Validate her concerns and her wide range of emotions as a normal part of mothering. Assure the mother that no question is silly or unimportant—she is the advocate for her child!

▼ Misconceptions That Interfere with Breastfeeding Management

There are numerous unfounded beliefs about breast-feeding that confuse parents and interfere with sound medical advice. Parents and caregivers alike are subject to these beliefs. You can assist both parents and care-givers in understanding these misconceptions and recognizing factors in sound breastfeeding management. Some of the more common misconceptions are given in the following list.

Bottles and artificial baby milk given to breastfeeding babies do not interfere with breastfeeding.

It is not necessary to feed breastfeeding babies with a bottle in order to train them to accept a bottle. Any artificial nipple given to an infant in the early weeks of establishing breastfeeding has the potential to create nipple preference for the artificial nipple (see Chapter 16). Additionally, infant formula exposes the infant to a greater risk of disease and sensitizes him to cow's milk protein (see Chapter 8).

Time at the breast needs to be limited in the early days to prevent nipple soreness.

Poor positioning is the major cause of sore nipples, as discussed later in this chapter. Babies need to be given unlimited access to the breast. Early, frequent feeds increase the mother's milk production and avoid complications (see Chapter 14). Enforced time limits increase the incidence of jaundice, engorgement, low milk production, and inadequate infant weight gain.

Even with time limits, most breastfeeding women will experience nipple soreness.

Breastfeeding should not hurt! As noted earlier, the vast majority of sore nipples are a result of poor positioning of the baby at the breast. Some women experience brief moments of latch-on tenderness that disappears within a few days. This is not pain that interferes with breastfeeding.

Newborn babies typically need to eat every 4 hours.

Breastfeeding babies may want to feed as frequently as every 1 or 2 hours in the early days. Enforced scheduling of feeds ignores infant feeding cues, interferes with the mothering process, and increases the incidence of jaundice, engorgement, low milk production, and poor infant weight gain. Mothers can trust their babies to determine the timing of feeds by learning how to read feeding cues. See Chapter 11 regarding infant feeding cues and the discussion of feeding frequency later in this chapter.

Water supplementation will help prevent jaundice in breast-feeding infants.

Water supplementation does not coat the gut as human milk does, nor does it have the laxative effect of colostrum to help with the excretion of meconium. Giving water to the baby can reduce effective suckling at the breast, increase the incidence of engorgement, and may cause nipple preference when given by bottle. It also reduces his caloric intake and his ability to self-regulate his intake. A jaundiced baby needs the increased stooling facilitated by receiving colostrum. Therefore, the correct response is to increase the number of breastfeeds. In fact, water supplementation can decrease the amount of human milk the baby takes in, thus increasing bilirubin levels (see Chapter 20).

Formula supplementation is necessary when the mother has low milk production.

Remedies for low milk production are to increase the frequency of feeds and to correct positioning and attachment (see Chapter 16). **Alternate massage** during a feed will help increase the volume of fat content. Giving an artificial substitute by a rubber nipple can result in nipple preference, difficulty with attachment, less time at the breast, inadequate milk removal, allergies, and doubts about competence or ability to breastfeed. Breastfeeding babies should be given no artificial substitute unless it is medically indicated. If supplementation is medically indicated, it should be given by a method that will interfere least with breastfeeding (see Chapter 19).

Weaning is recommended when mothers are taking most medications.

The American Academy of Pediatrics advises that most maternal use of medications does not require weaning (see Chapter 8).

Breastfeeding mothers and babies take more of the physician's time than do those who bottle feed.

When anticipatory guidance and appropriate teaching are provided to breastfeeding mothers, there is a lower incidence of sick calls and visits to the pediatrician (see Chapter 2). Mothers who remain unseparated from their babies in the hospital assume more care of their babies, which frees hospital staff for other tasks (see Chapter 10).

The best time to start breastfeeding is after the mother's milk "comes in."

Milk does not "come in." It is already present from 4 months of pregnancy onward. Delaying the start of breastfeeding can lead to engorgement, a delay in milk production, interference with the mother's instincts, and a decrease in milk production (see Chapter 10).

The best way to tell that a baby is getting enough of his mother's milk is that he sleeps for several hours after each feed.

Sleeping is not an indication of the baby receiving enough milk. The more calorically deprived a baby is, the more he will sleep. Mothers need to watch for the number of wet diapers and bowel movements, the baby's disposition during and between feeds, and other growth indicators (see Chapter 11).

After the mother's milk production is established, the baby will take most of the milk in the first 5 to 7 minutes.

Each baby's breastfeeding pattern is different. As babies become older, they will be able to remove milk more quickly from the breast. However, they should still be allowed to determine the end of the feed rather than being subjected to arbitrary time limits (see Chapter 12).

Mothers need to feed from both breasts at every feed; therefore, the mother should limit sucking time on the first side so the baby will take the second side.

Some babies nurse from only one breast at a feed and will follow this pattern for all feeds, whereas others may use one breast until late afternoon or evening when they use both. The amount of time it takes a baby to remove both foremilk and hindmilk from a breast varies. If a baby is removed from the breast before he receives hindmilk, he will ingest large amounts of foremilk. This could result in colic-like behavior or poor weight gain (See Chapter 14).

Artificial baby milk is just as healthy as human milk.

There are substantial differences between artificial baby milk and human milk. See Chapter 8 for a detailed discussion about the properties and health benefits of human milk and a comparison to infant formula.

Breastfeeding is essentially an alternative to infant formula.

Breastfeeding is much more than human milk. It is a dynamic process, a bonding relationship between a mother and her baby. Breastfeeding involves people, not simply infant food (see Chapter 3).

It is important to wait at least 2 to 3 hours between feeds so the breast can refill and the baby is not using the mother as a pacifier.

The breast is never totally empty. As milk is removed, more milk is produced. The shorter the period of time between feeds, the higher the fat content of the milk. Waiting a specified period of time between feeds can actually decrease milk pro-

duction and the amount of fat the baby receives (see Chapter 6).

ESTABLISHING MILK PRODUCTION

Milk is present in the mother from 4 months of pregnancy onward. At birth, the delivery of the placenta triggers a change in the woman's hormone levels that removes the inhibition of sustained milk production. Increased amounts of blood and lymph in the breast form the source from which the milk is produced. These fluids cause the breasts to become fuller, heavier, and perhaps slightly tender. As regular frequent breastfeeds progress, this normal fullness diminishes. By about 10 days postpartum, when lactation is well established, the breasts become comfortably soft and pliable, even when they are filled with milk. With regular frequent feeds, this condition is maintained.

A woman's production of milk requires a functioning letdown response and adequate milk removal on a regular basis. To a small extent, the quality and quantity of her diet are also factors. A 1993 study by DeCoopman supports the theory that milk production is determined locally, that is, by autocrine control. In other words, the removal of milk is just as important as nipple stimulation and letdown. When a baby nurses frequently, there is greater nipple stimulation and greater removal of milk. Consequently, milk production increases. To ensure good milk production, then, the mother will want to take care to avoid missed feeds, especially in the early months when she is still establishing milk production. Generally, women can be taught to allow the baby to remain at the breast until he spontaneously releases the breast on his own. If the baby tends to "linger" at the breast, the mother can watch for a change from nutritive to non-nutritive sucking. The non-nutritive sucking does not provide the stimulation necessary for increasing milk production. If the mother were to remove him from the breast at this time, it would not significantly affect milk production. However, mothers should be encouraged to gauge their baby's needs. Some babies will need more comfort sucking at the breast than others.

Signs of Sufficient Milk

There are a number of signs that indicate that a baby is receiving enough milk. Sufficient urine output—in the absence of supplemental fluids—to soak at least six or more regular diapers (fewer if superabsorbent diapers are used) indicates adequate milk volume. Stooling after day

5 is also an indicator of adequate milk transfer. In the first month the baby should stool four or more times each day. You may want to advise families to call their pediatrician at any time in the month when their baby does not have at least three yellow, seedy stools per day.

As long as a baby is not normally placid or fussy, a pleasant disposition generally is a sign of proper nourishment. A mother needs to understand that crying is not necessarily an indication that her baby is hungry. She should be alert to the other indications of adequate nourishment. Regular intervals of wakefulness, sleep, and feeding will reassure a mother that she is providing her baby with enough milk. Healthy skin tone and color are other signs of proper nourishment.

An infant's growth pattern also is evidence that he is thriving on his mother's milk. The most obvious signs are fat creases in his arms and legs, and the baby filling out his clothing. The mother should look for increases in length and head size, as well as regular weight gain. It is not uncommon for a breastfed baby to experience an initial weight loss of up to 7 percent of his birth weight during the first week. If feeds are restricted in the early days, this weight loss could be as high as 10 or 12 percent. With more frequent breastfeeds, weight should begin to increase so that the baby regains his birth weight by day ten. This pattern is less pronounced in babies who are nursed frequently from birth, with less initial weight loss and more rapid weight gain. Assure the mother that her baby's removal of her milk will create his own supply. When he experiences growth spurts he will want to nurse more frequently to meet his needs.

▼ One Breast or Two

In the first few days, when feeding times are shorter (about 10 to 15 minutes), the baby may nurse on only one breast at each feed, and then drift off to sleep. When he is put to the other breast, he may be too drowsy or too full to nurse. His drowsiness is due in part to the release of **cholecystokinin** (CCK) in his system during suckling. CCK is a gastrointestinal hormone that enhances digestion, sedation, and a feeling of satiation and well-being. It is released in both the infant and mother during suckling. The infant's CCK level peaks immediately after a feed and again about 30 to 60 minutes later (Riordan, 1999). During the time between these two peaks, if the baby is put to breast on the side that has not yet been nursed, he may arouse enough to nurse at that time.

As the days pass and the baby becomes more alert, feeding times will increase and he will be more likely to feed at both breasts at a session. Encourage mothers to remain flexible, especially in these early days while she and her baby are both establishing themselves in this new venture. Let the baby be the guide. If milk production is plentiful and the baby is gaining well, a mother need not be concerned about her baby's refusal of the second breast. This is common in the early days and may persist for many months. One-breast feeds can be adequate (Righard, 1993). Some babies never nurse on both breasts at a feed. If the mother experiences uncomfortable fullness of the second breast, she may encourage her baby to take that side to relieve the fullness and prevent engorgement. She can begin the next feed on the side that is fuller.

▼ Duration of Feeds

In general, feeding length should be determined by the baby's needs. When the flow of milk diminishes from one breast and the high-fat hindmilk has been extracted, the sucking rate will move from the long, drawing nutritive suck to a faster, more gentle suck. The baby's eyes will close, his fists will relax, and his hands will come away from his face. He may release the breast and let it slide out of his mouth. The mother can then nurse from the other breast and again permit sufficient nursing time for the baby to receive the hindmilk.

Limiting the time spent on a breast may result in the baby's receiving foremilk from both breasts and becoming too full to obtain a significant amount of hindmilk from either breast. This type of high-volume, low-fat feed can result in poor weight gain. As the baby matures, he will become more efficient at extracting milk, and the time spent at the breast will decrease. Flexibility on the mother's part will allow for variations in the baby's nursing style, hunger, and daily temperament.

Hospital procedures that restrict feeding frequency and duration are detrimental to the initiation of breastfeeding. In the hospital, the mother may be told to nurse for a few minutes on each breast initially, and to increase nursing times gradually thereafter. With your help, the mother will be able to work with her other caregivers to avoid such schedules and gain free access to her baby. She and her baby will then be able to enjoy the benefits of unrestricted feeds. You might also offer to give an inservice to the hospital staff on breastfeeding management!

Slaven (1981) demonstrated that unlimited suckling time beginning directly after birth improves breastfeeding. One group of women was on a timed regimen that began with 3 minutes on each breast, and increased gradually to 10 minutes over the next 4 days. The other group of women was allowed to nurse for any length of time that seemed suitable to them. When interviewed at 6 weeks, 80 percent of the second group were still breastfeeding, compared with only 57 percent of the timed group. Additionally, there were 10 percent fewer cases of breast engorgement in the untimed group, and no significant differences in the incidence of nipple problems between the groups. Other studies have shown that the removal of time restrictions has the added benefit of reducing bilirubin levels (Varimo, 1986).

Until breast tissue becomes accustomed to suckling, mothers may experience some initial nipple discomfort that peaks between the third and sixth day postpartum. Decreasing the time or frequency of feeds will not prevent this tenderness. Nipple soreness is caused primarily by improper positioning of the baby at the breast. Holding the baby with his body facing the mother and bringing the baby onto the breast so that the end of the nipple is not unduly stressed is the best insurance against soreness. With these techniques, the mother can be comfortable nursing for as long a period as her baby requires.

▼ Frequency of Feeds

During the first month, feeding frequency for a healthy, fully developed baby may range from 8 to 14 feeds daily, with most babies requiring 8 or 10. The baby who nurses more frequently may nurse as often as every 1 to 2 hours for part of the day and then with some feeds spaced 4 or 5 hours apart. The mother need not wake her baby at night for feeds unless he has fed less than 8 times in the past 24 hours or is gaining weight slowly. A mother need not be alarmed, however, if her baby wants to feed as often as every hour or hour and a half during the day or several times during the night. Every baby's needs are different. Encourage mothers to remain flexible to meet their own babies' requirements. Help them learn to watch their babies rather than clocks.

By 6 weeks of age, a baby has usually developed a pattern of feeding every 2 to 3 hours, with a longer stretch at night. This longer nighttime stretch may be balanced by a period of almost constant wakefulness and suckling at some other time of the day, generally the early evening. These are referred to as clustered or bunched feedings. As the baby matures and becomes a more efficient breastfeeder, he will obtain more milk in a shorter period of time and will begin to space his feeds farther apart.

Increases in Feeding Frequency

A mother may periodically notice an increase in the frequency with which her baby wishes to feed. All babies experience periods of sudden growth during their early months. They react to these growth spurts by feeding more frequently. Growth spurts can occur at any time. These periods of increased feeds usually last only a few days. Mothers have a reserve of milk to carry through during these times of feeding frequency until the growth

spurt has passed (Dewey, 1991). Some of the more common times for growth spurts are discussed in the next section.

First Days Home

If the baby was unable to nurse as frequently as he would have liked during his hospital stay, he most likely will nurse more frequently when he is allowed to establish his own routine. He may be overstimulated by eager parents or siblings during his first few days home and turns to nursing for comfort. He may also be reacting to the dramatic difference between the hospital environment (his first extrauterine experience) and his home, particularly at night.

During the first month of life, patterns of milk intake are established that will continue through the following 5 months (Allen, 1991). In these first few weeks, parents need to avoid strict scheduling of feeds and allow the baby to lead his feeds. This supports the individual nature of infant feeding and the importance of baby-led feeds. Each baby's own rhythm will reflect his feeding patterns.

10 to 14 Days

At about 10 to 14 days, the baby experiences his first growth spurt and will want to nurse more often. It is around this time that the mother also loses the initial fullness in her breasts. She may worry that the increased feeds and smaller breasts are indications that her milk production is dwindling. Anticipatory guidance will help avoid concerns that would cause her to question her ability to continue nurturing her baby.

3 to 6 Weeks

In addition to a second growth spurt that occurs at around 3 to 6 weeks the baby may nurse more often in response to an increase in his mother's activity level. At this time, mothers often resume many or all of their prepregnant activities, including a return to work or school. This increase in activity may lead to a drop in milk production. The baby's response is to feed more frequently to rebuild the supply. He may also nurse more frequently to reassure himself that his mother is still available to him.

3 and 6 Months

As the baby continues to grow, he will periodically nurse more frequently to increase milk production to meet his needs. These growth spurts typically occur at about 3 and 6 months. The mother may incorrectly interpret these increased feeds as a sign of her baby's readiness to begin solid foods. Again, anticipatory guidance will prevent mothers from misinterpreting these increases in feeds.

Other Times of Increased Feeds

Times of illness, overstimulation, emotional upset, or physical discomfort may cause a baby to turn to the breast for security and comfort. You can help the mother through these times by reminding her that babies nurse at the breast for comfort as well as for nutrition. Being able to comfort her baby at the breast is one of the wonderful benefits of breastfeeding.

Mothers who nurse in response to their babies' cues and are unmindful of schedules may never notice these growth spurts. Often, however, mothers are aware of fussiness in a previously contented baby, a baby who wants to nurse more frequently than usual, or a baby who has suddenly begun to nurse more vigorously. You can prepare the mother for these events before they occur, so that such incidents do not undermine her confidence or cause her to become so discouraged that she considers early weaning. Reassurance, support, and a listening ear can be crucial to a mother who finds herself with a fussy baby who requires a lot of attention. Encourage her to respond to her baby's needs during this growing time.

Decreases in Feeding Frequency

A mother often becomes concerned when her baby begins dropping feeds, especially if she has not yet begun giving him solid foods or other supplements. She may worry that he is not being nourished sufficiently if he had been nursing eight or nine times in 24 hours and suddenly drops to six or seven feeds. This schedule change frequently occurs when the baby reaches about 3 months of age. It is usually a result of his having become a more efficient nurser. Because he is able to obtain a greater amount of milk in a shorter period of time, he can go longer between feeds. He may also decrease the time he remains on the breast at a feed because he is able to obtain the milk he needs more quickly.

Encourage the mother to observe her baby's overall disposition and health. If he appears content, is voiding and stooling appropriately, is increasing his weight and body length, and has good skin tone, she can be assured that he is being well-nourished and that there is no cause for worry. If, however, his decreased feeds are accompanied by poor health or inadequate growth, advise the mother to consult her baby's physician immediately. You will need to assess her breastfeeding practices to help her make necessary adjustments.

▼

LEAKING

It is common for some women to experience milk leaking from their breasts during the first few weeks of breastfeeding. In most cases, it is caused by fullness in the breast or the milk letting down. Leaking is a normal part of the process of breastfeeding. It may occur during a feed from the breast not being nursed, just before a feed when the breasts are full, or when feeds are missed altogether. The range of leaking is extremely variable from one woman to another. Some women's breasts leak for as long as 3 months after delivery.

For many women, milk leaking from the breast is an encouraging sign that their milk supply is plentiful and that their letdown reflex is functioning well. In most cases, leaking will subside as harmony develops between the baby's needs and the mother's milk production. On the other hand, failure to leak milk is not an indication that milk production is low. Many women never experience leaking at any time while they are lactating. An absence of leaking in no way implies that milk production is low. It may indicate that the sphincter muscles within the nipple function well to close off the nipple pores.

▼

Causes of Leaking

Leaking may be a result of psychological conditioning of letdown. A woman may leak in response to hearing a baby cry, picking up her own baby to nurse, or simply thinking about breastfeeding or her baby. Because oxytocin is released during orgasm and because the release of oxytocin produces letdown, many women experience leaking during sexual intercourse. Leaking in response to lovemaking can be a sign that orgasm has occurred. It can be managed by nursing beforehand and covering bedding with towels. Milk leaking from the lactating breast can be caused by letdown, overfull breasts, stimulation during lovemaking, overuse of breast shells, frequent milk expression, clothing that rubs against the nipples, overproduction of milk, or hormone imbalances.

▼

When Leaking Poses a Problem

Although women generally consider leaking to be a nuisance, they usually accept it as a part of breastfeeding and use appropriate measures to control it. Some women cannot accept the inconvenience of leaking or the measures needed to control it, and may find weaning a more acceptable alternative. You need to assess carefully to what degree a woman is bothered by leaking, offering practical suggestions to those women who need help controlling leaking, and supporting those who decide to discontinue breastfeeding because of it (Morse, 1989). Morse noted that 66 percent of the breastfeeding mothers in her study were still leaking to some degree, and most of the mothers expressed negative feelings about leaking. Persistent leaking may be so inconvenient that the woman will consider weaning to avoid the restrictions on her social life and annoyance of continually having to change clothing and bedding.

Measures to Control Leaking

When leaking becomes a problem for the mother, you can suggest that she

- Press the heel of her hand over the breast or cross her arms and press.

- Wear absorbent breast pads and change them often.

- Feed the baby before lovemaking and use absorbent towels over bedding.

- Decrease pressure on the breast and elastic in the bra cup; loosen the bra or wear a larger size.

- Discontinue practices that may stimulate nerves in the nipple, such as clothing rubbing on the nipple, holding or cuddling the baby in a particular manner, sexual foreplay, or overuse of breast shells.

- Express or pump milk when feeds are missed or delayed.

- Wear dark, patterned clothing or a sweater to conceal moist spots.

- Check for the use of drugs that may stimulate milk production, and discontinue use.

Some women use a breast shell during a feed, wearing it on the breast that is not being nursed. The milk that leaks from the breast is referred to as **drip milk.** If the breast shells have been washed well and placed in the bra immediately before the feed, the drip milk can be saved for the baby. Because its fat content is low, drip milk should not be used regularly for infant feedings.

Excessive or Inappropriate Leaking

Occasionally, a woman's leaking is excessive, or she may experience leaking past the early weeks of establishing breastfeeding. Excessive leaking may be a sign of an imbalance in other body functions. In some women, milk production greatly exceeds the baby's needs. In others, leaking continues after the baby has been weaned or occurs at times not related to birth or breastfeeding. Such excessive or inappropriate milk production is termed galactorrhea, also referred to as *spontaneous lactation*.

Inappropriate milk production of the nonlactating breast may be due to the use of drugs such as thyrotropin-releasing hormones, theophyllines, amphetamines, or tranquilizers (MacFarlane, 1977). Chest or breast surgery, a fibrocystic breast, or herpes zoster may also stimulate nerves enough to induce milk production significantly. In some cases, the woman's body may be

especially sensitive to normal levels of prolactin. If no underlying disorder is found through medical examination, special efforts should be made to decrease the stimuli to the breast.

Galactorrhea is not a disease. It may be a symptom of an underlying health problem that causes elevated prolactin levels (**hyperprolactinemia**) and may be serious. Some possible causes of hyperprolactinemia that results in galactorrhea are hypothyroidism, psychosis and anxiety medications, hyperthyroidism, chronic renal failure, pituitary tumors, and uterine and ovarian tumors. Abnormal lactation can also be seen in connection with surgery and stress related to such tumors.

Any unexplainable excessive milk flow during lactation or milk production that continues beyond 3 to 6 months after the baby is weaned should be considered inappropriate. The woman should be encouraged to undergo a general physical examination. Infrequently, drugs may be used to suppress lactation, but they are often only temporary measures. Total treatment of galactorrhea is generally accomplished by treating the underlying cause (Lawrence, 1999).

NIPPLE SORENESS

Although sore nipples occur with relative frequency, they are not considered to be a normal part of breastfeeding. Initial tenderness, or **transient nipple soreness**, has been identified as a part of the typical postpartum course for the majority of mothers. It is often described as tenderness with the initial latch and first few sucks. The peak period of this tenderness occurs in the first week postpartum, particularly between the third and sixth days (Ziemer, 1990). It is possible that this period of tenderness is associated with the breast becoming accustomed to the frequency of use in breastfeeding a newborn.

Generally, pain is a sign that something is not right within the body. The same applies to nipple pain during breastfeeding. Nipple pain needs to be investigated if it occurs beyond the transient soreness of the first week or lasts after the first few sucks following attachment. Painful nipples can constitute a breastfeeding emergency because it is a common reason for early weaning (De Carvalho, 1984). This is much like using a scraped knee or knuckle. Untreated, nipple pain can progress to the development of a crack. The crack offers a portal of entry for bacteria and yeast that are present on the skin surface. This may lead to infection. The increased severity of pain, when untreated, may decrease the woman's desire to put her baby to breast. This problem may, in turn, lead to engorgement and reduced milk production.

Causes and Prevention of Nipple Soreness

Your role with regard to nipple pain needs to focus on prevention first. Prenatal education needs to emphasize correct positioning and attachment, the two most common causes of nipple soreness (Walker, 1989a). Postpartum caregivers need correct information regarding assessment of latch and positioning. Maternity policies need to reflect this as well.

Prevention efforts need to focus on proper positioning of both mother and baby. The baby needs a centered latch, with a mouthful of breast rather than just the nipple. Artificial nipples must be avoided in the early days of breastfeeding. Measures should be taken to prevent engorgement, identify women at risk for soreness, and educate those who care for women prenatally and early postpartum.

Many myths abound regarding the cause of nipple soreness. A long-held belief that a baby left too long on the breast would cause soreness led to time restrictions for early feeds. It has been found that restriction of feeds only prolongs the onset of soreness (De Carvalho, 1984) and additionally interferes with the baby's regulation of milk production (Woolridge, 1985). Women previously were taught to toughen their nipples prenatally with the hope of avoiding soreness. This often unpleasant and unnecessary chore is no longer recommended (Woolridge, 1986). Finally, it was suggested that fair-skinned women were prone to nipple soreness. However, with correct latch and position, they do not experience soreness at greater rates (Heat, 1987). You can give mothers correct information if they receive this outdated advice.

Positioning presents a problem when the baby's body is not in alignment with his head or when his head is not facing and level with the breast. Nursing is difficult for the baby when he does not face his food and must swallow with his head turned to the side or tipped back. Additionally, the mother's breast must deal with the extra tension and negative pressure exerted by a poor position. Other factors that may lead to nipple pain include nipple shape, engorgement, improper breaking of suction when taking the baby off the breast, sensitivity to a topical ointment applied to the breast, improper use of breast pumps, nipple shields, prolonged exposure of the nipple to moisture, and thrush (Walker, 1989a). A very eager nurser with little milk flow in the first 24 hours may also lead to pain.

Frequently, poor latch is evident after the introduction of an artificial nipple from a bottle or pacifier. The mechanism of suck on the bottle nipple is very different from that of the breast. Additionally, the rate of flow is considerably different. Milk flow in the breast is controlled by the infant's sucking. Conversely, milk flows from the bottle until the baby stops it. When the two are combined, it often produces an unenthusiastic and incorrect suck when the baby returns to the breast (Schlegel, 1983).

Assessment of Sore Nipples

When sore nipples have been identified, it is important to assess the situation thoroughly in order that the cause may be found and action taken immediately. As with any other condition, it is important to note the age of the baby and when the soreness began. The mother's description of the pain in relation to how it feels and at what times it feels a certain way may yield clues to the cause. For instance, burning pain may indicate thrush. Any chronic conditions of the mother as well as medication usage are notable. Even the use of soaps, creams, lotions, laundry products, and perfumes need to be discussed, particularly in terms of recent product changes. Nipple soreness may also develop when the baby begins teething, or if the mother begins menstruating or becomes pregnant. It is helpful in the assessment process to inquire about the baby's growth and development, and the mother's postpartum reproductive state.

The assessment of sore nipples requires an in-person visit. It is essential to see the baby's attachment and positioning during a feed. You need to observe the baby's alignment and closeness to the breast, the mother's position, and the mouth-breast connection, as described in Chapter 12. Note the appearance of the nipple before and after the feed. Blanching and flattening of the nipple may be clues to poor latch. If the mother is ending feeds, observe her technique. Pulling her baby off the breast without breaking suction will cause pain. Visually assess the baby's oral cavity, paying close attention to the tongue and frenulum. If no obvious cause can be found by observing the feed and the mother and baby, it may be necessary to perform a digital exam of the baby's oral cavity (see Chapter 19).

Treatment and Plan of Care

You can help the mother identify the cause of soreness and eliminate it. As previously noted, care must be given when positioning the baby at the breast. He should be level with and facing the breast, and his body aligned with his head. If the mother has been using only one position and has developed soreness, she may wish to choose another position to provide relief to the sore area. The mother's body position is also important. If her baby's head is not adequately supported, he may bite down reflexively. If her arms tire during a feed, the baby may not remain level with the breast. He may then exert more pressure on the nipple or slip off so that he latches only onto the nipple.

The baby's latch must consistently be correct in order for the baby to learn as well as for the mother's own relief. The baby's mouth must be wide open and centered at the level of the areola. To encourage the baby to open wide, he may be held in a position that allows gravity to aid him, such as the clutch hold. Some lactation consultants have found that gentle pressure on the baby's chin will help remind him to open wide. Babies will mimic other's facial expressions. Before latch attempts, the mother may demonstrate a wide open mouth for him and repeatedly say "open." She may then repeat "open" for him as he works to latch. This is also helpful for a baby who initially learned to latch by "chewing" his way onto the nipple. His lips must be flanged outward and the wide angle of the mouth maintained when the baby begins sucking. The mother can be taught to assess for correct lip placement and to help her baby flange either or both lips when needed.

Babies who bite at the breast often respond well to prone positioning, chin support, or **sublingual** pressure (gentle pressure under the chin). Jaw clenching may cause nipple **vasospasms** (spasms of the blood vessels within the nipple) identified by pain and blanching of the nipple. Relief can be obtained by working with the baby's latch, warm compresses to the nipple, and increased intake of calcium and magnesium in the mother's diet (Walker 1989a).

Vasospasms of the nipple during breastfeeding have also been identified with a **Raynaud**-like phenomenon. The pain was described as stinging and burning. The nipples simultaneously blanched as the mother prepared to nurse her baby. Initially, nursing aggravated the pain, and then it subsided during the feed. Moist heat provided a degree of relief (Coates, 1992). For babies with oral-motor difficulties, a referral to a qualified neurodevelopmental (NDT) therapist may be necessary. If the **lingual** frenulum is found to be tight and the tongue is unable to extend over the lower lip, consider that the frenulum may need to be clipped. The frenulum on the upper lip could also be tight and cause problems. A referral to an appropriate physician is necessary.

If the cause of nipple pain is found to be dried milk sticking to the mother's bra or breast pads, she can moisten them before removing them. If the mother has been pulling her baby off the breast without releasing suction, she can be taught how to break suction with her finger between the baby's gums before removing him. When her soreness is relieved, she needs to be instructed in the importance of baby-led feeds and allowing her baby to determine when to end the feed. Pain that has been connected to a retracted or inverted nipple may be relieved by techniques that gently encourage eversion of the nipple, as described in Chapter 6.

After a cause has been identified, it is important to institute a plan that also addresses **palliative care** (care that provides a measure of pain relief). The mother needs suggestions for immediate physical comfort. You might suggest a pain medication that is approved by the mother's and baby's physicians. The mother can also place ice in a wet cloth and apply the cloth to her nipples prior to a feed. (The ice should not be placed directly on the skin.) Starting a feed with the least sore breast first, initiating the milk ejection reflex before putting the baby to breast, and eliminating prolonged non-nutritive (comfort) sucking at the breast are other measures to relieve the mother's discomfort. For the duration of nipple soreness, when the baby is no longer actively feeding and has not yet released the breast, he may be removed gently. The mother may also try alternate massage to help sustain sucking and swallowing and relieve long periods of negative pressure. In alternate massage, the mother massages and compresses the breast each time the baby pauses during a feed. After feeds, the mother may apply her own expressed milk to the sore area and allow for air drying of the areola. If the mother is unable to tolerate any sucking, she may choose to pump her milk with a quality electric breast pump and, while she heals, provide her milk to her baby with an alternative feeding method.

Topical Creams and Ointments

Research comparing and evaluating the use of topical agents on sore nipples is inconclusive at this time. It is important to read the research with a critical eye before changing any clinical practice. Often topicals are investigated without giving sufficient consideration to proper positioning and latch technique. Discontinue the use of any topicals that need to be removed before a feed. The removal can further aggravate any existing nipple damage.

Some topicals that are suggested for nipples actually delay healing time, cause possible irritations or allergies, or contain harmful substances such as the pesticides found in regular lanolin (Walker, 1989a). Oils, including vitamin E, do not facilitate moist wound healing. They stay on the surface of the skin and do not provide the moisture that is lacking for healing (Huml, 1994). A further concern with vitamin E is that increased serum concentrations of vitamin E were found in breastfed babies after 6 days of ingesting milk from their mothers who were using topical vitamin E on their nipples (Hale, 1998; Marx, 1985).

Hypoallergenic medical grade anhydrous lanolin has been encouraged for use on sore nipples. The allergens and impurities of regular lanolin are removed, and it has been found to "provide a semi-occlusive moisture barrier that slows down internal moisture loss without clogging the pores, thus acting as a moist wound healer" (Huml, 1994). Spangler and Hildebrandt (1993) found that modified lanolin had an insignificant effect on nipple pain or damage during days 1 to 5 postpartum. They suggest that modified lanolin not be considered for routine use in all mothers. They did note a significant effect on nipple pain and damage during days 6 through 10 postpartum, and encourage its use as a treatment option.

Interruption of Breastfeeding

When all else fails and when identifying the cause with treatment provides little or no relief, in order to preserve breastfeeding, some mothers prefer to stop breastfeeding from several feeds to several days. When a mother experiences an interruption in breastfeeding, she will need to use a hospital-grade electric breast pump to maintain milk production. She can double pump for 10 to 15 minutes every 2 to 3 hours, closely matching her baby's feeding frequency. A bit of olive oil dabbed on the areola before pumping can lessen the pulling on the areola within the flange and make pumping more comfortable. The pump should be placed on a low setting at the beginning to avoid pain. As her condition improves, she can increase the pressure setting. The baby can be cup fed to avoid nipple preference during this time. When resuming breastfeeding, the baby should nurse at the breast initially every 12 hours. When she feels ready, the mother may put the baby to breast for every second or third feeding, increasing the frequency of feeds at the breast as tolerated.

Alternating Breastfeeding Positions

Advising the mother about various nursing positions may be helpful. In order to help her avoid further irritation to a sore spot, you can suggest that she keep the baby's chin, and thus his tongue, away from the sore part. Thinking of her breast as a clock can help the mother describe the location of the sore spot. In turn, you can suggest nursing positions to minimize further irritation. Figure 14.1 illustrates the relationship between the three most common nursing positions and the resulting sore spots. Other positions, such as with the mother and baby lying down with the baby's feet pointing above the mother's head, will also provide relief for the mother and distribute stress more evenly. Table 14.1 summarizes the treatment options for sore nipples.

Cracked Nipples

When soreness persists, cracks or fissures often develop on the nipples, appearing either crosswise or lengthwise along the nipple (Fig. 14.2). Infrequently a woman's nipple may fold over, causing a stress point at the fold. Bleeding may result at nursing times when the baby stretches the nipple to the soft palate. If the baby receives a significant amount of blood, he may vomit or have black stools. Sometimes the baby's physician may want to interrupt breastfeeding for a short time to rule out internal bleeding. If the black stools or vomiting are a result of blood from cracked nipples, the symptoms will cease when the baby stops nursing. If other methods of healing are not effective, the mother may wish to interrupt breastfeeding for a day or two until her nipples heal.

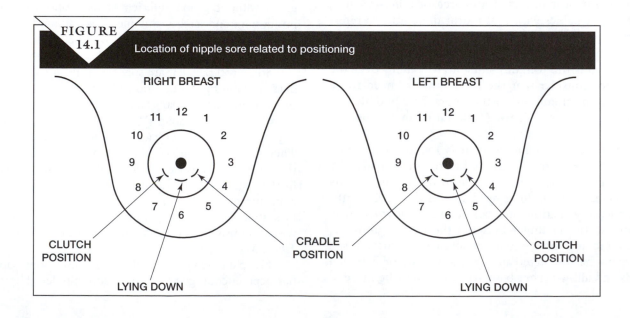

FIGURE 14.1   Location of nipple sore related to positioning

TABLE 14.1	
Sore Nipples	
Causes	**Actions for the Mother**
Soreness from newborn suckling	◆ Check to ensure that baby is put on and comes off breast properly. ◆ Check to ensure that nipple is back far enough in baby's mouth. ◆ Hold baby closely during nursing so nipple is not constantly being pulled.
Dried colostrum or milk causing nipple to stick to bra or breast pads	◆ Moisten bra or pads before taking off so as not to remove keratin.
Poor positioning	◆ Bring baby close to nurse, so he does not pull on breast. ◆ Bring baby to breast so that he has a big mouthful of breast tissue.
Baby chewing or nuzzling onto nipple	◆ Form nipple for baby. ◆ Set up pattern of getting baby onto breast, using rooting reflex.
Baby nursing on end of nipple	◆ Ensure that nipple is way back in baby's mouth by properly getting baby onto breast. ◆ Check for **flutter tongue**. ◆ Check for inverted nipple. ◆ Check for engorgement.
Baby is chewing his way off nipple or nipple is being pulled out of baby's mouth at end of feed	◆ Remove baby from breast by placing a finger between baby's gums to ensure suction is broken. ◆ End feed when baby's sucking slows, before he has a chance to chew on nipple.
Baby overly eager to nurse	◆ Respond to feeding cues promptly. ◆ Pre-express milk to hasten letdown and avoid vigorous sucking.
Inadequate letdown	◆ Use massage and relaxation before feeds. ◆ Condition letdown by setting up routine for getting baby onto breast.
Nipples not allowed to dry	◆ Check for leaking milk. ◆ Check that there are no plastic liners in breast pads. ◆ Eliminate synthetic fabrics in bra and clothing; wear cotton or cotton blends. ◆ Air dry breasts completely after feeds. ◆ Change breast pads frequently.
Improper use of nipple shield	◆ Use shield only to draw nipple out, then have baby nurse on breast. ◆ Avoid shields with inner ridges that irritate nipples.

TABLE 14.1 (CONTINUED)

Sore Nipples

Causes	Actions for the Mother
Inadequate milk supply; baby tugging or sucking on empty breast	◆ Nurse more frequently (every 1 to 1½ hours). ◆ Nurse long enough to facilitate good milk production.
Nipple skin not resistant to stress	◆ Improve diet, especially adding fresh fruits and vegetables and vitamin supplements. ◆ Eliminate or decrease use of sugary foods, alcohol, caffeine, and cigarettes. ◆ Check for use of cleansing or drying agents.
Natural oils being removed or keratin layers broken down by drying agents (soap, alcohol, shampoo, or deodorant)	◆ Eliminate irritants. ◆ Wash breasts with water only. ◆ Apply lubricant after air drying, if necessary.
Nipple irritated by going braless under rough clothing or by rubbing against bra during vigorous exercise	◆ Wear a bra or change to one with more support (jogger's bra). ◆ Wear softer fabric blouse.
Residue of laundry products on clothing	◆ Use less detergent, and rinse wash loads twice. ◆ Try different laundry products.
Teething causes increased feeds, chomping down on nipple, irritation by a change in baby's saliva, or medication used for baby's gums	◆ Wash breast after every feed in plain warm water to remove baby's saliva or other irritants. ◆ Breastfeed before giving solid foods rather than after. ◆ Use soothing techniques instead of nursing to comfort baby. ◆ Stop feed after the first incident of biting and resume when baby is more hungry. ◆ Keep finger ready to break suction and stop feed when sucking pattern changes.
Baby falls asleep at breast and clamps down on breast	◆ Remove baby before he falls asleep.
Teeth marks on breast (not usually cause for soreness but mother may say baby is biting)	◆ Alternate nursing positions.
Irritation from food particles in toddler's mouth	◆ Check toddler's mouth before feeds. ◆ Offer toddler a sip of water or wipe mouth with clean moist cloth before nursing. ◆ Breastfeed before offering solid foods.
Mother menstruating or pregnant	◆ If menstruating, discomfort will last only a few days. ◆ If pregnant, discuss plans for continued nursing or weaning.
Thrush (a yeastlike infection; see discussion of thrush)	◆ Have physician check and prescribe medication for both mother and baby. ◆ Discard or boil any items that baby puts in his mouth.

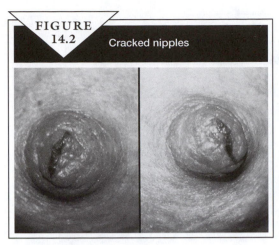

Printed by permission of Kay Hoover.

She can express her milk during that time. Table 14.2 summarizes the treatment options for cracked nipples.

Yeast Infections

A yeast infection is usually caused by *candida albicans,* a fungal organism that is commonly found in the mouth, gastrointestinal tract, and vagina of healthy persons. Under normal conditions, candida's growth is kept in check by the body's flora. Predisposing factors that may disturb the normal flora and lead to yeast infection include diabetes, illness, pregnancy, oral contraceptive use, poor diet, antibiotic therapy, steroid therapy, and immunosuppression. Also, local factors such as obesity or excessive sweating provide constantly warm, moist areas in which candida can thrive (Amir, 1996).

Candida is not normally found on skin such as the nipple. However, it may be present during lactation. A yeast infection has been associated with nipple damage early in lactation, mastitis, recent use of antibiotics in the postpartum period, long-term antibiotic use before pregnancy, and vaginal yeast infection (Amir, 1991). Von Maillot (1978) found that nearly two-thirds of mothers with vaginal yeast infections transmitted the infection to their infants. The baby contracts oral yeast as he passes through the birth canal and, in turn, transfers the infection back to the mother's nipple when he breastfeeds.

When a yeast infection is present in the baby's mouth, it is called thrush. Thrush presents as white patches that look like milk curds, as illustrated in Figure 14.3. Unlike milk, they cannot be wiped off. In the diaper area, yeast may present as a raised, very red area with a sharply defined border. Babies with a yeast infection often seem to be gassy and fussy. Symptoms of vaginal yeast are often difficult to miss. The vaginal area and vulva are tender, and very red with intense itching. There can also be a cheesy, white vaginal discharge.

Yeast on the nipple does not always present with visual symptoms, however. It is unusual to see white patches or redness on the nipple, although it is possible (Fig. 14.4). The most obvious symptom is usually breast and nipple pain. When a mother presents with severely sore nipples after a period of pain-free breastfeeding, a yeast infection should be suspected. Mothers often describe the pain as intense and burning, radiating through the breast

TABLE 14.2	
Cracked Nipples	
Causes	**Actions for the Mother**
All causes of sore nipples carried to extreme	◆ Consult physician about using ibuprofen, acetaminophen, or other pain killer.
	◆ Improve nutritional status, increasing protein, vitamin C, and zinc.
	◆ Refer to all above-mentioned actions for sore nipples.
Foldover nipple (crack may appear at fold)	◆ Air dry breasts after feed.
Local infection (baby with staph or other organism may have infected mother's nipples)	◆ Have physician check nipples, culture baby's throat and mother's nipples, and treat accordingly.
Baby overly eager at feeds	◆ Respond to feeding cues promptly.
	◆ Limit nursing times to 10 minutes per breast.
	◆ Pre-express milk to hasten letdown.
	◆ Nurse in a position which does not aggravate crack.
	◆ Soak nipple to soften before nursing.

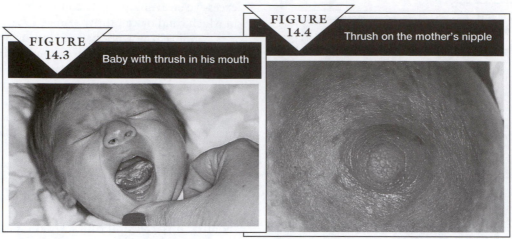

FIGURE 14.3   Baby with thrush in his mouth

Printed by permission of Chele Marmet and the Lactation Institute.

FIGURE 14.4   Thrush on the mother's nipple

Printed by permission of Kay Hoover.

during or after feeds (Lawrence, 1999). They may not be able to stand the feel of clothing on the nipple or water during a shower.

Treatment of a Yeast Infection

Usually, when a mother has a yeast infection on her nipples, her baby has oral thrush. The reverse is also true. It is imperative that both the mother and the baby be treated simultaneously, even if only one of them has symptoms. In addition to the baby's mouth and mother's nipples, treatment must be carried out on any other sites of infection. This includes the diaper area and vagina, as well as other family members who harbor the infection. It is important that the full course of treatment be followed, even after symptoms subside. A yeast infection recurs very easily. In one case, 6 weeks of treatment were needed (Bodley, 1997). The strain of yeast on the mother's nipples and the baby's mouth can be different from that found in a diaper rash.

Many strains of yeast are resistant to the common medications. Various treatment regimens exist for both oral and nipple yeast. A number of antifungal topicals are noted in the literature. They include nystatin; clotrimazole, 1 percent; miconazole nitrate, 2 percent; ketoconazole, 2 percent; ciclopirox, 1 percent; and naftifine hydrochloride. Although nystatin is often the first treatment suggested, the other topicals listed are noted to be more effective in treating yeast infections (Huggins, 1993; Lawrence, 1999). Clotrimazole, 1 percent, and miconazole, 2 percent, are available over the counter. The others listed require a medical prescription.

The usual treatment of oral yeast infection in the baby is to rinse his mouth with water after breastfeeding, shake and pour nystatin into a cup, and apply it to all surfaces of the baby's mouth with a cotton swab. The used swab should never be dipped again into the original vial of nystatin. The mother's nipples should be rinsed with a solution of one cup of plain, tepid water with one tablespoon of vinegar and then air dried. An antifungal cream is then applied. Breast pads need to be changed at least as often as every feeding (Hoover, 1995).

If the topical creams do not have an adequate effect, you may wish to discuss the use of gentian violet with the mother. Gentian violet has been identified as a very effective treatment for oral and nipple yeast infection. It is available over the counter and should be 0.5 percent (Huggins, 1993). A cotton swab is dipped in the gentian violet and is used to swab the baby's mouth. When the baby then latches onto the breast, this treats the nipple from direct contact. Some practitioners also advise that the mother's breasts be swabbed once a day. This is done one time per breast per day. Ulceration of the mucous membranes in the mouth may result with more frequent use or with a strength higher than 0.5 percent (Huggins, 1993). The course of treatment is usually 3 days.

Although you cannot legally prescribe the use of gentian violet, you may point out to the mother that others have found its use helpful in clearing a yeast infection from the breast. The mother should also be encouraged to have a dialogue with her own and her baby's physicians. This may be necessary, particularly with extremely persistent cases of yeast infection that do not respond to conventional topical medications. The mother may also need to investigate the option of an oral antifungal that works **systemically**.

Stopping the Spread of Yeast

Further considerations during the course of treatment focus on family hygiene. Good handwashing before and after diapering, before and after using the toilet, and before and after breastfeeding will help stop the spread of yeast. Anything that comes in contact with the mother's breast, such as a bra, breast shells, or breast pump parts, needs to be boiled once a day for at least 20

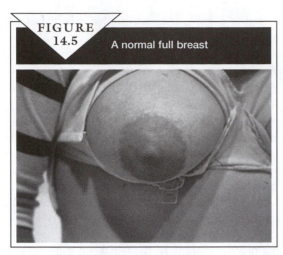

FIGURE 14.5 A normal full breast

Printed by permission of Kay Kutner.

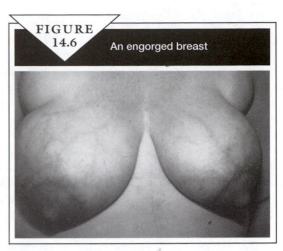

FIGURE 14.6 An engorged breast

Printed by permission of Debi Bocar.

minutes. These items are vehicles for reinfection, and boiling kills the candida. The same is true for anything that has come in contact with the baby's mouth, such as a pacifier, bottle nipple, or teething ring. Bottle nipples, pacifiers, and teethers should be discarded after 1 week.

If the mother is pumping, her fresh milk may be used, but it should not be frozen. Rosa (1990) states that freezing will not kill candida. Thus, it is possible that the milk may reinfect the baby when it is used later. If the baby is older, his toys need to be cleaned thoroughly with hot soapy water. All of the family's clothing will need to be laundered in very hot water. The mother's diet may also be a factor. If the yeast infection has been persistent, she may need to decrease dairy products and sugars while increasing acidophilus, garlic, zinc, and B vitamins in her diet (Baumslag, 1992). If the nipple soreness persists, a referral to a dermatologist is in order.

ENGORGEMENT

At birth, the delivery of the placenta triggers a change in the woman's hormone levels that helps stimulate the production of mature milk. Increased amounts of blood and lymph circulate in the breast and are the source from which the milk is produced. The enlarged blood vessels are often visible beneath the skin of the firmer, fuller lactating breast. These fluids cause the breasts to become fuller, heavier, and perhaps slightly tender. Figure 14.5 shows a breast that is normally full. As regular frequent feeds progress, this normal fullness diminishes. By about 10 days postpartum, when lactation is fully established, the breasts become comfortably soft and pliable, even when they are full of milk.

Engorgement, on the other hand, is a serious condition, and therefore, it is important to distinguish between it and the normal postpartum fullness. Engorgement is essentially overfullness, which occurs when milk is inadequately or infrequently removed from the breast. Engorgement is an **iatrogenic** entity, caused by medical interference with the natural process in the form of regulations, schedules, and poor management of lactation. After delivery, if the duct system is not sufficiently cleared of colostrum before milk begins to accumulate, the back pressure results in breasts that feel firm, hard, tender, and warm or hot to the touch. The skin may actually look shiny and transparent, as in Figure 14.6. Nipples may become flattened, or even disappear in extreme cases of engorgement owing to the inability of the skin to stretch any further. Table 14.3 characterizes four stages of breast fullness when describing engorgement (Kutner, 1996).

TABLE 14.3	
Four Stages of Breast Fullness	
Stage	**Definition**
+1	Breasts are soft. Milk flows freely.
+2	Breasts are firm and nontender. Milk flows freely.
+3	Breasts are firm and tender. Milk release is slow and relief is obtained quickly.
+4	Breasts are hard and painful. Milk release is slow and relief is not obtained quickly.

Engorgement can occur any time during lactation if feeds are missed or if milk is not removed from the breasts on a regular basis. The most common time for engorgement to occur is in the early days, when breastfeeding is beginning and nursing patterns are irregular. Engorgement can also develop when the baby begins sleeping through the night and whenever the mother and baby are separated so that feeds are missed. It is also a risk during the weaning process, especially if rapid weaning is necessary. Because engorgement can cause temporary and permanent problems with lactation, every attempt should be made to avoid it. Encourage mothers to remove milk from their breasts whenever they have a feeling of fullness, before they become uncomfortable. Figure 14.7 illustrates the causes and results of engorgement.

Problems Caused by Engorgement

Engorgement creates serious problems with milk production. Milk that is backed up in the breast increases pressure in the duct systems, which decreases the flow of blood and lymph. Consequently, less nutrients become available to make milk. The possibility of infection increases because bacteria are not being removed by the lymphatic system at the normal rate. Breast tissue elasticity allows milk storage for up to 48 hours before the rate of milk production and secretion begins to decrease rapidly. When milk remains there longer, the pressure on alveoli and ducts greatly decreases their effectiveness.

Engorgement also presents a danger of permanently harming breast tissue. The increased milk pressure can cause some alveolar cells and myoepithelial cells to shrink and die off. This atrophy of milk-producing cells can permanently compromise the milk-producing ability of the breast for that particular breastfeeding experience. Also, the **suppressor peptides** in human milk have a negative effect on milk production if the milk remains in the breast for extended periods. Suppressor peptides are inhibiting peptides in human milk that bring about the cessation of milk secretion during milk stasis and engorgement. Unrelieved severe engorgement can cause insufficient milk production by 6 weeks. These mothers and babies need to be followed closely.

Engorgement adversely affects the letdown mechanism as well. The flattened nipple of the engorged breast becomes difficult for the baby to grasp. Thus, the nerves within the nipple and areola may not be well stimulated and letdown may not occur. Without letdown, the baby cannot remove milk from the breast efficiently. Pressure then increases in the ducts even more. In addition, when engorgement causes flattening of the nipples, it allows the baby to grasp only the ends of the nipples. This often results in sore, cracked nipples, which can further inhibit letdown.

Preventing Engorgement

The practices promoted in Chapter 10 offer preventive measures for engorgement. Initiating breastfeeding within the first hour of life sets the stage for the prevention of problems. When mothers and babies are kept together 24 hours a day throughout their maternity stay, the mother becomes familiar with her baby's feeding cues and acts on them. Breastfeeding in response to baby cues, and for as long as the baby needs, must be encouraged as the norm. Eight or more feeds in 24 hours, including night feeds, will keep milk flow paced with production. If breast fullness increases, the mother can be encouraged to wake her baby and put him to breast for relief. For those situations in which the baby is very sleepy and not nursing adequately, mothers need to be taught how to express milk to maintain lactation. Each mother and baby must be assessed for correct latch and positioning, with help given as needed. Additionally, the use of artificial nipples is discouraged. They do not promote efficient suckling and may confuse the baby when he goes back to the breast. Education of the maternity staff must focus on these key areas for the postpartum period. Minimizing interference with breastfeeding is often the best prevention of engorgement.

Helping Mothers Relieve Engorgement

Treating engorgement involves a combination of identifying and correcting the cause and offering palliative measures. Engorgement can be a frightening experience for a mother. It is helpful for her to know it is temporary and that with proper treatment, engorgement usually is resolved within 12 to 24 hours. If the mother has been limiting feeds with respect to either frequency or duration, encourage her to breastfeed at least every 2 hours or sooner if her baby desires, and to allow him to nurse as long as he needs. After the engorgement is resolved, advise the mother to nurse her baby at least eight times every 24-hour period. If breastfeeding alone does not reduce the engorgement, she may need to express milk between feeds. See the guidelines for pumping later.

It is essential that you check the mother's positioning and the baby's latch. If they are not correct, it may lead to decreased milk removal. When engorgement has progressed to such a degree that the baby is unable to latch onto the breast, the mother can be encouraged to express milk before a feed to soften the areola. Expressing milk in the shower is enhanced by the relax-

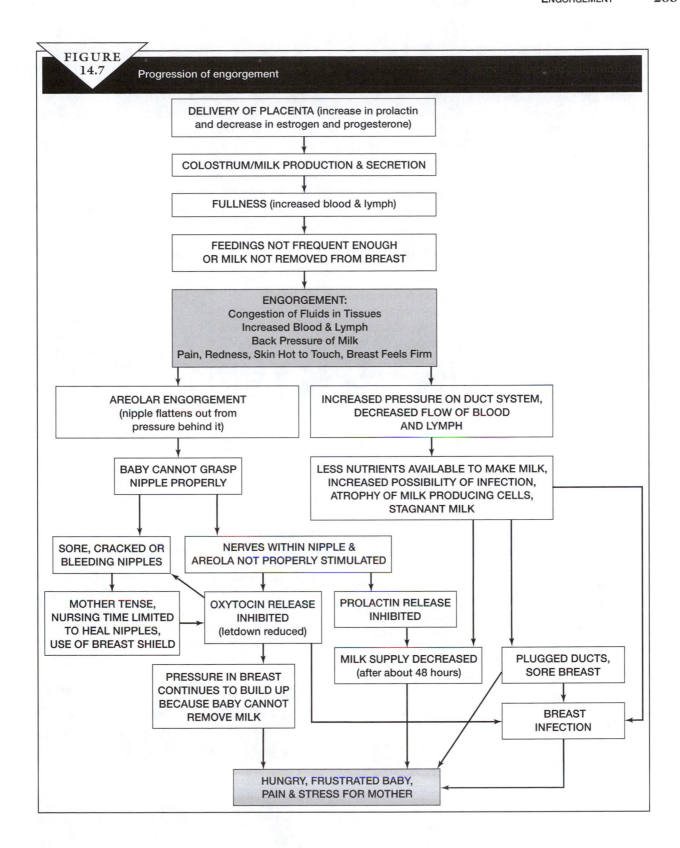

FIGURE 14.7 Progression of engorgement

DELIVERY OF PLACENTA (increase in prolactin and decrease in estrogen and progesterone)

COLOSTRUM/MILK PRODUCTION & SECRETION

FULLNESS (increased blood & lymph)

FEEDINGS NOT FREQUENT ENOUGH OR MILK NOT REMOVED FROM BREAST

ENGORGEMENT:
Congestion of Fluids in Tissues
Increased Blood & Lymph
Back Pressure of Milk
Pain, Redness, Skin Hot to Touch, Breast Feels Firm

AREOLAR ENGORGEMENT (nipple flattens out from pressure behind it)

INCREASED PRESSURE ON DUCT SYSTEM, DECREASED FLOW OF BLOOD AND LYMPH

BABY CANNOT GRASP NIPPLE PROPERLY

LESS NUTRIENTS AVAILABLE TO MAKE MILK, INCREASED POSSIBILITY OF INFECTION, ATROPHY OF MILK PRODUCING CELLS, STAGNANT MILK

SORE, CRACKED OR BLEEDING NIPPLES

NERVES WITHIN NIPPLE & AREOLA NOT PROPERLY STIMULATED

MOTHER TENSE, NURSING TIME LIMITED TO HEAL NIPPLES, USE OF BREAST SHIELD

OXYTOCIN RELEASE INHIBITED (letdown reduced)

PROLACTIN RELEASE INHIBITED

MILK SUPPLY DECREASED (after about 48 hours)

PLUGGED DUCTS, SORE BREAST

PRESSURE IN BREAST CONTINUES TO BUILD UP BECAUSE BABY CANNOT REMOVE MILK

BREAST INFECTION

HUNGRY, FRUSTRATED BABY, PAIN & STRESS FOR MOTHER

ation effect of water spraying on the mother's back and shoulders.

Cold compresses may be applied between feeds to help decrease the mother's discomfort. A frozen pack of vegetables such as peas or corn work well. They conform to the shape of the breast and may be refrozen for reuse as a compress. The mother may also lie flat on her back to elevate the breasts and help reduce the swelling. Cabbage leaves worn inside the bra, until milk begins to flow and excessive fluid in the tissues is reduced, is another simple remedy the mother may want to use.

▼ Guidelines for Pumping When Engorged

With appropriate guidelines, pumping or hand expressing when the breasts are engorged will preserve the mother's milk production. Pumping for engorgement is usually necessary for only 24 to 72 hours. Continuing to pump beyond that time can maintain the mother's milk production at a level that is higher than needed. For convenience, a double pump can be used to pump both breasts at the same time. This is especially important if the breasts feel hard and there is poor milk release.

It is not necessary to pump both breasts unless both are engorged. Only the affected breast needs to be pumped. Single pumping is usually recommended when there is +2 or +3 engorgement and the infant is still able to nurse (see Table 14.3 for definitions). If the areola is firm or hard, the mother will need to pump before nursing. She should pump only long enough to soften the areola so that the infant can latch on easily and not cause nipple trauma. The mother should then put her baby to breast to nurse. Following the feed, the mother should pump her breast again if needed. If milk was released from the breast easily and the infant was heard gulping, then she will need to pump only until the milk stops coming out quickly. If only periodic swallowing was heard, she should pump the breast for at least 10 minutes. If, at the end of 10 minutes, the milk begins to flow out quickly, she can continue to pump until it slows.

If the mother pumps only one breast at a time, she can use her other hand to massage the breast while she is pumping. She can apply cabbage or ice packs to her breasts between feeding and pumping sessions. She will want to stop pumping before nursing as soon as possible. She can then pump after nursing only when necessary. Soon she will not need to pump at all.

The Use of Cabbage for Engorgement

The use of fresh green cabbage leaves to treat engorgement is not a new phenomenon. The earliest written reference available is in a book called *The Glory of Woman*, published in 1896. It describes the application of fresh, young cabbage leaves to the "gathered" breast. An article

in 1987 was instrumental in reviving the practice (Rosier, 1987). The mechanism of action is not known. It seems that cabbage reduces swelling in the tissues. It has been used on other parts of the body for pathologic swelling, such as that which occurs in sprains and strains. Cabbage reduces the edema in breast engorgement and even the inflammation caused by plugged ducts and mastitis. It is speculated that cabbage contains a **phytoestrogen**. Prolonged application of cabbage can cause the milk to dry up entirely. It is for this reason that farmers are careful to keep their cows out of the cabbage patch because consumption of cabbage can decrease milk production.

Application of Cabbage to the Breast

To use cabbage for the relief of engorgement, the lactating woman places cabbage leaves on her breasts and can hold them in place with her brassiere (Fig. 14.8). The procedure for applying cabbage is simple. After discarding the outer leaves, pull off several inner leaves, wash them, pat them dry, and crush them slightly. Place the leaves on the engorged breasts and hold them in place with a bra. The remainder of the cabbage can be stored in the refrigerator to keep it cold for later use.

After a short period of time, women will sometimes report that their breast feels "different"—sometimes described as tingly and cool. When this sensation is experienced, when the milk begins to leak, or when there is evidence of softening of the tissues, the cabbage can be removed. The mother can then put her baby to breast, or she can pump if the baby still cannot latch on. With severe engorgement, because of the heat of the breast, the cabbage will actually wilt. It can be replaced with fresh leaves for as long as is required for relief, applying fresh leaves about every 2 hours. As soon as the infant or pumping provide the needed relief, use of the cabbage leaves should be discontinued. To dry up the milk completely, as in sudden weaning, the cabbage is left on the breasts around the clock, changing it as needed until the milk is gone.

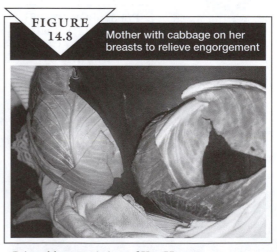

FIGURE 14.8 Mother with cabbage on her breasts to relieve engorgement

Printed by permission of Kay Hoover.

The amount of relief experienced by women varies. Some will get relief in as little as 20 to 30 minutes, whereas others may need to apply the cabbage over a period of 24 hours. In some cases, the decrease of edema is so pronounced that the milk ducts will stand out in bold relief on the breast after the cabbage is removed. The use of cabbage is included in the care plan in Figure 14.9. For plugged ducts or mastitis, the cabbage is used in the same way. It is washed, crushed, and applied to the plug or the area where the inflammation from the mastitis is evident, and it is left on the breast until relief is obtained. No untoward effects from the cabbage have been noted (Roberts, 1995a, 1995b). Table 14.4 presents treatment options for engorgement.

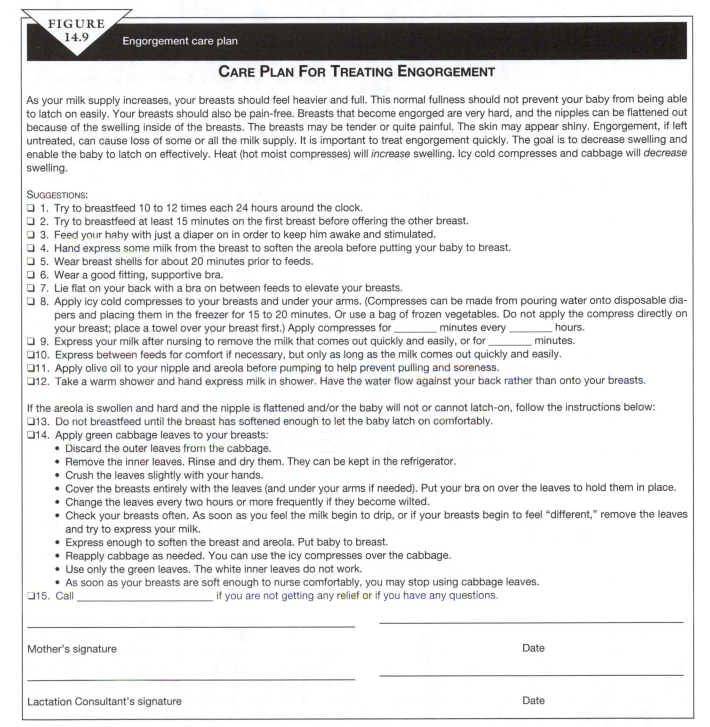

FIGURE 14.9 Engorgement care plan

CARE PLAN FOR TREATING ENGORGEMENT

As your milk supply increases, your breasts should feel heavier and full. This normal fullness should not prevent your baby from being able to latch on easily. Your breasts should also be pain-free. Breasts that become engorged are very hard, and the nipples can be flattened out because of the swelling inside of the breasts. The breasts may be tender or quite painful. The skin may appear shiny. Engorgement, if left untreated, can cause loss of some or all the milk supply. It is important to treat engorgement quickly. The goal is to decrease swelling and enable the baby to latch on effectively. Heat (hot moist compresses) will *increase* swelling. Icy cold compresses and cabbage will *decrease* swelling.

SUGGESTIONS:
☐ 1. Try to breastfeed 10 to 12 times each 24 hours around the clock.
☐ 2. Try to breastfeed at least 15 minutes on the first breast before offering the other breast.
☐ 3. Feed your baby with just a diaper on in order to keep him awake and stimulated.
☐ 4. Hand express some milk from the breast to soften the areola before putting your baby to breast.
☐ 5. Wear breast shells for about 20 minutes prior to feeds.
☐ 6. Wear a good fitting, supportive bra.
☐ 7. Lie flat on your back with a bra on between feeds to elevate your breasts.
☐ 8. Apply icy cold compresses to your breasts and under your arms. (Compresses can be made from pouring water onto disposable diapers and placing them in the freezer for 15 to 20 minutes. Or use a bag of frozen vegetables. Do not apply the compress directly on your breast; place a towel over your breast first.) Apply compresses for _____ minutes every _____ hours.
☐ 9. Express your milk after nursing to remove the milk that comes out quickly and easily, or for _____ minutes.
☐10. Express between feeds for comfort if necessary, but only as long as the milk comes out quickly and easily.
☐11. Apply olive oil to your nipple and areola before pumping to help prevent pulling and soreness.
☐12. Take a warm shower and hand express milk in shower. Have the water flow against your back rather than onto your breasts.

If the areola is swollen and hard and the nipple is flattened and/or the baby will not or cannot latch-on, follow the instructions below:
☐13. Do not breastfeed until the breast has softened enough to let the baby latch on comfortably.
☐14. Apply green cabbage leaves to your breasts:
   • Discard the outer leaves from the cabbage.
   • Remove the inner leaves. Rinse and dry them. They can be kept in the refrigerator.
   • Crush the leaves slightly with your hands.
   • Cover the breasts entirely with the leaves (and under your arms if needed). Put your bra on over the leaves to hold them in place.
   • Change the leaves every two hours or more frequently if they become wilted.
   • Check your breasts often. As soon as you feel the milk begin to drip, or if your breasts begin to feel "different," remove the leaves and try to express your milk.
   • Express enough to soften the breast and areola. Put baby to breast.
   • Reapply cabbage as needed. You can use the icy compresses over the cabbage.
   • Use only the green leaves. The white inner leaves do not work.
   • As soon as your breasts are soft enough to nurse comfortably, you may stop using cabbage leaves.
☐15. Call _____ if you are not getting any relief or if you have any questions.

_____   _____
Mother's signature   Date

_____   _____
Lactation Consultant's signature   Date

Printed by permission of Breastfeeding Support Consultants, 1998.

TABLE 14.4	
Treatment of Engorgement	
Causes of Engorgement	**Actions for the Mother**
◆ Missed feeds or infrequent feeds.	Room in with baby in the hospital. Breastfeed baby 10 to 12 times each 24 hours, or more if he is willing around the clock. Watch baby for feeding cues and respond to them. Use rousing techniques for sleepy baby. Increase skin-to-skin contact to encourage baby to nurse. Have the mother remove her shirt and bra, and hold her baby with only a diaper on. Pump breasts with a hospital-grade electric breast pump any time baby is unwilling or unable to nurse.
◆ Milk removal not adequate at feeds.	Check that baby's latch and position are appropriate. Stop the use of all artificial nipples. Increase skin-to-skin contact during feeds. Have mother remove her shirt and bra and hold baby with only a diaper on. Do breast compression during feeds to encourage baby to suckle. Pump breasts *after* the feed with a hospital-grade electric breast pump only to remove the milk that comes out quickly and easily. Pump breasts *between* feeds for comfort, if necessary, only as long as the milk comes out quickly and easily.
◆ Inadequate letdown due to edema and pain.	Relax in warm shower with water running over back, avoiding the breasts, and hand express to relieve fullness. Breastfeed *after* the breast has softened enough to allow baby to latch on comfortably. Use relaxation techniques and gentle breast massage during feeds. Lie flat on back between feeds to elevate breasts. Apply cool packs to the breasts and under arms. Frozen peas or corn work well. Do not apply directly on skin. Apply green cabbage leaves to breasts.

▼

PLUGGED DUCTS

Sometimes the ductwork in the breast becomes plugged with cells and other milk components that were shed within the ducts. The cause is incomplete milk removal or possibly outside pressure on specific areas of the breast. Pressure can be caused by any practice that does not allow free flow of milk in the ducts. The source may be a tight bra, underwires in a bra, or a baby carrier. It may be from consistently holding, carrying, or rocking the baby in the same position. Bunched up clothing under the arm (usually in the winter time), sleeping in a position that puts pressure on the breast, or pressure from a breast pump **flange** can also lead to plugs. Plugged ducts are characterized by localized soreness, swelling, lumpiness, or slight pain. Because a plugged duct is localized in the breast, it is not accompanied by a symptom in any other part of the body, such as fever or flulike symptoms.

Plugs may be broken up and worked down the ducts by regular frequent feeds and hand massage in the direction from the plug toward the nipple. Moist heat over the area of the plug may help move it along the duct. Plugs may also be encouraged to move by rotating the baby's position for feeds so that his tongue stimulates more milk flow in the area of the plug. Beginning a feed on the breast with the plug will help with removal

TABLE 14.5

Treatment of a Plugged Duct

Causes	Actions for the Mother
Poor positioning	◆ Try a variety of positions for better milk removal. ◆ Nurse baby with his chin pointed toward the plugged duct.
Breasts overfull due to missed feeds, irregular nursing patterns, engorgement	◆ If prone to plugged ducts, avoid missed feeds or pump to remove milk. ◆ If baby does not adequately remove milk from the breasts, pump or express milk after feeds.
Incomplete removal of milk from the breast	◆ Nurse long enough on each breast for the baby to remove sufficient milk. ◆ If baby does not remove milk, pump or express milk after feeds. ◆ While nursing on affected side, use massage and heat to encourage drainage. ◆ Nurse more frequently on affected breast. ◆ Gently roll, pull, and rub plug down while in warm shower. ◆ Use moisture to remove any dried secretions blocking nipple pores.
External pressure on the breast	◆ Avoid positions that put pressure on one spot for long periods, e.g., always sleeping on one side, always holding the baby one way, or baby sleeping on mother's chest. ◆ Use larger nursing bra or a bra extender. ◆ Avoid bunching up sweater or nightgown under arm during a feed. ◆ Use nursing bra instead of pulling up conventional bra to nurse in order to avoid pressure on ducts.

by taking advantage of the baby's more vigorous suck early in the feed.

Plugs may be absorbed quickly by the body and not appear in the milk. Sometimes, a plug that has been worked down the ducts and out the nipple will appear as a thick stringy mass on the nipple. This may be removed manually by the mother with no ill effects. If the plug is released and comes out with the milk, it may be brownish or greenish in color, as well as thick and stringy. Although the baby may reject the milk with the plug due to the taste or texture, most babies easily return to nursing afterward. There is no known danger to the baby.

The measures listed earlier for releasing a plug are helpful regardless of the reason for the blockage. In addition, the techniques in Table 14.5 may be helpful for specific causes of plugged ducts. Encourage the mother to make every effort to remove the plug quickly because plugged ducts can develop into larger blocked off areas

called a caked breast. This could then develop into a breast inflammation or infection. For any plug that does not respond to treatment, advise the mother to call her physician.

MASTITIS

A breast infection, also called mastitis, can develop from a crack in the nipple skin that provides a pathway into the breast for staph and other organisms. It is associated with milk stasis and engorgement, and can also result from a plugged duct that went unnoticed or untreated. The inflamed area of the breast becomes red, hot, and tender to the touch (Fig. 14.10). More than just a localized soreness, a breast infection also produces fever and flulike symptoms in the woman. Any time a breastfeed-

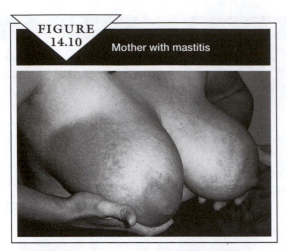

FIGURE 14.10

Mother with mastitis

Printed by permission of Sarah Coulter Danner.

ing mother feels like she is coming down with the flu, she needs to rule out the possibility of mastitis. If she has mastitis, she will want to begin treatment immediately in order to reduce the severity of the breast infection and protect her milk production. The incidence of breast infections is noted in the literature to range from 2 to 7 percent of lactating women. The possibility that mothers may have an infection and not seek medical treatment means that figure is probably much higher.

Causes of Mastitis

You can alert the women in your care to those times when breast infections are most likely to occur. Mastitis often occurs during the newborn period, a time when the mother is more likely to be tired. Until breastfeeding becomes established, milk may not be removed adequately from the breast. Any interruption in breastfeeding or change in nursing pattern can cause milk to remain in the ducts. An infection can also develop when the mother's time and energy become overextended, as with holidays, vacations, house guests, or when the baby is ill.

Riordan (1990a) noted that mothers ranked fatigue and stress as the most common conditions that preceded a bout of mastitis. Other factors identified in her survey include plugged ducts, change in feeding frequency, milk **stasis** (lack of flow), engorgement, sore or cracked nipples, an infection in the family, and trauma to the breast. Riordan also noted that the most frequent site of inflammation was the upper outer quadrant of the breast unilaterally, with near-equal distribution in the right and left breasts.

Most times, breast infections are a result of bacteria that come from the baby's mouth or the home environment. Recent work at the Vancouver Breastfeeding Centre showed that when pain was moderate or severe and

when cracks were present, mothers had a 54 percent chance of having an infection caused by *Staphylococcus aureus,* an easily transmitted organism of moderate virulence (Livingstone, 1996).

The organisms that cause a breast infection most frequently come from the baby or the home. Therefore, the mother is likely to have produced antibodies in her milk to fight the infection. Also, most breast infections are located outside the ductwork in surrounding breast tissue and do not enter the milk. Therefore, it is reasonably safe for the baby to nurse through an infection. Indeed, nursing is recommended for the mother's sake because milk can be removed more effectively by the baby nursing than by pumping or hand expression. Additionally, frequent feeds offer a cleansing effect on the breast rather than allowing milk stasis to develop (Melnikow, 1994).

Treatment of Mastitis

Treatments for mastitis include efficient milk removal, warm moist compresses to the site of inflammation, and an anti-inflammatory medication. Some clinicians have found relief from the application of cabbage leaves as well. Lawrence (1999) speculates that cabbage may work because it contains rapine, which some herbalists consider to be an antifungal antibiotic. The mother also needs total rest to help her body fight the infection. If she is employed outside the home, she might need to take sick leave.

An assessment of a breastfeed is recommended to ensure that the baby is latched and positioned for adequate milk removal. Advise the mother to breastfeed as frequently as her baby requires, and to express milk from the affected breast after every feed. Soaking the affected breast in warm water for short periods facilitates blood flow and drainage. Having her baby nurse on the affected breast first will allow the baby's more vigorous suck to drain the milk better.

When it has been determined that a mother has a breast infection, she is advised to contact her primary health provider. If she is running a temperature higher than 100° and the signs of breast inflammation have not resolved within 24 hours with the suggestions mentioned earlier, she will need to be placed on antibiotic therapy. Antibiotics are generally prescribed for a course of 10 to 14 days. In the absence of a fever, the physician may be willing to wait a few days to determine whether or not the other measures are effective.

Proper treatment of a breast infection includes the four important measures below. Other suggestions relative to specific causes are presented in Table 14.6.

Treatment of a Breast Infection

◆ Heat: Apply warm, moist compresses to the inflamed area before and during the feed.

◆ Rest: Go to bed and stay there for several days.

◆ Remove milk from the breasts: Continue nursing the baby with his chin pointed toward the inflamed area.

◆ Call the physician for an antibiotic: Follow through on the entire regimen, even if the infection seems to clear quickly.

If infection recurs within 2 months, the mother will need to be seen by her physician. Many physicians will prescribe over the phone without seeing the woman. If a third infection occurs, recommend that a culture be done on the mother's milk and nipple, and on the baby's throat to determine the appropriate antibiotic. Table 14.6 describes some of the possible causes of breast infections and actions to be taken by the mother in order to alleviate the infection.

Recurrent Mastitis

Some mothers seem to be prone to mastitis. After a mother has recovered from a breast infection, advise her to be watchful for signs of recurring infection. She will want to be especially careful to remove milk regularly from her breasts. If a feed is missed, she will need to express her milk. Caution her against becoming overly tired or overworked. At the first sign of an infection, warm compresses, more frequent feeds, and bed rest will help to shorten the length of the infection.

Anemia or other deficiencies predispose some women to recurrent mastitis. Recurring episodes are also seen when the mother has been treated with the wrong antibiotic or was not treated long enough. The mother may not have been compliant with the directions for

---

TABLE 14.6

Treatment of a Breast Infection

Causes	Actions for the Mother
Milk stasis: Poor milk removal from the breast	◆ Nurse as long as the baby desires. If breast is full after he is finished, express milk for relief.
Milk stasis: Breasts overfull due to missed feeds, irregular nursing pattern, or engorgement	◆ Avoid missed or delayed feeds. ◆ When feeds are delayed, pump or hand express to remove milk from breasts.
Overwork	◆ Rearrange priorities and daily schedule. ◆ Get help with all tasks.
Low resistance to infection due to anemia, poor diet	◆ Improve diet. ◆ Exercise. ◆ Reduce stress.
Lack of adequate sleep; fatigue	◆ Take daytime naps or rest periods (sleep rebuilds the immune system). ◆ Nurse lying down. ◆ Take baby to bed at night.
Failure to clear a plugged duct	◆ Work plug down manually, if it is not too painful. ◆ Have baby nurse with chin pointed toward plug.
Infection via cracked nipple	◆ Eliminate non-nutritive sucking. ◆ Briefly soak breasts in saline solution (¼ tsp salt in 8 oz water) after feed and air dry.
Infection passed from baby or other family member	◆ Treat primary infection in conjunction with mother's infection.

rest, breast drainage, and taking her antibiotic. Sometimes a woman will stop taking an antibiotic after several days because the symptoms of her breast infection are gone. However, without the full regimen of antibiotic, the infection may not be cleared and will recur as soon as her resistance is lowered again.

The baby is often the source of recurrent breast infections. You can also check for improper physical handling of the breast (e.g., hands not washed) as a possible source. The mother may want to evaluate her overall health (diet, rest, and exercise) and her daily activities and commitments (such as work, volunteer activities, and chauffeuring older children). She can work toward a more healthful and leisurely lifestyle, at least while she is breastfeeding.

▼ Abscessed Breast

An **abscess** is a localized collection of pus that forms from an infection that has no opening for drainage. In the breast, an abscess forms from a breast infection that was not treated or did not respond to treatment. The indications of mastitis—fever, flulike symptoms, nausea, extreme fatigue, and aching muscles—are also experienced with a breast abscess. However, the symptoms are less severe than with mastitis because the abscess is walled off. The infection site becomes red, swollen, and tender (Fig. 14.11). It is important to recognize that occasionally an abscess can occur in the absence of any systemic symptoms. If what seems to be a plugged duct or lump does not resolve with treatment within 48 hours, the mother needs to be seen and the lump evaluated by a physician.

An abscess can be a serious health hazard and should be treated by a physician immediately! The abscess usually is lanced and allowed to drain while the infection is treated with medication (Fig. 14.12). The mother may be able to continue to nurse on one or both breasts. This will depend on the location of the abscess, the pain associated with it, and the medication that is prescribed. If the mother is unable to nurse, she will need to express milk from the affected breast, or she may choose to wean from that breast. If she wishes to continue breastfeeding on the affected breast, she can implement the suggestions in Table 14.6 for treating a breast infection. A mother with an abscess may need more of your time while working through her options of treatment with her physician so that she can continue to breastfeed. Abscesses are a very rare occurrence in breastfeeding. They can be prevented by proper breastfeeding management and immediate treatment of mastitis.

▼ SUMMARY

You can provide much reassurance and assistance to the breastfeeding mother in the early weeks. Discussing common breastfeeding expectations can ease the mother through this time of great change. By being available to her when difficulties arise, and providing both support and guidance, you can be the catalyst for the mother reaching her breastfeeding goals. The anticipatory guidance you provide for early breastfeeds, care of the breast, and leaking will avoid unnecessary concern for the mother. Educating her about prevention and treatment of nipple soreness, engorgement, plugged ducts, and mastitis will make it less likely that these problems will arise or that they will be prolonged. You can help achieve consistency among caregivers in their approach to these events by educating them and being available as a resource.

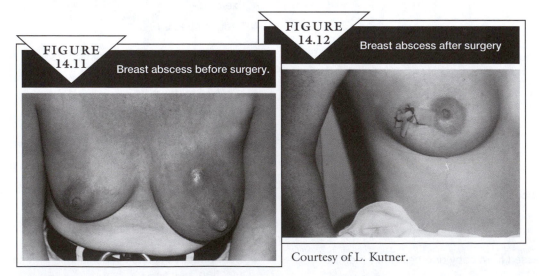

FIGURE 14.11 Breast abscess before surgery.

Printed by permission of Kay Hoover.

FIGURE 14.12 Breast abscess after surgery.

Courtesy of L. Kutner.

REFERENCES

ALCA News, Now Geraniums, 3(2); 1992.

Amir LH. Candida and the lactating breast: Predisposing factors. *J Hum Lact* 7:177–181; 1991a.

Baumslag N and Michels D. *A Women's Guide to Yeast Infections*. New York: Pocket Books; 1992.

Bodley V and Powers D. Long term treatment of a breastfeeding mother with fluconazole-resolved nipple pain caused by yeast: A case study. *J Hum Lact* 13:307–311; 1997.

Bottorff J. Persistence in breastfeeding: A phenomenological investigation. *J Adv Nurs* 15:201–209; 1990.

Coates MM. Nipple pain related to vasospasm in the nipple. *J Hum Lact* 8:153; 1992.

De Carvalho M et al. Does the duration and frequency of early breastfeeding affect nipple pain? *Birth* 11(2):81–84; 1984.

DeCoopman J. Breastfeeding after pituitary resection: Support for a theory of autocrine control of milk supply? *J Hum Lact* 9:35–40; 1993.

Dewey K et al. Maternal versus infant factors related to breast milk intake and residual milk volume: The DARLING study. *Pediatrics* 87:829–837; 1991.

Fetherston C. Risk factors for lactation mastitis. *J Hum Lact* 14:101–109; 1998.

Hancock K and Spangler A. There is a fungus among us! *J Hum Lact* 9(3):179–180; 1993.

Hewat R and Ellis D. A comparison of the effectiveness of two methods of nipple care. *Birth* 14:41–45; 1987.

Hoover K. The link between infant oral thrush and nipple and breast pain in lactating women; 1995.

Huggins K and Billon S. Twenty cases of persistent sore nipples: Collaboration between lactation consultant and dermatologist. *J Hum Lact* 9(3):155–160; 1993.

Huml S. Moist wound healing for cracked nipples in the breastfeeding mother. *Leaven;* 1994.

Kutner L. *Lactation Management Course*. Chalfont, PA: Breastfeeding Support Consultants Center for Lactation Education; 1996.

Lawrence R. *Breastfeeding: A Guide for the Medical Profession*. Philadelphia: C.V. Mosby; 1999.

Hale T. Medications and Mother's Milk. Amarillo TX, 1998.

Leff E et al., Maternal perceptions of successful breastfeeding. *J Hum Lact* 10(2):99–104; 1994.

Lindenberg C et al. The effect of early post-partum mother-infant contact and breast-feeding on the incidence and continuation of breast-feeding. *Int J Nurs Stud* 27:179–186; 1990.

Livingstone V et al. *Staphylococcus aureus* and sore nipples. *Can Fam Physician* 42:654–659; 1996.

Lothian J. It takes two to breastfeed: The baby's role in successful breastfeeding. *J Nurse Midwife* 40:328–334; 1995.

MacFarlane A. *The Psychology of Childbirth*. Boston: Harvard University Press; 1977; pp. 100–101.

Marx CM et al. Vitamin E concentrations in serum of newborn infants after topical use of vitamin E in nursing mothers. *Am J Obstet Gynecol* 152:668–670; 1985.

Melnikow J and Bedinghaus J. Management of common breastfeeding problems. *J Fam Pract* 39:56–64; 1994.

Morse JM et al. Leaking: A problem of lactation. *J Nurse Midwife* 34:15–20; 1989.

Righard L, et al. Breastfeeding patterns: Comparing the effects on infant behavior and maternal satisfaction of using one or two breasts. *Birth* 20:182–185; 1993.

Riordan J and Auerbach K. *Breastfeeding and Human Lactation*. Sudbury, MA: Jones and Bartlett Publishers; 1999.

Riordan J and Nichols F. A descriptive study of lactation mastitis in long-term breastfeeding women. *J Hum Lact* 6(2): 53–58 1990b.

Roberts K et al. A comparison of chilled cabbage leaves and chilled gel paks in reducing breast engorgement. *J Hum Lact* 11:17–20; 1995a.

Roberts K et al. A comparison of chilled and room temperature cabbage leaves in treating breast engorgement. *J Hum Lact* 11:191–194; 1995b.

Rosa C et al. Yeasts from human milk collected in Rio de Janeiro, Brazil. *Rev Microbiol* 21(4):361-363; 1990.

Rosier W. Cool cabbage compresses. *Breastfeed Rev* 13:28–31; 1988.

Schlegel AM. Observations on breastfeeding technique: Facts and fallacies. American *Journal of Maternal Child Nursing* 8:204–207; 1983.

Spangler A and Hildebrandt E. The effect of modified lanolin on nipple pain/damage during the first ten days of breastfeeding. *Int J Childbirth Ed* 8(3):15–18; 1993.

Stuchberry J (ed): Talking about . . . thrush. *Breastfeed Rev*, 9:22–24; 1986.

Varimo P et al. Frequency of breastfeeding and hyperbilirubinemia. *Clin Pediatr* 25:112; 1986.

von Maillot K et al. Candida mycosis in pregnant women and related risks to the newborn. *Mykosen* 246–251; 1978.

Walker M. Management of selected early breastfeeding problems seen in clinical practice. *Birth* 16:148–158; 1989a.

Woolridge M: Aetiology of sore nipples. *Midwifery* 2:172–176; 1986.

Woolridge M et al. The initiation of lactation: The effect of early versus delayed contact for suckling on milk intake in the first week postpartum. *Early Hum Dev* 12:269–278; 1985.

Ziemer M et al. Methods to prevent and manage nipple pain in breastfeeding women. *West J Nurs Res* 12(6):732–744; 1990.

BIBLIOGRAPHY

Allen J et al. Studies in human lactation: Milk composition and daily secretion rates of macronutrients in the first year of lactation. *Am J Clin Nutr* 54:69–80; 1991.

Amir L. Candida albicans: Is it associated with nipple pain in lactating women. *Gynecol Obstet Invest* 41:30–34; 1990.

Amir LH and Pakula S. Nipple pain, mastalgia and candidiasis in the lactating breast. *Aust N Z J Obstet Gynecol* 31:378–380; 1991b.

Barros F et al. Use of pacifiers is associated with decreased breast-feeding duration. *Pediatrics* 95:497–499; 1995.

Brooten D et al. A comparison of four treatments to prevent and control breast pain and engorgement in nonnursing mothers. *Nurs Res* 32(4):225–229; 1983.

Cable B et al. Nipple wound care: A new approach to an old problem. *J Hum Lact* 13:313–318; 1997.

Crook WG. The *Yeast Connection*. Jackson, TN: Professional Books; 1986.

Enzymatic Therapy: A comprehensive guide to Candida. Green Bay, WI: Enzymatic Therapy, Inc; 1988.

Horowitz BJ et al. Sexual transmission of candida. *Am J Obstet Gynecol* 69(6):883–886; 1987.

Johnstone HA: Candidiasis in the breastfeeding mother and infant. *JOGNN* 19(2):171–173; 1990.

Kaufmann R and Foxman B. Mastitis among lactating women: Occurrence and risk factors. *Soc Sci Med* 33:701–705; 1991.

Kutner L. Care plan for thrush. *J Hum Lact* 2(2):76–77; 1986.

Matheny R et al. Control of intake by human-milk-fed infants. Relationships between feeding size and interval. *Dev Psychobiol* 23:511–518; 1990.

Milsom I and Forsman L. Repeated candidiasis: Reinfection or recrudescence, a review, part 2. *Am J Obstet Gynecol* 152(7): 956–959; 1985.

Moon S and Humenick S. Breast engorgement: Contributing variables and variables amenable to nursing intervention. *JOGNN* 18(4):309–315.

Perez Escamilla R et al. Infant feeding policies in maternity wards and their effect on breast-feeding success: An analytical overview. *Am J Public Health* 84:89–97; 1994.

Pugh L et al. A comparison of topical agents to relieve nipple pain and enhance breastfeeding. *Birth* 23:88–93; 1996.

Riordan J. Mastitis: A new look at an old problem. *Breastfeeding Abstracts* 10:1; 1990a.

Rippon JW: *Medical Mycology* (2nd ed). Philadelphia WB. Saunders; 1992.

Roberts K et al. Effects of cabbage leaf extract on breast engorgement. *J Hum Lact* 14:231–236; 1998.

Sharp DA. Moist wound healing for sore or cracked nipples. Breastfeeding Abstracts 12(2); 1992.

Shrago L. Engorgement revisited. Breastfeeding Abstracts. 11(1); 1991.

Simkin P. Intermittent brachial plexus neuropathy secondary to breast engorgement. *Birth* 15(2):102–103; 1988.

Slaven S and Harvey D. Unlimited suckling time improves breastfeeding. *Lancet* 1(8210):392–393; 1981.

Trowbridge JP and Walker M. *The Yeast Syndrome*. New York: Bantam Books; 1988.

Utter AR. Gentian violet treatment for thrush: Can its use cause breastfeeding problems? *J Hum Lact* 6(4):178–180; 1990.

Walker M and Driscoll J. Sore nipples: The new mother's nemesis. *MCN* 14:260–265; 1989b.

Wilf R and Himeback S. Thrush, Presentation at the Eastern Pennsylvania Chapter of the International Lactation Consultant Association; Sept 27, 1988.

Ziemer M and Pigeon J. Skin changes and pain in the nipple during the first week of lactation. *JOGNN* 22:247–256; 1993.

Ziemer M et al. Evaluation of a dressing to reduce nipple pain and improve nipple skin condition in breastfeeding women. *Nurs Res* 44:347–351; 1995.

BREASTFEEDING BEYOND THE FIRST MONTH

Contributing Author: Carole Peterson

As babies mature beyond their first month, some aspects of breastfeeding change in response to their increased age and development. Babies are awake for longer periods of time and expand their world in the direction of physical and social development. Parents learn to adjust their childcare practices to accommodate breastfeeding management to these events. New challenges present themselves in the form of breastfeeding in public, traveling with a nursing baby, and managing breastfeeding as their baby grows.

Parents learn to recognize their baby's own unique means of communication. Waking and sleeping patterns, crying and cooing, and smiling and frowning all elicit responses and readjustments in routine. The baby progresses from an awareness of his mother as a satisfier of his needs, through the development of motor skills for self-amusement, and an awareness of his environment. He experiences teething, crawling and standing, **separation anxiety**, experimenting with vocabulary sounds, feeding himself, and drinking from a cup. Mothers face the challenges of nursing a toddler and, ultimately, weaning. You can help parents appreciate their baby's developmental milestones and recognize ways to adjust their approach to parenting accordingly.

PATTERNS OF GROWTH IN A BREASTFED BABY

During the first 3 months, babies usually gain 5 to 10 oz/week, and in the next 3 months, their gain is usually 2.5 to 4.5 oz/week (Dewey, 1993). Typically, they double their birth weight by 5 to 6 months, and triple it by 1 year. In the first few months, breastfed infants grow at about the same rate as their formula-fed counterparts. After this time, formula-fed infants begin to exceed breastfeeding infants in weight. Head circumference is similar, and breastfed babies tend to be longer. Formula-fed infants have been found to be less energy efficient. They take in more milk and use it less efficiently than infants who are breastfed (Dewey, 1992).

Body length and head circumference are indicators of appropriate growth. At 1 year of age, a baby's length should be approximately one and one-half his length at birth. Brain growth is quite rapid in the first year of life. Head circumference should increase approximately 7.6 cm (3 inches) by 1 year of age. Dewey's study on infant growth found comparatively that length and head circumference were not significantly different in breastfed and formula-fed infants.

Overfeeding a Breastfed Baby

Sometimes a mother may worry that her baby is nursing too frequently and for too long at a feed. This worry may result from a baby who seems to be overweight or one who spits up milk often. A baby is considered to be overweight if he is about two categories above the weight for his height, as determined by standard height and weight charts. A normal weight gain is 1 to 2 lbs/month for the first 4 or 5 months. This rapid weight gain should not continue into the second half of the first year.

Some families have heavier babies who thin down in the second year, regardless of whether they are breastfed or bottle fed. If the baby is much heavier than other family members were, he may be getting too much milk. In addition, a baby who often spits up or vomits from an overly distended stomach may be overfed. The mother can decrease feeds and substitute other activities for breastfeeding until the spitting diminishes.

It may be that the mother is responding to a baby who loves to nurse, who is calm only when nursing, or who seems to have a great sucking need. You can suggest alternate ways of comforting her baby so that she does not use feeding as a response to every cue. Encourage the mother to see the total picture of the developing mother-child relationship and help her refine her parenting skills to meet her child's needs. Babies are awake for longer periods of time as they grow older. As the months go by, the mother needs to occupy her baby with activities other than eating in order to expand his world in the direction of physical and social development.

Actions the Mother May Take

◆   Let the baby suck on his own thumb or finger.

◆   Nurse one breast per feed and allow the baby to continue sucking on the less full breast.

◆   Learn other ways of satisfying the baby—rock, carry, keep him within view of the mother, talk to him, change his position, play with him, or provide toys.

◆   Encourage the baby to amuse himself for short periods, lengthening the times as he grows.

◆   Interest the baby in other activities—a stroll, toys, baby exercises, and so on.

▼ INFANT DEVELOPMENTAL STAGES

A mother becomes acutely aware during the first hours and days after birth that her baby has already developed a distinct personality. As she becomes familiar with his waking and sleeping patterns, crying and cooing, and his smiling and frowning, she adapts her responses and her mothering to suit his individual needs. There are many characteristics and patterns that all babies exhibit as they develop mentally, emotionally, and physically. Caregivers who have experience with a large number of infants are able to identify ones who are not exhibiting age-appropriate reflexes and developmental milestones.

There are wide variations of normal, and each baby progresses at his or her own rate. Humans develop in a progressive manner, from head to foot and from the center of the body or torso out to the extremities. This progression aids us in attaining mobility. Parents often look forward to each new ability their baby exhibits as he develops. A mother who is aware of these developmental stages in advance is better prepared to respond appropriately to the changes in her baby as he grows. You can enhance a woman's mothering skills by preparing her for the typical developments in her baby's behavior. Help her establish ways of altering her nursing patterns and other caregiving to meet her baby's ever-changing needs.

▼ Newborn Development

Newborns are born with a set of reflexes that are necessary for survival. The mouthing reflexes such as suckling, swallowing, and rooting are all necessary to obtain food. Babies are born with a gagging reflex to protect them from choking as they learn to take in food. The startle and grasp reflexes are indications that the infant needs to hold onto the parent. They are also social reflexes that invite the parent to respond to the baby. The **tonic neck reflex**, or fencer position reflex, causes the baby to focus on the hand in front of him. The stepping reflex has no clear purpose but parents enjoy seeing their newborn appear to take steps. All of these reflexes remain in place until babies develop finer skills to replace them, sometime between 4 and 6 months.

▼ Two to Three Months

From the second to the third month, the baby's world broadens as he develops an awareness of his mother as a satisfier of his needs (Fig. 15.1). He behaves as though he and his mother are one person, and his need for her is absolute. The mother may have ambivalent feelings about such constant demands on her time and presence. She may enjoy the dependency because it helps her feel important and useful. At the same time, she may wish she had more time to herself for relaxation and recreation. The mother will continue to make adjustments as she defines her new role, enabling her to establish priorities in baby care without sacrificing her own needs.

During this period, the baby begins responding to stimuli, especially body contact. Babies become very social by 3 months as they learn to focus on objects around them. Their visual acuity becomes more clear by this time, and babies will bat at objects in an attempt to touch and move them. This is also the time for big smiles and recognition of voices of their caregivers. They learn to express unhappiness, delight, and excitement during this time.

The baby may show a preference for the parents, especially the mother, and may fuss when others care for him. He will respond more to high-pitched voices and may show interest in children while ignoring adults. This interest encourages siblings to entertain and continue to interact with babies as they grow. At this age, the baby is able to sense tension in his caregiver and will

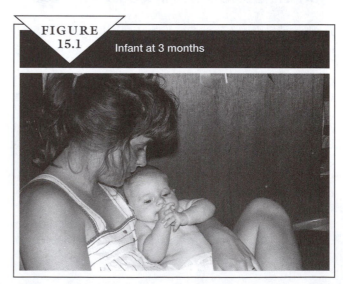

FIGURE 15.1 Infant at 3 months

Printed by permission of Debbie Shinskie.

respond with tension and fussiness, quieting down only after being held in a calm and relaxed manner. From the early weeks, and lasting up to 3 months of age, an infant may act fussy, screaming and contracting his arms and legs in response to digestive upsets. As the weeks pass and his system matures, he becomes calmer. His eating and sleeping take on a more definite pattern, which may be more easily integrated into the family schedule.

Although a baby typically experiences growth spurts at about 6 weeks and 3 months of age, growth spurts can occur at any time. Sometimes the baby may grow up to half an inch in just 24 hours! During this time, the baby eats much more frequently, in spurts that last 1 or 2 days. Encourage mothers to respond with frequent feeds and lots of snuggling.

As the baby gets older, less time will be spent at each feed. His suckling becomes more efficient as he matures, and he may also use methods other than nursing for self-comforting. Sometimes, the mother perceives this as her baby's decreased interest in breastfeeding. In addition, hormonal changes during this period cause the mother's breasts to be less firm. This may create worry that she has lost her milk. Coupled with her baby's growth spurt, her apprehension may increase even more. You can help mothers anticipate these as normal events in breastfeeding. Assessing her baby's disposition, appearance, number of wet diapers and stools, weight gain, and general health and vigor will be reassuring to her. This will encourage her to continue breastfeeding and help her feel secure in the knowledge that she and her baby are working in harmony to provide him with the precise amount of milk that will support his optimal growth.

As the baby approaches 3 months, his sleeping pattern usually shifts to at least one longer rest period and several naps each day. With the changes in sleep pattern, the mother may awaken with more fullness in her breasts than has been noted previously. Nursing her baby directly before she retires for the evening will help him sleep for the longest period at night and provide her with 5 or 6 hours of uninterrupted sleep.

At this age, the baby will be awake for more hours each day and will be much more alert and responsive. The mother will interact with him in ways other than breastfeeding, exposing him to everyday household sounds and providing bright colorful toys and decorations. Varying his positions and environment during the day will help provide the stimulation he needs for physical and mental growth. Help parents learn how to play with their baby. Many adults are uncomfortable with play. Assure parents that a baby at this age cannot be spoiled. By giving him the attention he needs now, they will be rewarded with a more emotionally secure and less demanding child later.

Around this time, the mother may be ready to leave her baby for short periods. Make sure she knows how to express milk from her breasts for these occasional absences. Encourage her to use a cup for feeding in order to avoid the potential for nipple preference. See Chapter 19 for a discussion of expressing and feeding milk to the baby.

▼ 4 to 5 Months

By 4 months after their baby's birth, most parents have learned to adapt their lives to the needs of their new baby and feel more confident in their ability to care for him. Their hours of patience, understanding, and love are beginning to be rewarded by his responsiveness and the development of elementary skills. By 4 months, he will have mastered the art of laughing out loud, to the delight of everyone around them. Their baby begins to gain independence through use of motor skills for self-amusement, and his demands on his parents will decrease accordingly (Fig. 15.2).

As babies gain head and neck strength, they learn how to hold their head up. Then they progress to mini-pushups as the torso becomes stronger. The baby becomes alert and persistent as he works toward more obvious goals such as reaching, touching, rolling over, and imitating sounds. He often displays a clear realization that he is different from his mother, exhibited by his desire for outside stimulation and his tendency to be distracted while at the breast.

During feeding times, the baby may strain his body away from his mother to have a better look at her or to scan his environment. Many mothers regard this as a sign of the baby's desire to separate himself from exclusive breastfeeding, or even as a rejection of them as

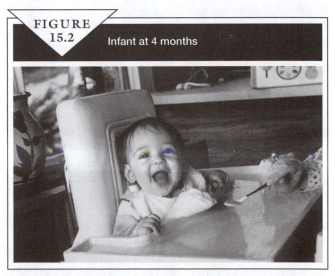

FIGURE 15.2 Infant at 4 months

Printed by permission of Carole Peterson.

mothers. The apparent loss of interest or tendency for being distracted is a positive step forward in the baby's growth and development. It shows that he is reaching out to learn more about the world around him. Breastfeeding can easily continue during this expansive period. Suggest that the mother reduce distractions during nursing times and that she feed her baby when he is most willing to nurse or is too sleepy to be distracted.

By the fourth month, teething may cause the baby to begin drooling, sucking on his fingers, or chewing on objects. Enzymes in the baby's increased saliva may irritate the mother's nipples. Suckling may induce pain in the baby's tender gums, causing him to pull off the breast abruptly. These fluctuations in the nursing pattern, coupled with those caused by the baby's distractibility, may result in less milk removal, with the potential for plugged ducts and mastitis. Limiting nursing time and wiping the nipples with clear water after feeds will help prevent skin irritation. Regular milk removal, either by nursing or expression, will keep milk ducts open, and prevent the development of plugs and infections.

By this age, the baby becomes noticeably more efficient at suckling. Feeds will be shorter in length and will occur less frequently. Because the baby will require less time at the breast to satisfy his hunger needs, the mother may consider feeding solid foods to him. You can remind her that her baby's swallowing mechanism and gastrointestinal tract will not mature enough to handle solid foods until 6 months of age or later. Assure her that her milk is still the ideal food to support his growth.

You can also assure the mother of her baby's continuing need for her attention, while at the same time needing to expand his world beyond the breastfeeding relationship. Reassure her that her baby is not rejecting her. She can share in his growth by providing opportunities for him to develop to his full potential. Breastfeeding will continue to serve as a quiet secure retreat from the stimulation of learning about the world apart from his mother.

▼ 6 Months

By 6 months, most babies babble, coo, and squeal, which marks the beginning of language. This is a very active and social period for babies. They have the head and neck control to be pulled to a sit, and most can sit if they are propped. They have the hand development to grasp a spoon and hold objects, and have mastered visually directed reaching so that they may grasp desired items and pull them toward their mouth. The tongue movement now allows them to take solid foods and begin to learn the social art of eating. Many begin reaching for foods when they join the family for meals. Large

motor development has also advanced to allow babies to roll over. The torso is strengthening to allow the baby to prepare for crawling.

▼ 7 to 9 Months

By 7 months, the baby is expanding his world further through physical movements. Babies become very active at this age (Fig. 15.3). They can roll over in either direction and can usually sit without being propped. By 9 months, they can sit well in a chair and pull themselves into a sitting position. The hands and arms become more developed, allowing the baby to wave bye-bye. He can transfer objects from hand to hand and use his thumb and forefinger to pick up objects, also called the **pincer grasp**. Many babies begin the early stages of crawling during this time, and will raise themselves onto their hands and knees and begin rocking back and forth. They know that the excitement of movement is just around the corner!

The baby's awareness of his mother's ability to be apart from him may bring on separation anxiety, which is expressing dismay when a loved one leaves the room. As a result, he may cry in anticipation of her leaving or while she is away. The baby makes a parent feel very guilty when they leave him for any length of time. He may wake during the night and cry out as a means of reassurance that his parents are nearby. The baby has learned that the parent is important but does not have the awareness that the parent will return. Parents need to recognize this as a part of their baby's development.

It is not uncommon for babies to prefer their mothers to their fathers during this period. Additionally, the baby's increased awareness of differences in people may cause him to react fearfully to a stranger. He may con-

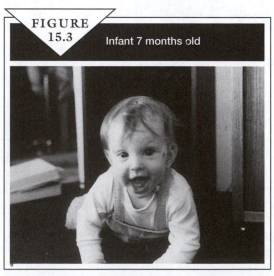

FIGURE 15.3 Infant 7 months old

Printed by permission of Carole Peterson.

tinue his checking-back behavior for reassurance. Exposure to new people need not be discontinued because of this reaction. Observing strangers will enhance the baby's awareness of his mother as a special person in his life.

10 to 12 Months

By 10 to 12 months, the beginning of locomotion has arrived! By this time, motor skills are mastered and regular meal patterns are firmly established. This is an expansive age for the baby. He vigorously and enthusiastically practices many new motor skills while he avidly explores his environment. Most babies will crawl during this time and some may crawl backward before they learn to crawl forward. Babies begin learning to cruise by using tables and chairs to balance them as they begin to learn to walk. (Fig. 15.4). As they progress, babies will use a combination of crawling, walking, stooping, and cruising as the world opens up to their exploration. By 1 year, they are interested in everything and will show their pleasure and displeasure easily.

This new maneuverability offers the baby the opportunity to discriminate further between himself and his mother, and to compare others with her. As he freely moves away from his mother to explore his environment, he continually checks back for assurance that she will be there when he returns. Because of these new comparisons, the baby may turn to his mother more frequently for comfort and reassurance. This may increase the number of feeds, which a mother may interpret as a sign that her baby is becoming overly dependent on her or on breastfeeding. This apparent dependence can be her baby's way of expressing his need for the reassurance

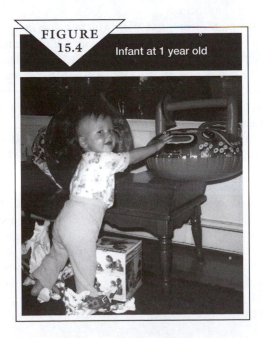

FIGURE 15.4 Infant at 1 year old

of the safe comfortable part of his world. It may indicate that he needs more time to adapt to his new experiences. You can let the mother know that her baby's need for closeness will eventually help him become more independent. What may seem like a step away from independence may actually provide the security that will give him confidence to move toward self-reliance.

The baby's recognition vocabulary (words that he understands and responds to) increases noticeably, and he begins experimenting with vocabulary sounds. He expands his sociability, often seeming to interact with others in a negative manner by repeatedly saying, "No!" During these months, the baby becomes so involved in physical achievements that he may be overwhelmed by outside stresses such as contact with strangers, separation from his mother, and changes in schedule. He may react with shyness or fear, or begin clinging to his mother like a much younger baby. He may climb into her lap to escape stresses as well as for emotional refueling. Although he may not appear tired, he will need several periods of rest from active exploration each day in order to renew his energy.

Because the baby's newly found freedom leads him into many new experiences, the mother may notice changes in his nursing pattern. Some days he may be too busy to nurse, whereas other days in which exploration becomes overwhelming, he may nurse more frequently. Some babies react to this developmental stage by increasing the frequency and duration of their feeds. The many new events and experiences in the baby's life seem to prompt a need for reassurance that there are safe and familiar aspects in his world. The constant need for reassurance and closeness, as well as increased feeds, may upset a mother who thought her baby was on the verge of weaning from the breast. She may be discouraged by his apparent lack of progress toward independence. However, you can assure her that satisfaction of his emotional needs now will lead to emotional growth and subsequent independence later. Around 7 months, when he has a tremendous development of motor skills, his breastfeeding may lag. It will then pick up afterward as the baby internalizes his new knowledge and gains confidence before reaching out again. Teething will also begin during this period, which may result in increased feeds for comfort and reassurance.

A mother can help satisfy her baby's strong desire to explore by giving him freedom to move within safe limits in the home. Parents need to be aware of a new set of rules in the household. Babies are able to reach many items that can pose a danger to them. Remind parents to examine their house for potential hazards. Babies can crawl up stairs but they cannot get down. Parents may want to place a baby gate in front of the stairs for safety.

The baby will be an eager participant in family activities and will especially want to take part in mealtimes.

He can be given finger foods that he can study, touch, turn over, and taste. Mealtime becomes a time of discovery and interaction. By participating in his own feeding, the baby can experience the independence he craves. He may then accept new foods more easily. He may also have a greater appreciation for the familiar closeness of nursing when he has had the opportunity to expand in other areas. Separation is less traumatic, and the baby may be ready to wean from the breast.

As the baby approaches his first birthday, renewed outside pressure may lead a mother to consider initiating weaning. Because her baby is now capable of obtaining his nourishment from solid foods, it may appear that he is outgrowing breastfeeding. However, you can assure the mother that he still needs the security and comfort of nursing as a stabilizing factor in his life. Also remind her that the American Academy of Pediatrics (AAP) recommends breastfeeding for the first year and beyond. Solid foods do not contain the special fatty acids present in human milk that are needed for continued brain growth. Mothers who breastfeed older babies continue to need support and encouragement, even when all seems to be going well. If the mother should decide to wean at this time, support her decision. Help her replace her usual nursing periods with other types of close interaction.

▼ Beyond 1 Year

The expansion of the baby's world carries over to mealtimes. He will enjoy using a spoon to feed himself and will practice picking up and drinking from a cup. As with all other tasks that the baby attempts, the mother will want to encourage exploration and practice. She can accept mistakes and spills as a part of learning. This attitude is especially helpful for parents to adopt in regard to their child's eating habits.

In his second year of life, a child no longer requires as much food as he did previously. His interest becomes directed toward other things. This shift in focus contributes to a decrease in his appetite. Although he may gain as much as 16 pounds in the first year, he may not double his weight for another 3 years. His food preferences are becoming better defined, and a low-key approach to feeding—not pressuring him to eat certain foods—may be the most effective method of ensuring an adequate diet. A detailed discussion of how to introduce foods to the baby appears later in this chapter. The mother can be satisfied if her 1-year-old baby eats one balanced meal a day plus two other partial meals and nutritious snacks. Mother's milk will continue to supply significant calories, vitamins, and minerals (Slusser, 1997).

As his needs change during this expansive age, the baby's breastfeeding patterns will fluctuate. He may decrease feeds when he is busy experimenting with new skills. Alternatively, he may breastfeed more frequently because of an increased need for security. Sometimes breastfeeding becomes the baby's primary means of getting his mother's undivided attention. The breastfeeding mother will learn to recognize her baby's needs when he seeks her attention. He may need assistance, recognition, companionship, cuddling, or breastfeeding. Testing all other possibilities first, before putting the baby to breast, will ensure that breastfeeding is not used as a solution to all bids for attention. This will ease the transition to a more mature relationship between mother and child. Setting aside several special times during each day for total interaction with her baby will result in fewer interruptions at other times. These times will help a mother fulfill her baby's need for attention and social interaction in a positive manner.

Sometime between 12 and 15 months, the baby may again develop a fear of strangers and a dislike for separation from his mother. He may regress to earlier behaviors in order to make emotional adjustments to such incidents. A working mother may be especially aware of these regressions. She will want to make certain that her baby's caretaker will provide the attention and caring he needs to develop emotional stability.

Owing to overstimulation during the day or because of separation anxiety, the baby may return to waking at night. He may especially appreciate the closeness of breastfeeding to soothe him back to sleep. Love and reassurance that are freely given when needed are likely to be the best cure for insecurity. Recognizing this may appease the mother of a baby who clings and nurses more frequently than she would like. Soon, the baby's outside interests will become more important than breastfeeding. The mother's love, patience, and understanding will be rewarded when she sees her child as a secure and independent individual.

Communication and play will become increasingly important as the baby grows older. He extends his world primarily to increase his interaction with his father, who presents the novelty of another personality with different ideas and responses. The working mother who returns home at the end of the day may present this same type of diversion. When the baby begins to develop a close relationship with another person, the mother may worry that her role is diminishing. In reality, her baby needs her in new ways as he reaches out to others. This positive step in his development will eventually lead to the beginnings of his ability to identify and understand the separate interests of his parents. Eventually, he will learn that absent parents will return. This may prevent him from becoming emotionally upset over temporary separations. Allowing the baby opportunities to become self-reliant and to proceed at his own pace will provide him with an atmosphere that will encourage his growth. The mother can provide opportunities for breastfeeding as she perceives her baby to need them, neither encouraging nor discouraging breastfeeding as a means of controlling him.

▼ Developmental Factors Associated with Sleep

A baby's physical development will determine when he will be able to sleep through the night. As the central nervous system develops, the ability to sleep for longer periods increases. Butte (1992) speculates that the differences in sleep organization and energy expenditure between breastfed and formula-fed infants may indicate that breastfeeding enhances maturation of the infant's central nervous system. A baby's personality may determine which part of the 24-hour cycle he chooses to sleep for a longer period. Babies exhibit sleep patterns similar to those of adults. Some will rise early and retire early, and others will rise late and retire late. Their sleep patterns may be adjusted to a slight degree.

At around 5 to 8 months of age, a baby may experience separation anxiety if he awakes during the night and realizes that his mother is not nearby. Even after they have developed the ability to sleep for longer periods, babies may find their sleep disturbed by dreams. The need to nurse may also cause disturbed sleep. This is common during growth spurts, increased activity during the day, and stages of rapid mental growth. In his book *Touching*, Ashley Montagu (1972) states that, it "...is in his second year that a child experiences the need for close physical contact that will enable him to fall asleep." The mother or father may want to lie with their child until he falls asleep.

▼ BREASTFEEDING AS BABY GROWS

As the baby grows and breastfeeding progresses, many events occur that require a mother to expand her child care and parenting techniques. You can help her identify ways that breastfeeding management fits into these events. The mother may need to make choices about how she will nurse in front of others or in public places. As she becomes more comfortable in her role as a mother, she may take her baby traveling with her. She may require suggestions for comforting her baby when he is teething or ways of coping with his biting. At some point, her baby may lose interest in nursing, or develop a preference for one breast over the other. As the mother resumes outside activities, she may wish to consider the option of leaving a substitute cup or bottle for her baby. If she finds that she is still nursing her baby beyond the point at which she had planned to stop, you

can help her re-evaluate her goals. Each of these events are examined in this chapter, with suggestions on how to help the mother progress through breastfeeding in a rewarding and positive way.

▼ Breastfeeding in Public

Each individual mother acts according to her own attitudes and philosophies to make her breastfeeding experience unique. Some mothers prefer to nurse only in the privacy of their homes. Others are comfortable breastfeeding in the homes of their friends and family. Many women enjoy taking their babies along with them shopping and dining out, and are comfortable breastfeeding in public places. Women are often uncomfortable breastfeeding in the presence of other people. They may feel that they are the center of attention and worry that others may disapprove. Several states have passed legislation protecting a mother's and baby's right to nurse anywhere. Pointing this out may provide reassurance to mothers who question the acceptance of public breastfeeding. When a mother learns nursing techniques that eliminate awkwardness and obscure her body from view, she will often become more comfortable nursing in public.

A mother can gain confidence by watching other women nurse their babies, observing practical methods and the reactions of other people. She will also feel more sure of herself after she practices discreet nursing in front of a mirror or another person. The baby's father is often a great "mirror" for the mother. He may be more likely to give candid comments of what others might see. Another excellent place to try discreet nursing is within breastfeeding support groups, where other mothers share the same concerns and observations. Such practice will decrease nervousness and awkwardness, helping the mother to appear less noticeable.

If the woman knows she will be away from home, she can prepare for discreet nursing by selecting her clothing carefully. Wearing loose-fitting clothes will allow easy access to the breast. A sweater, jacket, or other such garment worn over her shoulders will conceal her breast from those who may view her from the side. She may want to use a baby sling to provide support and extra cover, as well as ease in mobility. To avoid attracting attention, she will want to feed her baby before he is overly hungry and starts to fuss. She will need to allow time for this feeding in her schedule, as well as time to look for an appropriate place to nurse if she is unfamiliar with her location.

Each individual woman will decide how to manage her own breastfeeding and choose those locations for nursing in which she can be relaxed and comfortable. When in the company of acquaintances, the mother may want to ask politely if they mind if she nurses her baby.

If objections are raised, she can nurse in another room where her baby will probably feed better because she is relaxed and there are fewer distractions. You can present the ideas and options discussed later and let the mother decide which ones suit her needs. Offering her suggestions before she begins taking her baby out in public will increase her self confidence.

A spot that is out of the way of aisles and walkways is ideal for breastfeeding. The mother may be more comfortable and the baby will be less distracted. Such places may be a corner table or booth in a restaurant, a bench next to a wall, sitting next to her mate or friends, in a department store dressing room, in a parked car, or in a restroom lounge. Breastfeeding in any restroom is not recommended since it is a highly unsanitary environment. A restroom is not an appropriate place for any type of eating!

▼ Traveling with a Breastfeeding Baby

Sometime after her baby is about 6 weeks old, and the mother's physical recovery is nearly complete, she may be ready to travel for extended periods. A baby between the ages of 6 weeks and 6 months of age is usually an excellent traveler. He has a fairly predictable routine, is not yet eating solid foods, and is not very mobile. Often, babies of this age will sleep through the monotony of an automobile, train, bus, or airplane ride, making the trip that much easier for the parents. Traveling with a baby also decreases the worry a mother might experience were she to be apart from her baby.

Planning for the Trip

Although traveling with a baby is more cumbersome than traveling alone, careful planning and preparation can help to make it both convenient and enjoyable. In order not to be overburdened, parents can confine baby care items to those that are absolutely essential. Breastfeeding works out nicely in this respect. It eliminates the need for supplemental foods or an artificial baby milk, as well as the equipment necessary to prepare and transport them. It also eliminates the worry about the possibility of contaminated water to reconstitute formula.

Because she will not need an insulated bag to carry formula, the mother may choose a lightweight diaper bag, which can double as a purse. Using disposable diapers will further decrease baggage and can be purchased conveniently along the way so that only a few need to be carried. At least two changes of baby clothing in the diaper bag, as well as plastic pants worn over diapers to contain potentially messy stools, will decrease the need to open suitcases in search of clothing while en route.

Parents will want to take along simple objects to keep the baby amused during the trip. Colorful pictures, rattles, and toys that can be tied onto a string attached to the car seat will capture the baby's attention temporarily. However, if the baby is awake for long periods during travel time, he may quickly become bored with his toys.

Traveling by Foot

A baby sling is indispensable for traveling with a baby. It is more versatile than a stroller, especially in crowded shops, on stairways, on hiking trails, and in the sand. Wearing the baby in a sling also keeps little hands from touching things in stores. The comfortable position and motion in which the baby is carried often lulls him to sleep. A lightweight cloth sling will fit easily into the mother's bag, ready to be used at any time. For added protection in cold weather, the baby can be carried in the sling under the parent's coat.

Traveling by Automobile

For safety, a baby should be strapped securely into an approved infant car seat when traveling by automobile. Infant car seats are also effective when used in other modes of travel and are more comfortable for the baby than adult seats. An infant should never be held in a parent's arms in a moving automobile. A sudden stop may result in the parent losing hold and the baby being hurled through the windshield or against the car's interior. Caution parents against carrying their baby in a sling or baby carrier of any kind while they are riding in the car. The force of the parent's body can cause serious injury to the baby in the event of a sudden stop.

A mother should be discouraged from breastfeeding during an automobile ride unless she is able to nurse her baby while he remains in his rear-facing car seat and she has her own seat belt fastened. A bottle of water or expressed milk may help stretch out nursing times. Parents can be encouraged to stop every 2 or 3 hours to allow for nursing and to let the baby move around freely. While this will mean a longer trip, ultimately it will be more enjoyable when everyone arrives safely and comfortably at their destination.

At times, parents may need to endure the baby's crying if they cannot find a suitable distraction. This is probably the most difficult part of traveling with a child. It usually occurs near the end of the trip, when the parents are pushing to arrive at their destination. You can help parents understand that babies are not able to tolerate very long periods of travel. Encourage them to relax their schedule to accommodate their baby.

Traveling by Air

When planning a trip by air, a mother can request the roomier seat behind the bulkhead. For safety, babies should ride in their car seats strapped into a regular seat in the event of a difficult landing. Strollers and other baby equipment should be well marked and can be checked with the luggage, leaving the mother free to carry her baby and only those few baby items she will need during the flight. As a courtesy, airline attendants often allow parents with small children to board the plane before the other passengers so that they can get settled and avoid waiting in lines. Mothers need to be aware that changes in cabin pressure may affect the baby's ears. If the mother breastfeeds during takeoff and descent, she can help prevent this discomfort.

▼ Teething and Biting

As a baby matures, he may experience physical discomforts like teething, that make him irritable and unhappy. The average baby cuts his first tooth between 6 and 8 months of age, although teething can occur anywhere from 4 to 14 months of age. As a tooth erupts, it causes swelling and irritation of the gums. When the baby sucks, blood rushes to his gums, which adds to the swelling that is already present and causes immediate discomfort. Thus, when the baby begins to nurse, he may quickly pull away from the breast and cry out with pain. The mother may notice additional clues that her baby is teething. He may become irritable, begin drooling more than usual, and occasionally spit up or develop loose stools for no apparent reason. He may also begin waking during the night to seek comfort. Some mothers have reported that their babies experienced a slight fever when teething.

Overcoming Teething Pain

Often, the baby discovers that chewing and rubbing his gums reduces the pain. A teething baby may be observed rubbing his jaw or pulling on his ear to relieve discomfort. The same nerves to the teeth branch out to the face, cheek, and outer ear. If the baby cries out when the mother rubs his gums, she will know that he may be teething. Continued rubbing on the gums should comfort him and help him to settle down. Providing the baby with a cooled teething ring, or rubbing ice or a cold cloth on his gums before breastfeeding can relieve the soreness long enough for him to nurse. Providing suitable objects and hard foods, such as toast for the baby to chew on, helps relieve the pain and promote tooth eruption. Teething pain can also be overcome by the use of over-the-counter pain relievers, as well as by locally acting over-the-counter preparations that temporarily numb gum tissue. The mother will want to consult her baby's physician before using such medications.

Breastfeeding Issues with Teething

Teething has the potential to interfere with breastfeeding and may lead to biting. This is a habit that parents can quickly discourage. The mother will want to be more observant at this time and watch for signs of the end of the feed. When there is a slowing of the suck-swallow rhythm, she can remove the baby from her breast. If biting occurs during a feed, the mother can remove her baby from the breast immediately and wait a few minutes before resuming the feed. If the baby bites again, she can end the feed promptly.

Because of the sucking mechanism involved during breastfeeding, it is impossible for the baby to suckle and bite at the same time. Clamping down tightly will interfere with the stroking of the tongue as it compresses the nipple from base to tip. If the baby is biting, it can be assumed that he is not hungry enough to nurse at that time. The mother can end the feed and try again later when his hunger returns. If she suspects teething pain to be the cause of biting, she can try some comfort measures and then resume nursing.

Biting at the end of a feed may occur as the baby falls asleep and closes his jaw. The mother can prevent such clamping down on her nipple by inserting her finger in the baby's mouth between his gums and removing her breast when she perceives the baby is nearly finished. Then her finger can be withdrawn slowly to break suction and avoid discomfort. When a mother is bitten for the first time, she may react with an outcry and a startled jerk away from her baby. Let her know that this is a common reaction. She can be cautious not to respond so strongly in the future so that the baby does not interpret this as a sign of rejection and discontinue nursing because of it. Assure her that biting can be overcome and that it need not be a reason to wean.

Sustaining Breastfeeding Beyond One Year

There are a number of techniques you can suggest to mothers to help them continue breastfeeding beyond 1 year. As the baby becomes more alert and is distracted easily, she can breastfeed in a quiet place to limit distractions. When supplemental foods are added to her baby's diet, she can breastfeed first and then offer the other food to her baby. A baby who has begun eating other foods may wish to breastfeed less frequently, and his frequency and duration of breastfeeds will continue to diminish as more foods are added to his diet. The mother can continue to put her baby to breast and respond to his wishes. As she approaches weaning, she will want to allow him to lessen the number of feeds gradually and be sure he gets plenty of other foods each day.

Supplementary Feeds

Some breastfeeding women choose to provide their babies an occasional substitute for their milk by cup or bottle. The decision whether or not to introduce substitutes as **supplementary feeds** is up to each individual mother. The most common definition of a supplementary feed is a food other than human milk that is fed to the infant following or in place of a breastfeed. It is also referred to as "topping off" the breastfed infant with liquids other than mother's milk. This may be done with either water or infant formula. Some sources refer to these substitutes as complementary foods. See the discussion later in this chapter regarding complementary feeds.

Many mothers take their babies with them or plan activities around the baby's feeding times and never have a need for supplementary feeds. Other mothers wish to have time away from their babies without the worry that feeds will be delayed or that they must rush back in time for the next feed. Mothers may experience an accident, illness, or other unforeseen happening, such as getting stuck in traffic or having an automobile breakdown. A substitute feed can eliminate the worry of an unhappy and hungry baby.

Supplementary feeds must be introduced in such a way that the baby does not receive a substantial amount of supplements that would interfere with his breastfeeding pattern. This can be accomplished by limiting the amounts of fluids given. It is best to delay any supplementary feeds until the baby is at least 3 weeks old and has firmly established good nursing habits. The mother can begin by arranging for someone else to feed her baby about one ounce of fluid, in a cup or bottle, once or twice a week. She will want it to be offered by someone other than the mother because babies often refuse if the mother is even in the same room. It should also be done at times when the baby is not fussy or too hungry. Many fathers and grandparents enjoy feeding the baby. They can be relied on not to overfeed the baby when they understand the relationship between the amount of milk the mother produces and the amount the baby needs.

Cup feeding is the preferred method for supplementary feeds, because it does not cause the nipple preference associated with bottle feeding. Most babies will accept feeding by a cup. Because it is the preferred method, you will want to encourage the mother to feed with a cup rather than a bottle. If she prefers a bottle, the baby's acceptance of a bottle may require several attempts. Sometimes a baby will accept a bottle, reject it the next few times, and then accept it again later. You can encourage the mother not to give up after several refusals. She can continue to offer the bottle until her baby accepts it. Many times, bottles are unnecessary because the baby is able to drink directly from a cup. Breastfeeding babies find the transition to a cup to be easier than do bottle-fed babies. Similarly, the baby can be fed from a medicine dropper or spoon. Because of the potential for nipple preference, bottles should be avoided when other feeding methods are possible.

Some consider the mother's milk to be a supplementary feed when it is expressed rather than nursed out by the baby. This is certainly preferred over water or formula. Encourage the mother to plan ahead and to express milk on a regular basis for these feeds. She may use formula if there is no history of allergies in the family and if she has discussed with her baby's physician which type to use.

When supplementary feeds are given, the mother will need to consider the care of her breasts, which may become full as a result of a missed feed. She could nurse or express milk just before departing, or she can express her milk while she is away. If she would rather wait and let the baby nurse when she returns, she may need to wear a larger bra to avoid pressure on her full breasts, which can cause blockage of her milk ducts. Mothers who work outside the home or return to school or an active social life soon learn how to manage such absences without experiencing discomfort from full breasts. Having prepared supplementary feeds ahead of time, they feel secure in their babies' willingness to accept substitute nourishment.

Breastfeeding a Toddler

Breastfeeding patterns in other cultures show that with loving patience from their parents, children will outgrow their need to nurse in their second, third, or even fourth year of life. Most often, cultural practices set the standards for weaning times in a society, without regard for the baby's biologic need. Within social groups where early weaning is common, the mother who chooses baby-led weaning is often pressured by lack of acceptance and misinformation about breastfeeding her older baby.

This misinformation takes several forms. Some people may believe that breastfeeding a baby beyond infancy will make him more dependent on his mother. However, many studies have shown that satisfying a baby's emotional needs will encourage his self-reliance. Normal sucking needs can last for several years, and babies may require a substitute for sucking if weaning occurs before sucking needs subside. Some people believe that nighttime feeds cause the baby to continue waking during the night. In reality, sleep patterns most often are the result of neurologic development and environmental factors, not the availability of breastfeeding.

A 1994 study found that women who breastfed longer than 12 months were older, better educated, and had exclusively breastfed longer. About a third of the mothers slept with their babies (Hills-Bonczyk, 1994). Mothers who want to breastfeed into and through the toddler stage need reassurance that it is perfectly natural and normal to do so. The support of others within their social structure will validate their choice. They will be empowered further by informed professionals who can answer their questions. These mothers will benefit from the emotional support and practical suggestions of other

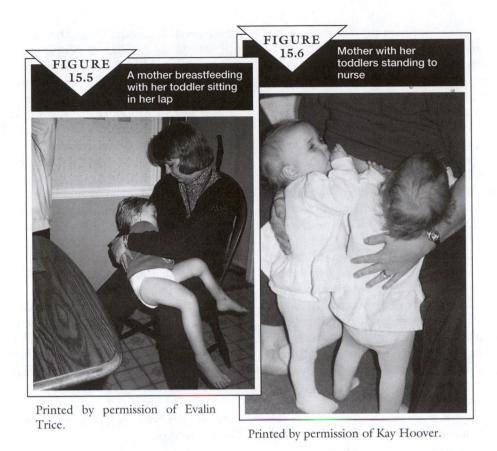

FIGURE 15.5 A mother breastfeeding with her toddler sitting in her lap

Printed by permission of Evalin Trice.

FIGURE 15.6 Mother with her toddlers standing to nurse

Printed by permission of Kay Hoover.

mothers who understand their circumstances and are willing to listen to them.

The concept of breastfeeding a baby beyond infancy can be presented to mothers in a gradual way, so that they can consider this parenting option objectively. The term "older baby" when used in the context of breastfeeding is defined differently by each society. Many American women will respond that 18, 15, or even 9 months fits this description. Most women in the United States do not expect to continue breastfeeding their infants into the toddler years. They simply respond to their babies' breastfeeding needs on a daily basis as a natural part of mothering. Describing breastfeeding a toddler as an extension of the warm infant-mother relationship will help women view it positively.

Breastfeeding a toddler is rewarding and satisfying for the mother who recognizes that she is meeting her child's needs (Fig. 15.5). It can be a source of great comfort and stability to the child, especially in times of stress, when he is injured, has his feelings hurt, is feeling shy, or is in a new and strange environment (Wrigley, 1990). Breastfeeding is a comforting way for the active child to touch base with his mother between explorations. Particularly during the toddler period, breastfeeding offers the mother a reassuring way of communicating her love even though she and her child may be at odds over his behavior. A child who is able to communicate verbally can bring his mother great joy by expressing his feelings about breastfeeding. There can be love and humor in this relationship with both mother and child being the giver and receiver. These are some of the aspects of the breastfeeding relationship that serve as a transitional parenting technique from infancy to childhood.

Challenges to Breastfeeding a Toddler

Although breastfeeding a toddler can be very rewarding, it may also cause inconveniences and conflicts that rival those of the newborn period and that often cause mothers to consider weaning. The physical act of nursing a toddler can be quite different from breastfeeding an infant. The older baby may not wish to be held and will assume a position that allows him to conveniently view the room, including standing or straddling (Fig. 15.6). For a time, his developing teeth may leave pressure marks on the areola until he learns to hold the breast with his lips. Crumbs or food particles left in the child's mouth may irritate the mother's nipples during feeds.

Some women may consider weaning because they feel that they have lost control of their bodies or that their babies are manipulating them. The child may insist on nursing at inconvenient or embarrassing moments. He may tug at the mother's clothing, even partially disrobing her. He may enjoy fondling her body, which embarrasses her when others notice. She may feel trapped and controlled by her child, resenting that she was not prepared for this phase of breastfeeding.

The mother can prevent such ill feelings by guiding her child in his use of breastfeeding, just as she guides him in other aspects of his life, such as eating, sleeping, and playing. She can limit breastfeeding to certain times and eliminate overindulging him or allowing him to use breastfeeding as a power tactic. Feeds can be limited to coincide with her own needs so that breastfeeding continues to be a source of pleasure for both of them. Help her adopt a balanced view of breastfeeding as an integral part of parenting that is appropriate when not overused. She can then continue to enjoy this special relationship with her baby as he matures.

Whenever a woman expresses dissatisfaction with nursing her toddler, allow her to discuss her feelings freely. Help her work out with her baby some signals and times for breastfeeding that are reasonably acceptable to both. The family may adopt a special name for nursing, so that when the toddler asks to breastfeed while out in public the mother can avoid embarrassment. Rather than arguing with him at every request, she might try to stretch the intervals between feeds. He may, for example, be satisfied with a drink or treat just before the usual time for nursing. The mother may also suggest other activities to take his mind off breastfeeding. Encourage her to remain flexible enough to adjust her approach if she sees this causes stress in the child. The concept of time is often difficult for a child to comprehend. She can link the time to nurse to a special location. For instance, he will understand if she says, "Let's nurse when we get home in Mommy's chair." Being consistent in restricting breastfeeding to a particular place is the key to making this technique work.

Opposition from Others

Sometimes the baby's father will object to his older baby being nursed. He may believe that the child appears to be too dependent while nursing or he may worry about the social and sexual implications of breastfeeding an older baby. If the mother complains about breastfeeding, the father may wonder why she continues. Help the mother learn precisely what the father's objections are. Work with her to develop a breastfeeding plan to resolve the issue. She can discuss with him the baby's physical and emotional needs at this stage in his development, as well as her desire to continue breastfeeding. If he continues to object, she can avoid nursing in his presence. He may accept the situation better if he does not actually see the toddler nurse. The mother will benefit from your support if she decides to continue breastfeeding despite the father's objection.

People other than the baby's father are often uncomfortable seeing a woman breastfeed a toddler. To avoid this situation mothers can be encouraged to breastfeed discreetly. A mother can also refrain from breastfeeding in front of people who are critical so as not to intensify their reactions and to avoid being intimidated by them. She will need to remain firm in her conviction that she is doing what is best for her child. You can refer to Chapter 18 for suggestions on helping the mother handle criticism about breastfeeding her toddler.

Siblings may appear to resent the special attention the breastfeeding child receives from his mother. Re-evaluating her children's needs and setting aside special time with each child may eliminate such resentment. The mother may inadvertently be responsible for prolonging breastfeeding by picking up and nursing her toddler in order to keep him from disturbing her older children's toys or disrupting their play. Providing storage places and play areas that are inaccessible to the baby can prevent him from interfering with siblings, so that the mother does not resort to breastfeeding to keep him occupied.

You can try to listen to the mother's concerns with a sympathetic ear and help her work out solutions that fit her situation. She may not know another person who will praise her for her efforts and reassure her that she has chosen the right action for her child and family. Whether she chooses to wean or to continue breastfeeding, she needs an accepting listener who will support her in her decision.

▼

COMPLEMENTARY FEEDS

Parents are often told that their baby would sleep through the night if he had more to eat. There is no conclusive evidence to indicate that any particular feeding method promotes longer nighttime sleep. Because human milk is digested more quickly than cow's milk, it seems reasonable that a breastfed baby would naturally wake up hungry in the middle of the night. However, a baby who is still exclusively breastfed at 5 months may sleep 8 hours at night. That same baby may have been up every 3 or 4 hours during the night at one month. It seems more likely, then, that the reason for longer sleep at 5 months is due to a more fully developed nervous system and is unrelated to nutritional factors.

When a baby receives his first complementary food, the weaning process is initiated. A complementary feed refers to new foods added to the growing breastfed infant's diet that are intended to meet the energy and nutrient needs that are not met by the mother's milk alone. Some use this term interchangeably with "supplemental feed" and interpret it as "topping off" the breastfed infant with liquids other than the mother's milk (i.e., water or infant formula).

As solid foods are introduced to the child's diet, he begins to establish eating patterns that will last a lifetime. Parents recognize this as a giant step in their baby's development that requires many decisions on their part. They wonder when to begin introducing solid foods to their baby, what types of food are best, how to offer the food, and how to make sure he is receiving adequate nutrition.

Some people will tell parents that a baby should be given cereal just before going to bed in order to "fill him up." Macknin and colleagues (1989) found evidence that sleeping through the night is a developmental event that cannot be changed by feeding cereal. When adults experience restless sleep, most physicians will recommend a light snack such as warm milk, not a heavy meal, before retiring. Too much food can cause indigestion and further encourage wakefulness. Warm milk is usually suggested because it is thought to have a **soporific** (sleep-inducing) agent in it that helps people fall asleep. It seems, then, that human milk is the ideal food for encouraging a baby to sleep. Everyone's system is different, and just as some adults seem to need a snack in the middle of the night, so, too, will some babies.

When there is a family history of allergies, parents want to know what they can do to prevent allergic reactions in their children. Sometimes parents' ideas on how to manage feeding may vary from what their baby's physician advises. In such cases, they may need to make compromises. You can give parents the information that will help them make responsible decisions about foods for their baby.

Pressure to Begin Solid Foods

New parents are deluged with advertising from baby food manufacturers who proclaim the many advantages of commercially processed foods. They may also receive an overabundance of advice from family and friends on when and how to introduce these foods. Books, magazines, and newspapers contain articles written by medical and lay persons who advocate various methods and times for starting solid foods. Parents must evaluate this assortment of facts and opinions against their own backgrounds and their baby's needs. This may be one of the first times that parents are motivated to function as informed consumers to search out, evaluate, and act on the surplus of information available to them.

Counseling Implications

You can be a valuable source of information for parents on introducing solid foods to their breastfed baby. Provide them with clear, accurate, well-documented facts to eliminate their possible confusion due to contradictory advice. Presenting ideas and literature to parents in the early months will give them time to consider the options. It will provide them with the opportunity to discuss questions with the baby's physician well in advance of when their baby will require such foods.

A mother needs encouragement and a high level of self-esteem in order to continue exclusive breastfeeding despite being pressured to start solid foods. She needs to hear that her baby looks and acts healthy and is getting enough sustenance from her milk alone. She also needs to be reassured that she has an adequate milk supply and the capacity to increase that supply to meet increased needs. You can be an active force in helping her delay solid foods if you give her the kind of support that will build her confidence in her mothering skills.

Sometimes the baby's physician will suggest that a mother start her baby on solid foods when it does not seem appropriate or when the mother does not feel ready. You can encourage her to ask the physician to clarify why solid foods are suggested. Was the physician merely saying that the mother may begin solid foods if she wishes? Or were solid foods recommended for a specific reason? She can reinforce her breastfeeding goals and discuss such pertinent aspects of her baby's health as weight gain and family weight patterns, allergies, and anemia. Offering solid foods in small quantities after breastfeeding or postponing offering solid foods and increasing feeds may satisfy the physician's requirements for her baby.

Choosing the Appropriate Time to Introduce Solid Foods

The introduction of solid foods expands a baby's dietary choices and serves as a complement to the mother's milk during the process of weaning. There are many factors to consider in deciding when to add solid foods to a baby's diet. In general, the ideal time falls somewhere between the age when the baby's system is mature enough to handle solid foods and when he needs more nutrients than he can obtain solely from his mother's milk. For babies of average birth weight with adequate fetal stores of fat and iron and whose mothers' pregnancy diet was nutritionally sound, mother's milk serves well as the only food until about 6 months of age. Human milk provides all the calories, vitamins, and minerals in the proper proportions needed by the baby. In addition, its protective factors help prevent allergy and illness. Introducing other foods before the baby's body is ready can lead to frequent digestive upsets, increased upper respiratory infections, poor nutrient absorption, and excessive weight gain due to increased calorie consumption.

A 1993 study showed that early introduction of solid foods correlated with higher weight at 8, 13, and 26 weeks of age. At 14 to 26 weeks of age, early solid foods related to increased respiratory illness (Forsyth, 1993). Excessive weight gain in infancy can lead to lifelong obesity. Not all babies will be able to wait until 6 months of age to start solid foods, however. Some babies who begin nursing constantly at 4 or 5 months and never seem to be satisfied may be indicating a need for further nourishment from solid foods. Every baby will be ready for solid foods at a slightly different age and will need to be watched for signs of readiness.

Signs of the Baby's Readiness for Solid Foods

The baby displays obvious outward signs that he is ready for solid foods just when his internal functions have developed to the point where they can efficiently handle a more diverse diet. As he approaches 6 months of age, the baby's neuromuscular development allows for proper chewing and swallowing of nonliquid foods. As his intestinal maturation permits more complete digestion and absorption of a variety of foods, his body becomes able to handle the waste products from solid foods. The baby's immunologic system has also begun to function so that he no longer must depend on all of the protection provided by his mother's milk. At the same time, the child indicates his readiness for additional foods through the eruption of teeth, the ability to sit up, the disappearance of the tongue extrusion reflex, improved eye-hand coordination, and the ability to grasp objects with his thumb and forefinger (Fig. 15.7).

The most obvious indication of a baby's interest in starting solid foods is his behavior when others are eating. He may watch them intently, imitate their chewing, and reach for food while loudly vocalizing his desire for it. An intensified demand to nurse that is not satisfied after several days of increased feeds may be an additional clue to the mother that it is time to introduce solid foods to her baby.

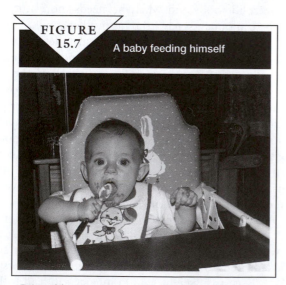

FIGURE 15.7

A baby feeding himself

Printed by permission of Debbie Shinskie.

The mother needs to understand that the introduction of solid foods will decrease milk production. Her baby will require less milk, and therefore, she will produce less. If solid foods are started during the first 3 months when milk production is being established or during the crucial growth spurt times, milk production will be seriously compromised. A mother who plans to start her baby on solid foods at any age needs to understand that she will be nursing less because of it.

Breastfeeding should diminish slowly as solid foods are increased, to the point that they are the primary source of nutrition. During the second 6 months of life, the mother's milk can still meet three-fourths of her baby's nutrient needs. Even during the baby's second year, human milk is nutritionally valuable (Slusser, 1997).

Sometimes, parents express an interest in starting their baby on solid foods in order to solve an unrelated problem. Misconceptions about breastfeeding or about the baby's behavior patterns may cause parents to believe the negative aspects of their relationship with their baby are feeding related. Such misconceptions may involve frequency of feeds, milk production, richness of the mother's milk, sleep, crying, and infant development. By clearing up these misconceptions you can help parents avoid starting solid foods early unnecessarily. In the DARLING study (Davis Area Research on Lactation, Infant Nutrition and Growth), the age of starting solid foods was not related to the frequency of night feeds. Early solid feeders actually had lower intake of their mother's milk at ages 6 and 9 months (Heinig, 1993).

Supplementing to Provide Iron

Sometimes, parents will start solid foods in order to supply their baby with iron. In a healthy full-term baby, this is not usually necessary. The mother's milk supplies sufficient iron for the baby until he triples his birth weight. Human milk contains lactoferrin, an iron-binding protein that increases the absorption of the normal amounts of iron that are available in the milk. This process may be disrupted when outside sources of iron are introduced. Adding iron too soon can also interfere with the disease protection qualities of lactoferrin. Lactoferrin binds iron and increases its absorption. This robs some microorganisms of the iron that they require in order to grow and multiply. Premature infants and infants of anemic mothers will need iron supplementation whenever a simple hemoglobin blood test determines that iron stores are low. It can be given in the form of drops.

How to Introduce Solid Foods

The introduction of solid foods should be a pleasant experience for a mother and her baby, and needs to be handled with a positive attitude. The process should be very gradual so that the baby will not be overwhelmed by this new way of eating. His digestive system also will have a chance to get used to each change in diet. In the beginning, solid foods will be considered complementary foods, being offered after the baby has nursed. This practice will maintain milk production, and it will allow the mother and baby to rely on breastfeeding as a means of relaxation and comfort during this time of change. With breastfeeding as a stabilizing factor in his life, a baby will be better able to adapt to the new experience.

Parents will want to start at a slow pace, with one complementary feeding every one or two days. The best time to initiate this is at times when the baby is still hungry after a breastfeed. Often, the afternoon and early evening hours are times when the baby will accept additional foods. This coincides with the time when the mother is most tired and busy with meal preparation. It provides an opportunity for the father or other family member to interact with the child and relieve her of baby care.

By the age of 7 to 9 months, one or two feeds a day plus regular breastfeeding will satisfy the baby's nutritional needs. As he becomes a real participant in family mealtimes, he can be patterned into a schedule of three meals a day by around 9 to 12 months. He will still require nutritious snacks several times a day, as well as several separate nursing times. Breastfeeding can gradually be eliminated from mealtimes as the baby learns to eat balanced meals and drink from a cup.

Initially, foods will need to be highly puréed and diluted with liquid. These foods can be spoon fed, and they should not be given in a bottle. As the baby becomes accustomed to eating solid foods, the liquid content can be decreased and the texture can be more coarse. This will help in the transition to chunky foods and finger foods and then table foods. If solid foods are delayed until 8 or 9 months, the baby can be started out on finger foods and chunky foods, saving the bother of preparing puréed foods. The texture of foods needs to be compatible with the infant's ability to chew and swallow. Table 15.1 provides guidelines for a child's ability to feed himself as he develops and matures. As illustrated in the table, the average baby will be eating chunky finger foods by 9 months. By 1 year of age, he will be eating regular table food, cut up to sizes appropriate for the child's age and capabilities, along with the rest of the family.

Types of Foods Given

According to some authorities, when solid foods are delayed until 5 or 6 months of age, the order of introduction of various foods seems to be of little importance. One exception with the early foods is that the breastfed infant will need to receive foods relatively high in protein (AAP, 1985). The protein requirement in the baby's diet is beginning to exceed that which human milk provides. Single-grain infant cereals, such as rice or barley, will provide additional energy and iron. Therefore, these cereals are often the pediatrician's choice for the first complementary food. The mother can express some of her milk or use warm water to mix with the cereal. Vegetarian diets are considered to be inadequate for infants (Birkbeck, 1992).

The introduction of specific foods can be based on the parents' or pediatrician's personal preferences and acceptance by the infant. These foods may vary according to the baby's age. It is common practice to introduce rice cereal first. For taste preference, vegetables and

TABLE 15.1

Self-Feeding Characteristics by Age

Age	Characteristics
6 to 9 months	Holds, sucks, and bites finger foods.
9 months to 1 year	Enjoys finger foods, eats most table foods, drinks from cup with help, will hold and lick spoon after it is dipped into food.
15 months	Begins to use spoon, turns it before it reaches mouth; may no longer need bottle; may hold cup; likely to tilt cup rather than head, spilling contents.
1 to 2 years	Eats with spoon, often spilling; turns spoon in mouth; requires assistance; holds glass with both hands, size of glass is important.
2 years	Puts spoon in mouth correctly, occasionally spilling; holds glass with one hand; distinguishes between food and inedible materials.
2 to 3 years	Feeds self entirely, with occasional spilling; uses fork; pours from pitcher; can obtain drink of water from faucet without assistance.

Excerpted from *Child Health Encyclopedia: The Complete Guide for Parents* by The Children's Hospital Medical Center and Richard Feinbloom, M.D. Reprinted by permission of Delacorte Press/Seymour Lawrence.

then fruits usually follow. Meats will be the last food introduced. Juices can also be introduced one at a time, preferably from a cup to avoid nipple preference, although babies do not require juice.

Single-ingredient foods are the best choice. They can be started one at a time at weekly intervals. This allows an opportunity to identify food sensitivity and avert development of food intolerance or allergies. If the baby has a reaction and several foods have been given together, the mother will be unable to identify the one causing the reaction. When a food sensitivity is identified, the mother can discontinue the food and reintroduce it at a later time as recommended by the baby's physician. She may find that small amounts of a food can be tolerated, whereas larger amounts will cause reactions.

If the baby objects to a particular food, the mother can withhold it for several weeks before offering it again. The experience of trying new foods should be pleasant for the baby. He should not be forced to eat something that he finds unpleasant. New foods should not be introduced when the baby is ill or has recently had an inoculation. Food reactions may be mistaken for signs of illness or medication reactions and vice versa. Babies require no desserts or sweeteners added to their foods. Sweet foods are a poor substitute for those that have greater nutritional value because they cause tooth decay and promote poor eating habits.

Infants can be given water as a supplement to solid foods, to allow them an opportunity to fulfill fluid needs without taking in extra calories. Babies who cry from thirst can be given water rather than other fluids. Additional water is often required by the baby in order to help rid his body of the waste products in solid foods. This is especially the case with meats and egg yolks. Fruits, fruit juices, and vegetables pose less of a problem for the baby.

In the second year of life, a child no longer needs a special infant diet. At that time, he can begin sharing family meals that are reasonably modified. To modify regular family meals for infants, parents can prepare them without excessive salt or spices, cut them into appropriate-sized pieces, and serve them at a moderate temperature.

Amount of Food Given

Mothers often wonder how much food they should offer to their babies. When first presenting a food, the mother will frequently prepare a small dishful, only to find that her baby scarcely tastes it. Suggest that she begin with a teaspoon or so of creamy consistency food. She can then work up to a few tablespoons, at a rate determined by the baby's appetite. It is unfortunate that many babies are overfed because parents expect them to consume an entire jar of commercially prepared baby food in one sitting. Parents need to be aware of their

baby's signals that he has had enough. At first, the mother can expect to see more food running down the sides of her baby's mouth than is getting into his stomach. This will change as he learns to use his newly developed swallowing mechanism.

Messiness is a normal part of this new experience. It will be evident again when the baby starts feeding himself. Some babies are not very interested in solid foods until they can handle the food themselves. Others love to eat right from the start. Caution the mother not to overfeed an eager baby. Solid foods contain more calories per volume than milk. A young baby's mechanism for determining hunger is by volume of food. Overfeeding may be discovered as constipation, spitting up, excessive weight gain, or a rapid decrease in the number of feeds.

▼ Allergy Considerations

When babies are breastfed exclusively, components in the mother's milk coat the intestinal tract. This prevents foreign proteins from entering the baby's system and causing allergic reactions. Eventually the baby's body develops the ability to protect itself without human milk. However, children of parents with a history of allergy appear to have a more prolonged dependence on the protective factors in human milk. These children have an increased susceptibility to ingested food proteins. Therefore, it follows that the hereditary risk of food allergy seems to be reduced when the baby is breastfed exclusively for 6 months (Saarinen, 1979). In addition, avoidance of the most potent allergenic foods during the first year of life is effective in reducing allergic reactions in children.

The degree of response to foreign proteins varies widely from one baby to another. Some babies exhibit sudden and clear-cut allergic reactions, whereas others may behave slightly fussy or irritable. The signs of food reactions that may help a mother to recognize an intolerance in her baby are listed in the following section. Of course, these symptoms may also be caused by illness in the baby, and they need to be brought to the attention of his physician if they persist.

Signs of Food Intolerance

◆   Runny nose, stuffiness, and constant cold-type symptoms.

◆   Skin rashes, eczema, hives, and sore bottom.

◆   Asthma.

◆   Ear infections.

◆   Intestinal upset, gas, diarrhea, spitting, and vomiting.

◆   Fussiness, irritability, and colic-like behavior.

◆   Poor weight gain due to malabsorption of food.

◆ Red itchy eyes, swollen eyelids, dark circles under the eyes, constant tearing, and gelatin-like fluid in the eyes.

Foods in the Mother's Diet

If there are allergies in the family, a mother can be careful about her diet during pregnancy and limit milk and egg consumption, especially during the last month. Other foods can be substituted to ensure a balanced, nutritious diet. She can breastfeed her baby exclusively for at least 6 months, although 8 or 9 months is even better. The baby should receive no artificial baby milk unless it is prescribed by the physician. Even the hypoallergenic products can trigger allergic reactions because they are based on cow's milk. If vitamin or mineral supplements are required, only those that are prescribed by the baby's physician should be given. Some of these supplements may contain ingredients that will sensitize the baby.

Sometimes, foods that the mother ingests will pass through her milk to her baby and cause allergic reactions. This is usually a problem only when the mother eats an excessive amount of a particular food, and it can be avoided by eating a variety of foods in moderation. In order to completely eliminate a reaction, a mother may need to exclude a food from her diet totally. Cow's milk, citrus fruits, eggs, corn, and wheat are common offenders. By experimenting with other foods that are known allergens, the mother can identify and eliminate the offending foods. If the mother suspects that a food is causing problems and notices repeated symptoms after she has eaten the food and fed the baby, perhaps the food is the cause.

Mothers do not need to eliminate foods arbitrarily from their diets unless they suspect that a particular food is causing problems. Otherwise, they can continue to consume in moderation any foods they have been accustomed to eating. If a mother does eliminate a food from her diet, especially one such as cow's milk, which is high in protein and calcium, she will need to substitute another food or supplement to obtain the necessary nutrients to support lactation.

Family History of Allergies

When the potentially allergic baby is started on solid foods, the mother will need to be especially cautious about introducing one food at a time and waiting at least 1 week for a possible reaction. Foods that need to be avoided in the first year of life include cow's milk and milk products, citrus fruits and fruit juices, eggs, tomatoes, chocolate, fish, pork, peanuts and other nuts, and wheat. Honey should never be given to an infant younger than 1 year of age because it has the potential to cause infant botulism.

Parents can limit the baby's exposure to other allergens as well by keeping his room free of dust and mold, and their home free of dogs, cats, birds, and other pets for at least 6 months. Wool clothing and blankets, as well as lanolin products, should not come in contact with the baby's skin. There should be no smoking near the baby and preferably none in the home.

Parents need to inform their baby's physician when there is any family history of allergies. They will want to notify the physician whenever they suspect an allergic response in their baby. The physician can help them pinpoint the offending allergen and may provide medication to relieve the symptoms. Although the regimen for avoiding allergies may seem bothersome, many mothers report that a healthy, pleasant, clear-skinned baby is worth the effort.

▼

WEANING

It is far too impersonal and arbitrary for a mother to allow cultural influences to dictate how long she will nurse her baby. The suitable time for weaning will define itself, provided that the mother is well read and well informed about breastfeeding and the process of weaning. With the appropriate information, she will be confident that her decision is based on consideration of her baby's physical and emotional needs. Your practical suggestions for implementing weaning can help make weaning problem free, enabling the mother to view it as a natural step toward her baby's maturity.

When weaning is allowed to take place buffered from societal pressures, natural times for ending breastfeeding seem to fall between the periods of the baby's greatest developmental activity. Common ages for weaning are 12 to 14 months, 18 months, 2 years, and 3 years. Most mothers in the United States wean before 9 months. Ending breastfeeding between 3 and 6 months is largely a matter of physical management. Weaning a 3-year-old may involve a challenge to expand mothering techniques and actual bargaining with the child to establish acceptable substitute activities. It is important that you adopt a nonjudgmental attitude and support the woman's decision to wean. Your role is to educate and advise her about weaning. Once the mother has made the decision, your role is to support that decision and help her through the weaning process.

Weaning may be initiated by either the mother or the baby, or mutually when the baby sends signals that indicate readiness to wean and the mother responds accordingly. The baby may act more self-reliant and go for long stretches without nursing, perhaps accepting a drink or snack as a substitute. He may show his disinterest in breastfeeding by being easily distracted at the breast, spending less time at feeds, frequently refusing the breast, and showing a greater interest in solid foods. These signs indicate to the mother that her baby may be ready to wean. Too often, however, women wean before their babies are ready, frequently due to misconceptions or pressure from others.

Pressured Weaning

It is hoped that weaning will be initiated when both the mother and baby are ready. If the baby no longer desires to nurse, encourage the mother to accept this sign of his maturity and discontinue putting him to breast. When the mother decides to end breastfeeding, she can find other ways of satisfying her baby's needs. In both of these situations the mother usually learns to accept weaning without guilt or resentment. Unfortunately, weaning is often carried out because of misconceptions, outside pressure, or a change in personal circumstances. When this happens, the mother may become angry and resentful, with feelings of guilt because she was unable to continue breastfeeding.

Crying

A mother may have a baby who cries a lot, and she may doubt that she is satisfying his hunger. She may be so distressed by his behavior that she decides to wean, thinking this will avoid further aggravation. You can help her explore the reason for his crying. It may be due to allergies, his normal temperament, a means of getting attention, or hunger. You can teach her comforting techniques and explain how she can increase milk production, if necessary. She may need some successes with her mothering skills to build her confidence so that she can continue to breastfeed with confidence.

Teething, Biting or Illness

When breastfeeds are not going well because of teething, biting, or illness, the mother may become frustrated and fatigued with trying to manage breastfeeding and also comfort her baby. She may decide to wean in an effort to decrease tension or so that someone else can feed the baby while she rests. You can help her understand that this is a temporary situation. Bottle feeds are not likely to improve the situation. Weaning at this time can produce the additional discomfort of engorgement and the inconvenience of trying to decrease milk production. In times of stress, a baby needs the closeness and reassurance of the breastfeeding relationship.

Nighttime Feeds

Continued nighttime feeds may cause a mother to consider weaning. She may be so fatigued from lack of sleep that she does not function well during the day. If her baby is older, weaning may be the answer. It may be possible to simply drop night feeds. Help her explore the reasons for her baby's wakefulness. It may be caused by separation anxiety, habit, not enough daytime feeds to satisfy hunger, or a need for attention. Perhaps her outlook will improve and she can accept the night feeds if she gets into the habit of napping during the day or cosleeping with her baby at night. Additional suggestions are discussed in Chapter 14.

Changes in the Family

At times, a family's life may become complicated with moving, job changes, illnesses, marital problems, or other stressful situations. It might appear that weaning would make life simpler for the mother at such a time. However, she will want to weigh the apparent benefits against the effect weaning has on her baby. His needs for security and continuity are even greater when there are significant changes in his life. Ending breastfeeding at this time could lead to fussiness and increased demands for attention. These responses are not at all what the mother envisions when she decides to wean. You can guide the mother in developing ways to integrate breastfeeding into her lifestyle so that she feels less hassled. She may choose to wean gradually, so that her baby has time to adjust to his new environment.

The mother may see weaning as a necessity because she fears pregnancy and wants to resume taking oral contraceptives. You can give her some information about other methods of contraception (see Chapter 17) that are compatible with breastfeeding. Encourage her to discuss them with her physician. It is hoped that she will find one that is acceptable to both her and her partner.

Sadly, there are cases in which breastfeeding babies have become emotional "footballs" between parents who are involved in a divorce. In one case, a mother who continued to breastfeed her older child was accused of child abuse by the child's father. In other cases, mothers have been pressured to wean in order to allow extended visitation between the father and child. However, visitation can take place in such a way that it accommodates breastfeeding. You can provide the mother with information and help her achieve this goal.

Societal Pressure

Pressure from family members or friends can prompt a mother to consider weaning. They may tell her that her baby is becoming too dependent because of breastfeeding. She might worry that this is actually the case. If this is a concern, the mother may want to examine her nursing pattern. Perhaps she needs to take care not to initiate nursing in response to all of her baby's bids for attention. Her baby will become self-reliant if given the opportunity, and when he can rely on his mother for comfort and security when he really requires it. She can continue to breastfeed, clearly understanding that it is providing emotional benefits to her baby.

Sometimes the baby's father encourages weaning when he views the mother and baby constantly together and he feels left out. Perhaps he misses evenings out with his mate or simply would like more of her attention. She can explore his reasons for wanting her to terminate breastfeeding and try to find a suitable compromise. Special times together for the couple or fewer feeds when he is home may satisfy the father. Ultimately, the mother may decide to wean to maintain harmony in the home. Your role is to support her in her decision.

A mother may be criticized for breastfeeding an older baby and may begin to wonder if breastfeeds are still beneficial. Let mothers know that their milk still has nutritional advantages for the toddler. Furthermore, the emotional security of breastfeeding can be a stabilizing factor in a child's life. In order to decrease criticism, she can avoid nursing in front of those who disapprove and keep a toy or snack ready as a distraction to postpone feeds. Or, she can avoid taking her child places when she anticipates that he will be hungry or tired and wish to nurse.

Often, the mother wishes to continue breastfeeding, and she will need help in responding to those who oppose breastfeeding an older baby. If she senses that they are receptive, she can attempt to educate them about the continuing benefits of breastfeeding. She may simply need to indicate her determination to continue nursing by standing firm and nursing discreetly. She will benefit from your encouragement and support to offset the negative influences around her. You can put her in touch with other women who are breastfeeding older babies. This will help build her confidence and maintain her perspective.

Baby-led Weaning

When a mother is relaxed about breastfeeding and has no pressures or problems that lead her to wean, she can allow her baby to nurse at his own pace and establish his own weaning time. Through baby-led weaning, the baby will drop feeds gradually if he is put to breast only when he indicates a need for it. By neither denying nor initiating breastfeeding, the mother follows her baby's feeding cues and subsequent pattern for weaning.

Sometimes, the mother overlooks her baby's signs of readiness to wean and may initiate feeds that could be eliminated. She may initiate nursing as soon as her baby awakens instead of preparing breakfast for him. She may nurse to keep the child quiet while she talks on the telephone or is engaged in other activities. If the mother wishes to change these patterns, you can encourage her to develop other mothering skills to replace breastfeeding. Suggest that she read stories to her baby, offer him a snack, or provide him with toys and activities to fill usual nursing times. Rocking, cuddling, singing, and holding can effectively replace the coziness and comfort of breastfeeding.

Sometimes, a baby will start to wean when his mother does not want or expect it, and she may respond by trying to entice him to nurse more frequently. She may find it difficult to accept that he is growing and maturing. You can help her learn to appreciate his maturity by stressing his new achievements and showing her new ways of interacting with him and continuing their close relationship.

Mother-led Weaning

Mother-led weaning occurs when the mother attempts to end breastfeeding without having received cues from her baby. Some mothers become impatient for their baby to wean. If a mother has begun to resent feeds, it may be time for her to initiate weaning. Your use of guiding skills will help her explore her goals and her baby's needs. She may be feeling pressure from others or has received poor information or advice. She may be planning to return to work and believes that she must wean in order to do this. Perhaps she senses that her baby is no longer satisfied with breastfeeding.

Help her determine what is best for her and her baby. Mothers rarely set exact unalterable dates for weaning. A new mother may have a vague idea about when she would like to wean. When that time comes, her relationship with her baby has changed and she may put off weaning until a later date. Many women eventually set a flexible deadline for weaning.

Weaning is a transitional period that needs to be managed with appreciation for the baby's needs. A baby younger than 9 months to 1 year of age needs to be weaned to a bottle. He will still have strong sucking needs if breastfeeding is ended completely. Many mothers wait a little longer to wean so that they can avoid bottles and offer fluids directly from a cup. When the mother brings up the topic of weaning, it may not mean that she wants to begin, rather only that she is curious about it and would like information. The mother may approach the subject with hesitation because she knows you advocate breastfeeding. Try to be sensitive to her cues and let her know that you will help her whether she chooses to wean or to continue breastfeeding. Your nonjudgmental attitude will encourage her to express her concerns freely and to define her questions clearly so that she can understand the nature of weaning.

Gradual Weaning

If the mother wishes to initiate weaning, she can eliminate the least preferred feeding first. Advise her to allow at least 3 days for her baby and her breasts to adjust to this dropped feeding. In its place, the mother can substitute a drink, snack, cuddling, or a favorite activity. If she is dropping an early morning feed, she may want to have breakfast ready when the child awakens. If she is dropping a late night feed, she can consider alternate ways of getting him to sleep.

If weaning is proceeding too quickly, her child may react by demanding more attention, requesting more feeds, or exhibiting physical changes such as allergic reactions, stomach upsets, or constipation. The mother will need to slow the weaning process. When she and the child are comfortable with the substitution, she can proceed to drop another feeding, continuing in this manner for several weeks or months. The child may wish to continue one preferred feed and will decrease his frequency to once every few days until he stops breastfeeding entirely.

Weaning too quickly may cause the mother's breasts to become uncomfortable. She can express her milk to relieve the discomfort while being careful not to express her milk so much that she actually increases milk production. She will want to watch for any symptoms of plugged ducts or mastitis, and can wear a supportive bra that is not binding. She may want to consider other comfort measures such as a pain reliever, ice packs, or cabbage leaves. The mother and baby both adjust better when weaning is gradual and tailored to their needs. By allowing several months for weaning, any physical and emotional discomforts can be minimized.

Minimal Breastfeeding

Many women find that **minimal breastfeeding** provides an attractive compromise to total weaning. Minimal breastfeeding describes a pattern of breastfeeding between one and three times a day, with complementary feeds providing the remaining nourishment. This may be an option when the mother and baby are separated for regular periods, as when the mother returns to work or school. Breastfeeding two to three times a day can help women still feel the special connection to their baby that accompanies breastfeeding. A 1989 study showed that 49 percent of mothers used minimal breastfeeding (feeding one to two times per day) for an extended period as a comfortable transition to weaning (Williams, 1989).

Untimely or Emergency Weaning

Mothers must sometimes wean their babies abruptly, with no time for preparation or forethought. If emergency weaning is unavoidable, the mother must put aside her ideal vision of gradual, comfortable weaning and work within the confines of her situation. If she is able to take several days to wean, she can drop every other feed the first day. She can express just enough milk from her breasts to relieve discomfort but not so much that she causes further milk production. She can then eliminate the remainder of the feeds, making sure she includes extra cuddling and attention for her baby.

If she must wean immediately, she will experience about 24 hours of painful engorgement. This will subside gradually. She can wrap her breasts in cabbage leaves to reduce swelling. See Chapter 14 for guidelines in applying cabbage to engorged breasts. Acetaminophen can relieve her pain and help reduce swelling. In addition, she can use ice wrapped in a towel on her breasts to reduce pain. She will want to avoid heat because it promotes lactation. Plugged ducts or mastitis could occur as a result of the lack of milk flow. Your kind attention and availability will be invaluable to her as she experiences this period of stress. A word of caution: Some outdated medical literature recommends breast binding, a practice that can lead to plugged ducts and intensify the mother's discomfort. Mothers should never be advised to bind their breasts!

Sometimes a mother inadvertently weans her young baby while actually wanting to continue nursing. Perhaps she started giving occasional bottles and before she realized the consequences, her milk production had diminished. She may feel as though breastfeeding has slipped away from her, and that when it got so far out of hand, she was unable or unwilling to turn back. She will especially need your acceptance and support at this time to help her through her disappointment.

Should the mother indicate an interest in relactating, you can refer to the discussion of relactation in Chapter 22. Untimely weaning can shake a woman's confidence in her ability to mother. Encourage her to continue giving her baby the same cuddling and attention she gave him when she was breastfeeding, always holding him close and providing good eye contact during feeds. Help her realize that what she has experienced with this baby will not necessarily repeat itself with the next baby.

Some circumstances that the mother cannot control may lead to weaning. Breastfeeding may be contraindicated if the mother contracts a serious illness or requires medication that would pass through her milk and harm her baby. Also, she may return to work or school and no longer be able to manage breastfeeding. Her baby may go on a **nursing strike** and not resume breastfeeding. She may become pregnant and her history of miscarriages or premature births may preclude breastfeeding. The discomfort of sore nipples during pregnancy, coupled with a decrease in milk production, may suppress her desire to nurse any longer.

After such forced weaning, the mother may grieve over the loss of breastfeeding. She may feel guilty or incompetent because she could not continue this part of her mothering role. Your listening to and accepting her feelings will help her work through this personal loss. You can stress the benefits she provided her baby during the time she breastfed and teach her other mothering skills to substitute for the closeness of breastfeeding.

After Weaning

It is very common for mothers to feel some regret or sadness when breastfeeding ends, even if they had wanted to wean. Every woman will benefit from support and understanding by those close to her in order to overcome these feelings. Help the mother recognize that she will learn new skills for comforting her baby that will replace breastfeeding. Help her regard weaning as another step in her child's development, and encourage her to look forward to new stages.

The mother may experience several physical adjustments after weaning. Anticipatory guidance will help her expect these changes. Most women need to adjust their diets to eliminate calories that were supporting milk production in order to avoid gaining weight. Some are pleased to find a sudden weight loss of a few pounds resulting from a loss of fluid and fat from the body's fat stores. The breasts may also change, becoming soft, flat, or droopy for a few months. If menstruation did not resume until after weaning, menstrual cycles may be somewhat irregular for a few months, with skipped periods, light flow, or spotting. Many women find that their breasts gradually return to their prepregnancy size. Some observe that their breasts never fully regain the fatty layer that was present before conception. The Montgomery glands recede and the areola may remain darker than before she was pregnant. Stretch marks may still be apparent on her breasts.

Some mothers may experience milk secretion for several months after weaning. This will gradually diminish and turn to a colostrum-like consistency. If the mother is spontaneously secreting milk 6 months after weaning, she might evaluate any circumstances that may be stimulating milk production. Perhaps she is holding her baby against her chest, wears clothing that rubs the nipples, or is sensitive to sexual foreplay that involves her breasts.

The cessation of milk secretion varies greatly from one woman to the next. It may last several weeks or as long as 1 year after weaning. After milk secretion has stopped completely, if the mother notices the appearance of a discharge, she will want to consult her physician to determine the cause. Sometimes old milk works its way out, and other times fluid may result from an infection or growth.

SUMMARY

Anticipatory guidance will help parents know the changes to expect as their babies develop throughout their first year and beyond. They can then make adjustments in routines and practices in order to accommodate breastfeeding management to these developmental stages. The baby will expand his world and develop both physically and socially, and will learn that certain cues elicit responses from his parents. Thus, he will at times cry, coo, smile, or frown depending on his needs. Whereas his mother first represents his whole world, he expands to an awareness of others and to his environment. Motor skills will develop further as he begins to crawl and walk. Teething, shorter feeds, separation anxiety, experimenting with vocabulary sounds, feeding himself, and drinking from a cup all will evolve during this period. Mothers will find creative ways to nurse their toddler and eventually will wean him from the breast. This expansive time can be both exhilarating and challenging at the same time. Your advice and support will be appreciated by parents as they learn to make the necessary adjustments to meet their baby's needs.

REFERENCES

Birkbeck J. Weaning: A position statement. *N Z Med J* 105:221–224; 1992.

Butte N et al. Sleep organization and energy expenditure of breast-fed and formula-fed infants. *Pediatr Res* 32:514–519; 1992.

Dewey K et al. Growth of breastfed and formula-fed infants from 0 to 18 months: The DARLING study. *Pediatrics* 89:1035–1041; 1993.

Forsyth J et al. Relation between early introduction of solid food to infants and their weight and illness during the first two years of life." *Br Med J* 306:1572–1576; 1993.

Heinig M et al. Intake and growth of breast-fed and formula-fed infants in relation to the timing of introduction of complementary foods: The DARLING study. *Acta Paediatr* 82:999–1006; 1993.

Macknin M et al. Infant sleep and bedtime cereal. *Am J Dis Child* 143:1066–1068; 1989.

Montagu A. *Touching: The Human Significance of the Skin*. New York: Harper Row; pp. 291–292; 1972.

Saarinen UM et al. Prolonged breast-feeding as a prophylaxis for atopic disease. *Lancet* 2(8135):163–166; 1979.

Slusser W and Powers NG. Breastfeeding Update I: Immunology, Nutrition and Advocacy. *Pediatri Rev* 18(4): 111–119; 1997.

Williams K and Morse J. Weaning patterns of first-time mothers. *American Journal of Maternal Child Nursing* 14L:188–192; 1989.

Winchell K. *Nursing Strike: Misunderstood Feelings. J Hum Lact* 8(4):217–219; 1992.

Wrigley E and Hutchinson S. Long-term breastfeeding: The secret bond. *J Nurse Midwife* 35:35–41; 1990.

BIBLIOGRAPHY

American Academy of Pediatrics. *Pediatric Nutrition Handbook.* Elk Grove Village IL; 1985.

American Academy of Pediatrics. Breastfeeding and the use of human milk. *Pediatrics* 100:1035–1039; 1997.

Beatty J. *Observing Development in the Young Child.* Columbus, OH. Charles Merrill; 1990.

Bee H. *The Developing Child.* New York, NY: Harper and Row; 1989.

de Bruin, N et al. Energy utilization and growth in breast-fed and formula-fed infants measured prospectively during the first year of life. *Am J Clin Nutr* 67:1256–1264; 1998.

Dewey K. Effect of age of introduction of complementary foods on iron status of breast fed infants in Honduras. *Am J Clin Nutr* 67:878–884; 1998.

Goldman A. Association of atopic diseases with breast-feeding: food allergens, fatty acids, and evolution. *J Pediatr* 134:5–7; 1999.

Hendricks K and Badruddin S. Weaning recommendations: The scientific basis. *Nutr Rev* 50:125–133; 1992.

Hills-Bonczyk S et al. Women's experiences with breastfeeding longer than 12 months. *Birth* 21:206–212; 1994.

Hill P et al. Effects of parity and weaning practices on breastfeeding duration. *Public Health Nursing* 14:227–234; 1997.

Hughes FP et al. *Child Development.* St. Paul, MN: West Publishing Co; 1988.

Isolauri E et al. Breast-feeding of allergic infants. *J Pediatr* 134:27–32; 1999.

Jiang Z et al. Energy expenditure of Chinese infants in Guangdong Province, south China, determined with use of the doubly labeled water method. *Am J Clin Nutr* 67:1256–1264; 1998.

Judd J. Assessing newborns from head to toe. *Nursing,* Dec. 1985.

Keener M et al. Infant temperament, sleep organization, and nighttime parental interventions. *Pediatrics* 81:762–771; 1988.

Kendall-Tackett K and M Sugaman. The social consequences of long-term Breastfeeding. *J Hum Lact* II (3):179–184; 1995.

Lloyd B et al. Formula tolerance in postbreastfed and exclusively formula-fed infants. *Pediatrics* 103(1):E7; 1999.

Lorick G. Untimely weaning: Assisting the mother who may grieve. *Int J Childbirth Education* 8:41; 1993.

Maekawa K et al. Developmental change of sucking response to taste in infants. *Biol Neonate* 60 (supp 1):62; 1991.

NAACOG. Physical assessment of neonates. *Practice Resources;* Oct 1986.

Rowe L et al. A comparison of two methods of breastfeeding management. *Aust Fam Phys* 21:288–294; 1992.

16

PROBLEMS WITH MILK PRODUCTION AND TRANSFER

Contributing Author: Linda Kutner

The most common reason women give for stopping breastfeeding is that they believe they do not have enough milk. This is also why most women give their babies supplements. The information presented in this chapter will assist you in helping a mother identify when her milk production is truly low. You will learn to recognize signs when a newborn is receiving sufficient amounts of his mother's milk, as well as when he is not. Measures for increasing milk production and for efficient milk transfer are presented as well. With appropriate teaching and follow-up, you and the mother can maximize the outcome of adequate milk production with the result being a baby who thrives on his mother's milk.

THE PERCEPTION OF INSUFFICIENT MILK SUPPLY

When a mother says that she has insufficient milk for her baby, you first need to determine why she believes this. Although it may be a case of low milk production, it might actually be lack of confidence or lack of knowledge about normal newborn behavior. A mother may perceive her milk to be inadequate for her baby for a number of reasons. She may believe it is not rich enough or satisfying enough. She may worry that her milk is causing an allergic response or excessive gas in her baby. By far, the most common concern is that she has an inadequate amount of milk. Therefore, helping the mother identify whether she actually has a problem and reassuring her when you have determined that her production is fine will have a tremendous influence on her breastfeeding duration.

Reasons for a Perceived Low Milk Supply

Why do so many women believe there is a problem with their milk? Hill (1991) cites some of the differences between women who perceived they had insufficient milk versus those who did not. She also identified the most common reasons reported by mothers who perceived their milk production to be insufficient. Some worried that the infant did not seem satisfied and was fussy after feeds. Frequent feeds and poor infant weight gain were also concerns. And mothers reported that their milk supply dried up after they had introduced infant formula or solid foods. Lactation consultants and other caregivers need to be aware of some of these differences and bring them to the attention of the mother, so that she can be given special help or information.

Some women lack confidence in their bodies to do what they were meant to do. The medical profession's use of negative terminology in women's health could be a contributing factor. The imagery associated with such terms as lactation failure, failure to progress and incompetent cervix can undermine a woman's self-confidence and self-esteem. Subliminal messages perhaps, but ones that can eat away at their confidence at a vulnerable time in their lives. Mothers are extremely sensitive to negativism during the postpartum period.

Because many young parents live quite a distance from their nuclear families, they may lack a strong support system and positive role models for birthing and parenting. Women who choose to breastfeed in a culture that is saturated with bottle-feeding messages face many societal challenges. Other women who are considered role models usually have bottle fed their babies. The expectations of society, and especially the media, are that babies are fed by bottles. Often, caregivers either lack correct information regarding breastfeeding management or are noncommital to avoid making mothers "feel guilty" if they choose not to breastfeed.

The stress of becoming a new mother can fuel a woman's worries about competence. Parents want to know they are doing the best for their baby. A mother's misconceptions about the realities of motherhood can cause her to question her choices and doubt her mothering abilities. Her preconceived notion of babies may not match the reality of her baby or her baby's needs. Misconceptions of normal baby behavior can create anxieties in inexperienced parents. Consequently, they may blame their choice to breastfeed as the cause for fussiness, wakefulness, or other normal behaviors.

▼
Recognizing Sufficient Milk Production

Worries about inadequate milk production can be minimized when mothers understand the role of milk removal in triggering further milk production, as well as what to expect in normal newborn behavior. Make sure that mothers have a clear understanding of how to determine if their baby is receiving sufficient milk and is well nourished. This will prevent unnecessary early weaning due to a mother's perception that she is not providing adequate amounts of milk for her baby. Signs that indicate to the mother and caregiver that breastfeeding is going well are listed in the following section.

Signs That Breastfeeding is Going Well

◆ By day 6, the infant has at least six wet diapers in each 24-hour period.

◆ The infant has pale dilute urine.

◆ By day 6, the infant produces four or more stools that are yellow or at least are turning yellow. He continues to have at least four stools in each 24-hour period until he is about 1 month old.

◆ The infant routinely breastfeeds at least eight times in a 24-hour period.

◆ The mother's breasts feel softer after a feed (although for some women, there is not a dramatic difference).

◆ The mother's nipples are not painful during or after feeds.

◆ The infant is gaining 5 to 10 oz a week.

◆ The infant has regained his birth weight by 10 to 14 days.

◆ During the feed, the infant's sucking rhythm slows as the milk is released, and swallowing or gulping can be heard.

◆ The infant is alert and active, and his skin appears healthy.

◆ The infant is content between feeds, and is usually able to rest for 1 to 2 hours before signaling to feed again. (Although well-fed infants may be fussy for other reasons, leading mothers to believe that they do not have enough milk.)

It is important that the mother feel confident in her ability to feed her baby. Help her feel assured that she can produce the necessary milk for her baby. If she and her baby were discharged from the hospital in 48 hours or less, advise that the baby be seen by the primary care physician within 2 to 4 days of life (AAP, 1997). A second visit to the baby's physician is advisable at approximately 2 weeks for a physical assessment and weight check, or sooner if the baby's condition warrants. These safeguards will help ensure a healthy baby and a confident mother.

▼
IDENTIFYING PROBLEMS WITH INFANT GROWTH

Several factors contribute to the total picture of a baby's adequate growth. Birth weight should have doubled by 4 months and tripled by 12 months (Lawrence, 1999). Body length is a significant indicator and should have increased by 50 percent at 1 year. Head circumference, which indicates brain growth, should have increased by 7.6 cm (3 inches) at 1 year. Other signs of healthy growth are sufficient voids and stools, which will be frequent in the first month and less frequent thereafter. Also, bright eyes, an alert manner, and good muscle and skin tone should be present. Family history is a consideration that is sometimes overlooked. If the parents are small in stature, or gained weight slowly as infants, the same pattern can be expected for their children. Be sure this is taken into account before it is determined that there is a problem.

To ensure the health of every infant in your care, be alert to weight gain and to the factors that could contribute to low milk production. Being aware of each mother's nursing schedule and her baby's feeding pattern will help you assess whether breastfeeding may be contributing to inadequate growth. Consider all growth indicators and possible causes of poor growth as you and the mother develop a care plan for improvement. Very few mothers actually have insufficient milk production. Further, most cases of insufficient milk result from breastfeeding mismanagement, which can be corrected. Be careful not to confuse the very rare maternal inability to produce adequate amounts of milk with the lack of opportunity to produce the milk. The lack of opportunity to produce milk is a breastfeeding management issue.

▼
Newborn Dehydration

When a baby does not receive enough fluids, he can become dehydrated. Dehydration can occur when a breastfed baby is not receiving an adequate amount of his mother's milk. Many mothers and babies are discharged from the hospital before someone who is knowledgeable about breastfeeding management has evaluated their breastfeeding technique. Consequently, some mothers will not have established milk production nor had a good breastfeed before they are sent home. Sofer (1993), after following six case studies, reported that high milk sodium levels, rather than being the cause of dehydration, seem to occur after milk production slows.

All mothers must be taught to assess adequate breastfeeds, wet diapers, and stools. There is never any reason for a healthy newborn to progress to the point of dehydration. In the hospital, a mother can be taught how to recognize when her baby achieves an effective latch. Before discharge, teach her the warning signs of potential breastfeeding problems (see Fig. 10.3 in Chapter 10). Teach her, as well, the signs that breastfeeding is going well (see Fig. 10.3 in Chapter 10). Just because a baby's jaw is moving up and down does not mean he is taking in milk. Give the mother a diary to document breastfeeds, voids, and stools (See Figure 11.3 in Chapter 11). This information will indicate milk intake.

It is imperative that mothers and babies who are discharged early are followed up shortly after discharge. If the mother has not established effective breastfeeding at the time of discharge, the physician's office must be notified. Office staff must be educated to understand the impact of number of feeds, voids, and stools. Recognizing the symptoms of dehydration will help you and other caregivers identify infants at risk.

Symptoms of Dehydration

- Sunken fontanels
- Weight loss greater than seven percent of birth weight
- Poor skin turgor
- Dry mucous membranes
- No tears
- Lethargy
- Weak cry
- Infrequent feeds
- Infant sleeps at the breast
- Scant urinary output
- Few or no stools

◤ **Concerns with Infant Weight Gain**

Concerns about the infant's weight gain usually surface within the first month of life. As discussed in Chapter 11, weight loss of over 7 percent in the first week of life warrants an evaluation and assistance with breastfeeding. The weight should have stabilized by the end of the first week. By 10 to 14 days, the infant should return to birth weight. If birth weight has not been regained by 14 days, you need to explore the mother's breastfeeding management to ensure that weight does not become an issue.

In order to assess milk transfer, you can weigh the infant before and after feeds. Test weighing should be done only on a digital electronic scale to ensure accuracy (Meier, 1994). It should not be done routinely or in the first 48 hours in the hospital. Reserve this assessment for problems associated with milk intake.

Breastfed and formula-fed infants consume dramatically different amounts of calories. The question has been raised whether breastfed infants are not consuming enough calories or if formula-fed infants are actually fed too many calories. Garza and Butte (1990) looked at several possible explanations for the lower intake of the breastfed infant. They found that by 4 months of age, gross energy intakes by exclusively breastfed infants are significantly less than current recommendations, which are based on artificial feeding. Additionally, breastfed infants were found to have normal growth rates that differed from the growth rates of formula-fed infants. They also had lower total daily energy expenditure, sleeping metabolic rates, rates of energy expenditure, rectal temperature, and heart rates.

A later study by Butte and colleagues (1993) supports this theory. They found that in unfavorable environments, infants may have higher than usual energy requirements. Rather than low milk production or intake, they suggest that the infant's environment could explain the growth differences. This may be an issue for babies who live in high-poverty areas. Infection is usually the concern that gets mentioned as a cause. However, if babies are subjected to less restful sleep or multiple care providers, this may also increase their need for calories. Because of the difference in growth in exclusively breastfed infants and those fed an artificial baby milk, the need for growth charts for breastfed infants has been expressed.

Slow-Weight-Gaining Infant

Every child develops at his own rate. An adolescent may experience a growth spurt and grow 6 inches in 1 year. The same is true for babies. Some babies simply gain weight more slowly than others. It is important to distinguish between a baby who is not gaining weight adequately and one who is simply gaining weight slowly. A slow-weight-gaining infant will show slow but steady growth over time; growth proportional for weight, length, and head circumference; and appropriate development for his age.

Remember the rule, if it's not broken, don't fix it! In the absence of other risk factors, minimal intervention, if any, is required. You can observe a breastfeed to evaluate the mother's breastfeeding techniques. Ask about her baby's feeding pattern and suggest any necessary changes. Make sure that the baby is not receiving pacifiers or bottles that would limit his sucking time at the breast. Review feeding cues with the mother to be sure she is responding to her baby at appropriate times. Suggest that she have her baby weighed twice a week and record his weights to monitor his gain. These measures may be all that is necessary for the slow-weight-gaining infant.

Poor-Weight-Gaining Infant

A newborn who is still below birth weight by several ounces at day 14 may need a greater degree of intervention. The same is true of an older infant who is not gaining or is gaining less than 3 oz. per week. Make sure he receives a minimum of 8 to 12 feeds per day around the clock. Feeds should last 20 to 40 minutes with a lot of audible swallowing. The baby may be an inefficient feeder. The mother can give him the cream portion of expressed milk that has been stored (the cream will rise to the top). Warn against the use of any pacifiers or bottles. Suggest that she have her baby weighed at least twice a week and record his weights to monitor his gain. The mother will also probably need to express milk with a breast pump to increase milk production.

A baby who is gaining weight poorly because of low milk production may need to be supplemented with an artificial baby milk until the mother's milk production becomes sufficient to return to exclusive breastfeeding. Discuss the need for supplementation, the type and amount of formula the physician may recommend, and the method to be used for supplementing her baby. With these infants, it is imperative that they receive the supplementation that they need. This can be accomplished with minimal disruption to breastfeeding.

The goal is twofold. First and foremost, the baby needs to receive calories. Increasing his weight is essential. If the mother's milk production is low, the baby will need to be supplemented with formula. The second goal is to increase the mother's milk production to the level that it can sustain her infant. Only then can supplements be discontinued. In order to accomplish both goals at the same time, the baby can be supplemented through a tube at the breast. This provides the baby with nourishment and the mother's breasts the stimulation they need for milk production. Pumping with a hospital-grade electric breast pump between feeds will further help increase milk production.

Infants who are not gaining well must be followed by their physician. You will want to send a detailed report of your consultation with the mother to the primary care physician. Your follow-up of the mother will also be an important factor in helping to turn this situation around. As the baby begins to gain weight, the mother can slowly decrease the amount of supplement he is receiving. Caution the mother that if her baby begins to catch up on his weight rapidly and then slows down, she may be decreasing the supplementation too quickly. It is difficult to know the pattern of growth one should expect from an individual child. It is suggested that the weight at 4 to 8 weeks be used as a child's baseline. Caregivers should become concerned when the growth deviates downward by two major percentiles on the growth chart.

Identifying Mothers at Risk for Low Milk Production or Transfer

Your role in the case of low milk production or transfer revolves around helping the mother explore the possible causes of the situation. Usually, there are multiple factors involved when a baby is not gaining adequate weight, factors that relate to the mother, to the infant, or to the management of breastfeeding. Some factors are more significant than others, such as in the case of a mother who is hypogalactic (unable to produce sufficient milk). When multiple factors are present at birth, the mother and baby must be followed closely after hospital discharge. Table 16.1 identifies potential dyads who may have problems establishing either adequate milk production or a positive milk transfer. You can work with the mother and infant while they overcome their problems, in a manner that is both safe and supportive of the breastfeeding experience.

Mismanagement of breastfeeding may be the cause of slow or poor weight gain, and the mother may need help to correct her breastfeeding technique. Some feeding-related causes are the baby's inability to suck well, improper positioning, inadequate time at each breast, supplemental bottles, prolactin inhibitors, and an inhibited or unstable letdown. A specific cause may not always be apparent. When the mother and baby are both more proficient at nursing, problems that are causing low milk production may diminish.

Warning Signs That a Baby Is Not Gaining Adequate Weight

The above-mentioned factors will help you identify mothers and babies who are at risk for low milk production or transfer. Unfortunately, you may not always have the opportunity to see these mothers and infants before an actual problem has developed. You need to recognize signs that will alert you to problems.

There are many indications that an infant is compromised, and some of these factors conflict. In general, infants who are not gaining adequately will frequently sleep for long periods of time to conserve energy. They may fuss when removed from the breast and then go back to sleep as soon as they are put back to breast. The mother may tell you that she is nursing all of the time because the infant cannot be laid down without fussing. Other infants are reported to be "good" babies and nurse only infrequently. These infants usually are reported to sleep through the night, and few have periods of quiet alert time.

Infants with poor weight gain often have a worried or anxious look on their face. They hold their body in a

TABLE 16.1

Factors That May Influence Milk Production and Transfer

Maternal factors	
	◆ Primipara
	◆ Gained less than 18 pounds during pregnancy
	◆ History of low milk production or breastfeeding problems with previous infants
	◆ Flat or inverted nipples or taut, tight breast tissue
	◆ Epidural
	In place longer than 3 to 4 hours before delivery
	Administered more than one time
	Received more than one bolus of epidural medication
	◆ Induction of labor with Pitocin
	◆ Received excessive intravenous fluids; on magnesium sulfate; edema present in ankles that was not present before labor
	◆ Pain medication in labor, more than 1 hour before delivery
	◆ Had a cesarean delivery
	◆ Breastfeeding initiated more than 1 hour after delivery
	◆ Sore nipples throughout feeds at the time of hospital discharge
	◆ Embarrassed or unsure of her ability to breastfeed her baby
	◆ Using a nipple shield for breastfeeds
	◆ Sleeps far from her baby, which interferes with easy access to her baby and response to feeding cues
	◆ Is taking medications, especially contraceptives, that affect milk production
	◆ Is fatigued or ill
	◆ Had previous breast trauma, or either reduction or augmentation surgery
	◆ Has hypothyroidism (rare)
	◆ Has hypoprolactinemia (rare)
	◆ Has an anatomic problem with the position of the lactiferous sinuses (rare)
	◆ Has an extremely low food and fluid intake (rare except in food crisis)
	◆ Experienced little or no breast change in size or color during pregnancy, indicating lack of sufficient functioning breast tissue (extremely rare)
Infant factors	
	◆ Less than 37 weeks' gestation
	◆ Weighs less than 7 pounds at birth
	◆ 7 percent or greater weight loss at time of hospital discharge
	◆ Male infant
	◆ Vacuum or forceps used for delivery
	◆ Has a tight frenulum
	◆ Has a cleft lip or palate or both
	◆ Fetal distress; meconium expelled during delivery
	◆ Insult to the oral cavity, as with a laryngoscope and deep suctioning
	◆ Is kept in nursery instead of with mother
	◆ Is SGA or LGA

TABLE 16.1 (CONTINUED)	
Factors That May Influence Milk Production and Transfer	
	◆ Is jaundiced
	◆ Is sleepy and difficult to wake, and fails to give clear feeding cues
	◆ Has difficulty latching on consistently
	◆ Has not established effective breastfeeding before hospital discharge
	◆ Has a medical condition such as a **metabolic** disorder, **neuromotor** problem, **congenital** heart disease, respiratory infection, urinary infection, hypothyroidism, or other disorder (The baby needs to be seen by someone who can give special care in these areas)
Factors associated with breastfeeding management	◆ Circumcision done before infant established an effective breastfeeding pattern
	◆ Feeding restrictions placed on infant, such as with timed feeds or not being allowed to receive anything by mouth (NPO)
	◆ Bottles or pacifiers given during hospitalizations
	◆ Other foods and drink are being given to the baby, decreasing his appetite and time spent at the breast
	◆ Night breastfeeds were stopped too early (prolactin response is higher at night)
	◆ Breastfeeds are not long enough. Inadequate removal of milk leads to a buildup of the suppressor peptides in milk that signals the breast to reduce milk production
	◆ Baby is not attached at the breast for effective suckling
	◆ Breastfeeds are infrequent
	◆ Breastfeeds are short and hurried. The baby is being removed from one breast too soon and is not receiving enough hindmilk

LGA, large for gestational age; SGA, small for gestational age.

flexed fetal position to help maintain their temperature. If the infant has lost a large amount of weight, he will have hanging folds of skin on his thighs and buttocks. His cry may be a high-pitched sound like the "mew" of a cat.

Infants who are not gaining well usually have decreased urinary output. What urine they do pass may be concentrated. In the older infant, the urine may smell strongly of ammonia. In the infant younger than 5 to 6 weeks of age, few stools are passed. In the very young infant, the parents frequently report that he is still passing meconium after the fourth day of life.

▼

FAILURE TO THRIVE

The condition in which an infant's weight is seriously compromised is referred to as failure to thrive (FTT). Neville (1983) defines an infant with FTT as one who fails to regain birth weight by 3 weeks of age, has a weight loss of greater than 10 percent of birth weight by 2 weeks of age, or has a deceleration of growth from a previously established pattern of weight gain. Finally, there is evidence of malnutrition on examination, such as minimal subcutaneous fat or wasted buttocks. In older infants, a weight that is two standard deviations or more below where it should be on a standard growth chart is an indication of FTT. A growth chart that shows normal weight for each age is a tool for determining if an infant is growing within established guidelines. The growth chart can be used to plot the infant's predictable growth curve as a means of assessing progress.

A baby with FTT may be lethargic, hypertonic, irritable, and difficult to soothe. He may sleep excessively or be fussy continuously. His compromised status may be caused by his physical condition or that of his mother. The causes related to the mother and infant are identified in Table 16.2. In many cases, FTT is a consequence of mismanagement of breastfeeding. It is important to realize that even a breastfeeding baby who appears to be satisfied can fail to thrive. An easy, placid baby is vulnerable to FTT because he does not give appropriate hunger cues. Below are issues you can address with the mother.

Issues to Address with the Mother

◆ How much weight did you gain during pregnancy?

◆ Describe the changes that occurred in your breasts during pregnancy. (This may give you a clue to determining if she has sufficient mammary tissue.)

◆ Do you have a history of infertility?

◆ Are you aware of having any thyroid dysfunction?

◆ Have you had any breast surgery?

◆ During delivery, was there excessive blood loss or the use of Pitocin or intravenous fluids?

◆ Are you using oral contraceptives?

◆ Describe your diet.

◆ Do you smoke cigarettes?

◆ Have you experienced any engorgement or mastitis?

◆ Describe your management of breastfeeds.

Reversing the Trend of Failure to Thrive

If FTT is suspected, measures must be initiated immediately to reverse the pattern of weight loss. Weichert (1979) reported a four-step approach designed to force an immediate reversal of growth insufficiency. Mothers provided formula in a nursing supplementer during feeds, nursed in a place protected from distractions and disturbances, and were encouraged to groom their infants while they nursed. They were also given chlorpromazine, 25 mg three times a day for 7 days. Anxiety, pain, and fatigue can raise the mother's level of **dopamine,** which is a prolactin inhibitor. Chlorpromazine decreases dopamine levels and, therefore, improves milk production. Weichert found that removing maternal anxiety about milk supply improves outcomes.

Your assistance can be pivotal in helping the mother turn her baby's weight pattern around. Make sure that she understands that interventions may be required for a long time. Help her form realistic expectations, and be available to her for emotional support. It is very easy for the mother of an infant with FTT to be-

TABLE 16.2		
Causes of Failure to Thrive		
Maternal causes	◆ Previous breast surgery, either reduction or augmentation	
	◆ Hypothyroidism	
	◆ Hypoprolactinemia	
	◆ Anatomic position of the lactiferous sinuses	
	◆ Insufficient mammary tissue	
	◆ Sheehan's syndrome	
	◆ Disrupted neurohormonal pathways	
	◆ Use of a nipple shield	
	◆ Retained placental fragments	
	◆ Mismanagement of breastfeeding	
Infant causes	◆ Neuromotor problems	
	◆ Tight frenulum	
	◆ Systemic illness	
	◆ Sleepy infant	
	◆ Inability to compress lactiferous sinuses	
	◆ Mother's anatomy versus infant oral cavity	
	◆ Disorganized suck	
	◆ "Good" baby who does not exhibit hunger cues	

come overly stressed. As things begin to improve, caution the mother to proceed slowly with decreasing the amount of supplement and frequency of milk expression. Sometimes interventions, as described in the following section, are required the entire time the infant is exclusively breastfed.

Interventions for the Infant with Failure to Thrive

◆ Assess the baby's sucking technique, and observe how he is held at the breast.

◆ Breastfeed the baby 10 to 12 times in 24 hours around the clock until he has four stools per 24 hours for 3 days in a row.

◆ Alternate breasts when the baby's suckling pattern changes and swallowing ceases.

◆ Use alternate massage during feeds.

◆ Limit feeds to 40 minutes per session no matter which feeding methods are used.

◆ Supplement with formula at every feed.

◆ Express milk with a hospital-grade electric breast pump to help stimulate milk production.

◆ Make certain that the baby's caloric needs are being satisfied by frequent feeds and supplemental formula as recommended by the physician or determined by an International Board Certified Lactation Consultant (IBCLC) experienced in working with FTT infants.

◆ Discontinue the supplements that are given at night first when things improve.

◆ Build the mother's confidence in her ability to breastfeed her baby.

◆ Ensure that the baby is checked by his physician frequently.

◆ Weigh the baby frequently and record any weight changes.

◆ Advise the mother to stay in close contact with you and her baby's physician.

▼ ### Measures to Increase Milk Production

The need to increase milk production can occur at any time during the lactation period. It may occur in the early days of breastfeeding, at times of growth spurts, or whenever the number of feeds is reduced. The mother may have weaned and now wishes to relactate, or she may plan to breastfeed an adopted baby. The baby may have a weight gain problem that requires the mother to increase milk production. Supplements may have been introduced, and the mother wishes to increase milk production in order to reduce or eliminate the amount of supplement her baby is taking.

The degree to which the mother is able to increase milk production depends on the age of her baby, his willingness to nurse at the breast, and the stage of involution of her breasts. It will also depend on the condition of the baby and any medical factors that would interfere. Whether or not the baby is taking a supplement and the amount of supplement taken will influence the length of time it takes to increase milk production. A mother's success will also depend directly on her attitude and motivation. Her baby needs to feed at least 10 to 12 times in 24 hours. She needs to be willing to give her time and energies fully to breastfeeding her baby. Hill (1993) found that mothers who experienced no insufficiency were ones who fed more frequently and longer at each feed. She also found no ethnic differences.

You can help the mother increase milk production by offering some of the suggestions presented in Table 16.3. Just as with other aspects of breastfeeding management, there are a variety of measures to consider when developing a plan with the mother to increase her milk production. Be careful not to overwhelm the mother with too many suggestions. Each mother's needs are different. One mother may respond well to a **galactogogue** (foods, drinks, or herbs believed to increase milk production), whereas another can achieve results simply by altering her management of feeds. Select only those measures that apply and with which the mother can cope. The mother will need close contact and plenty of emotional support from you. This is especially the case in the first few days, when she is trying to sort out the methods that work most effectively for her.

Supplementing the Baby

It is crucial that the baby receive adequate calories at the same time the mother is working at increasing her milk production. If milk production is too low to provide sufficient calories, she may need to give her baby formula until her milk production increases. The use of any feeding bottles and pacifiers must be stopped. Supplements should be given by cup or with a tube feeding device at the breast. At feeds, she must nurse first, and offer supplements afterwards when necessary. If her breasts feel full after a breastfeed, she can express and feed the milk to her baby with a cup or a supplementer. Advise the mother to weigh her baby often. When her milk production improves, she can reduce supplements slowly and continue to increase breastfeeds.

Supplements need to be regulated and offered only in measured amounts so that the baby is not filled with supplement to the detriment of nursing. Suggest that the mother plan the number of ounces to feed her baby during a 24-hour period. The standard instruction to nurse first and supplement afterward may be misleading. Some babies nurse as few as six times a day, whereas others may

TABLE 16.3

Measures to Increase Milk Production

Actions for the mother	◆ Rest as much as possible, and relax during breastfeeds to help the milk flow.
	◆ Spend 100 percent of her time with the baby for 48 hours, concentrating on increasing feeds and resting. Get help with all other tasks.
	◆ Take special precautions to prevent sore nipples.
	◆ Use local galactogogues (foods, drinks, or herbs believed to increase milk production).
	◆ Keep a record of feeds (both breastfeeds and any supplements). This can show how quickly the milk production is increasing and help the mother find a workable feeding pattern.
	◆ Use a hospital-grade electric breast pump to provide additional stimulation to the breasts.
	◆ Improve diet by eating more protein, fresh fruits and vegetables, and B vitamins.
Management of breastfeeds	◆ Encourage letdown by relaxation techniques and following a daily feeding routine.
	◆ Prepare the baby so he is alert and ready to nurse by rousing or soothing him as needed.
	◆ Make sure the baby is attached for effective suckling at breastfeeds.
	◆ Put the baby to both breasts at a feed, several times each, to increase stimulation.
	◆ Encourage the baby to feed more frequently and longer, both day and night.
	◆ Nurse long enough for the baby to receive hindmilk. This will vary from one baby to another.
	◆ Nurse for comfort if the baby is fussy.
	◆ Get into bed with the baby for feeds to increase skin contact.
	◆ Resume night feeds if they had been dropped.

nurse as many as 12 times. The baby could consume so much formula this way that nursing may never resume.

The mother can ask her baby's physician how much supplement he wants the baby to receive. The recommended number of ounces can be divided into two, three, or four feeds, depending on the amount. Advise that she offer it at predetermined times. Supplements can be put into a supplementer and dispensed at the end of a breastfeed. If the baby does not take it all at one feed, he may not need as much supplement in his daily diet. On the other hand, he may need those few ounces sometime later within that 24-hour period. Advise the mother to watch her baby carefully for signs of hunger and to respond accordingly.

Performing a feeding assessment will help you determine the amount of supplementation that an infant needs. The infant should not have nursed, nor should the mother have expressed her milk, in the 2-hour period preceding the assessment. Weigh the infant before and after a feed on a digital scale to determine how much he takes in during the feed (Fig. 16.1). Then ask the mother to pump her breasts after the feed to ascertain the amount of residual milk the infant left in the breast. The amount of milk the infant took in from the breast, plus the residual milk, will give you a good indication of the mother's milk production over the preced-

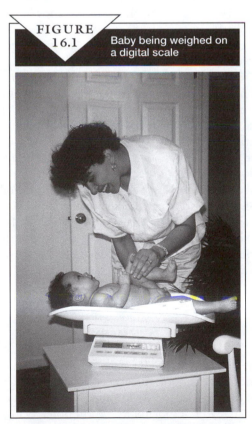

FIGURE 16.1 Baby being weighed on a digital scale

Courtesy of Medela, Inc., McHenry, IL.

TABLE 16.4	
Determining the Number of Ounces an Infant Needs	
Example for an Infant Weighing 4 pounds and 2 ounces	
Convert infant's weight to ounces.	4 lb × 16 oz = 64 oz
	64 oz + 2 oz = 66 oz
Divide total ounces by the number 6.	66 oz ÷ 6 = 11 oz (for a 24-hour intake)
Divide the 24-hour requirements by the number of feeds per 24-hour period.	11 oz ÷ 8 feeds = 1.37 oz per feed
	11 oz ÷ 6 feeds = 1.83 oz per feed

ing 2 or 3 hours. Using the calculations in Table 16.4, you can then determine the infant's total 24-hour requirements and divide it by the number of feedings he takes or should take in a 24-hour period. Knowing what the infant took in from the feeding assessment, compared to what he should have taken in, will give you and the mother a fairly accurate measurement of the amount of supplement her infant will require.

You can encourage the mother to keep a record of how much supplement the baby is getting, as well as the number of feeds, wet diapers, and stools that occur. If the mother increases the amount of supplement, the baby's time at the breast will diminish. Instead, she needs to increase both the number and duration of breastfeeds as she gradually reduces the amount of supplement. She needs to do this with the knowledge of her baby's physician.

Suggest that the mother make goals in her record book, such as, "Today 10 oz, next week 7 oz." The goals for decreasing supplements must be realistic and may plan for dropping only one-half to one ounce every few days, or faster if the baby is doing well. She should never dilute formula in an attempt to cut back on supplements, as this may lead to insufficient nourishment for the baby. The mother needs to know that the task of totally eliminating formula and increasing her milk production to replace it may take several weeks of concentrated effort. Following a consistent pattern of nursing, while offering supplements and watching for small daily successes, will aid her in reaching her goal of breastfeeding her baby exclusively. Your close contact with her will give her the support and objectivity she needs in order to succeed.

SUMMARY

It is the caregiver's responsibility to give mothers the information and support they need in order to be confident in their ability to provide adequate amounts of milk to their baby. The possibility of a mother being physically unable to establish milk production or an infant being physically unable to achieve milk transfer is extremely rare. Problems with milk production and transfer usually result from inappropriate breastfeeding management. Identifying these problems early and taking appropriate action will prevent serious consequences for the baby. No breastfed baby should get to the point that he becomes dehydrated or fails to thrive. Breastfeeding dehydration and FTT occur because someone failed to give the mother appropriate advice and support. Also, they failed to recognize significant barriers to milk production or positive milk transfer. It is hoped that the issues presented in this chapter will help practitioners avoid such serious consequences.

REFERENCES

American Academy of Pediatrics, Breastfeeding and the use of human milk. *Pediatrics* 100:1035–1039; 1997.

Garza C and Butte N. Energy intakes of human milk-fed infants during the first year. *J Pediatr* 117 (Suppl): S124–S131; 1990.

Hill P. The enigma of insufficient milk supply. *American Journal of Maternal Child Nursing* 16:316–316; 1991.

Hill P and Humenick S. Insufficient milk supply. *Image* 21:145–148; 1989.

Hill P and Aldag J. Insufficient milk supply among Black and White breast-feeding mothers. *Res Nurs Health* 16:203–211; 1993.

Sofer S et al. Early severe dehydration in young breast-fed newborn infants. *Isr J Med Sci* 29:85–89; 1993.

Weichert C. Lactational reflex recovery in breastfeeding failure. *Pediatrics* 63:799–803; 1979.

BIBLIOGRAPHY

Butte N et al. Higher energy expenditure contributes to growth faltering in breast-fed infants living in rural Mexico. *J Nutr* 123:1028–1035; 1993.

Edwards A. et al. Recognizing failure to thrive in early childhood. *Arch Dis Child* 65:1263–1265; 1990.

Frantz K and Fleiss P. Ineffective suckling as a frequent cause of FTT in a totally breastfed infant. In Freier S. and Eidelman AL. (eds.) *Human Milk, Its Biological and Social Value*. Amsterdam: Excerpta Medica; 318–321; 1980.

Frantz K. The slow-gaining breastfeeding infant. Clinical issues in perinatal and women's health nursing. *Breastfeeding Nurses' Association of the American College of Obstetricians and Gynecologists* 3(4):647–655; 1992.

Grossman L et al. The effect of postpartum lactation counseling on the duration of breastfeeding in low-income women. *Am J Dis Child* 144:471–474; 1990.

Hill PD. Insufficient milk supply syndrome: Clinical issues in perinatal and women's health nursing. *Breastfeeding Nurses'*

Association of the American College of Obstetricians and Gynecologists 3(4):605–612; 1992.

Kaplan J et al. Fatal hypernatremic dehydration in exclusively breast-fed newborn infants due to maternal lactation failure. *Am J Forensic Med Pathol* 19:19–22; 1998.

Lawrence R. *Breastfeeding: A Guide for the Medical Profession*. St. Louis, MO: Mosby; 1999.

Meier P et al. A new scale for in-home test-weighing for mothers of preterm and high risk infants. *J Hum Lact* 10:163–168; 1994.

Neville M and Neifert M. *Lactation Physiology, Nutrition, and Breastfeeding*. New York: Plenum Press; 1983.

Stutte P et al. The effects of breast massage on volume and fat content of human milk. *Genesis* 10:22–25; 1988.

CHAPTER 17

CHANGES IN THE FAMILY

One who bears her children is a mother in part,
But she who nurses her children is a mother at heart.
Jacob Cats (1577–1660)

The one job almost every person shares in common at some point in their life is that of being a parent. Although we receive special instruction to qualify us for driving an automobile, for employment, and other life skills, our society does little to prepare us for the important job of parenthood. At the same time, fewer and fewer couples live near their extended families and, in many cases, have no family support system for everyday parenting. Increasingly, couples are left to their own devices as they use trial and error in establishing themselves as parents. This as well as other changes in the family that result from the birth of a new child are explored in this chapter. Mothers, fathers, and siblings have their own unique set of adjustments. You can provide assistance and support as the family settles into newly defined roles and relationships.

ACQUIRING THE PARENTAL ROLE

Parents learn their roles with their babies as an on-the-job training venture. No amount of preparation can totally prepare them for their interactions and parenting style with their unique children. However, most parents progress through predictable stages as they are preparing for and caring for their first child. The four stages of role acquisition are anticipatory, formal, informal, and personal (Bocar, 1987; Mercer, 1981).

The **anticipatory stage** is a time when parents begin to learn about their new roles. They may take classes, read books, and subscribe to parenting and child care magazines. They often begin asking questions of their own parents and other family or friends who already have children. After taking in and considering new information, they move into the **formal stage**. It is during this time that they begin to view their roles as parents more personally. They often strive for "parenting perfection" and aim to do it "just right." The frustration of this goal and the realization that "just right" is very individual leads them into the **informal stage**. This stage is a time of modifying, blending, and individualizing their roles to fit their unique family. Finally, as they

become more comfortable in their own parenting role, they move into the **personal stage**. At this time, their style of parenting evolves to be consistent with their personalities—parenting that fits them like an old glove.

The roles of the mother and father are developed in response to the needs of their baby, their family backgrounds, and the couple's own interaction. These roles are defined gradually through experience, and they are enhanced and made more enjoyable through open communication between both partners. Bonding to the baby by both the mother and father in the first hours and days of life seems to encourage the acceptance of their roles as parents and ensures their attachment to the baby. The mother's physical recovery and the development of realistic expectations can help her maintain a positive perspective. This enables her to make a smooth transition from the role of wife to mother, just as her partner redefines his role as a new father. The couple will learn to work together to support one another through this transition by helping each other adjust to the changes occurring in their lives.

Occasionally, new parents find it difficult to move beyond the formal stage of parenting to develop their own style. This is particularly evident in parents who have taken formal parenting classes or read books that are based on a rigidly structured approach to child-rearing. A program that espouses a rigid, rule-oriented, scheduled approach to parenting may be characterized by scheduled feedings, scheduled naps, high chair manners, playpen and room time, and chastisement for real or imagined infractions (such as banging the high chair tray). Such a program promises parents that if they follow it, the baby will be sleeping through the night at an early age. Concerns about this type of program have been raised by health professionals who see infants of these parents who present with slow weight gain, untimely weaning, and even failure to thrive. The American Academy of Pediatrics (AAP) passed a resolution in 1998 to continue to investigate and monitor these programs. There are concerns not only about the potential physical problems that can ensue from parents following the rules of the program but of the psychological outcome of children who are left to "cry it out" (Aney, 1998). As a lactation consultant, you need to be aware of these programs in order to tailor your advice to parents appropriately.

▼ Emotional Adjustments to Becoming a Mother

All women react differently to motherhood. Most new mothers have one characteristic in common, however. They have little or no idea of what to expect in their babies' behavior and development! They may have formed opinions on child care and find that these ideas do not work with their own baby. They may have had preconceived ideas about types of babies and find that theirs is another type entirely. Many parents eventually realize that even though their love for their baby is great, they need to develop special skills in order to be effective parents. They need to be reassured that these parenting skills are learned, not innate. Their competence and confidence will grow with practice, experimentation, observation, and self-education.

Every mother has some adjustments to make after her baby is born, whether she is having her first child, second, or fifth. These adjustments can affect her both physically and emotionally. A mother may not be prepared for the fact that caring for her baby is a round-the-clock job. She cannot return to her life as she knew it before. This is a wonderful phase in a family's life. At the same time, it can be frustrating to some women.

One of the pitfalls of counseling is to assume that the experienced mother does not need your support. She is constantly making adjustments, and although her questions and concerns will be different from those of a first-time mother, they are just as significant. Having a supportive person with whom she can share her concerns can be especially important for a mother who is often called on to help others in the family, such as siblings and grandparents, make their own adjustments. Her source of support may be a family member, a friend, or a support group.

The postpartum period is laden with emotions that rival the adolescent years. Hormonal shifts are dramatic within the first 24 hours after giving birth. Suddenly, a new little person is totally dependent on the mother. She is also coping with extraordinary body changes. Her emotions will be ruled by a combination of biochemical, psychological, and societal factors. Her birth experience may have been exhilarating, confusing, exhausting, or devastating. Her ideas about parenting and her expectations of herself, her baby, and her family may not reflect the reality of the situation. With some or all of these charged circumstances, it is an understatement to say that postpartum is a time of emotional adjustments!

The Lactation Consultant's Role with the Mother

You can offer valuable support to a mother by encouraging her to express her feelings. Show empathy, help her develop mothering skills, and encourage her to develop friendships with other new mothers. Praise and sympathy may help her see that her reactions are normal and that the blissful image of the perfect TV mother is far from reality. Encourage the mother to develop realistic expectations about her baby and about motherhood. Help her see that not all problems with her baby are a result of breastfeeding. If she is considering weaning, remind her that weaning may not solve her other problems. Her baby will still cry, and she will still feel tired and tied down at times. Bottle-feeding mothers have these problems, too!

The way in which a mother accepts and adjusts to the changes caused by parenthood, and how she interacts and communicates with others—her partner, family, friends and caregivers—are all a part of maturing. Some mothers, and some fathers, too, will breeze through trying times (Fig. 17.1). Others will have difficulty coping with relatively simple challenges. This is all a part of growth. Your role as a support person is to accept these parents where they are and to help them grow. Be patient, and encourage them to improve their situation one small step at a time. Help them focus on areas in which they can realistically make improvements.

Normal Postpartum Adjustments

Normal postpartum adjustments involve a variety of factors. Women often feel unprepared for their new role as mother. They may lack personal experience in caring for a baby and may not have family close by to support them and care for them in the early weeks. Often, it is assumed that because a mother is highly educated, she is

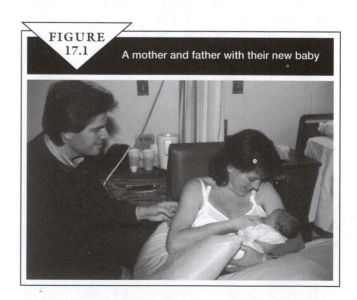

FIGURE 17.1 A mother and father with their new baby

comfortable and adequately prepared for parenting (Pridham, 1991). Sometimes, a mother's feelings of uncertainty in her role may show up as a specific concern or worry. Perhaps she believes her milk production is inadequate (Buttorf, 1990). Alternatively, she may be worried about how to handle her fussy baby.

If the mother has quit work, she will experience a loss of additional income and decreased contact with adults. The lack of adult contact can often result in feelings of isolation and loneliness. The mother may have no contact with other new mothers with whom she can share her feelings, or may receive little support from family or friends in her new role as mother. All of these factors can cause her to feel an absence of any sort of support system.

Baby Blues

The ability of women to adjust emotionally to motherhood varies greatly during the postpartum period. Some women need do no more than make room for the new baby. Many women, however, will have a few rough days, balanced by high moments. Some may feel blue for several weeks. Such reactions are considered perfectly normal. Such depression may be minimized by a positive birth experience and an abundance of emotional support and practical help following the birth. This brief depression, often called the **baby blues**, frequently appears around the third day postpartum. The mother may have bouts of tearfulness and sadness, mingled with happiness and excitement. These emotions are more common in women who are having their first baby.

Motherhood is a new job, and the stress of the new expectations may seem overwhelming at times. The mother may have a baby who is continually fussy and never sleeps, one who does not live up to her expectations of a happy responsive baby. She may have had a disappointing or unpleasant birth experience, or may have experienced an unwanted pregnancy. Poor nutrition and lack of rest can also cause emotional depression in the new mother, especially when coupled with the many adjustments to a new baby.

Depression may be expressed through a mother's tone of voice or by a lack of confidence in her ability to breastfeed. She may say she is lonely, has no visitors, and has no place to go. She may not answer her telephone or may stay away from home in an attempt to keep busy. She may demonstrate a lack of tolerance for other family members. One significant indication of depression may be that the mother does not refer to her baby by name.

Postpartum Depression

A small number of women become clinically depressed for several months following birth. They will require professional help that is outside of your role as lactation consultant. Typically, the mother will be depressed from 1 to 6 weeks postpartum. **Postpartum depression,** which is a mild to moderate depression, is characterized by mood changes, sleep disturbances, and fatigue. The mother feels unable to cope with life and may have unexplained physical symptoms such as abdominal pains or headache. She feels no attachment to her baby and worries that something is not "right." The mother may even entertain occasional thoughts of harming herself.

Loss of control is a significant emotion experienced after the birth of a baby. Beck (1993) found it to be at the core of postpartum depression. Other risk factors identified for postpartum depression include single marital status, low educational level, low income, and pregnancy complications (Burger, 1993). At present, there is no research that identifies a link between postpartum depression and physiologic changes such as postpartum hormonal shifts (Beck, 1993).

You should never attempt to counsel an emotionally distressed mother alone. Gently urge the mother to contact her physician for a referral to a professional therapist. In addition to counseling, treatment may involve medications, some of which are not compatible with breastfeeding. You can be a source of information for the mother by citing current medication information and providing her with resources. Premature weaning has been found to occur more frequently among depressed women (Cooper, 1993).

Postpartum Psychosis

Rarely, during the postpartum period, a psychosis develops that involves symptoms more serious than baby blues or depression. The mother's responses will go beyond insomnia, fatigue, and depression. **Postpartum psychosis** occurs on a much more intense level than postpartum depression. It can lead to a loss of control, rational thought, and social functioning. The mother may experience overwhelming confusion and hallucinations. She may even attempt to harm herself or her child. The priority for this mother is to keep her and her child safe and to get her into effective treatment immediately.

Survivors of Sexual Abuse

Survivors of sexual abuse are more common than you may think. Bass and Davis (1998) state that one in three women has been sexually assaulted in their lifetime. Long-term effects of the abuse will affect the functioning of at least 20 percent of adult survivors. Because of the intimate nature of breastfeeding, past sexual abuse may cause a disruption or disturbance of the breastfeeding process.

Pregnancy and childbirth are common times for a sexual abuse survivor to become aware of or be reminded of her abusive situation. Lactation consultants need to be aware that memories, flashbacks, and feelings from the abuse may interfere with the mother's ability to breastfeed. Memories may be triggered by the sounds or feelings of giving birth, the feeling of the baby at the breast, the loss of control felt in the early days of parenting, or even the sight of milk during letdown. Any of these events can trigger a flashback that causes the woman to feel uncomfortable with breastfeeding.

Identifying a Sexual Abuse Survivor

In some instances, a woman may tell you that she is a sexual abuse survivor. She may feel comfortable telling this to you because you take the time to listen to her concerns. You are assisting the mother with an intimate topic, and because of the nature of your role, you listen intently with warmth and caring. Your role as a lactation consultant requires you to be open and accepting. These are the attributes the survivor may look for in a confidante.

You may suspect the mother is a survivor by the way she positions herself when you assist her with latch on. Or she may seem to be uncomfortable holding the baby while she is discussing breastfeeding. Some warning signs that may indicate a history of abuse are late prenatal care, substance abuse, mental health concerns, eating disorders, poor compliance with self-care, or sexual dysfunction. She may feed expressed milk to her baby with a bottle and not put him to breast. Although these signals may not necessarily indicate a history of sexual abuse, they are signs that will alert you to possible problems.

Breastfeeding Implications for the Survivor

The most stressful time in the breastfeeding experience for the survivor will be during the early postpartum period, when the new mother is stressed, tired, and vulnerable. Although all new mothers can be affected at this time, survivors may be more emotionally fragile with memories of the abuse or depression. Nighttime breastfeeding can be a difficult time, because assault happened most often in the night at bedtime. Having someone feed her milk to the baby for the nighttime feed may help this situation. When the infant gets older and becomes more playful, the mother may seem reluctant to continue breastfeeding. Assuring the mother that her infant needs and desires her milk may help her breastfeed longer. You may need to support the mother in her decision to wean.

The mother will benefit from the positive experiences of breastfeeding. You need to be aware of situations that can provoke emotional or psychological discomfort. Be prepared to meet the mother's needs whatever they may be. Her choices in breastfeeding, which may mean expressing her milk and giving it by bottle, may not be what you would choose. Remember that those choices are best for her. The mother's reactions to a situation may vary widely. This is truly a situation in which you must meet the mother from her perspective. Some mothers have found breastfeeding to be too uncomfortable for them to continue. Others have found the breastfeeding experience to be quite healing. Be alert to the mother's feelings and provide support when possible including support for weaning if that is the mother's choice.

As a lactation consultant, it is not your role to treat or investigate sexual abuse situations. You will need to find a counselor who specializes in sexual abuse, preferably one who is familiar with breastfeeding mothers. Or you could meet with a counselor in your community to provide appropriate breastfeeding information.

▼ ## The Mother's Physical Recovery Following Birth

After a woman gives birth, there are many changes that take place within her body to return it to its prepregnant state. The early postpartum period can be a difficult time for a mother. Having just completed 9 months of pregnancy, she may feel disappointed that her abdomen still protrudes because of stretched muscles. Her walk may be more of a waddle because of loosened pelvic ligaments and stitches or pads. The fullness in her breasts may be slightly uncomfortable, and she will have little energy left to cope with her appearance and the stresses of daily life.

Assure mothers that this is normal! For the first 6 weeks, new mothers need rest for physical recovery. A mother who is getting insufficient rest may develop excessive bleeding, exhaustion, possible dizziness, or weak pelvic floor muscles. Add breastfeeding to the mix, and she may experience sore nipples or a breast infection. You can encourage her to get as much bed rest as possible. Staying in her bathrobe for the first few weeks will decrease her activity level and discourage visitors from staying too long. The mother can also nap when her baby naps and nurse while lying down to catch up on needed rest. A reminder of the need for moderation is especially helpful in the first weeks following delivery. By this time, the mother is beginning to feel energetic and restless at home, and may be more apt to overexert herself. Caution her to minimize household tasks and to take care not to resume strenuous activities too quickly. Her partner can help by limiting visitors during that time.

Familiarize the mother with the normal physical changes that occur during the weeks following delivery. As her body recovers, the new mother will want to be conscious of any unusual pains or sensations and report them to her physician. In addition to the usual postpartum characteristics involving the **uterus** and **perineum,** the new mother may experience some special problems with body functions or other minor physical irritations. The resumption of menstruation and the possibility of another pregnancy are also concerns for many new mothers. Lactation consultants who care for mothers in the early postpartum period can weave these matters into their teaching and include information about the helpfulness of breastfeeding to the healing process. Uterine recovery, more time for rest while nursing, relief of breast fullness, and delaying the return of fertility and menses are all benefits of breastfeeding.

Uterus

The uterus, which has attained a weight of about 2.5 pounds by delivery, begins to diminish in size soon after the birth of the baby. By 1 week postpartum, it has decreased to about 1 lb, and at 6 weeks, it is usually down to a size and weight of approximately 2 oz. During this time of involution, there is a discharge composed of blood, mucus, and tissue called **lochia,** which is the gradual sloughing off of the extra tissue lining the uterus. Its color transforms from red to pink, and then to white in about 3 weeks. A change in color from pink to white and back to red again may indicate that the mother's level of physical exertion is too high. Advise mothers to report this to their physician and to cut back on their activity level.

There is often an increase in lochia flow during some feeds, as a result of uterine contractions caused by the release of oxytocin. Sometimes, these contractions of the uterus may cause what is commonly referred to as afterpains. Afterpains usually last for only a few days to one week. Mothers who have had other children may find that these contractions are more severe. If it is too painful for the mother and she does not ask for help, it could affect her milk letdown. You can provide the mother with anticipatory guidance related to afterpains. Assure her that afterpains are normal. Encourage her to perform deep breathing exercises or possibly use pain medication approved by her physician. Reassure the mother that the pains last for only a few days after delivery and are nature's way of limiting blood loss.

Perineum

After a vaginal delivery, there is swelling and tenderness in the perineum, the region between the vagina and the rectum. Often, an **episiotomy**, which is a surgical incision between these two points, is performed to enlarge the vaginal opening during delivery. An episiotomy can increase postpartum swelling and cause a pulling sensation. Ice packs, sitz baths, sprays, cooling cotton pads, and medications can provide comfort for the mother.

Perineal floor exercises, known as **Kegel exercises**, will help the mother regain muscle tone in the pelvic floor, where stretching is most pronounced during labor. If these muscles remain weak, the uterus may tip or sink down into the vagina. The mother may also have difficulty controlling urination. To perform Kegel exercises, the woman inhales and then tightens the muscles surrounding her vagina, **urethra**, and **rectum** as she exhales. Such exercises can be performed regularly throughout the day. They will help return muscle tone, enabling the mother to maintain control of urination.

Body Functions

In the first few days postpartum, the mother may notice changes in her body functions. She may need to urinate frequently as she loses extra fluids accumulated during pregnancy. Many mothers have difficulty urinating, especially those who have had a **catheter** inserted in the bladder to keep it empty. It is not unusual for a mother to not have a bowel movement for a while after birth.

Initially, a woman who delivered vaginally may find it unsettling to assume a position that is similar to the position in which she had recently delivered her baby. She may fear that her uterus might be expelled or that her episiotomy will rupture or become more painful. A mother who had a cesarean delivery may have difficulty with bowel movements because her intestines were anesthetized during surgery and will need some time to resume normal functioning. The manipulation of the intestines during cesarean deliveries also causes gas and bowel dysfunction. Deep breathing exercises, rocking back and forth in a rocking chair, and alternate abdominal tightening and relaxation will help. She will also need a lot of bulk and fluids in her diet, and may require a stool softener if other methods fail. Some hospitals also offer antigas medication, which has not been shown to cause problems for breastfeeding babies.

Minor Irritations

There are a variety of other common minor irritations that women may experience during their early postpartum days. Some women experience backaches in the early weeks as a result of the hormones that had softened or loosened the sacroiliac ligaments and allowed more flexibility of the pelvic structure for birth. Backaches are also associated with the use of epidural anesthesia (MacArthur, 1993). Heat, massage, pelvic rock exercises, and correct lifting and breastfeeding positions will help. Another change women experience is heavy perspiration, particularly at night. This is the body's way of removing surplus fluid that has accumulated during pregnancy. Encourage the mother to wear cool, loose clothing and to take frequent showers to help her feel better.

Although less common today than in the past, shaving of the woman's pubic area before delivery is still practiced in some hospitals. Such a practice does not improve the outcome of the delivery. The decision to elect this type of preparation before delivery needs to be made jointly between the woman and her caregiver. If she has had a complete shave, the new mother may experience itching and chafing as the pubic hair grows back. Some women's hair follicles may become infected as a result of shaving practices (Brewer, 1981). The extra large sanitary pads used postnatally may be irritating. As the lochia discharge subsides, the mother may be more comfortable with a minipad.

Changing Priorities

Encourage the mother to evaluate her priorities concerning household chores. We all have different levels of tolerance for dirt, dust, and disorder. Some of us welcome the opportunity to relax our standards! A mother must work things out so that she and her family are satisfied. Pet peeves such as unwashed dishes or daily clutter are the chores to do first, because it takes less energy to do the chore than to become frustrated by it. Help the mother realize that the intense amount of time her baby now consumes will diminish rapidly. As the baby becomes efficient in expressing and meeting his own needs, the mother's schedule will become more relaxed and time for housework, hobbies, and relaxation will steadily increase.

Caution mothers that overdoing today results in a fussy baby tomorrow (if not tonight) and an exhausted mom, too! An overactive lifestyle may lead to a breast infection or a decrease in milk production. Each mother will make her own decision whether or not the importance of the task outweighs the consequence. If she has responsibilities such as a job, volunteer work, or transporting older children to activities, perhaps she can make some compromises or tradeoffs that will allow her the time she needs for herself and her baby. She can resume obligations slowly and watch the baby and other family members for signs of distress. If it is not working, she may need to cut back some of her outside commitments.

You can encourage the mother to be imaginative in developing arrangements to return to her previous obligations. She could work at home, employ a teenager, or trade favors with another mother. She might participate in only those activities where her baby is welcome, arrange to take her baby with her, or work out some other method to suit her needs. She may want to read some of the books available on how other mothers balance their demands. There are also organizations of mothers who have made a variety of lifestyle decisions. Searching the Internet may lead to connections with other mothers who are also awake at odd hours and find it hard to leave home for some adult conversation.

The mother's ability to adapt her lifestyle to motherhood will depend on her emotional well-being, her physical recovery, her maturity, and the support she receives from family and friends. You may be able to hasten the mother's recovery and her return to a workable schedule by encouraging her to rest during the early weeks. Help her form realistic expectations, and point out options she may have with household chores, child care, and obligations outside the home.

▼ Becoming a Father

Although there are no comparable physical adjustments to parenthood for the father as there are for the mother, there are a variety of social, emotional, and behavioral adjustments that he must make in redefining his role in terms of fatherhood. The father will be adapting to a new relationship with his mate, now a mother, and to the changes brought about by a new family member—a newborn baby who poses a very serious responsibility. On becoming a father, a man's role is usually expanded to one of supporter and helpmate, as well as one of protector and provider for his newborn infant. This represents an awesome responsibility to many men, and each will adjust in his own way. It is important that the mother accept her mate's definition of his role in parenthood. Encourage the couple to share their feelings with one another, both positive and negative, in an open and honest manner.

Like mothers, fathers learn their role through many factors. Society's definitions, experience with their own fathers, and peer pressure from other men will influence their approach. Pressure or encouragement from within their own family is also an issue. Each father will choose his own level of involvement in the care and nurturing of his baby. His level of participation seems to be enhanced when he is actively involved in the pregnancy and the labor and birth process.

Fathers and Common Parenting Issues

There are a wide range of opportunities for anticipatory guidance to help fathers ease into the parenting role. Even before the childbearing years, boys and girls alike deserve exposure to discussions of infant feeding and the importance of breastfeeding. Often, you have an opportunity to provide such education in your community schools. This is very important for planting the seed for future generations to make knowledgeable choices regarding infant feeding. Such early education results in breastfeeding becoming more acceptable, and therefore the norm.

When a couple discovers that they are expecting, frequently they seek out prenatal classes to prepare for their parenting role. You can be sure that the advertisement for your infant feeding class stresses that both the mother and father are invited. Further encouragement can be given for the father's participation through telephone contact with either parent. It is helpful to include a role model in the class. A new father who has "survived" the first weeks and months of parenting may be excited to share his experience. You can provide a realistic picture of life with the new baby. Learning what to expect and strategies for coping will help both parents ease into their roles.

Much focus in prenatal breastfeeding education is on the mother's needs. However, researchers have identified a need for educating fathers, as well as mothers, regarding the realities of breastfeeding. This will strengthen their involvement and validate their feelings in the early postpartum period (Freed, 1992; Gamble, 1992; Jordan, 1990). Jordan (1990) further notes that fathers often cite concerns related to breastfeeding such as limited opportunity to develop a relationship with their children initially, feeling inadequate, and feeling separated from their mates. Sensitivity to these concerns and appropriate guidance can be reflected in classes.

Walker (1991) suggests encouragement of other infant caregiving tasks such as bathing, burping, and diapering the baby. He can help the mother with positioning to breastfeed and can carry the baby in a sling and provide skin-to-skin contact. Fathers benefit from learning about infant cues and responsiveness in order to recognize what is normal and how to interact with their young infants (Delight, 1991).

Although the baby initially may show a preference for the mother, the father needs to have some time alone with the baby in order to develop his own parenting style and closeness to his child. Although he will have different strategies from the mother, his strategies are no less important or effective. He needs to be given encouragement in his new role (Eidelman, 1994; Graham, 1993; Jordan, 1993). Fathers may be further encouraged by the fact that they are the first person in their baby's life who teaches him that food and love must not always come from the same person!

Understanding the basics of breastfeeding will enable fathers to provide their wives with practical help. Fathers who attend prenatal classes may be better able to assist mothers in tangible ways such as helping the mother get comfortable. In more abstract ways, they can fill in pieces of information the mother may have forgotten and provide encouragement when she is having a bad day. Prenatal classes expose fathers to the normalcy of breastfeeding and the reasons why breastfeeding is important for babies. They learn practicalities of breastfeeding such as the economics, the ease of night time feeds, health issues, and overall convenience. These influences may further cement their support of their wives' decisions to breastfeed.

Finally, lactation education needs to address issues related to the mother and father as a couple. The father often feels as though he has lost his mate, because she seems immersed in the care of their new baby. Early parenting is very intense both physically and emotionally, whether the baby is breastfed or not. Fortunately breastfeeding simplifies some aspects of these early days. Nighttime feeds are easier, there is no special preparation for feeds, and the baby's food is always available.

Other aspects of life with a new baby—physical recovery from childbirth and changes in roles of the couple as new parents—will benefit from anticipatory guidance. Although physical recovery from childbirth is enhanced by breastfeeding, the reality remains that the mother will experience fatigue, discomfort, and breast changes in the early days. Parenting expands the couple's relationship to a wonderfully new dimension. This change is not without periods of stress and uncertainty. You can acknowledge these points when educating clients and stress that they are normal. Encourage parents to communicate with one another regarding their feelings and keep a focus on the couple aspect of their family through this time of great change.

Support Person for the Mother

A breastfeeding mother benefits from an abundance of emotional support from those close to her. Ideally a major portion of this support will come from her partner. Discussing plans for breastfeeding will enable them to share their opinions and concerns, and arrive at a mutual decision. Many mothers certainly can breastfeed without their mate's support. However, the experience is much more rewarding and fulfilling when it is shared by the entire family in a positive and accepting atmosphere.

Support by the father takes many forms. It can range from physical care of the baby, to helping with household chores, to a strong philosophical support of what the mother is doing. Often, the lack of sharing of tasks becomes a focus of the mother's complaints. She may wish that her mate would take more initiative in helping or that he were more competent with baby care and household chores. You can help her understand that learning these tasks is like learning a new job. Her partner needs time and encouragement to develop confidence and competence. Because she probably spends much more time with the baby than he does, she has learned very quickly how to interact with and care for him. She needs to be patient and give her mate the same opportunity to learn what works for him and how he fits in. When the mother encourages the father in his new role, she often finds that he becomes her best supporter and an outspoken advocate of breastfeeding.

Father's Interaction with Baby

Each father will choose his own type and level of involvement with his baby. Ideally, a father will participate in the birth process and begin to bond with his baby immediately after birth. He is likely to respond more openly and readily to the baby than a father whose first interaction occurs after the baby is brought home. It is helpful if the father devotes the first hours and days to becoming familiar with his newborn child and learning the skills necessary in comfortably caring for him. Mothers and fathers both need to learn these parenting skills. They do not come naturally as some parents expect.

A father can be invaluable in helping to soothe a fussy baby in such ways as walking, rocking, singing, and cooing. He can help the mother by sharing in the baby's care and by providing her some free time alone. He can bathe, burp, diaper, and play with his baby. Some fathers choose to bring the baby to the mother for nighttime feeds. Others prefer to limit their contact to when the baby is alert and pleasant.

Many mothers find that their mates' involvement increases as the baby gets older and responds to his attentions. Whatever type of interaction the father chooses, the mother wants to be careful not to discourage his efforts by criticizing the way he does things to the point that he limits his involvement. She can offer instructive guidance, particularly when a certain practice might be harmful to the infant (e.g., not supporting the infant's head when carrying or holding him). However, unwarranted criticism should be avoided. Although the father may do things differently from the mother, it may still be very satisfying for him and the baby.

The importance of the father-infant bond should be stressed to new parents. Many times, the father feels left out or ignored as this new person enters his life. Babies whose fathers interact with them on a continuing and consistent basis show an eagerness for learning. They may have a more confident self-image and show more confidence in relating to males. These babies are more likely to have a sense of humor and a longer attention span. Fathers benefit as well by interacting with their babies. By doing so, they attain permission to learn their new role and new job as a father. Fathers can learn how to care for the baby, can read to him, and can be supportive in easing the intensity of motherhood for both the parents and the baby. You can encourage fathers in their new role by emphasizing the importance of their interaction.

CHANGES IN FAMILY RELATIONSHIPS

The responsibility of being parents presents a major adjustment to many couples. At times, some new parents may feel resentful toward their baby for disrupting their lives and interfering with their freedom. Help them understand that such negative reactions are normal and are often balanced by deep feelings of affection and love for their infant. Parents need not feel guilty about their reactions. Encourage them to share their feelings honestly and openly with one another.

The need for open and honest communication is especially great during the first few months of parenthood. Both partners will feel inadequacies and a need for support in establishing their new roles as father and mother. They may react strongly to the ways in which the other performs his or her role. They may resent the fact that the baby now receives a lot of the affection and intimacy that was previously monopolized by the other partner. Remaining sensitive to one another's needs will help them to make compromises and adjustments.

▼ Sexual Adjustments

Re-establishing enjoyable sexual relations is an important part of the total adjustment for new parents. Effective communication between the man and woman and the passage of time will be major factors in their achieving this adjustment. By reassuring the mother that the need for sexual adjustment is common to most new parents, you can make it easier for her to discuss her feelings with her partner.

New babies consume a great deal of time and energy, and at the end of a tiring day, lovemaking may seem like just one more chore. As the mother becomes settled into her new role, she may be encouraged to look for ways to boost her energy level. She can nap when her baby naps, nurse while lying down, and sleep with her baby at night. Fatigue may also be related to her diet. You can help the mother look at her dietary practices and offer her suggestions for improvement through quick and healthy food choices (see Chapter 7). The mother can also explore ways to streamline her household tasks and ask for help to maximize her efficiency.

As a result, it is hoped that she will have time to enjoy companionship, conversation, and lovemaking with her partner. New fathers, as well as new mothers, need to be reassured that they are good parents. A woman may need to be reminded to praise her partner. Fatherhood is a part of manhood, and a confident man is more likely to inspire an enthusiastic sexual response from her. Her partner also will need to be understanding about the physical demands of motherhood and, at times, compromise his own needs.

Resuming Sexual Intercourse

Although the recovery period following birth may take several months, many physicians advise women that they may resume sexual intercourse after the 6-week checkup. This checkup indicates how the mother's recovery is progressing and whether any complications exist. Some couples are able to resume sexual relations before the 6-week checkup. The mother will want to listen to her body before resuming intercourse.

Emotional Factors

There are both physical and emotional factors involved in a woman's desire in or response to lovemaking in the months following childbirth. It may take several months for a new mother to regain her desire or for her responses to return to normal. This may be due, in part, to the fact that her baby is providing her with sufficient affection and emotional gratification, and she does not feel a need for further intimacy. You can assure the mother that this response is normal and that it usually subsides as she adjusts to her new role.

A woman may find that her breasts are oversensitive during foreplay or, at the other extreme, she may experience no sensual response at all to her partner's touch. Her responses will return to normal, usually within several months after delivery, although a few women may experience this throughout lactation. Some women describe themselves as becoming sexually aroused or experience an increased sensuality when nursing the baby. This may frighten them and cause them to wonder if this is an acceptable reaction. The sensation is a result of the hormone oxytocin, which is released during both lactation and orgasm. Women who experience this sensation need reassurance that nothing is wrong or inappropriate. This is part of the enjoyment of breastfeeding!

Either partner may be reluctant to engage in foreplay that involves the woman's breasts for fear of passing on germs. In a normal situation, in which the skin of the breast is healthy and unbroken, chances of transmitting an infection are minimal. The woman most likely has previously been exposed to any germs her mate may carry and she has produced, and will continue to produce antibodies to them in her milk. Thus, the baby will automatically be protected from infection. Parents need not let this fear hinder their lovemaking. The mother can cleanse her breasts with plain water before the next feed, if she desires.

Physical Discomfort

A new mother may experience some physical discomfort when she first resumes sexual intercourse. The hormones involved with lactation cause a decrease in vaginal lubrication, which may result in discomfort during intercourse. The discomfort can be relieved by an artificial lubricant, such as K-Y jelly. Interventions the mother experienced during birth often interfere with her desire for intimacy in the postpartum period. Intercourse may be painful because of pressure on an episiotomy or abdominal incision from a cesarean birth, or due to internal injury related to the use of forceps. A mother who experiences pain from a birth injury can explore ways to enhance intimacy that do not aggravate the injury. If she is not healing at a comfortable rate, she should be encouraged to seek advice from her physician.

Perineal floor exercises (Kegel exercises) are very important for general toning as well as for facilitating entrance in intercourse. If either partner does not experience physical sensations during intercourse, it may be the result of stretched pelvic floor muscles. If the muscles surrounding the vagina are not toned up sufficiently, then neither partner will feel much of anything. Perineal floor exercises will help retone these muscles.

Overfull or leaking breasts may be a source of discomfort for the mother. Sexual orgasm releases the hormone oxytocin, which also facilitates the letdown of the mother's milk. For this reason, leaking during intercourse is very common and indicates a positive response to lovemaking. If the couple is uncomfortable with the wetness that results, a towel can be used to protect the bed linens. An adjustment in positioning can alleviate pressure on the woman's breasts. Nursing the baby before intercourse will decrease fullness as well as leakage.

Adjusting Sexual Routine

As discussed earlier, adjustments in positioning can help alleviate physical discomfort caused by painful incisions or full breasts. An adjustment may also be needed in the couple's timing for their lovemaking. They may be tense if lovemaking begins at a time when the baby usually wishes to nurse or even if the baby is pleasantly awake. Nursing the baby immediately before bedtime and taking advantage of moments alone during nap time may provide the parents with an opportunity for intimacy.

Variations in technique or routine may also enhance lovemaking. If the mother experiences discomfort or lack of response in her breasts during foreplay, developing new patterns of foreplay can be an enjoyable solution. The stresses of discomfort and demands of the baby are easier to cope with when there is tenderness between the partners. Often it is effective for couples to have a period of rekindling their tenderness for each other by spending time just holding and cuddling.

The Lactation Consultant's Role

It is important for the mother and father to understand that their need for sexual adjustment is normal and common to new parents. This information can be imparted to them in a number of ways. You might routinely give mothers a piece of literature with pertinent points or address the issue of sexual adjustment at a group discussion. It is very reassuring to mothers to learn that some women experience the need for sexual adjustment after birth and that other breastfeeding mothers have vaginal dryness. For many, this reassurance is all that they need in order to realize that what they are experiencing is normal and that coping requires simply a little understanding and willingness to adapt.

▼ Menstruation and Fertility

Menstruation and fertility are delayed for varying periods of time during lactation. Studies demonstrate that the delay occurs as part of the mother's physiologic response to suckling and other infant stimuli. This changes the release of brain hormones and reproductive hormones, thus disrupting the ovulation and menstrual cycle. The single most important factor in suppression of ovulation in normal lactating women is the early establishment of frequent and strong suckling stimulus of the baby (McNeilly, 1993; Tay, 1996). Prolactin was thought to play the major role in this suppression of ovulation. However, current research shows that a variety of hormones are involved, and that prolactin is not an essential mediator. Researchers have noted a link between levels of growth hormone, leutinizing hormone, follicle-stimulating hormone, and estrogen (McNeilly, 1993).

Initially in the postpartum period and for some months thereafter, the breastfeeding mother experiences a phase of amenorrhea (lack of periodic vaginal bleeds). The menstrual cycle may be delayed for several months, followed by a period of resumed menstrual cycles that may be **anovulatory** or produce an inadequate ovum. The length of amenorrhea and infertility is linked to breastfeeding frequency, short intervals between feedings, (Gray 1993) duration of feedings (Diaz, 1991; Gellen, 1992; McNeilly, 1994; Vestermark, 1994), the presence of nighttime feeds, (Vestermark 1994), and the absence of supplemental feeds in the baby's diet (Diaz, 1992).

Menstruation may resume at any time for a breastfeeding mother and is greatly dependent on her overall breastfeeding pattern. The rate of return of menses is between 19 and 53 percent by 6 months postpartum in women who breastfeed exclusively (Lawrence, 1999). Although a very small percentage of women may resume menstruation as early as 6 to 12 weeks, others may not menstruate until breastfeeding has ceased totally. Some women experience a scanty show before their true menstrual cycles resume. The onset of menstruation should not be confused with any normal or abnormal postpartum bleeding. If the mother suspects abnormal bleeding, she should consult her physician.

Some women report a bleed around day 42 to 56. This may signal an end to lochial discharge, or it may reflect a change in the mothers' activity level (Visness, 1997). Other bleeding, or bleeding with breastfeeding difficulties, is a sign to seek immediate health care advice. Mothers can continue nursing during menstrual cycling because menstruation causes no significant changes in the composition of the mother's milk. Hormonal changes, however, may cause a change in the taste of her milk, which can prompt the baby to be fussy during a feed or even refuse to nurse. The infant's reaction may also be due to added tension in the mother or to swelling in the breast caused by menstrual edema. All of these factors can affect letdown.

Contraception

During the postpartum period, parents face important decisions about birth control methods. They may gather information about various contraceptive devices through reading, talking with friends, and consulting their physician. Often, a woman may ask you about the methods of birth control that are compatible with breastfeeding. Options available to a breastfeeding woman include

◆ Sterilization

◆ Lactational amenorrhea method (LAM)

◆ Foam and condom in combination

◆ Diaphragm

◆ Natural family planning methods

◆ Jellies and creams

◆ Oral contraceptives

◆ Injectable medroxyprogesterone (Depo-Provera)

◆ Implants of levonorgestrel (Norplant)

Of these contraceptive methods, the ones that are controversial with regard to breastfeeding mothers are the hormonal contraceptives. It is important to be aware of the whole of a woman's life when helping her choose among contraceptive options. Some, who fear another close pregnancy most of all, will not breastfeed if they cannot use a method that involves some mechanism outside themselves. These women need to have in-depth discussions with their prenatal care providers. If you first encounter such women postpartum, it may not be appropriate to encourage them to rely on breastfeeding and their own body's signals for family planning. You are not responsible for a mother's final choice; you are responsible only to ensure that your counseling is based on scientific evidence and that it supports her goals. Referral to other providers may help the mother find the solution that is best for her.

Lactational Amenorrhea Method (LAM)

The absence of ovulation and menstruation is not merely a convenience to the mother during lactation. Research has demonstrated that lactation can delay the return of fertility during the postpartum period. Women who are breastfeeding fully (that is frequently day and night), and are experiencing lactational amenorrhea, are more than 98 percent protected from pregnancy for 6 months after birth (Hight-Laukaran, 1997; Kennedy, 1998; Labbok, 1994, 1997). This fact has given rise to the lactational amenorrhea method (LAM) of contraception (Fig. 17.2).

LAM has three conditions: The mother's menses has not yet returned, the baby is breastfed around the clock without significant amounts of other foods in the diet, and the baby is younger than 6 months of age. This also implies that the baby is not given a pacifier and that all sucking is at the breast. If any one of these conditions is not met, the mother is at increased risk of pregnancy and should supplement with another method to ensure an adequate interval between births. For LAM to be most effective, it is recommended that the baby breastfeed optimally, beginning soon after birth and continuing to breastfeed exclusively day and night for 6 months. The use of artificial nipples, such as a bottle or pacifier,

interferes with frequency and duration of suckling at the breast and therefore is not recommended.

LAM offers a method of protection from pregnancy at a vulnerable time in the mother's life—the first 6 months postpartum. It does so with no side effects to either the mother or child. Many mothers find this an excellent opportunity to be in tune with their bodies and to work with their own natural tendencies. There is no need to purchase contraceptive items, so the mother's economic resources are not drained. Nor does she need to worry about availability. LAM requires only that the mother learn the three signs, and that she breastfeed her child in an optimal manner. Such a method that allows a mother to meet both her needs and her baby's needs in a safe manner deserves to be included in the repertoire of family planning options that are often part of prenatal and postpartum education. Mothers need to understand that as soon as there is a decline in breastfeeding, either

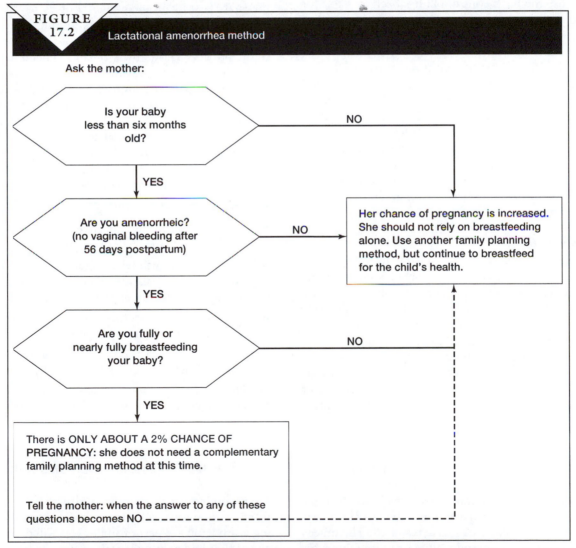

FIGURE 17.2   Lactational amenorrhea method

Ask the mother:

Is your baby less than six months old? — NO →

Her chance of pregnancy is increased. She should not rely on breastfeeding alone. Use another family planning method, but continue to breastfeed for the child's health.

↓ YES

Are you amenorrheic? (no vaginal bleeding after 56 days postpartum) — NO →

↓ YES

Are you fully or nearly fully breastfeeding your baby? — NO →

↓ YES

There is ONLY ABOUT A 2% CHANCE OF PREGNANCY: she does not need a complementary family planning method at this time.

Tell the mother: when the answer to any of these questions becomes NO - - - - - - - - - - - - - - - -

Reprinted by permission of the Institute for International Studies in Natural Family Planning from *Guidelines for Breastfeeding in Family Planning and Child Survival Programs,* Washington, DC, Georgetown University, Labbok M, Koniz-Booher P, Cooney K, Shelton J, and Krasovac K(eds); January 1990.

because the baby is receiving other foods regularly or is nursing less often, the contraceptive protection decreases.

Oral Contraceptives

Combination oral contraceptives contain both estrogen and progesterone. They appear to cause the most difficulty in lactating women, especially in the early postpartum period, before lactation is well established. Oral contraceptives may affect milk volume, and concerns related to milk composition have also been raised (Erwin, 1994). Long-term effects of oral contraceptive use on babies are not known—although none have ever been seen.

Current research into the long-term effects of oral contraceptives is limited both in terms of quantity and length of study, reaching only to puberty of the exposed children (Pardthaisong, 1992). No account has yet been taken of the effects that this hormonal exposure will have on the reproductive potential of these children. However, because the birth control pill has been available for nearly 40 years, one would expect that any adverse effect would have been noted. Generally, it is recommended that breastfeeding women delay taking combined oral contraceptives for at least 6 months postpartum.

Progestin-only oral contraceptives (i.e., the mini pill) do not appear to interfere with milk production, and therefore are deemed more acceptable to use during lactation (Dunson, 1993; Speroff, 1993). However, the long-term effects, as previously described, remain unknown. Generally, it is not recommended to begin this method before 6 weeks postpartum. Women who are familiar only with oral contraceptives may find this information daunting.

Other Methods

Periodic abstinence, or natural family planning, is another contraceptive option. It includes charting the **basal body temperature,** (temperature taken on waking around the same time each day) or checking vaginal secretions and keeping a careful calendar record of menstrual periods to predict fertile days. This method is not to be confused with the rhythm method, which is less effective in many settings. That method involves estimating the fertile period from the calendar records of menstrual periods alone. In total natural family planning, the changes in cervical mucus before ovulation help signal the beginning of the fertile days.

Women who are familiar with natural family planning will probably have more success with it postpartum than new users, because the signs can be quite different during lactation. Cervical mucus patterns in the first few breastfeeding months postpartum may be less clearly defined than after regular cycles have resumed. The mucus changes from a scant semisolid white or yellowish matter to an abundant thin, clear, watery and slippery fluid that allows the sperm to penetrate the canal of the cervix easily. Also, fluctuations in the woman's basal body temperature aid the couple in determining fertile periods. During menses and up to ovulation, the basal body temperature is at its lowest phase. After the time of ovulation, the temperature will rise. It will stay at about that level until just before the onset of menses. Couples use the combination of mucous and temperature changes to identify the 5 to 7 days per month when infertility cannot be confirmed and conception is possible.

Points for Parents to Consider

You can direct couples to sources of more detailed information without becoming involved in the details of their sexual relationship. Most physicians' offices provide pamphlets and leaflets on topics such as family planning, sex education, parenting, and sterilization. Literature on each of the individual birth control methods is also available free of charge. Lactation consultants who teach prenatal classes can encourage couples to discuss contraception with their providers during pregnancy to provide sufficient time for careful consideration. The obstetric provider knows the woman's general medical history, family history, and other needs for medication that may influence which options are contraindicated for her. The choice of contraceptive method is the parent's responsibility. Restrict your help to that of offering counseling concerning options that are compatible with breastfeeding, rather than giving advice.

The following considerations may be helpful to parents in selecting a form of contraceptive:

◆ Religious or ethical feelings about birth control.

◆ Concerns regarding effectiveness. How disruptive would a pregnancy be at this time in their lives?

◆ Choice of who will take responsibility for contraception. Will they share responsibility by alternating methods or by mutual participation?

◆ Most convenient method in terms of remembering to use it and desiring to use it every time.

◆ How closely they want their method to be associated with actual intercourse.

◆ How they feel about expense, inconvenience, foreign objects, messiness, and loss of spontaneity.

▼

SIBLING REACTIONS AND ADJUSTMENTS

Homecoming for the parents and new baby may range from a very smooth adjustment to a distant or demanding attitude on the part of siblings. It will depend on the age of the child and the length of time he has been separated from his mother. Prepare the mother for possible

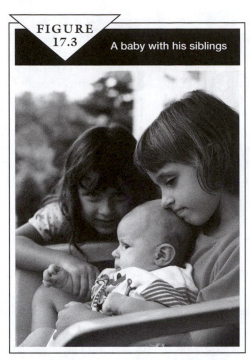

FIGURE 17.3 A baby with his siblings

Reprinted by permission of Debbie Shinskie.

changes in her older children and let her know that these are common reactions. She may be engrossed with the baby and feel less close to her other children for a while. This may cause the children to show some jealousy and perhaps develop a closer relationship with their father or other relative in the early weeks, while appearing distant to the mother. Relationships will mend as all family members learn to love the baby in their own way (Fig. 17.3).

Helping Siblings Prepare for the New Baby

Parents can begin preparing their children for the baby's arrival by sharing the events of pregnancy with them. They can discuss the development of the fetus, visits to the physician, and what will take place at the hospital or other birth environment. Parents can read books to the sibling that depict a new baby in the family. Children can also be involved in preparing for the baby. They can help with getting clothes and baby equipment ready, as well as packing the mother's suitcase. If the child's sleeping arrangements must be changed, parents will want to do this early and in such a way that the older child does not feel crowded out by the new baby.

Perhaps the mother could make a construction paper booklet with magazine pictures about what it is like in the hospital (physicians, nurses, nursery pictures), coming home, with the baby at home—bathing, sleep-

ing, nursing, crying—and the new family. Looking at their own family's baby pictures can be fun, too. She can prepare the child for what new babies do—such as nursing, sleeping, and crying—and the fact that they are not yet able to play. Any changes in usual activities and the reasons for those changes can also be discussed. The mother can tell her child that she will need his help in caring for the new baby, with such things as bringing diapers and clothing to her, holding the baby, talking to him, and getting him to smile. Siblings can also be prepared by visiting a family with a new baby to see what a new infant looks and sounds like. The parents and siblings of that infant may also be of help in explaining to the child some of the changes in their family.

Preparing for the Mother's Absence

It is important that the older child be prepared for his mother's absence during her hospital stay. He will want to understand where the mother is going, why, for how long, and what she will do while she is there. It may help to visit the hospital with him during the pregnancy, so he can better understand what will take place. Many hospitals offer sibling classes and tours, and sibling visitation during the mother's postpartum stay can be worked out at that time. The mother can also plan to maintain contact with her family through phone calls, notes, and instant photos while in the hospital.

Some parents choose to have siblings present at the baby's birth. Such a choice requires preparation about what birth is like and how the mother will act. When siblings are present at the birth, a caregiver needs to be present just for the children in order to meet their needs during the experience. The sibling should be given the choice about whether or not to be present at the actual time of delivery.

Adjusting to the New Baby

Whenever a new baby is brought into a family, the role of each family member is redefined and expanded. An older child who previously had been the "baby of the family" will lose his position as the center of attention. He may need to assume responsibility for tasks that had previously been performed by his parents. He may be expected to dress himself, help with household chores, and generally fend for himself instead of always relying on someone being there to help him.

Each child needs time and understanding in assuming his new role. The parents can help him adjust by making him feel special in new ways. The mother can begin fostering her older child's emotional growth by giving him her undivided attention the first time she sees him following the birth of the baby. She can have another adult hold the baby while she renews physical contact with her older child and expresses her love for him. After the family is settled, the parents can create situations where each child can look at, touch, or hold the baby. Suggest that the mother set aside special moments during each day for the other children, to let each one know how she appreciates his unique qualities.

During feeds, a sibling may want to be included in the closeness and interaction he observes between his mother and the new baby. To accommodate this the mother could nurse her baby where there is ample room for all family members, such as the bed, couch, or floor. She can plan activities during nursing times which she can share with her toddler, such as reading books, playing simple games ("I spy something red"), and activities (paper and crayons, tea party, puzzles, record playing).

A toddler who had weaned may ask to nurse again. If the mother gives him the opportunity to do so, he will be reassured by his mother's awareness of his needs and her willingness to respond favorably. He may want only to taste the milk, in which case the mother can put some of her milk in a cup to satisfy his curiosity. This renewed interest in breastfeeding is usually temporary. However, occasionally a toddler might resume nursing on a regular basis and the mother may need your support (see Chapter 23).

Despite the parents' efforts toward a smooth adjustment, some toddlers and young children may exhibit regressive behaviors when a new baby arrives. These behaviors can include such things as whining, baby talk, bed wetting or accidents from a previously toilet-trained older child, waking during the night, clinging to the mother, or hitting the baby. Such behavior may be the child's way of asking for attention. Often, a child will develop mixed feelings about the new baby. He may enjoy cuddling and talking to the baby and, at the same time, may find it difficult to share his mother's attention with him. The mother can reassure her child that she understands and accepts his feelings and him. She can help him find his new position in the family by giving him special opportunities to demonstrate his capabilities in caring for the baby. Also, she can emphasize his importance as an older child in protecting and amusing the baby. She can point out the many benefits and privileges of being more independent and self-reliant.

SUMMARY

Your availability and support to couples will help them as they evolve into their new role as parents. Mothers will experience both emotional and physical adjustments following birth. Understanding typical postpartum adjustments and the aspects of physical recovery will help

them avoid needless worrying. Fathers have their own unique adjustments as they learn how to interact with their new baby and provide support to their mate. As a couple, the mother and father will experience adjustments in their sex life and will need to consider contraceptive options that are compatible with breastfeeding. Siblings will benefit from preparation for the mother's absence during the birth, as well as understanding as they adjust to the new baby. This is an exciting time for the family as they welcome a new baby into their home and learn to respond to one another in new ways.

REFERENCES

Aney M. Babywise linked to dehydration, failure to thrive. *AAP News*, April; 1998.

Bass E and L Davis. *The Courage to Heal*. New York; Harper Collins; 1994.

Beck C. Teetering on the edge: A substantive theory of postpartum depression. *Nurs Res* 42:42–48; 1993.

Bocar DL and K Moore. *Acquiring the Parental Role*. Lactation Consultant Series #16. New York: Avery Publishing Group; 1987.

Brewer G and JP Green. *Right from the start: Meeting the challenge of mothering your unborn and newborn baby*. Emmaus, PA: Rodale Press, p. 52; 1981.

Burger J et al. Psychological sequelae of medical complications during pregnancy. *Pediatrics* 91:566–571; 1993.

Buttorf J and Morse J. Mothers perceptions of breast milk. *JOGNN* 19:518–526; 1900.

Cooper P et al. Psychosocial factors associated with the early termination of breastfeeding. *J Psychosom Res* 37:171–176; 1993.

Delight E et al. What do parents expect antenatally and do babies teach them? *Arch Dis Child* 66:1309–1314; 1991.

Diaz S et al. Relative contributions of anovulation and luteal phase defect to the reduced pregnancy rate of breastfeeding women. *Fertil Steril* 58:498–503; 1992.

Diaz S et al. Early difference in the endocrine profile of long and short lactational amenorrhea. *J Clin Endocrinol Metab* 72:196–201; 1991.

Dunson T et al. A multicenter clinical trial of a progestin-only oral contraceptive in lactating women. *Contraception* 47:23–35; 1993.

Eidelman A et al. Comparative tactile behavior of mothers and fathers with their newborn infants. *Isr J Med Sci* 30:79–82; 1994.

Erwin P. To use or not use combined hormonal oral contraceptives during lactation. *Fam Plann Perspect* 26:26–30; 1994.

Fly A et al. Major mineral concentrations in human milk do not change after maximal exercise testing. *Am J Clin Nutr* 68:349–351; 1998.

Freed G, et al. Attitudes of expectant fathers regarding breast-feeding. *Pediatrics* 89:224–227; 1992.

Gamble D and Morse J. Fathers of breastfed infants: Postponing and types of involvement. *JOGNN* 22:358–365; 1992.

Gellen J. The feasibility of suppressing ovarian activity following the end of amenorrhea by increasing the frequency of suckling. *Int J Gynecol Obstet* 39:321–325; 1992.

Graham M. Parental sensitivity to infant cues: Similarities and differences between mothers and fathers. *J Pediatr Nurs* 8:376–384; 1993.

Gray R et al. The return of ovarian function during lactation: results of studies from the U.S. and the Philippines. In Gray R (ed). *Biomedical and Demographic Determinants of Reproduction*. Oxford: Colorado Press, 428–445; 1993.

Hight-Laukaran V et al. Multicenter Study of the Lactational Amenorrhea Method (LAM) II. Acceptability, Utility, and Policy Implications. *Contraception*, 55:337–346; 1997.

Holz KA. A practical approach to clients who are survivors of childhood sexual abuse. *J Nurse-Midwife* 39(1):13–18; 1994.

Jordan P and Wall V. Supporting the father when the infant is breastfed. *J Hum Lact* 9:31–34; 1993.

Jordan P. and Wall V. Breastfeeding and fathers: Illuminating the darker side. *Birth* 17:210–213; 1990.

Kendall-Tackett K. Breastfeeding and the sexual abuse survivor *J Hum Lact* 14(2)125–130; 1998.

Kennedy K et al. "Consensus statement on the use of breast-feeding as a family planning method." *Contraception* 39:477–496; 1989.

Kennedy K et al. Users' understanding of the Lactational Amenorrhea Method and the occurrence of pregnancy. *J Hum Lact* 14:209–218; 1998.

Kennedy K et al. Concensus Statement: Lactational Amenorrhea Method for family planning. *International Journal of Gyn/Ob* 54:55–57; 1996.

Labbok M et al. Multicenter Study of the Lactational Amenorrhea Method (LAM) I. Efficacy, Duration, and Implications for Clinical Application. *Contraception* 55:327–336; 1997.

Lawrence R. *Breastfeeding: A guide for the medical profession.* New York: Mosby; 1999.

MacArthur C and Knox G. Association with backache is real. *Br Med J* 307:64; 1993.

McNeilly A et al. Physiological mechanisms underlying lactational amenorrhea. *Ann NY Acad Sci* 709:145–155; 1994.

McNeilly A. Lactational amenorrhea. *Endocrinol Metab Clin North Am* 22:59–73; 1993.

Mercer R. A theoretical framework for studying factors that impact on the maternal role. *Nurs Res* 30:73–77; 1981.

Pardthaisong T et al: The long term growth and development of children exposed to Depo-Provera during pregnancy or lactation. *Contraception* 45:313–324; 1992.

Pridham K, et al. Early postpartum transition: Progress in maternal identity and role attainment. *Res Nurs Health* 14:21–31; 1991.

Speroff L. Postpartum contraception: Issues and choices. *Dialogues in Contraception* 3:1–3, 67-; 1992–1993.

Tay C et al. Twenty-four hour patterns of prolactin secretion during lactation and the relationship to suckling and the resumption of fertility in breast-feeding women. *Human Reprod* 11:950–955; 1996.

Vestermark V et al. "Postpartum amenorrhoea and breastfeeding in a Danish sample. *J Biosoc Sci* 26:1–7; 1994.

Visness C et al. The duration and character of postpartum bleeding among breastfeeding women. *Obstet Gynecol* 89:159–163; 1997.

Walker M. Breastfeeding and fathers: The darker side: Reply. *Birth* 18:175; 1991.

BIBLIOGRAPHY

Beck C. A checklist to identify women at risk for developing postpartum depression. *JOGNN* 27:39–46; 1998.

Blume ES. *Secret Survivors: Uncovering Incest and its After-effects in Women,* New York: John Wiley & Sons; 1990.

Bohn DK. Domestic violence and pregnancy. Implications for practice. *J Nurse-Midwife* 35(2):86–98; 1990.

Mullen PE et al. Impact of sexual and physical abuse on women's mental health. *Lancet* 16:841–845; 1988.

Murphy S. Siblings and the new baby. Changing perspective. *J Pediatr Nurs* 8:277–288; 1993.

Newton N. Psychologic differences between breast and bottle feeding. *Am J Clin Nutr* 24:993–1004; 1971.

Simkin P. Memories that really matter. *Childbirth Instructor* 4(1):20–23, 39; 1994.

C H A P T E R

18

SPECIAL COUNSELING
CIRCUMSTANCES

Contributing Author: Carole Peterson

Lactation consultants meet women with a rich variety of lifestyles and choices. Sometimes, these circumstances affect the mother's options and decisions. As a counselor to many types of women, you need to be conscious of culture and lifestyle choices. Your ability to counsel and establish rapport with a mother could be affected by lack of knowledge or assumptions that are made about a mother. This discussion deals with some of the situations you may encounter in which your counseling technique may be altered by the mother's lifestyle choice or influence from others who are close to her.

OPPOSITION TO BREASTFEEDING

Despite the strong endorsement of breastfeeding by the American Academy of Pediatrics (AAP, 1997), there are still widespread negative attitudes toward breastfeeding in this country. When the number of women breastfeeding increases, it will gain wider acceptance and public approval as the natural and normal way to feed a baby. However, today mothers often receive questions and comments that prompt them to explain and defend their decision to breastfeed. Such remarks can undermine a mother's confidence and cause her to doubt her decision or her capability to breastfeed. It may help the mother realize that most of these people do not truly oppose breastfeeding. They simply may not understand it. When the mother is confident in her decision to breastfeed, she may be able to educate some of these people and familiarize them with the feeding patterns of a breastfed baby.

Opposition to breastfeeding often manifests itself, not as blatant remarks, but as subtle undermining of the mother's efforts. Professionals and laypersons alike are often quick to state that breastfeeding is "the best" infant food. However, when the baby cries or the mother expresses a concern, breastfeeding is blamed. The mother is encouraged to "rest" and give a bottle, as though breast and bottle were interchangeable. Mothers

will benefit from your education and support to get them through those challenging times when doubts are raised and the mother's confidence is undermined.

As a lactation consultant, you cannot control the pressures a mother may encounter while she is breastfeeding. You can, however, provide positive support, suggest ways for her to cope with the opposition, and personally make an extra effort to boost her morale and self-confidence. Questions or remarks mothers often receive are

- How long do you plan to nurse?
- Are you *still* breastfeeding?
- Isn't he getting a little old to nurse?
- Does he want to nurse again so soon?
- He seems hungry all the time; maybe your milk isn't rich enough or maybe you don't have enough milk.

A mother may receive opposition from a variety of people. It may come from strangers, friends, her employer, her physician, the baby's grandparents or other relatives, or even the baby's father. Some of these are more difficult to cope with than others. Having sources of support for breastfeeding has been identified with a more successful outcome (Buckner, 1993; McNatt, 1992). You can help mothers identify the various breastfeeding supporters within her network of friends and family. The support will help the mother through the challenges she may face when others oppose or question her choice to breastfeed.

Opposition from Strangers

A mother who is confident and knowledgeable about her decision to breastfeed is less likely to be affected by the opinions or rude remarks of a total stranger. In order to minimize the potential for such comments, she can ensure that she is discreet when she is breastfeeding in public. She will want to wear clothing that allows easy access to her breast while still providing coverage. Practicing discreet breastfeeding in front of a mirror will help her become confident with techniques that work for her.

Opposition from Friends

Opposition from friends may prove more difficult for the mother to handle. Depending on the nature of the friendship, a mother may attempt to educate a friend who opposes breastfeeding. She needs to find a comfort level with such a friend in order to maintain both their relationship and her breastfeeding. Developing friendships with people who are supportive of breastfeeding or who are breastfeeding mothers themselves may help her become more confident with breastfeeding.

Opposition from the Mother's Employer

Many women who return to work while they are still breastfeeding experience negative reactions from their employers. Although there are numerous employers who are supportive of breastfeeding women, there are many more who make it difficult for women employees to combine working and breastfeeding. The stress and tension created by an unsupportive work environment can be avoided if the mother speaks frankly with her employer about her plans to breastfeed. She can discuss any special needs she will have in terms of either breastfeeding her baby at work or expressing milk for her baby, as well as her desire to continue working.

The mother may need to convince her employer that she will make every effort possible to ensure that breastfeeding will not interfere with her job performance. She may also point out to her employer the health benefits of breastfeeding that result in less use of time off and less need to use medical benefits. Employers who have had experience with breastfeeding employees often have more positive attitudes about combining employment with breastfeeding. Negative attitudes have been shown to be related more to lack of experience than to outright opposition (Bridges, 1997). Lactation consultants could approach employers in their communities about breastfeeding's contribution to infant and maternal health and the implications of that for employment. Many would probably be more responsive if they were aware of breastfeeding's importance to society.

Some women are uncomfortable approaching their employer, especially those in a male-dominated profession or those with little job security. They may worry that their position will be jeopardized by such a "feminine request." These mothers need to look at their job and decide which aspects could be compatible with breastfeeding. In some cases, the woman may be unable to resolve the lack of support from her employer. If she finds that the situation is undermining her breastfeed-

ing, she may need to re-evaluate her priorities and motives regarding working and breastfeeding. Unreasonable and unfair treatment by an employer can be referred to a local labor relations board. However, there are work environments that are not conducive to breastfeeding. You can help the mother by assisting her in developing a plan within the parameters of her employment. See Chapter 22 for further discussion of combining breastfeeding with employment.

Opposition from a Physician

It is often difficult for a mother to deal with her physician's lack of support for breastfeeding. She values her physician's opinions and trusts his judgments about the care of her baby. If the physician does not seem very committed to breastfeeding, he may be unsupportive and give her misinformation about its management. If the mother has a good rapport with her physician, she may be able to work out differences about breastfeeding. Telling her physician how important it is to her and to her baby is a first step. If the mother does not have a good rapport with her physician, she may need to consider whether this relationship is good for her.

A mother with an unsupportive physician needs a lot of extra contact and confidence building. She may be the patient who provides information to the physician that helps him understand the importance of breastfeeding. Sharing of information in order to provide anticipatory guidance will help this mother through times of change and uncertainty. It may help to provide her with information, such as research articles, to share with her physician to back up her efforts. Sometimes, a perceived lack of support by a physician may actually stem from lack of knowledge and experience with breastfeeding. The topic of physicians, mothers, and breastfeeding is also discussed in Chapter 2.

Opposition from Grandparents and Other Relatives

In many cultures, the baby's grandmother has a pivotal role in a mother's breastfeeding experience. Often, a new mother will turn to her own mother for encouragement and wisdom as she develops into her own parenting role. This is true particularly if she is a first time mother. Breastfeeding is a part of the feminine identity. During their mother's childbearing years, many women were discouraged from breastfeeding for a multitude of poor reasons. However, these reasons remain as part of their understanding of the childbearing continuum. It is difficult for mothers to disregard these beliefs without feeling guilty.

A grandmother may see the choice to breastfeed by her daughter as a reflection on her own parenting choice. Some grandmothers and grandfathers express real sympathy for the strains of early parenting—lack of sleep, coping with crying, and physical recovery from birth. They may perceive that breastfeeding makes those strains even harder. Consequently, they will encourage the mother to decrease stress by supplementing breastfeeding or weaning.

A mother who receives negative comments from her own mother or mother-in-law needs to understand the grandmother's concern for both the mother and baby. She does not want her daughter to be disappointed by the same failure she may have experienced. On the other hand, she may be envious that her daughter can do something she was not able to do. Additionally, the grandmother may be experiencing her own guilt about not breastfeeding her own children.

You can help the mother recognize that her own mother did the best she could at the time for her child with the information and support that she had at hand. She may even be encouraged to share gently with her mother that she understands that she did her best and that she herself is also doing the same today for her child with the information we now have. Because the grandmother may not understand the typical feeding pattern of a breastfed baby, she may worry that his frequent feeds indicate that he is not being properly nourished. This concern may undermine the new mother's confidence and come through as lack of support for her daughter's breastfeeding.

You can encourage the mother to be patient and understanding of any relative, especially a grandparent, whose opposition stems from a genuine concern for the mother and baby. Perhaps she can attempt to educate the grandmother and enlist her support by giving her some literature to read or urging her to talk with a supportive physician or lactation consultant. She may simply need to accept the grandmother's point of view and not allow it to affect her breastfeeding. She will need to stay firm in her resolve while remaining kind and considerate.

▼ Opposition from the Baby's Father

It is especially difficult for a mother to encounter opposition from the baby's father. Often, the father's preference is significant in the mother's choice for infant feeding. Thus, his opposition will weigh greatly on her decision to initiate or continue breastfeeding (James, 1994). Sometimes, a father may seem to be unsupportive of breastfeeding because he wants his child to be independent and worries that breastfeeding will make the baby too dependent on the mother. You can give the

mother reading material on child development and explain how meeting a child's needs in the present will actually make him less dependent in the future. Encourage her to share this information with the baby's father. She can use facts about the importance of breastfeeding as a springboard to discuss her feelings surrounding the issue.

If the father believes that breastfeeding interferes with the couple's sex life, help him see that having a baby interferes with all parents' sex lives no matter how the baby is fed! If he seems jealous, you can suggest that the mother spend some special time alone with him. The father's opposition may stem from the same concerns as those of grandparents and other relatives—the health and well-being of his partner and baby. You can point out the positive aspects of this concern and suggest ways for the mother to reassure and educate the father that breastfeeding is beneficial to the entire family and that *not* breastfeeding increases many health risks for both the mother and baby.

Point out how the emotional benefits of breastfeeding have enhanced their baby's pleasant disposition and how that contributes to family harmony. The father can also be given literature about the nutritional benefits of mother's milk. Help him recognize the evidence of health benefits in his own baby's growth and development. If the baby's father feels left out of his care because he is not able to feed him, the mother can suggest ways for him to be involved other than with feeds. See Chapter 17 for more discussion of the father's interaction.

As the man's role changes from mate to father, it may be difficult for him to regard the woman's breasts as something other than sexual. In Western culture, women's breasts are promoted in a sexual manner in all forms of media. The father may subconsciously believe that the baby is invading his territory. The couple needs to discuss the man's concerns openly. Throughout evolution, the purpose of the female breast has been to nurture babies. Encourage the couple to discuss these issues with sensitivity and understanding.

As the baby grows older, a previously supportive father may question the need or appropriateness of continuing to breastfeed an older baby. This is true especially if the baby is male. Society's sexual preoccupation with the breast may cause worry of a loss of masculinity due to an over dependence on the mother. The mother can gently and patiently remind the father of the benefits of breastfeeding for the baby both nutritionally and developmentally at any age. She can help him understand the baby's needs and her desire to continue breastfeeding.

In some cases, a mother may never resolve the father's opposition to breastfeeding. She will need a great deal of support and will benefit from frequent contacts. If the mother decides to wean her baby because of the father's opposition, you need to accept this decision and help the mother wean gradually and with love. As a lactation consultant, avoid placing yourself in the middle of a conflict between a breastfeeding mother and an unsupportive partner. You can serve as a listening ear for the mother, perhaps suggesting reading material for the father and offering the mother extra support. You can help a mother understand that her partner's not choosing to be involved in certain areas of care, such as diapering or bathing the baby, may not mean that he is unsupportive of her mothering or breastfeeding. A referral to a mother-to-mother group such as La Leche League or Nursing Mothers may provide the additional support that she needs at this time. It is important that you accept the father's position and help the mother cope without making any judgments or becoming involved in any conflicts that may arise.

Mother's Confidence

Breastfeeding is a confidence game! The mother who is confident in herself and her commitment to breastfeeding, will continue despite setbacks or problems. O'Campo and associates (1992) found maternal confidence to be a determining factor in the duration of breastfeeding. Although the lactation consultant may not be able to *give* the mother self-esteem, a positive breastfeeding experience can (Locklin, 1993). You can build the mother's confidence by pointing out her baby's positive aspects and showing her how well he is growing. Positive feedback helps the mother understand that breastfeeding really does work. Her decision to do so is then validated.

MOTHER'S ENVIRONMENT

Some mothers in your care may have an environmental situation that detracts from breastfeeding. Such issues may interfere with understanding and rapport between you and the mother. Mothers who live in the inner city differ in their frame of reference from those who live in suburbia or a more rural setting. Low-income families and those from other cultures may have values that differ from those of a typical middle-class American family.

It is important that you not assume the lifestyle choices of others. You also cannot assume that the mother is married or that the father is living with the mother and baby, or even that there is enough food for the family to eat. Single-parent households are common, and a breastfeeding woman who is solely responsible for her baby's care may have many obstacles to overcome. In many cases, a teenage mother will be coping with single parenthood as well as the usual adjustments of ado-

lescence. All of these circumstances present special counseling concerns. Your manner of approach and availability to the mother can have a great influence on her mastery of the situation.

Being realistic in your expectations for each mother and her goals for breastfeeding are important. Beliefs and practices vary widely among cultural groups. Breastfeeding, especially exclusive breastfeeding, may be more than some mothers can handle or even desire. Learn about cultural differences and trends in your own community so that you can respond to the individual needs of mothers. Remaining flexible and objective in your approach will help mothers fit breastfeeding into their own lifestyles. Working with the mother as a team, you can develop innovative approaches for providing accurate information and support to ethnic women.

Low-Income Mother

Most lactation consultants are likely to encounter mothers whose financial status is below that of the average American family. For those whose income is near or below the poverty level, more factors come into play. They may have lower self-esteem, more limited expectations, and lower educational and occupational levels. In addition, they may live in an area in which many unfavorable conditions exist. This includes overcrowding, run-down housing, crime, physical and mental health problems, broken families, relocation problems, inadequate community services, isolation, alienation, and language problems. For these individuals, life may be a series of one crisis after another, such as unemployment or illness.

Psychosocial Issues

The low-income mother may have barriers present that impede her decision to initiate or continue breastfeeding. Lack of support and lack of accurate information are factors, as well as a need to deal with survival and crisis issues in her life. You can tell the woman that her baby will be healthier, and therefore happier, if she breastfeeds. Let her know that more women are breastfeeding now so that she will not feel as different. Praise her for making an intelligent decision, one that is based on sound medical fact rather than fads or advertising claims. Medical personnel can be instrumental in encouraging low-income women to continue breastfeeding. They are seen as the experts, and their advice is to be respected. By advocating breastfeeding to these women, they are giving valued information.

Low-income women may not take childbirth classes for reasons of cost, availability, or lack of interest. They may receive medication during labor and delivery that delays or interferes with breastfeeding in the first few days of life. Early introduction of artificial baby milk, particularly when introduced on the maternity unit, undermines the mother's confidence in her ability to breastfeed (Grossman, 1988; Michaelsen, 1994). She may believe that a substitute is just as good or perhaps better because it is more "scientific." Its use is implicitly advocated when it is freely given by postpartum hospital staff as gift packs. Your support during their hospital stay and the first week postpartum may be critical to their success in breastfeeding.

As breastfeeding continues, you can capitalize on their mothering achievements. Emphasize the mother's ability to nurture her baby and to persevere with the sometimes demanding task of breastfeeding. A mother whose baby cries often may doubt that he is being satisfied by her milk. This can become a self-fulfilling prophesy. Worry may inhibit letdown, which, in turn, will lower milk production. Lavish praise from you, as well as learning about other signs of adequate milk production, will help the woman continue.

More than for other groups, the low-income woman may find that breastfeeding builds her self-confidence and self-esteem. When she realizes that breastfeeding is a wonderful contribution to her child's well-being, which she has been able to accomplish with her own resources, her self-image will be enhanced. This can improve her parenting skills and encourage her to share her success with other women. Some women report that child-rearing was the experience that enabled them to become active learners because they had become advocates for their children's health (Belenky, 1986).

In addition to advising the mother about breastfeeding, you may need to help her locate other health services and act as the single thread of continuity in her health care. She may have received prenatal care in one place and delivered her baby in another; she may seek attention for her sick children from a clinic and for her well children from a child health station, and so on. In the United States, you can make her aware of local health services and suggest that she take advantage of the local WIC (Women, Infants, and Children program) to obtain supplemental foods. See Chapter 2 for further discussion about the WIC program.

Breastfeeding Challenges for Low-Income Women

Low-income mothers often feel out of control of their own lives and surroundings, which may break down their sense of attachment to society. A sense of despair or stress can prevail. The mother may feel that her immediate circle of relationships is not comfortable or supportive. She might distrust you because her life is insecure and you represent the "system" that has been so unkind to her. She may believe that breastfeeding is one more stress in her life. Also, she may worry that because she has heard this so many times from others, breastfeeding will be one more failure in her life.

The task of overcoming these obstacles in order to approach and communicate effectively with the mother may seem overwhelming. The suggestions given in the following sections may help you make your efforts acceptable and meaningful to the mother. Although many community resources are available to low-income women, the mother may be unaware of them. A public health nurse is a good resource for you to contact regarding referral processes. Communities vary in their use of public health nurses. Although they may not always make home visits, they might be able to suggest agencies or people that the mother could contact.

Some mothers believe that they need an immediate resolution to a crisis in their lives (Hardy, 1989). You will need to put aside theoretical and background information for the moment and concentrate on the problem or issue at hand. You can focus on external factors rather than such unchangeable ones as personality or the shortcomings of an individual's lifestyle. Suggestions need to be practical rather than general. Simply advising that she nurse her baby more often will not be as useful as helping her figure out times and ways she can actually do this. Help her as well with practical solutions to improve nutrition for herself and her family, and refer her to the local WIC clinic for nutritious foods to supplement her diet.

The mother's literacy level could impede her ability to absorb the information that is provided. Offer attractive, simply written brochures with illustrations that cover only the essential points that she needs to know. Make sure that the literacy level of the material you use is appropriate and be sensitive to the visual images and the amount of words on each page. If too many words make a brochure overwhelming, it will not be read or absorbed. In teaching the mother about breastfeeding techniques, use visual aids rather than verbal explanations whenever possible. Provide her with a checklist of the suggestions you discussed as a reminder. If you are assisting her over the telephone, reinforce the basic points of your conversation and try to get some feedback from the mother to indicate that she has understood your message and will act on your suggestions. Mothers need to understand the consequences of a negative practice, such as drug use while breastfeeding. If such a situation presents itself, do not hesitate to be firm with your information. Be patient and persevering in areas of importance. The mother and baby will both benefit from your sincerity and concern.

Reaching Out to Low-Income Women

Although breastfeeding discussion groups can serve as an effective teaching arena, attendance may often be minimal for low-income women. Many women feel that their lives are overwhelmed with work, child care, and obtaining the necessities of life. Adding a class to the mother's agenda may be more than she can handle. Try to conduct meetings in surroundings that will be comfortable to the women. Some may prefer a private residence, whereas others would rather meet in a church or community center. When the participants take a major role in planning and organizing such meetings, they believe that they are part of the process. They can also determine the day, time, and topics that are most relevant to them.

A low-income woman may be very isolated with no support system at home and may not know anyone who breastfed. Discussion groups with other mothers who share the same concerns can provide the peer support she needs to succeed and help build trust in your services. In order to make the meetings enjoyable, keep presentations short and to the point. Address issues that are relevant to the mother's needs. A casual, informal approach will help encourage discussion.

Make sure the women understand that you are available to them at all times. Trying to reach out to mothers in their own neighborhoods and freely giving them your telephone number will encourage mothers to contact you. Realize that many families may not be able to afford telephone service and that you may need to make home visits to stay in touch with them. If you make home visits a part of your availability to mothers, it is important that you be conscious of safety issues. Plan visits during daylight hours. Leave behind information with a colleague or family member that includes where you will visit, times you expect to arrive and leave, and the route you will take. A cellular telephone is helpful for the home visiting lactation consultant. Recognize, too, that circumstances may arise in which it is not in your best interest to make a home visit. Arrangements can be made to have someone accompany you on the visit, or perhaps, you can arrange to meet with the mother in a different location. Be sensitive when you discuss these arrangements with the mother. You are discussing her home and her neighborhood, and will need to present your concerns or change in plans in a positive and tactful manner.

It is often difficult convincing low-income mothers that they should and *can* breastfeed. Research has shown a greater likelihood for the low-income mother to choose breastfeeding if she has a higher level of education (MacGowan, 1991; Michaelsen, 1994), is married, (MacGowan, 1991) or has greater ego maturity and is thus more able to deviate from community norms (Jacobson, 1991). However, the greatest motivator seems to be a support person she respects who had a positive breastfeeding experience. The low-income mother's need for access to support and accurate information play a vital role in her breastfeeding experience. Her perception of family and peer support, particularly that from another woman with whom she is close, is another factor (Locklin, 1993).

Several studies have demonstrated an increase in breastfeeding rates among low-income women when their local health care clinics increased breastfeeding support to include classes, one-on-one instruction, and peer counselors. Grossman (1988) noted that only 17 percent of a nonintervention group (those receiving no extra education or support) chose to breastfeed at delivery. The group receiving the greatest intervention (classes, one-on-one education, and peer counselor support) chose to breastfeed at a rate of 66 percent at delivery. Kistin's study showed that peer counselor support had a positive effect on breastfeeding initiation and duration, as well as the mother's choice to breastfeed exclusively (Kistin, 1990, 1994). See Table 18.1 for a summary on counseling the low-income mother.

TABLE 18.1

Counseling Summary—Low-Income Mother

◆ Listen to the mother and actively acknowledge her view of her situation.

◆ Determine whether the mother has any sources of support for, or interference with, breastfeeding from a partner, family, or peers.

◆ Keep instructions simple and use visual aids whenever possible.

◆ Praise the mother, letting her know she is making the intelligent choice, is doing the best for her baby, and is doing well at breastfeeding.

◆ Use outreach counseling and contact the mother frequently to help prevent problems.

◆ If the mother lacks support at home, encourage her to focus on major priorities, especially employment, child care, nutrition, breastfeeding, rest, and major household tasks.

◆ Become knowledgeable of a mother's nutritional habits and offer suggestions if improvement is needed.

◆ Help the mother locate supplemental food programs and make the best use of her food dollars.

◆ Ensure that the mother is aware of contraceptive methods that are compatible with breastfeeding.

▼ Single Mother

You are likely to encounter a mother who has sole responsibility for her baby. This may be due to divorce, separation, death of her mate, a choice to remain unmarried, or a situation that requires the baby's father to be away from home for extended periods of time. The mother may be living alone or residing with her own parents or a friend. Each situation presents its own unique challenges. The single mother typically lives alone and is juggling a job, schooling or training, household responsibilities, and parenting. Work affords her the opportunity for adult companionship, instills a sense of independence, and furnishes necessary income. When she returns home from a long day of work, she has other responsibilities waiting for her.

If the single mother returns to live with her own parents, she can benefit from their support and security. At the same time, she may feel a need to maintain her own identity as an adult and a mother, and to preserve an identity as a family unit for her and her baby. It can be difficult for two family units to live harmoniously under one roof. The mother may find herself dealing with criticism about her parenting, as well as other family members disciplining her child. A lack of privacy, can interfere with her breastfeeding. Many mothers view their return home as a temporary situation until they secure other living arrangements.

When a mother's single status has resulted from the death of her spouse, emotional stress may cause a decrease in her milk production. Her baby may tune in to her emotional state and want to nurse more frequently. Breastfeeding can provide comfort to both the mother and baby in times of stress. Any increase in frequency will certainly help maintain milk production. The mother will benefit from your support as well as that of professional counseling.

A single mother may have no support system among friends or family, and no one with whom she can share concerns or parenting responsibilities. Her attempt to be a "supermom" in order to meet her baby's needs as well as those of every day life may leave little time for herself. Help the single mother think of ways she can meet her own and her baby's needs at the same time. She can take a walk with her baby in a backpack or stroller, or take baby swim classes or exercise classes with other moms and babies. The mother's nutritional status may be poor because of a lack of desire or time to prepare well-balanced meals for one person. Single mothers are likely to appreciate your caring and frequent contact. They might also contact a local Parents Without Partners or other support group for single parents. See Table 18.2 for a summary on counseling the single mother.

▼ Teenage Mother

Nine out of 10 pregnant teenagers elect to keep their babies. Some of these young mothers will want to breastfeed (March of Dimes, 1980). Many pregnant teenagers under the age of 18 choose not to get married. They do not feel pressured socially into having a mate or a father for their babies. They may not complete high school because of the demands on their time, and they may be unable to care for their babies because they lack the skill or income. They often have no job skills and are dependent financially on their families and society. These young mothers wish to be treated as adults and will not respond well to lecturing, advice, or any patronizing manner that suggests an adult-child relationship. Remember that they are adolescents first and parents incidentally and, many times, accidentally. They need you to listen to their concerns and to respond.

Prenatal Issues

There is a frequent pattern of inadequate prenatal care and poor nutrition among pregnant teens. This factor decreases their chances for a healthy baby. Teens have a higher incidence of premature, low-birth-weight infants, still births, and neonatal death than do postadolescent mothers. Some young mothers attempt to hide or deny their pregnancy in the early months. Consequently, they

---

TABLE 18.2

Counseling Summary—Single Mother

- ◆ Become knowledgeable of the mother's nutritional habits—meal patterns, who cooks, consumption of fast foods, and so on.
- ◆ Become aware of the mother's responsibilities with home and job.
- ◆ Become aware of the mother's living arrangements—living with parents, partner, or alone.
- ◆ Determine the mother's sources of support for breastfeeding—partner, family, and peers.
- ◆ Refer the mother to a support group for single parents.
- ◆ Help the mother think of ways she can meet her own and her baby's needs at the same time.

begin prenatal care much later than usual, many times as late as the end of the second trimester.

A pregnant teenager may be fearful and unhappy about the physical changes that are happening to her body. She may also be apprehensive about the impending labor and delivery. She may be concerned about the reactions of people close to her, such as family, friends, teachers, and her baby's father. Depending on the degree of her emotional adjustment to pregnancy, she may doubt her self-worth and have a poor self-image.

Many times, teenagers have poor eating habits. The pregnant teenager needs to understand the importance of good nutrition to her developing fetus and to her own body. Pregnancy compromises the health of a young mother whose own growth needs compete with the growth needs of her fetus. She will be reluctant to gain weight and lose her thin body. She may, therefore, be encouraged and comforted by hearing praise for the weight she gains and its benefit for her baby. She may actually need to consume more food than older mothers and will benefit from ongoing individualized advice regarding her diet. The adolescent who has just experienced puberty may require even more calories to support the rapid growth that follows. If she is living at home with her parents, the teenage mother may not have much influence on meal planning. Nutrition education is a primary achievement for all pregnant teenagers.

After the Baby is Born

Adolescent mothers may be less likely to arrange for immediate or prolonged contact with their babies following birth. They often feel threatened and overwhelmed by the hospital environment and will be reluctant to ask for anything from the nursing staff. Teens may not understand the importance of this early contact and consider the social aspect of visitors to be more important. Hospital personnel need to be sensitive to this situation by inviting interaction between the mother and her baby, and not relying on the mother to ask for her baby to be brought to her. The young mother's confidence is very fragile. Childbirth is a time of vulnerability for all new mothers. For the teen mother, it may be the first realization of the task she has just undertaken.

After she is at home with her baby, the young mother may question her adequacy as a parent and have difficulty coping with the daily responsibilities of parenthood. In some cases, the teenager's mother raises the baby as a sibling, with the baby's own mother having little to do with his care. The mother's maturity and attitude will be determining factors in how she copes with parenthood and breastfeeding. The less mature teenager may have difficulty giving love and attention to her baby at a time when she still desperately needs such nurturing herself. However, many young mothers are ready to accept the responsibilities of motherhood and respond in much the same way as an older mother.

Some teens find themselves in a power struggle with their mothers over the care of the baby. The teen may want to show her maturity by caring for her baby, whereas her mother thinks that she is too young to care for a baby. Providing the mother with accurate information on baby care may prove helpful to the teen in this situation. The teen's mother may feel threatened by her daughter's desire to breastfeed. Perhaps she did not breastfeed and is concerned that the baby will not receive proper nutrition. She may also worry that her daughter's choice to breastfeed reflects negatively on her own child-rearing techniques. Ironically, some teens choose breastfeeding in order to maintain a voice in the care of their babies in this power struggle. They see breastfeeding as the one thing that only *they* can do for their baby.

Breastfeeding Issues

Not suprisingly, breastfeeding rates among teenage mothers are much lower than those of adult mothers. This poses a special urgency for you to reach out to this population. The need is further amplified when one considers that the babies of teens are the ones who most need to receive the health benefits of breastfeeding. Teens tend to deliver earlier, have lower birth weight babies, and have more delivery complications. They typically live in less healthful environments, and their children are more at risk for cognitive and behavioral problems (McAnarney, 1993). All of these factors can be influenced positively by breastfeeding.

Some of the factors identified earlier for lower breastfeeding rates among teens are often the same factors that present with adult mothers who choose not to breastfeed. They are less likely to be married, and will be at lower educational and income levels (Peterson, 1992). Unique to teen mothers, however, is the influence of their own emotional development on the decision of whether or not to breastfeed. The teen mother is struggling with her own growth, independent of pregnancy and motherhood, often with a very egocentric outlook. She may have difficulty seeing beyond her own overwhelming needs in order to tend to her baby's needs. This applies to both general adolescent concerns and those related to her pregnancy.

In order to encourage teens to breastfeed, it is crucial that you understand the motivations involved in the decision to breastfeed for a teen mother. Lizarraga (1992) found that older teens who were married and no longer in school during their pregnancy were the most likely to choose breastfeeding. Those teens who were exposed to other women breastfeeding or who were breastfed themselves also were more inclined to breastfeed. Conversely, teens who need the most outreach to encourage breastfeeding are the younger, single teens who are enrolled in school and not exposed to breastfeeding in general. Generally, teens have issues about their own sexuality and body image that may interfere with the desire to breastfeed (Peterson, 1992).

Neifert (1988) looked at the motivating factors for teen mothers who choose breastfeeding. She found that 83 percent of the teens in her study made the decision to breastfeed before the third trimester of pregnancy. This demonstrates the need to reach teens in early pregnancy regarding infant feeding. Additionally, you can capitalize on opportunities to introduce breastfeeding within school curricula for all students. Neifert also found that 65 percent of the teen mothers "chose breastfeeding because it was 'good for the baby,' and 67 percent identified the 'closeness' of the nursing relationship as the most enjoyable part of breastfeeding." Obstacles to breastfeeding for the teen mothers in her study included concern about modesty and the need to return to school within 2 months postpartum.

In addition to psychosocial issues surrounding adolescence, pregnancy, and breastfeeding, physical factors may arise related to puberty. It is important to note that ductwork within the breast proliferates during pregnancy, refuting an earlier belief that adolescent mothers have difficulty producing milk (Stout, 1992). Teens have the potential to breastfeed with the same outcome as older mothers. When difficulties are encountered, however, they are less likely to overcome them and continue breastfeeding. This may be due to their being overwhelmed by parenting responsibilities, coupled with a lack of support for breastfeeding among family and friends. It may also be due to teens' lack of futuristic thinking, because many fail to see future consequences of their actions. They have difficulty, as well, understanding that a problem will be resolved "in the moment." This will, of course, vary with each individual mother. Some may have an excellent support system and will breastfeed for the same amount of time as the average breastfeeding mother.

Interactions With Teenage Mothers

A teenage mother usually has a great need for a one-to-one relationship with someone who cares about her and understands her needs. She also wants consistency and personal involvement in this relationship. It is important to get to know her as an individual and not just as the baby's mother. Ask her about herself—how she is adjusting, how the birth went, how she feels, and what her needs are. Recognizing that teens often maintain a more egocentric view, such interest in her as a person will help build rapport and develop trust in the relationship. This egocentric thinking lends itself to discussing what the advantages are of breastfeeding for the mother. She wants to know what is in it for her.

Often your interaction with teens will take place in a class setting. New information needs to be presented in simple, clear terms that do not overwhelm. Learn what the teens already know so that you do not present repetitive information. After 15 minutes of new information, teens may lose interest, so you need to make the time together both humorous and informative. Allow for nonthreatening participation and make time for interactive, hands-on learning during class. To demonstrate the consequences of positioning the baby at the breast, for example, teens can be asked to swallow some water looking straight ahead and then to swallow looking to the side. This will demonstrate how difficult it is for a baby to swallow if he must turn his head in order to latch on. A doll can be used to practice positioning, and a golf ball to show the size of a newborn's stomach. Use audiovisual aids and handouts that depict other teens, rather than adults, in breastfeeding situations.

Find out what the teens know about breastfeeding already as well as what they would like to know. This can be a challenge, because the teen mother will often not volunteer information and is less likely to ask questions. These are important considerations in a group setting in which fear of peer ridicule inhibits such interaction. One way of dealing with these dilemmas is to ask teens to write out their questions or concerns anonymously on paper. This encourages them to think about the situation and protects their privacy. Because teens may not attend every educational offering or appointment, you will need to cover breastfeeding basics whenever possible. When offering education to teens in a group setting, you also need to make yourself available for individual time.

Recognize that it is possible the teen mother does not have help or support available to her at home with regard to breastfeeding. Her own mother may not have breastfed, and her peers are much less likely to have breastfed than an adult woman's peers. Interactions between the teen and her mother while breastfeeding may or may not be positive. Her mother may have unresolved issues about her own breastfeeding experience or lack of it. Convey your support to the teen mother and be accepting of her situation. She may already be in disfavor with her family because of her pregnancy. Encourage her to bring any family or friends with her to classes in order to help build the teen's support system. Give her friends and family information about why breastfeeding is important and ways that they can be supportive. See Table 18.3 for a summary on counseling the teenage mother.

Finally, be sure to become familiar with organizations that provide assistance to teen mothers. Some agencies that reach out to teenage mothers are WIC, the March of Dimes, the American College of Obstetricians and Gynecologists, and the United States Government

<table>
<tr><td colspan="2" align="center">**TABLE 18.3**</td></tr>
<tr><td colspan="2" align="center">Counseling Summary—Teenage Mother</td></tr>
</table>

◆ Become knowledgeable of the mother's nutritional habits and influencing factors—eating with her family, body image, and so on.

◆ Determine whether the mother has any sources of support for, or interference with, breastfeeding—family, peers, and partner.

◆ Determine the mother's reactions to pregnancy, hospital environment, and becoming a parent—self-worth, body image, and interaction with baby.

◆ Determine who is the primary caretaker of the baby.

◆ Determine the mother's sources of emotional support.

◆ Refer the mother to a support group for teenage parents, when appropriate.

◆ Look for signs of adequate milk production.

Department of Health and Human Services. See Appendix A for source information for these organizations.

▼ Mothers with Cultural Differences

Families who have left their native environment have several characteristics in common when they work toward becoming part of a new culture. They all experience a sense of loss of their own culture. Culture, the environment that surrounds us in our beliefs and attitudes, is a strong structure to our being. The degree to which people become **acculturated** (integrated into a new culture) depends on many factors. Some individuals cling to certain values. Others, especially in succeeding generations, replace old values with new ones as cultural differences become more diffuse. Other factors that impact on behavior are age, educational and social exposure, the intent to return to their country of origin, economic status, contact with older relatives, and the part of the country in which they reside. The lower classes tend to hold onto their traditional values. The middle and upper classes have incorporated other cultural practices into their own value system. Practically speaking, this means that women from other cultures exhibit a very wide range of value systems, family support, and interest in breastfeeding.

Family Dynamics

In many Western cultures, the individual is considered to be the basic social entity, the building block of all social relations and institutions. In other cultures, the family may be the dominant unit, with decision making the responsibility of the family rather than the individual mother. It may also be the responsibility of the eldest male or other male figure in the family group. A dwelling that houses an extended family of parents or other guardians often provides its own support system for raising the child. In order to counsel effectively in this or similar situations you must take care not to interfere with family and peer support. A woman's cultural beliefs are more important and ingrained in her being than you are, the new person in her life. Instead, you can strengthen family support by providing clear, accurate information in a climate of acceptance.

Health and Illness Behaviors

Mothers of different cultures may have health and illness behaviors that vary significantly from your own. Ignorance of these differences can alienate the mother and run the risk of your offering recommendations that will be irrelevant or ignored. Culture affects the way a mother regards health and the measures she will take to prevent or treat illness. She may place considerable reliance on cultural patterns as a method of coping. Indeed, magical and religious practices can be therapeutic and can bring about social support from the community of persons of like culture. In order to counsel a woman from another culture effectively, you will need to understand her values and cultural practices and learn how they can influence her breastfeeding.

Cultural Beliefs Regarding Breastfeeding

Your approach in helping mothers will need to be a flexible one that involves learning about their beliefs and adapting your suggestions to meet their needs. Do not try to change culturally based practices unless they are very detrimental. Inappropriate advice from you may upset the mother and cause friction with other family members. You will lose credibility and rapport with the mother if you discredit beliefs she has held her entire life.

Instead, you can seek ways to work around culturally based practices. Use them to benefit rather than harm breastfeeding. For example, some Mexican American women who work outside in the heat believe that their milk will spoil in their breasts during the day and so they wean before returning to work. One caregiver found a way to use this belief as a motivating factor to continue to breastfeed. She instructed the women to express out the "bad" milk and throw it away, and then nurse their babies when they return home. In this way, the mothers were able to continue breastfeeding, with formula supplements being given to the babies during the daytime, similar to the way many other working mothers manage breastfeeding.

You can work in similar ways, keying into what is important to each mother and offering practical suggestions. A woman who has breastfed from the culture you encounter is the best method of promoting breastfeeding. She can assist you in learning the beliefs and child rearing choices that are predominant in a certain culture. She can also help you be supportive and can research suggestions that will assist the mother.

The cultural heritage and economic standing of a particular mother will have a direct bearing on her breastfeeding experience. It will affect how long she chooses to nurse, as well as her ability to deal with negative input from her partner, family, or friends. Values and priorities vary greatly among women of different cultural backgrounds. Some may regard health care providers and the scientific community with great respect. Others may put more faith in self-care or folk medicine. Many cultures regard colostrum as valueless or undesirable and do not encourage breastfeeding until the second or third postpartum day. You can inform these mothers about the medical value of colostrum, realizing at the same time that their cultural beliefs may predominate.

Some cultures discourage the consumption of cold foods and beverages by new mothers for a period of weeks or months. Hot teas and soups may be helpful to these mothers in meeting their fluid requirements. Cultural beliefs may also place limitations on activity for the postpartum mother that may be interpreted as a lack of compliance in the mother by uninformed caregivers. Recognizing this, you can encourage the involvement of extended family in the mother's care. Cultural restrictions may carry over to how one relates to the baby as well. It is possible that certain ways of touching the baby or referring to the baby may be considered taboo. Always ask permission when you wish to touch the baby. Gentle, honest inquiries about the mother's customs will help you learn appropriate responses.

Language Differences

Cultural barriers may be even more pronounced when they are accompanied by a language difference. In order to establish effective communication, you will need to develop a sensitive understanding of the woman's culture and language. Speak slowly and clearly, and provide simple explanations. It would be helpful to have the services of a colleague who can speak comfortably in a second language, especially Spanish, which is the predominant second language in the United States. If you have no one available in your practice who speaks the language of a particular mother, you can ask the woman if she has a bilingual friend or relative who can assist.

You might also contact a local high school or university to request a volunteer to serve as interpreter. It is important that the interpreter be another woman, because the mother may be reluctant to share intimate information with a male other than her partner. Also be certain that the interpreter is communicating accurately and not adding her own opinions or values that may differ from yours or those of the mother.

Communication is especially important if the mother has a breastfeeding problem that she needs to discuss. A woman with a limited understanding of English can usually converse well enough about the general management of breastfeeding. When she has a specific problem, however, she may need to converse in her own language in order to be understood and to comprehend your advice.

Women who have difficulty reading the English language cannot take advantage of books on breastfeeding. Brief pamphlets with simple themes and illustrations can help these mothers, especially if they are written at an appropriate reading level. You might also arrange to have some of your literature translated so that the mothers can benefit even more. Demonstrations with visual aids and the use of flash cards with translations may be helpful. Bilingual aids are available through La Leche League International and other sources. A parent book, *Bestfeeding* by Renfrew, contains a Spanish language picture and verbal section (Renfrew, Childbirth Graphics 1990) carries a small book of breastfeeding words and phrases in many languages. (See Appendix A.) Various journals such as *Birth* carry advertising for films and literature in other languages. A multilingual source of common expressions related to health care is *Taber's Cyclopedic Medical Dictionary*. Local social services and library materials may be helpful as well. The telephone company also has a translation service for medical professionals.

Body Language as a Communication Tool

Because body language is an important communication tool, personal contact is preferable to telephone contact. In some cultures, nodding and smiling do not denote understanding as they do in Western society. You cannot assume that a mother comprehends what you are saying because of these gestures. Watch for nonverbal cues of hidden messages given by facial and body expressions. A nod of the head accompanied by a bland or puzzled look can imply confusion. To ensure that the woman understands your instructions, you can ask her to repeat them. You can also demonstrate the procedure and summarize the important points at the end of your conversation. Use of listening skills is critical in determining the woman's motivation to breastfeed and cultural factors working for or against her breastfeeding.

You may wish to visit the woman in her home in order to obtain a more complete picture of her physical and emotional environment. If you do so, recognize that many families may be reluctant to invite strangers into their homes. Others may be embarrassed by their current living arrangements. They may respond to a friendly and sincere interest in their welfare. Learn cultural customs of greeting and inclusion of others in the discussion before you make this visit. Doing so will show your interest and respect for the woman and her culture. Remember that the Western way is not the best or only way for breastfeeding to be successful. Many other countries and cultures have better breastfeeding rates than the United States. Western culture has much to learn. Open yourself up to learn the ideas and choices that work in other places.

Promoting Breastfeeding to Women of Other Cultures

Your role with women of another culture goes beyond learning to function within the culture. It also involves actively promoting breastfeeding, which is often forsaken by women of many ethnic groups in favor of infant formulas. Lack of education and economics play key roles. Among mothers immigrating to the United States, Ghaemi-Ahmadi (1992) noted a great reduction in breastfeeding rates and duration between siblings born in the home land and those born in the United States. This decrease correlated with the mother's need to return to work or school, as well as the availability of free infant formula. Ghaemi-Ahmadi's research advises that breastfeeding education needs to provide information regarding the feasibility and practicality of breastfeeding while the mother is employed or in school.

James (1994) noted the correlation between free formula and decreased breastfeeding rates among women living in the United States who were originally from other countries. It was found that the providing of free samples while in the hospital undermines the mother's confidence in her body's ability to produce milk. This sends a message to the mother that her caregivers do not take her decision to breastfeed seriously. Providing free infant formula to a mother at discharge also says that this is the American way. If a mother wishes to become acculturated in her new home, she may believe that formula feeding is the way to achieve it. Further, James found that familial support for breastfeeding needs to be an integral part of breastfeeding education. When an extended family is absent, the mother tends to rely heavily on the father's preference for infant feeding. Prenatal education, early in pregnancy, should actively seek to include the father and any members of the extended family.

Most women wish to do what is best for their babies. They often will follow your suggestions after they fully understand the reasons for doing so. While learning about the woman's culture and her unique beliefs, you may become more aware of your own beliefs. You need to leave your beliefs and assumptions outside the door when counseling these women. Intercultural experiences can be tremendous eye openers. They provide an opportunity for personal growth by enabling you to view yourself and others more objectively. See Table 18.4 for a summary on counseling mothers with cultural differences.

TABLE 18.4

Counseling Summary—Mothers with Cultural Differences

◆ Investigate the mother's income level and apply suggestions for the low-income mother, if applicable.

◆ Become knowledgeable of the mother's cultural heritage:
  Practices relative to breastfeeding
  Degree of acculturation
  Practice of religious or superstitious beliefs
  Family support system
  Health and illness practices

◆ Bridge the language barrier by using an interpreter, visual aids, body language, and translated literature.

◆ Ensure that the woman has understood your message by having her summarize or demonstrate important points.

◆ Assess the woman's need and desire for a personal relationship with a counselor.

◆ Accept cultural practices if they are not detrimental to the mother or her baby. Provide applicable information in order to eliminate harmful practices.

◆ Adapt your counseling approach to meet the woman's special needs.

◆ Include family members in your consults with the mother.

▼ MOTHER-TO-MOTHER SUPPORT GROUPS

With the rise in popularity of breastfeeding, a majority of babies leave the hospital being breastfed, either partially or exclusively. However, many of the mothers who start out breastfeeding fail to continue because they lack the necessary support and information to do so. Regardless of your specific role with mothers, it is important to become aware of and involved in all lactation services and support available within your community. Mother-to-mother support groups supply this support through written materials, counseling services, regular discussion groups, and special programs. (Fig. 18.1.)

In a support group, women's traditional patterns of seeking and receiving advice from relatives and friends are reinforced. Mothers can seek help at any time, day or night, and help is usually available in the mother's own community. Discussion groups and mutual help are given by experienced mothers. New mothers gain the feeling of self-reliance and are reassured. Starting a mother-to-mother support group can be a rewarding and challenging venture, providing a needed service to women in your community and furthering the cause of breastfeeding. See the discussion in Chapter 2 regarding your relationship to mother-to-mother support groups.

▼ Outreach Counseling

A mother-to-mother support group provides anticipatory guidance to breastfeeding women in the community. Mothers who are contacted before a problem arises will learn more of what to expect. They avoid potential problems and can begin to resolve issues before they become obstacles. Providing regular group discussions and personally inviting women to such meetings are also effective. It is important that mothers who have had a problem are contacted as frequently as the situation warrants. Initiating phone calls is one aspect of outreach counseling. Other ways of actively reaching out to women include speaking at childbirth classes and clinics, sharing information with professionals, and visiting high school health classes.

▼ Meeting the Needs of the Mothers

The goal of a mother-to-mother support group is to educate women about options and help them choose what will fit their particular needs. Counselors in the group should inform and support mothers in their choices. Continuous contact between a counselor and the mother is encouraged from the baby's birth through the weaning process. Exclusive breastfeeding for at least 6 months, baby-led weaning, and limiting separation of mother and baby are usually emphasized; these goals, however, may not always be possible. Helping mothers manage breastfeeding and working, weaning at an early age, and other variations in breastfeeding styles that require compromises will reflect the group's flexibility and acceptance. It is important that counselors remain flexible and prepared to make such changes when necessary. The mother-to-mother support group should accommodate the style and needs of the women and the community it serves.

Because of the large number of breastfeeding mothers and the endorsement of breastfeeding by the American Academy of Pediatrics, physicians and other health professionals want mothers to breastfeed. The development of a positive working relationship between you, the lay counselor, the mothers they counsel, and their caregivers is essential to effective counseling. It is important that you not place yourself, counselors, or mothers in opposition to other members of the medical community. This will discourage health care providers from referring mothers to you and will diminish your credibility in the community. Open communication and cooperation between the medical community and breastfeeding professionals is essential, with the mother making her own decisions based on information from both.

▼ Regular Meetings for Mothers

Regular meetings for breastfeeding mothers in the community provide a valuable counseling opportunity.

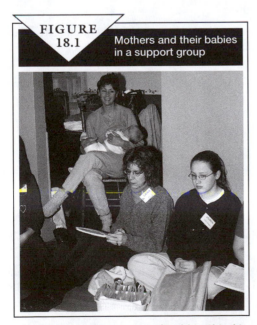

> **FIGURE 18.1** Mothers and their babies in a support group

Reprinted by permission of Debbie Shinskie.

Meeting formats should encourage friendly and informal discussion, and provide a supportive environment for a mother who lacks contact with other breastfeeding women. The primary factors influencing meetings should be the needs of the women who will be attending. The goal should be to involve mothers as much as possible and help them feel comfortable in taking part. This may be accomplished by such techniques as posing questions, demonstrations, small group discussions, and book reviews.

When No Support Group Is Available

If a support group is not available in your community, you may need to pay closer heed to details in your role with the mothers in your care. In the absence of community support, you can provide ongoing support and appropriate written materials. Referrals for other areas of support are still important and should be made. In the absence of lactation support in the community, it is especially important that you provide follow-up contacts to mothers after hospital discharge and after counseling a mother through a difficulty. Lack of community support may lead you to develop a mother-to-mother support group, train group leaders, and be available as a resource to the group.

SUMMARY

Often, a mother's breastfeeding experience involves special circumstances. You can provide valuable support and guidance to help the mother navigate through the rough waters. When the mother experiences opposition to her choice to breastfeed, she will greatly value a listening ear, praise, and practical suggestions, particularly when the opposition is from one who is close to her. You can also be a valuable resource to the mother who is experiencing challenges such as low income, single parenthood, or teen parenthood. Such mothers often bear very great burdens that go well beyond the scope of lactation issues. They are in need of thoughtful suggestions and referrals that take their special needs into account. The mother whose culture differs from the mainstream culture of her locale will also have a greater need for you to remain open and flexible so that you may gauge suggestions accordingly. Mother-to-mother support groups often provide the greater degree of support needed in these special circumstances. These groups will benefit from your support as well.

REFERENCES

American Academy of Pediatrics. Breastfeeding and the use of human milk. *Pediatrics* 100:1035–1039; 1997.

Belenky M et al. *Women's Ways of Knowing*, New York: Basic Books, Inc; 1986.

Bridges C et al. Employer attitudes toward breastfeeding in the workplace. *J Hum Lact* 13:215–219; 1997.

Buckner E and Matsubara M. Support network utilization by breastfeeding mothers. *J Hum Lact* 9:231–235; 1993.

Ghaemi-Ahmadi S. Attitudes toward breastfeeding and infant feeding among Iranian, Afghan, and Southeast Asia immigrant women in the United States: Implications for health and nutrition education. *J Am Diet Assoc* 92:354–355; 1992.

Grossman L et al. Prenatal interventions increase breastfeeding among low-income women. *Am J Dis Child* 142:404; 1988.

Hardy J and Streett R. Family support and parenting education in the home: An effective extension of clinic-based preventive health care services for poor children. *J Pediatr* 115:927–931; 1989.

Jacobson S et al. Incidence and correlates of breastfeeding in socioeconomically disadvantaged women. *Pediatr* 88:728–736; 1991.

James D et al. Factors associated with breastfeeding prevalence and duration among international students. *J Am Diet Assoc* 94:194–196; 1994.

Kistin N et al. Effect of peer counselors on breastfeeding initiation, exclusivity and duration among low-income urban women. *J Hum Lact* 10:11–15; 1994.

Kistin N et al. "Breastfeeding rates among Black urban low-income women: Effect of prenatal education." *Pediatr* 86:741–746; 1990.

Lizarraga J et al. Psychosocial and economic factors associated with infant feeding intentions of adolescent mothers. *J Adolesc Health* 13:676–681; 1992.

Locklin M and Naber S. Does breastfeeding empower women? Insights from a select group of educated, low-income, minority women. *Birth* 20:30–35; 1993.

March of Dimes/National Foundation. Adolescent pregnancy. *Leaders Alert Bulletin*; 1980.

MacGowan R et al. Breastfeeding among women attending Women, Infants, and Children clinics in Georgia, 1987. *Pediatrics* 87:361–366; 1991.

McAnarney E and Lawrence R. Day care and teenage mothers: Nurturing the mother-child dyad. *Pediatrics* 91:202–205; 1993.

McNatt M and Freston M. Social support and lactation outcomes in postpartum women. *J Hum Lact* 8:73–77; 1992.

Michaelsen K et al. The Copenhagen cohort study on infant nutrition and growth: duration of breastfeeding and influencing factors. *Acta Paediatr* 83:565–571; 1994.

Neifert M et al. Factors influencing breastfeeding among adolescents. *J Adolesc Health Care* 9:470–473; 1988.

O'Campo P et al. Prenatal factors associated with breastfeeding duration: Recommendations for prenatal interventions. *Birth* 19:195–201; 1992.

Peterson C and DaVanzo J. Why are teenagers in the United States less likely to breastfeed than older women? *Demography* 29:431–450; 1992.

Renfrew M. *Breastfeeding: Getting breastfeeding right for you.* Berkeley, CA: Celestial Arts; 1990.

Stout R. Composition of milk in adolescents. *J Adolesc Health* 13:261; 1992.

▼ BIBLIOGRAPHY

Abramson R. Cultural sensitivity in the promotion of breastfeeding. Clinical issues in perinatal and women's health: Breastfeeding. *NAACOG* 3(4):717–722; 1992.

Bocar D. "Combining breastfeeding and employment. Increasing Success." *J Perinat Neonat Nurs* 11:23–42; 1997.

Brent N et al. "Breast feeding in a low-income population. *Arch Pediatr Adolesc Med* 149:798–803; 1995.

Bryant C et al. A strategy for promoting breastfeeding among economically disadvantaged women and adolescents. *NAACOGs Clin Issues* 3:723–730; 1992.

Clark AL (ed). *Culture and Childbearing*. Philadelphia. F.A. Davis Co; 1981.

Corbett-Dick P and Bezek S. Breastfeeding promotion for the unemployed mother. *J. Pediatr Health Care* 11:12–10; 1997.

D'Avanzo C. Bridging the cultural gap with Southeast Asians. *MCN* 17:204–208, 1992.

Editorial. A warm chain for breastfeeding. *Lancet* 344:1239–1241; 1994.

Ellis J. Southeast Asian refugees and maternity care: The oakland experience. *Birth* 9(3):191–194; 1982.

Faught P. Special people, special needs: The adolescent challenge. *Int J Childbirth Ed* 10:15–17; 1995.

Fullar S. Care of postpartum-adolescents. *MCN* 11:398–403; 1986.

Gunnlaugsson G and Einarsdottir J. Colostrum and ideas about bad milk: A case study from Guinea-Bissau. *Soc Sci Med* 36:283–288; 1993.

Hoddinott P and Pill R. Qualitative study of decisions about infant feeding among women in east end of London. *Br Med J* 318:30–34; 1999.

Hopkins-Kavanaugh K and Kennedy PH. Promoting Cultural Diversity: Strategies for Health Care Professionals; 1992.

Humphreys A et al. Intention to breastfeed in low-income pregnant women: The role of social support and previous experience. *Birth* 25:169–174, 1998.

Ibrahim M et al. Breastfeeding and the dietary habits of children in rural Somalia. *Acta Paediatr* 81:480–483; 1992.

Julion B. Letter. *J Nurse Midwife* 38:179–180; 1993.

Kanashiro H et al. Consumption of food and nutrients by infants in Huascar (Lima), Peru. *Am J. Clin Nutr* 52:995–1004; 1990.

Kannan S et al. Cultural influence on infant feeding beliefs of mothers. *J Am Diet Assoc* 99:88–90; 1999.

Kendall Tackett K. Breastfeeding and the sexual abuse survivor. *J Hum Lact* 14:125–133; 1998.

Kyenkya-Isabirye M and Magalheas R. The mothers' support group role in the health care system. *Int J Gynecol Obstet* 31 (Suppl 1): 85–90; 1990.

Levitt M. et al. Social support and relationship change after childbirth: An expectancy model. *Health Care Women Int* 14:503–512; 1993.

Locklin M. Telling the world; Low income women and their breastfeeding experiences. *J Hum Lact* 11:285–291; 1995.

Lynch and Hansen MJ. *Developing Cross Cultural Competence.* Baltimore MD. Paul H. Brookes Publishing Co; 1992.

Morse J et al. Initiating breastfeeding: A world survey of the timing postpartum breastfeeding. *Int J Nurs Stud* 27:303–313; 1990.

Motil K et al. Lactational performance of adolescent mothers shows preliminary differences from that of adult women. *J Adolesc Health* 20:442–449; 1997.

Naeye PIL. Teenaged and preteenaged pregnancies: Consequences of the fetal-maternal competition for nutrients. *Pediatrics* 67(1):146–150; 1981.

Riordan J and Auerbach K. *Breastfeeding and Human Lactation.* Sudbury, MA. Jones and Bartlett Publishing; 1999.

Romero Gwynn E and Carias L. Breastfeeding intentions and practices among Hispanic mothers in southern California. *Pediatrics* 84:626–632; 1989.

Romero Gwynn E. Breastfeeding pattern among Indochinese immigrants in Northern California. *Am J Dis Child* 143:804–808; 1989.

Sciacca J et al. Influences on breast-feeding by lower income women: An incentive based partner-supported educational program. *J Am Diet Assoc* 95:323–328; 1995.

Serdula M et al. Correlates of breastfeeding in a low-income population of whites, blacks and Southeast Asians. *J Am Diet Assoc* 91:41–45; 1991.

Spector R. *Cultural Diversity in Health and Illness.* Stamford, CT: Appleton and Lange; 1996.

Stuart-Mccadam P and Dettwyler K. *Breastfeeding Biocultural Perspectives.* New York: Aldine de Gruyter; 1995.

Thomas RG and Tumminia PA. Maternity care for Vietnamese in America. *Birth* 9(3):187–190; 1982.

Tyler VL. *Intercultural Interacting.* Provo, UT: Brigham Young University Publications; 1987.

Waxler-Morrison et al. *Cross Cultural Caring: A Handbook for Health Professionals.* Vancouver, BC, Canada: UBC Press; 1990.

Williams E and Pan E. Breastfeeding initiation among a low-income multiethnic population in Northern California: An exploratory study. *J Hum Lact* 10:245–251; 1994.

19

BREASTFEEDING TECHNIQUES AND DEVICES

U.S. culture seems to be enamored with gadgets and gizmos. Breastfeeding is no exception, with a variety of devices available that are intended to facilitate feeds. In such a climate, it is important for caregivers and parents alike to ask themselves what is truly needed for a woman to breastfeed. Indeed, what is truly needed to care for an infant? Advertisements for baby care items often focus on separation of the mother and baby, and treat separation as the desired norm. This trend is evident in breastfeeding devices as well. Breast pumps, for example, are often sold on the assumption that the mother and baby will need to be apart. Each individual consultation must start with the basic premise that under normal circumstances, no special aids are needed. First and foremost you must be an advocate for the mother and baby remaining together. When feeding alternatives are required, you can help the mother decide the method that will best suit her needs.

BREASTFEEDING TECHNIQUES

There are some simple techniques that are helpful to women prenatally and in the early weeks of breastfeeding. Performing a pinch test will help the mother determine whether her nipple will evert for feedings. Learning how to massage her breasts will help her prepare for early feeds and, if necessary, for removing milk from her breasts through pumping or hand expression. Supporting her breast during feeds will help the baby maintain a good latch during the early days of nursing.

Pinch Test

The **pinch test** can be used prenatally to assess a mother's nipples for protrusion. This can be part of the mother's prenatal assessment. A mother who is identified as having retracted or inverted nipples near the end of her pregnancy may begin manipulating her nipples to help increase protraction. Figure 19.1 shows a mother's breast before performing the pinch test. To test the protractility of the nipple, the mother grasps the base of the nipple with her forefinger and thumb, as in Figure 19.2.

She then presses the thumb and forefinger together several times around the base. If the nipple moves forward, it is considered a normal, protracting nipple and needs no special intervention. A retracting nipple moves inward rather than forward, as depicted in Figure 19.2. It may benefit from the use of an inverted syringe prenatally or a breast pump after the baby is born. A nipple may appear to be inverted on visual inspection and then protracts when pinched. Although this nipple may need shaping before latch-on, it will most likely not interfere with breastfeeding. The nipple that appears inverted on visual inspection and does not respond to stimulation is considered to be completely inverted and will benefit from nipple manipulation. See Chapter 6 for a discussion on differences in nipples.

Breast Massage

Mothers will find breast massage to be beneficial at various times and for a variety of reasons. Any form of massage encourages the mother to relax. Because touch causes myoepithelial cells to contract, breast massage helps stimulate the milk ejection reflex (letdown). Massage also affects the release of oxytocin, which is released in a pulsating manner when the baby suckles. During breast massage, oxytocin levels increase and will remain high while the massage continues (Yokoyama, 1994). Working in coordination with oxytocin and the myoepithelial cells, massage helps "push" the milk down the lactiferous sinuses, thus making it more available to be removed by the baby or by expression. Squeezing increases the positive pressure inside the breast. This makes a more efficient pressure gradient for the movement of milk from an area of high pressure to an area of low pressure (the baby's mouth).

Breast massage is especially useful to mothers who are in the process of relactating or initiating lactation to nurse an adopted baby. The mother can massage her breasts just before a feed, hand expression, or pumping in order to stimulate letdown. The massage may be done in conjunction with relaxation techniques such as deep breathing and visualization.

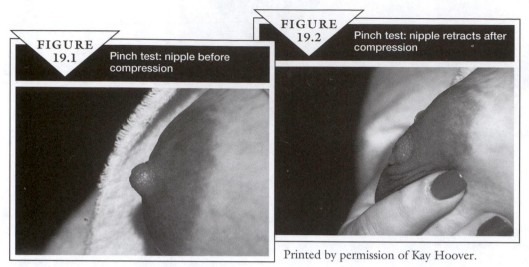

FIGURE 19.1   Pinch test: nipple before compression

FIGURE 19.2   Pinch test: nipple retracts after compression

Printed by permission of Kay Hoover.

Printed by permission of Kay Hoover.

Breast massage is helpful as well for a mother whose baby seems impatient for the milk to flow. She can massage to enhance letdown before putting her baby to breast. Performing massage before manual expression or pumping will help initiate letdown in these instances. When the mother has engorgement, a plugged duct, or mastitis, massage will help flow in these situations in which milk stasis increases difficulties. Alternate massage can also be done when the baby pauses during the feed to sustain sucking in a sleepy baby or inefficient feeder. Alternate massage increases the volume of fat content per feed.

Breast Massage Technique

The technique for breast massage is easy for mothers to learn (Fig. 19.3). Beginning at her chest wall, the mother uses the palm of her hand to exert a gentle pressure on the breast, massaging in a circular motion from the chest wall toward the nipple. Note that she uses the palm of her hand and not her fingers. She will continue in this manner, working her hand around the breast. Encourage her to focus on the areas of greatest milk duct development, which are under the breast and along the side under the arm. If the mother is large breasted, she may need to support her breast with the other hand while she is massaging it. Keep in mind when teaching breast massage, that women from a culture other than your own may have variations in breast massage that accomplish the same purpose. A culturally sensitive approach is needed. You may learn a different method to use in your practice!

▼ C-Hold

In the early days of breastfeeding, the mother is advised to support her breast for feeds by cupping it with her hand in the form of the letter "C." Referred to as the C-hold, this technique helps form the breast and nipple, thereby easing the baby's latch onto the breast. This hold also supports the weight of the breast and keeps the nipple from slipping out of the baby's mouth. With the C-hold, the mother cups the breast in her hand, placing her thumb on top and her fingers below (Fig. 19.4). It is similar to the hand placement used for hand expression. Her hand needs to be placed well behind the areola so that her fingers do not interfere with the baby's latch. Her fingers and thumb may slightly compress the breast to help form it for her baby. This is most helpful for the mother to use in the beginning when her baby is just learning to latch. When the mother feels that her baby no longer needs assistance, she can discontinue holding her breast at feeds.

▼ Dancer Hand Position

A slight variation of the C-hold can be used with premature infants and other babies who have weak muscle development and find it difficult to hold their jaw steady while they suck. This position, the **Dancer hand position**, begins in the C-hold position. The mother then brings her hand forward so that her breast is supported with the first three fingers. The baby's chin is supported by the crook of her hand between her thumb and index finger (Fig. 19.5). The mother may bend her index finger slightly so that it gently holds the baby's cheek on one side, with the thumb holding the other cheek. This hold helps decrease the available space in the baby's mouth and increase negative pressure. When the mother uses steady, equal pressure while holding her baby's cheeks, she will avoid interfering with the rooting reflex. As muscle tone begins to improve, the thumb can be placed back on top of the breast, and the index finger can support the baby's chin.

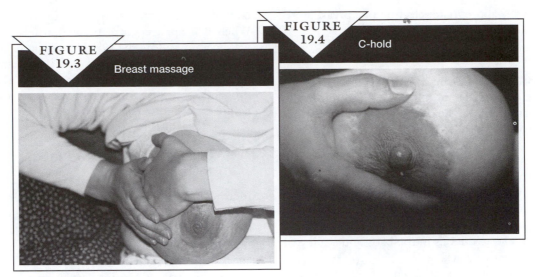

FIGURE 19.3   Breast massage

FIGURE 19.4   C-hold

Printed by permission of Kay Hoover.

BREASTFEEDING DEVICES

Occasionally, a mother may have a special need for a breastfeeding device to assist her with feeds or for the care of her breasts. After careful assessment of a situation, you can make appropriate suggestions, ideally ones that will have the least negative impact on breastfeeding. Starting with the least invasive methods for approaching the problem will lead to fewer complications and difficulties at a later time. Mothers who need to use breastfeeding aids will benefit from special counseling suggestions and close follow-up during their use. The products discussed in this chapter are available from numerous sources. The *Breast-feeding Products Guide* cited in the Suggested Reading in Appendix A identifies these sources.

Lubricants on the Breast and Nipple

Glands within the areolar skin normally keep the nipple area soft and pliable. An artificial lubricant is necessary only if this natural lubrication has been disturbed and needs to be replaced. Prenatally, a lubricant may be indicated when a mother has excessively dry skin, eczema, or other dermatologic condition. It will also replace moisture when natural lubrication has been removed by the improper use of drying agents or other practices. After breastfeeding has begun, mothers may apply a lubricant if their nipples become sore or cracked. Although research does not totally support the therapeutic effect of breast lubricants, mothers generally believe that topical treatments will reduce soreness. You can

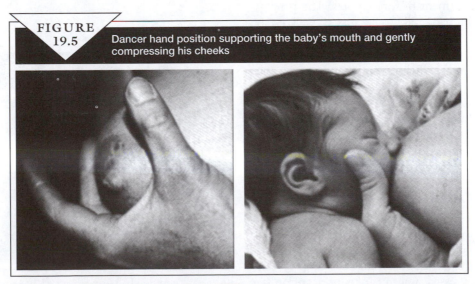

FIGURE 19.5   Dancer hand position supporting the baby's mouth and gently compressing his cheeks

Courtesy of Childbirth Graphics Ltd., 1985.

guide them in the appropriate selection of a breast lubricant or none at all!

What To Avoid

The choice of breast lubricant must take into consideration its potential effects on the health of both the mother's breast skin and her baby. Any lubricant that contains petroleum should be avoided, because it will inhibit skin respiration and actually prolong nipple soreness. Such petroleum-based products include baby oil, Vaseline petroleum jelly, Vaseline Intensive Care Lotion, cocoa butter, A and D ointment, and dimethicone. Products that contain alcohol are drying to the skin and should be avoided as well. Vitamin E oil should be avoided due to elevated levels in the baby and sealing of an open wound with a crack.

If the baby's mother or father has a family history of allergies, he should not be exposed to any substance such as peanut oil or Massé cream that is a potential allergen. Some lubricants contain wool derivatives, and although they are beneficial to most mothers, they should be avoided by those with a family history of wool allergy. Additionally, some lubricants with wool derivatives have been found to contain pesticides, which may pose a threat to the baby (Walker, 1989). Any product that must be washed off should not be used, because rubbing will further irritate sore nipples. Several types of breast creams are distributed to mothers in the hospital and are available in most pharmacies. Generally, although these products do no harm, they are ineffective in the prevention of sore nipples and may prevent a mother from seeking early help for the cause of the soreness.

Recommended Lubricants

Many lactation experts suggest the use of the mother's own milk in the treatment of sore nipples. The prophylactic benefit of human milk to infants is well established. Perhaps it holds promise in the treatment of nipple soreness as well. Hypoallergenic medical grade anhydrous lanolin may be helpful for severely dry or sore nipples. This form of lanolin does not contain the concerning levels of pesticides. Owing to removal of the alcohols that contribute to allergic response, this lanolin is reported to be less of a risk in allergic patients. See Chapter 14 for an in-depth discussion of the use of lubricants for treatment of sore nipples.

Application of Lubricants

Lubricants should be applied only after the mother's skin is thoroughly dry in order to avoid trapping excess moisture on the nipple. The mother can express a bit of her milk and gently massage it around the nipple. Caution her to avoid excessive amounts of a lubricant on the end of the nipple, where pore openings are located. When it is applied correctly after a feed, the lubricant will be absorbed by the skin before the next feed. Moist healing with lanolin or other topical preparations should be discussed with the mother, as well as the use of hydrogel dressings. Warm water soaks have also shown relief for some mothers.

▼ Inverted Syringe for Flat or Inverted Nipples

Many clinicians suggest the use of an inverted syringe to help mothers evert a flat or inverted nipple. This technique can be performed prenatally as well as before a feed. In the prenatal period, the mother first will want to check with her primary caregiver to determine whether or not this type of nipple stimulation is safe during her pregnancy. Nipple stimulation has been suggested to lead to preterm labor in a mother who is at risk.

To use an inverted syringe to evert the nipple, the mother will need a syringe with a barrel that is slightly larger than her nipple. Usually a 10- to 20-ml syringe will work well. The tapered end of the syringe is cut off and the plunger direction is reversed so as to provide a smooth surface next to the breast. The cut end should never be placed against the mother's breast because the sharp edges may damage her breast tissue. The mother places the smooth end of the syringe over her nipple and pulls gently on the plunger (Fig. 19.6).

It is important that the mother do the pulling on the syringe and not you or another caregiver. She will best be able to assess her own comfort level. Instruct her to hold the pressure for about 30 seconds and release. The pressure should be gentle and not painful. If pain is experienced, the mother should stop the procedure. She should never pull hard enough to cause pain or color

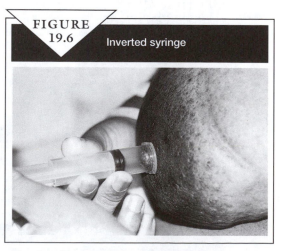

FIGURE 19.6   Inverted syringe

Reprinted by permission of Kay Hoover.

changes in the nipple. After each use of the syringe, it should be washed in hot, soapy water and air dried for the next use (Kesaree, 1993).

Prenatally, the mother can use the syringe two or three times a day until the baby is born. She can hold the plunger out for 30 seconds two or three times in each session. After the baby is born, if he has difficulty latching on, the technique may be used before putting him to breast to help evert the nipple and improve latch.

Breast Shells

It is widely believed that wearing breast shells inside the woman's bra will improve nipple protractility by gently placing pressure on the skin, stretching and pushing the nipple forward (Fig. 19.7). It should be noted that prenatal wearing of breast shells has not been shown to be beneficial to breastfeeding. Studies indicate no changes in the nipples and even show a decrease in breastfeeding rates.

The mother's bra should be one cup size larger to avoid pressing the shell too tightly against the breast. The shells should have several openings for air circulation in order to keep the skin from becoming softened and susceptible to chapping. A similar effect to that produced by the shell can sometimes be achieved by cutting a small hole in the bra, allowing only the nipple to protrude. Breast shells should not be worn when the mother is sleeping. Caution mothers about excessive use of shells as well. When breast shells are worn for long periods of time, the pressure on the lactiferous sinuses can cause or prolong leaking.

When used prenatally, the shells are worn for 8 to 10 hours or more per day intermittently for short times until they are comfortable. When inversion is first discovered after delivery, breast shells can be worn between, or for short periods before, feeds to help shape the nipple.

Breast shells have been found to help relieve engorgement when they are worn for about 20 minutes before feeds. Any milk that has accumulated in a breast shell worn between feeds cannot be saved. However, a breast shell can be worn inside the bra during a feed on the breast that is not being suckled. Milk that leaks from that breast during the feed can be saved. If the mother plans to save the drip milk, she must be sure that the shell is clean when it is put on the breast and is applied immediately before the feed.

Nipple Shield

Few methods of intervention in breastfeeding management strike more discord among lactation professionals than nipple shields. This is with good reason. A nipple shield is placed over the mother's nipple so that the baby latches onto the shield to feed (Fig. 19.8). The older nipple shields were thick and shaped more like a bottle teat than a device to aid breastfeeding. The data regarding these shields demonstrated diminished milk transfer. At least one out-of-court settlement against a nurse and the hospital where she was employed cited the potential negative outcome of reduced milk production with shield use that was coupled with possible inappropriate use or inadequate instruction (Bornmann, 1986). Even the modern, thinner silicon shields are reported to demonstrate a reduced milk transfer (Auerbach, 1990b). In addition to concerns related to milk transfer and volume, nipple shields may present the dilemma of nipple shield addiction. This will lead the baby to refuse to suckle on the soft breast in preference for the rigid texture of the shield or other such rigid shape (DeNicola, 1986).

As with any other tool used to aid breastfeeding, the nipple shield does have its place in certain situations when appropriate follow-up care is given. For instance,

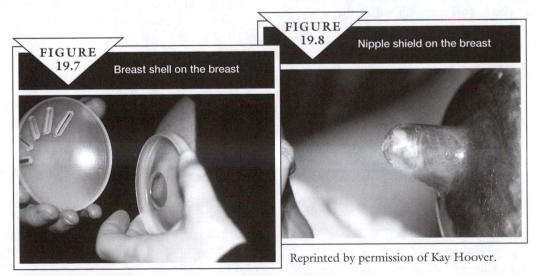

FIGURE 19.7 Breast shell on the breast

Reprinted by permission of Kay Hoover.

FIGURE 19.8 Nipple shield on the breast

Reprinted by permission of Kay Hoover.

shields are sometimes used with preterm infants to assist the infant at the breast. The shield should not be the first choice for intervention with latching difficulties or sucking concerns. Techniques such as proper positioning, forming the nipple, reducing breast fullness, eversion with an inverted syringe, and encouraging more sucking need to be tried first.

In situations in which the baby is refusing the breast and the mother has exhausted other techniques, you may suggest the use of a nipple shield. Before presenting this option to the mother, consider whether or not the benefits of the shield's use outweigh the risks. The mother must determine whether its use will fit in her breastfeeding plan and whether she will accept the risks and comply with careful follow-up. If a mother is considering weaning because of her breastfeeding difficulties, a shield may be appropriate. The nipple shield may buy the mother and baby time to work through a difficulty and preserve breastfeeding (Wilson-Clay 1996).

Proper Method for Using a Nipple Shield

If a mother wishes to use a nipple shield, be sure that she is aware of its appropriate use and follow-up. When used appropriately, the shield is removed after the baby begins the feed. He is then quickly put back to breast to suckle without the shield. The mother needs to be instructed that she will experience less stimulation to her breasts when the shield is in place. Reduced stimulation can lead to reduced milk production. It is for this reason that the mother should try to remove the shield during the feed so that the baby suckles directly on the breast and stimulates milk production.

The baby's intake and output need careful monitoring during the shield's use. A daily record of the baby's feeds, voids, and stools should be monitored, along with periodic weight checks. The mother may need to pump during the nipple shield's use to maintain milk production. She also needs to understand that the shield is meant to be a temporary measure to work through a breastfeeding difficulty. Encourage her to wean from the shield as soon as possible. She can put her baby to breast periodically without the shield when it "feels right" to see whether or not he will feed without it.

Nipple Shield Consent Form

Because of the risks, it is recommended that you require a signed consent form specifically for the use of a nipple shield. A consent form for use of a nipple shield may contain the warning below.

> I wish to use a nipple shield as a device to help my infant learn to latch onto my breast. I understand that improper or continuous use of this nipple shield can cause a 22 percent to 50 percent decrease in my milk supply and that it may inhibit my milk ejection reflex. These ef-

fects can result in little or no weight gain for my infant. I understand that while I am using this nipple shield I must use a large hospital-grade electric breast pump to stimulate and maintain my milk supply. I understand that while using this nipple shield my infant's weight will need to be checked once or twice a week. I understand that improper or continuous use of this device can lead to my infant becoming dependent on it in order to nurse from my breast. I understand that this device is to be used as a temporary breastfeeding aid and that the use of it should be discontinued as soon as possible.

Printed by permission of Breastfeeding Support Consultants.

Weaning the Baby From the Shield

When you and the mother decide that the time is right to work toward weaning from the shield, the mother will benefit from practical suggestions. In the past, it was suggested that the shield be trimmed back gradually to facilitate weaning. This is not advisable because the trimmed edges may lacerate the baby's mouth or the mother's nipple. Rather, the mother can watch for times when her baby offers cues that he may nurse without the shield. Often, a sleepy baby is less likely to resist the change from shield to breast. Some babies will accept the breast without the shield after the initial fullness at the beginning of a feed has decreased. Increased skin-to-skin contact with the mother will aid in the transition from shield to breast.

If a baby is particularly resistive to feeding without the shield, it may be made less attractive to him by stuffing a small piece of damp cloth inside the teat cavity so that milk no longer flows out. The baby is then allowed to suck with no results. The breast with dripped milk is quickly offered in place of the stuffed shield. If all else fails, the mother may choose to continue nursing indefinitely using the shield rather than weaning from the breast totally. A mother who chooses to do this will benefit from ongoing support. Her baby will need periodic weight checks, and the mother may need to pump to ensure continued milk production.

▼ Pacifiers

Pacifiers are often at the center of debate concerning their usefulness for babies. This is true particularly for babies who are breastfeeding. What may be an appropriate avenue for meeting the sucking needs of a bottle-fed baby is often the cause of difficulty when used with a breastfeeding infant. Pacifier use correlates with a higher incidence of early weaning (Barros, 1995; Victoria, 1993); particularly when sucking technique is incorrect (Righard, 1997). Pacifier use also increases the incidence of candida and ear infections. They can cause malocclusion, and some can suppress the central grooving of the baby's tongue.

Pacifiers offer no nutritional benefit to the infant. They expend calories and, in some instances, may contribute to slowed infant growth. The time a baby spends sucking on a pacifier is time spent away from the breast. This interferes with the cooperative relationship of the baby increasing the mother's milk production through suckling. Therefore, pacifiers may negatively affect the mother's milk production in relation to her baby's needs (Newman, 1990). If a pacifier is used too often, the baby may show a poor weight gain from having inadequate time at the breast. Less time at the breast can also cause insufficient drainage of the mother's milk, which, in turn, can result in engorgement or mastitis.

Pacifiers frequently are used by the mother in response to her baby's crying. You can help parents learn other ways to comfort their baby. (See the discussion of crying in Chapter 11.) It has been shown that babies whose parents "wear" them against their bodies (as with baby slings or snugglies) will cry less often and also are given a pacifier less often (Hunziker, 1986). Teaching parents options that are more appropriate than pacifiers for helping their crying babies will help them make better choices and decrease breastfeeding difficulties.

Appropriate and Safe Use of a Pacifier

One instance in which pacifiers have a positive use is in the case of premature infants. Preterm infants have been shown to benefit from sucking on pacifiers during **gavage** feeding (Bernbaum, 1983; Drosten, 1997). Accelerated maturation of the sucking reflex, decreased intestinal transit time, and increased rates of weight gain were positive effects that were identified. The pacifier is also useful in calming infants who must undergo painful procedures. It may be especially important in reducing testing stress in cases of severely ill babies.

Caution mothers to use pacifiers judiciously. A pacifier should never replace a feeding. Should a mother decide to use a pacifier, she needs to be instructed not to offer it until she is certain that her baby's other needs such as the need for food, comfort, and human contact are fully met. When offering the pacifier, she needs to tune into her baby's cues. If he settles when being held, then he was in need of cuddling comfort. If he remains unsettled and roots, urge the mother to put him to breast before offering a pacifier. If he does not want to nurse and continues to demonstrate a need to suck, a pacifier may help pacify him.

Use of the pacifier should be accompanied by plenty of skin contact. Additionally, mothers need to receive instructions on safe pacifier use. The pacifier should not be connected to a cord around the baby's neck. Recalls are abundant owing to the danger of parts separating. A 1998 recall of one brand of pacifier was initiated because of phytalates in the material.

EVALUATOR TECHNIQUES

There will be times when a caregiver needs to place a finger in the baby's mouth to calm the baby, assess the oral cavity, or improve the baby's suck. At times, clinicians will need to determine whether or not an infant has a dysfunctional suck. Before any manual manipulation is attempted, however, it must first be determined whether or not the baby's uncoordinated sucking can be resolved with the passage of time and with increasing the baby's caloric intake. Fluid flow regulates suck. Therefore, some babies' sucking improves when fluid is introduced in the mouth while sucking. The initiation of a more intrusive intervention in the hospital for the healthy full-term infant is rarely indicated.

Putting your finger into the baby's mouth for evaluation purposes should be done only in special circumstances and should be performed very carefully by a trained person. The baby's oral cavity is extremely sensitive, with many nerve innervations. Too much inappropriate manipulation can result in an aversion to anything going into the mouth, including the breast. Barger (1998) identifies four levels of digital intervention for infants who have difficulty suckling. When assistance is indicated, the caregiver should start with the least interventive method and progress to the highest degree of intervention only when other less interventive methods have failed. Refer to Chapter 13 for further discussion on the four levels of digital intervention.

Finger to Pacify Baby

The evaluator or parent may insert the index finger in the baby's mouth to pacify him or to initiate suckling. Insert your index finger, pad side up, very gently into the baby's mouth and wait until he begins sucking on the finger (Fig. 19.9). This technique can also be used in conjunc-

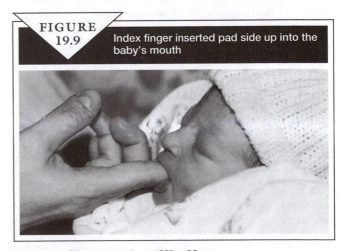

FIGURE 19.9 Index finger inserted pad side up into the baby's mouth

Reprinted by permission of Kay Hoover.

tion with a tube feeding system at the breast to increase the baby's calorie intake, referred to as finger feeding. This is considered to be a minimal level of intervention.

Finger to Evaluate Oral Cavity

Evaluating the infant's oral cavity is regarded as a low level of intervention. You can assess the infant's oral cavity and suck with your index finger. When he is relaxed and ready to receive your finger, insert your index finger, pad side up, very gently into the baby's mouth. Feel the inside of the oral cavity and the palates. Is the palate normal, flat, or excessively high? When the baby suckles, does the tongue cover the alveolar ridge? Does his tongue cup around the bottom of your finger to form a trough? Does the tongue move rhythmically from front to back? Assessing these elements will help you determine if a problem exists.

Suck Reorganization

Notice that in the two previous interventions, the baby was in control. Suck reorganization involves more control by the caregiver through manipulation of the finger in the mouth. It is considered to be a moderate level of intervention. With your finger in the baby's mouth, pad side up, place slight pressure on the midline of the tongue, pulling the finger out slowly to encourage the baby to suck it back in. Give verbal reinforcement when the baby sucks appropriately.

Suck Training

The incidence of a need for suck training intervention is extremely rare. It is considered to be a high level of intervention. Suck training involves tapping, stroking, and massaging the baby's tongue, gums, and palate. There may be "walking" of the fingers back on the tongue almost to the point of the baby gagging. The therapist places his or her index finger in the baby's mouth and stimulates certain portions of the baby's oral anatomy to train him to suck. This technique is highly active and controlling on the part of the therapist.

A baby who needs suck training must be referred to a professional who is trained and skilled in this field, such as a physical or speech therapist with further specialization as a neurodevelopmental therapist (NDT). This is beyond the scope of most nurses or lactation consultants. If there is a need for suck training, there are often other neurologic problems (such as cerebral palsy) and the suck is often the first area in which the problem is manifested. You need to work in concert with the baby's physician and other specialists. A referral to the Easter Seals organization may also be necessary.

MILK EXPRESSION

There are times in most women's breastfeeding when they need to remove milk from their breasts. No matter what method of milk expression a mother chooses and no matter how diligent she is in expressing her milk, she cannot remove milk from her breasts as efficiently as her baby can. The baby combines suction and rhythmic compression of the areola with his gums to suckle out the milk. Just as a mother and baby need time to learn how to nurse, a mother may express several times before she becomes proficient and is able to obtain the desired amount of milk. Gentle breast massage will encourage the flow of milk and help relax and soothe the mother so that more milk is obtained.

Manual Expression

Every mother needs to know how to hand express her milk, regardless of her breastfeeding situation. This enables her to be self-reliant no matter what circumstances may arise in the course of breastfeeding. She will be able to extract milk despite a broken pump, power failure, natural disaster, or low battery. Learning to be independent and function without a need for devices can help instill further confidence in her abilities. With manual expression, the mother is able to express anytime and anywhere, without waiting. It is cost free and quiet and she is in charge of the pressure applied. Milk collection by hand expression shows no difference in contamination rates as compared with milk collection using a breast pump (Pittard, 1991). Even though no differences were found in this study, manual expression often is cleaner than pumping because women do not always clean their pumps adequately.

Technique for Manual Expression

In preparing to express by hand, the mother should first wash her hands well. She may choose to gently massage her breast and possibly apply a warm, moist washcloth to the breast for several minutes. Both techniques will help promote milk flow. If she wishes, she may continue to massage her breast throughout her expressing session. Instruct the mother to lean slightly forward, with her nipple aimed at the collection container, as shown in Figure 19.10. Grasping her breast as she would when using the C-hold, she will place her thumb on the areola above the nipple and her first finger on the areola below the nipple. Next she will press her thumb and first finger inward toward her chest wall a short way and then firmly press on the lactiferous sinuses beneath the areola between the finger and thumb.

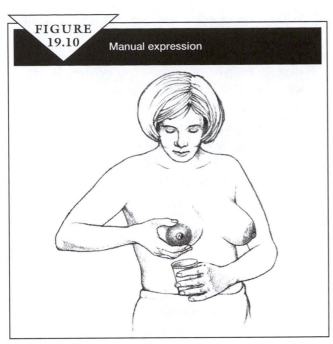

FIGURE 19.10 Manual expression

Illustration by Marcia Smith.

The mother will then continue the cycle of pressing and releasing the thumb and forefinger throughout her expressing session. Initially it may take several attempts until milk begins to drip. Milk will spray out with greater force after the milk lets down. The mother needs to rotate her thumb and forefinger around the areola to compress all the lactiferous sinuses. Caution her not to squeeze the nipple itself and not to move her fingers along her skin. Such actions have little or no benefit to expressing milk and may damage her breast tissue.

Many mothers find a method of hand expression quite different from this technique that works equally well or better for her. In fact, most women report that they find it difficult to master the technique as it is usually described in the literature. Some women express by cupping the breast with the C-hold, gently massaging and applying pressure on the lactiferous sinuses. Encourage mothers to experiment with various hand positions until they find what works best for them. There is no one perfect way for this or many other techniques. Honor these individual choices by not insisting on the mother's conforming to a certain technique. Practice and adaptation are keys to making hand expression work for the individual mother. Once hand expression is mastered, it can be faster and more efficient than a pump.

Use of a Breast Pump

When a mother is using a breast pump, close contact with a lactation consultant will enable her to share any anxieties and frustrations. The close contact will also help you determine whether or not she is having any difficulties in pumping or maintaining milk production. Her needs are especially great when she is using a mechanical device to empty her breasts and maintain milk production without the emotional gratification of her baby nuzzling at her breast. Her reactions may range from fear of possible pain, to embarrassment, to irritation, or to passive acceptance. If the need for a pump has resulted from a health problem in her or the baby, she may be anxious about the outcome and need to share her concerns with someone. If she will be pumping for several days, or perhaps even weeks or months, she may experience periods of discouragement and will benefit from your reassurance and support.

The mother who is preoccupied with the situation that required that she pump may not pay close attention to the information you provide her. Make a special effort to offer her clear instructions and explanations. In addition, take time to review any action plans at the end of your conversations in order to avoid misunderstandings. Written instructions, presented clearly and simply, will help her deal with the situation when you are not available. Although her present circumstances may be stressful, you can help a mother view pumping as a positive force in the resolution of her problem. Encourage her to regard pumping as more than a means of obtaining milk. It is her lifeline to breastfeeding her baby. By pumping regularly, she can maintain the potential ability to provide her baby with both the ideal food and protection from illness, as well as the benefits of a warm and loving relationship. It is something that only the mother can do for her baby. In a situation in which she can do little else, pumping can help her to feel involved and essential.

Conditioning Letdown for Pumping

When a baby suckles at the breast, the stimulation on his mother's nipple triggers the letdown of her milk. A breast pump or manual expression does not provide the same degree of stimulation as that of the baby. Therefore, the mother may need to condition her milk externally to let down. The mother's emotional state is a factor in her ability to establish letdown. She will want to prepare herself mentally for pumping and arrange to pump at times when she is rested and unhurried.

The mother can create a conducive atmosphere by arranging to pump her milk in a place where she has privacy, a comfortable chair, and a picture of her baby. She may want to make a tape recording of her baby's sounds to listen to while pumping. Other techniques for establishing letdown are outlined in Chapter 6.

When a mother has difficulty establishing letdown while pumping, she may become tense, agitated, and emotionally upset, thereby inhibiting her letdown even further. When you have confirmed that she is using a quality pump and good technique, you can encourage the mother to continue pumping her breasts gently to obtain the milk that is readily available and to persist in her efforts to relax. The routine of pumping may help her in establishing letdown. Often, a regular routine itself helps the mother relax and patiently work toward increasing her milk production. Another factor that will contribute to successful pumping is ensuring that the mother's nipple has contact with the side of the flange so as to provide the stimulation needed for her milk to let down.

Selecting a Breast Pump

Choosing a pump that best meets the mother's needs is essential. There are many types of breast pumps available, and each has its own particular advantages that best serve certain situations. In selecting a pump, the mother will want to consider her baby's age and condition, and how long she will need to pump. If she is pumping while at work, her options may be limited by the type of pump (if any) that is available. The amount of time she has available for pumping, facilities for pumping, affordability and her own personal preference are other factors to be considered.

You need to be familiar with the types of breast pumps that are available in your community, as well as the ease with which mothers can obtain them. Being able to offer practical information, such as descriptions and prices of various pumps, how they are used, and their advantages and disadvantages, will help mothers in deciding which pumps to select. Breast pumps that are manufactured by companies that sell artificial baby milk or feeding products may not be the best choice. Advise mothers to select a pump that is manufactured by a company whose primary mission is the support of breastfeeding. If she is using a manual pump or battery or electric pump that does not have autocycling suction, she must avoid long periods of uninterrupted vacuum, because this may damage her breast tissue. For this reason, autocycling pumps are recommended. Some guidelines that may help mothers in their selection of a breast pump are listed in the following section.

Criteria For Selecting A Breast Pump

◆ Does it cycle quickly, similar to the rhythm of an infant's suck?

◆ Is the flange shape comfortable and an appropriate size for the mother's breast?

◆ Can standard size bottles be used for collecting the milk?

◆ Are the breast pump parts dishwasher safe?

◆ Is the pump easy to assemble, with few parts?

◆ Is the pump easy to use with the type of hand or arm motion required?

◆ If the pump is electric, will the power source be adequate (i.e., type of outlet—two or three prongs—and amount of voltage)?

◆ Is the pump quiet?

◆ Is the pump easy to transport?

◆ Is the pump affordable for the length of time it is required?

◆ Is service readily available?

◆ Are written instructions available?

◆ Is there someone knowledgeable in breastfeeding to answer questions and resolve problems?

◆ Is there a toll free number to call with questions?

Hand-Held Breast Pump

Many mothers use a hand-held breast pump as an occasional supplement to breastfeeding. (Fig. 19.11). A hand-held pump consists of a collecting bottle and a flange that fits over the breast. A piston, trigger, or motor provides the suction. There is a wide variety of styles and prices available. Hand-held pumps may be either manual, battery, or a combination of battery and electric. A manual pump that uses natural movements will be the most comfortable for mothers. One of the earliest hand-held breast pumps, still found in some stores today, was the bicycle horn pump. The name de-

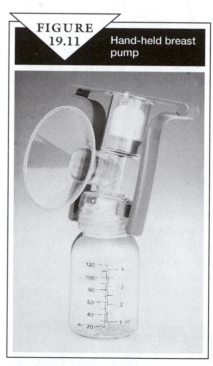

FIGURE 19.11 Hand-held breast pump

Courtesy Hollister/Ameda-Egnell, Cary IL.

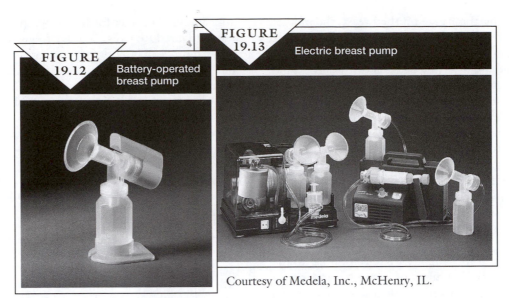

FIGURE 19.12   Battery-operated breast pump

FIGURE 19.13   Electric breast pump

Courtesy of Medela, Inc., McHenry, IL.

Courtesy of Medela, Inc., McHenry, IL.

rives from its resemblance to a bicycle horn. This pump can cause damage to the mother's nipple and also harbors bacteria that could be dangerous to the baby. Hand pumps that use a bulb to generate suction should not be used. Motorized hand pumps provide suction with either a control button for the mother to regulate pressure or with an autocycling motor that does all of the suction work (Figure 19.12)

Electric Breast Pump

Electric breast pumps are usually used in the regular absence of nursing when the mother and baby cannot be together (Fig. 19.13). Electric breast pumps are the best option for mothers who need the most efficient pumping, such as with an ill baby. Some women use them for other lengthy or regular separation such as full-time employment. Electric pumps are the most costly, with the most expensive models usually obtained through rental rather than purchase. They most closely mimic the baby's suckling rhythm and provide the stimulation that is necessary to maintain the mother's milk production. Electric pumps also offer the option of pumping both breasts at the same time, as shown in Figure 19.14, thus saving time and increasing breast stimulation. In some cases, simultaneous double pumping has been found to obtain higher milk yields (Auerbach, 1990a).

Pumping Technique

Because the use of breast pumps is accompanied by an interruption in breastfeeding, the mother may need specialized counseling. For this reason, many lactation consultants choose to carry various pumps and accompanying equipment to have it readily available for demonstration and hands-on teaching. Mothers need complete instructions that include a demonstration of proper equipment use. No matter what type of pump is used, appropriate written instructions should be given to the mother.

To begin pumping, the mother needs to wash her hands first. She will then want to get comfortable and may find it helpful to do breast massage. Expressing a few drops of milk by hand before pumping will help the milk let down before pumping is begun, thus enabling the mother to see faster results. She can also moisten the flange of the pump with her milk for a better seal. Some clinicians suggest that the mother use olive oil on the flange to obtain a good seal and decrease skin friction.

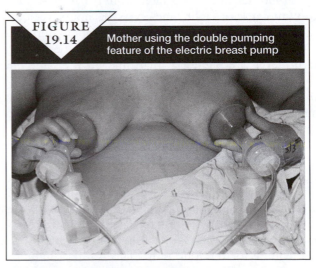

FIGURE 19.14   Mother using the double pumping feature of the electric breast pump

Printed by permission of Kay Hoover.

When securing the flange on the breast, the mother needs to center her nipple so that her breast tissue touches the sides of the flange. Special inserts that rest inside the flange are available to achieve the proper fit. However, they may cause sore breasts or nipples in some women. The mother will want to use only as much suction as is needed to maintain milk flow throughout her pumping session. Advise that she begin with the suction on the lowest setting and increase suction strength gradually as necessary.

A mother who is single pumping will find it helpful to alternate between breasts several times throughout her pumping session to capitalize on the multiple letdowns that occur simultaneously. She may pump 5 to 7 minutes on one breast and then switch to the other breast for another 5 to 7 minutes. She can return to the first breast for 3 to 5 minutes of pumping and repeat that time on the second breast. Finally, she may finish on the first breast with 2 to 3 minutes of pumping and then the second breast for the final 2 to 3 minutes. If the mother is double pumping with an electric pump or two battery pumps, 12 to 15 minutes total pumping time may be sufficient.

Encourage mothers to tailor pumping times to their specific needs and situations. Mothers can expect to pump varying amounts of milk on different days and at different times of the day. Morning pumping frequently yields more milk than does pumping in the afternoon or evening. If her baby is breastfeeding some or most of the time, pumping can be adapted to their breastfeeding schedule. Pumping may be done in place of a missed feed, between feeds, or one breast may be pumped while feeding the baby on the other breast. The mother can experiment to find which arrangement will best suit her and her baby's needs.

Pumping for a Hospitalized Baby

A mother who is separated from her baby will need to pump at least eight times every 24 hours, regardless of the amount of milk she obtains. Pumping during the night will produce larger quantities of milk because prolactin levels are highest at that time. At the same time, the mother needs a 4- or 5-hour stretch of sleep to maintain her own health and energy. She can be encouraged to pump during the night whenever she wakes naturally. As the time for her baby to come home grows closer, she can begin to pump more regularly at night. For a more gentle nighttime waking, she may drink extra fluids just before bedtime to facilitate her waking.

Regular milk removal will help the mother build and maintain milk production so that she has sufficient milk when her baby is able to nurse. Initiating copious milk production helps establish milk production that will endure for the long term. This is especially important in times of stress. If the mother needs to collect large amounts of milk for her baby, she can pump more frequently, reduce stress, and try to get adequate rest.

A mother may find that one breast produces more milk and lets down more easily than the other. This is normal and is seen in most women. Both breasts need regular milk removal in order to establish milk production and to avoid complications caused by overfullness. The most efficient means for milk removal via pump will vary from mother to mother.

▼ Collecting and Storing Human Milk

Mothers collect their milk for a variety of reasons. Milk may be stored in the freezer for emergencies and for a regular separation such as working or attending school. They may wish to provide stored milk for a short-term separation such as a shopping trip, wedding, or other social outing. Expressed milk may also be necessary for the infant who tires out or cannot manage every feed at the breast. Some mothers donate their milk to be given to other babies.

Encourage the mother to contact you if she has any doubts about whether or not to use her expressed milk. If a mother expresses her milk to relieve breast fullness, or collects drip milk during a feed, she can save it for later use. Milk that has accumulated in a breast shell worn between feeds should not be saved, because it has been against the mothers skin for a lengthy time. When the mother is taking a medication that would be potentially harmful to her baby, the milk cannot be given to her baby. If she or her baby has a yeast infection, any collected milk may harbor the infection and should be discarded. Another instance that may require varying guidelines for human milk storage is milk for a baby in a multiple child care setting. In this case, the mother needs to review safety issues with the care provider. You can assist them by providing up-to-date guidelines and possibly educating the child care staff about human milk storage and use.

Storage Container

Milk must be stored properly in order to preserve its quality and keep it from spoiling. Collection containers and any parts of a pump that have contact with the mother's milk must be cleaned after every use with soapy water and thoroughly rinsed. Washing in a dishwasher is also appropriate. The equipment may then be air dried. Glass containers have been shown to be the best choice for milk storage. Glass does not absorb the milk's antibodies or other proteins. It is cleaned more easily and offers protection against contamination of the milk during storage. The next best choice for storage would be a hard plastic (polypropylene) container. A drawback to this container is that the interior surface may scratch and make cleaning difficult.

A storage container frequently used but not recommended is a soft plastic (polyethylene) baby bottle liner. Certain antibodies in human milk are dramatically reduced in concentration when the milk is stored in soft plastic containers such as bottle liners. Additionally, such soft plastics are difficult to seal and may puncture easily. Some mothers have even reported that their milk stored in these bags smelled and tasted bad, rendering it unusable (Goldblum, 1981; Hopkinson, 1990).

Another factor that will affect the choice of container is the amount of milk to be stored. The amount may vary as the mother determines how much her baby will consume in her absence. Until studies determine the safety of using the leftover milk, it is suggested that mothers discard any milk left in the bottle at the end of a feed. Therefore, it is suggested that the mother initially store her milk in small amounts, usually 2 to 4 oz, in order that less milk is wasted at feeds. No matter what amount is stored, if it is to be frozen, the mother needs to leave space for expansion of the milk in the container during freezing.

The container should be labeled, using a waterproof marker, with information that will assist the mother and any other caregivers in the milk's proper use. At the very least, the label should include the date and time the milk was expressed, and possibly the amount of milk contained. If the milk is given to the baby by another caregiver with multiple children, the mother's and baby's full names must also be indicated. Their last names are important, because some babies will have last names that are different from their mothers'. In the case of day care providers with multiple children, the mother may want to transport the milk in a container that is ready for feeding. This reduces the possibility of the caretaker contaminating the milk while pouring.

Storage Time

Storage times vary depending on how soon the baby will by given the expressed milk. One study suggests that if the milk will be used within 5 days, it can be placed in the refrigerator immediately after it is collected (Sosa, 1987). However, milk banking experts recommend a shorter time—3 days—because it is so hard to control for contamination. An expert work group that met in August 1996 concluded that the recommendation for the storage of refrigerated milk be 3 days rather than the 5 days cited in the Sosa study (Wellstart, 1996). If refrigeration is not immediately available, Pittard (1985) suggests that milk may remain at room temperature for up to 8 hours without a significant increase in the bacteria count. Hamosh (1996) recommends that milk be stored at room temperature for no more than 4 hours. This conservative approach accounts for the variables inherent in milk collection such as amount of con-tamina-tion and definition of "room temperature." If a mother is not sure that she will use her milk within 3 to 5 days, she will need to freeze it. If she wishes, she can place her expressed milk directly in the freezer after collecting it, provided it is not being added to milk that is already frozen (see discussion later).

Human milk may be stored in the freezer for up to 1 year depending on the type of freezer. In a freezer that is part of a refrigerator unit and has a separate door, the milk will keep for 3 months. A deep freezer will keep the milk for 6 months to 1 year depending on the temperature. To avoid extremes of temperature, milk should not be stored on the door of the refrigerator or freezer, or near the freezer's defrosting unit. The optimal temperature in the freezer is 0°F or minus 18 to 20°C. If the freezer does not contain a thermometer, one can be placed there.

Special Guidelines for the NICU Infant

Human milk collection and storage guidelines will vary slightly depending on the reason the mother is collecting her milk. Guidelines often focus on mothers with well babies who are collecting milk for convenience or employment. Such guidelines cannot be applied to all situations. A mother who is collecting milk for her baby in the intensive care unit will need to follow more strict guidelines to ensure the safety of her baby, who may be preterm or ill. Whenever possible, the milk should be expressed just before feeding the baby. Expressed milk that is not to be used within 1 hour must be refrigerated immediately. If the milk will not be used within 48 hours, freezing is recommended for milk that is being stored for an ill or preterm baby. Milk for a preterm infant needs to be placed in a separate storage container for each pumping session to minimize handling and contamination of the milk (Human Milk Banking Association of North America 1993.)

Combining Containers of Milk

Mothers often have questions regarding the procedure for storing their milk from more than one pumping session, or from both breasts at the same pumping session. When a mother pumps both breasts at the same time, both bottles of milk can be combined for storage. Milk from different pumping sessions may be combined for storage, with the label stating the date and time of the earliest pumping. That is the date that is used in selecting which container to use. Newly pumped milk may be added to previously pumped milk after it has been cooled. Newly pumped milk may be added to frozen milk after it has been chilled for at least 2 hours. Caution mothers not to add more milk to the container than what has already been frozen, in order to prevent the freshly pumped milk from partially defrosting the frozen milk. In all cases, the storage time for such combined milks will be based on the expiration date of the earliest expressed milk.

Defrosting and Warming Human Milk

With appropriate labeling, the mother will be able to use milk based on the date it was expressed. Encourage her to use her oldest milk first. If she has a large stock of milk in her freezer, it may help to arrange the milk with the oldest containers most easily visible. If the milk is frozen, it may be thawed by placing it in the refrigerator. The thawed milk may remain refrigerated for up to 24 hours before using it (Pierce, 1992). It must then be discarded if it is not used. Refreezing is not an option.

Milk may be thawed either by placing it in the refrigerator overnight or by thawing it rapidly in a pan of warm water or under a stream of warm tap water. Milk should be used within 24 hours of thawing, or it should be discarded. Refrigerated milk may also be warmed in this manner. Mothers often ask about the use of a microwave oven for warming milk. They should be discouraged from this practice. Microwaving liquids results in hot spots that may pose a danger to the baby's mouth (Nemethy, 1990). Additionally, microwaving has been found to cause a marked decrease in activity of anti-infective properties in human milk (Quan, 1992).

When human milk sits in the refrigerator or freezer, the fat in it will rise to the top of the milk. Reassure the mother that this is perfectly normal. Shaking the milk throughout the warming process will mix the fat. After stored human milk has been warmed, it needs to be used immediately and only for that feed. If any milk remains after the baby's feed, it cannot be saved because it will harbor bacteria from the baby's saliva.

▼ Human Milk Banks

A mother's own expressed milk is more appropriate for her baby than is any other alternative feeding choice. It is produced in response to this particular baby, in response to his suckling and his environment. Occasionally, a mother may not be able to provide her own milk through either breastfeeding or expressing. In such cases, a mother's own milk can be replaced by donor milk from other women, in preference to infant formulas. Milk banks offer this safe alternative to mothers who cannot breastfeed.

A milk bank is a collection point for human milk that is donated by healthy nursing mothers. All donors are screened for infectious diseases. The milk is processed and pasteurized, and is dispensed only by prescription to infants, children, and occasionally, adults with a medical need for human milk. A processing fee is charged to recipient families, but no recipient is denied access to donor milk for inability to pay. Recipients are also asked to cover the costs of shipping the frozen milk.

There has been a decline in the number of milk banks in the United States owing to the use of preterm formulas and the isolation of human immunodeficiency virus (HIV) from human milk (Balmer, 1992). However, donor milk can be shipped anywhere in the country overnight. It is important that lactation support providers know how to access this service so that parents with critically ill infants do not have to search for it (Arnold, 1998).

Babies may need donor human milk for a variety of reasons. They may be unable temporarily to breastfeed, intolerant of human milk substitutes, or suffering from digestive disorders or severe diarrhea. Some preterm or very ill infants need donor milk until their mother's own production can be increased to meet their needs. Sometimes, a condition that demands human milk does not show up until several weeks or months after birth. The mother may be unable to relactate and, therefore, turns to a milk bank to help her baby survive. In many cases, the cost of production exceeds the cost to the recipient. Therefore, depending on the volume of milk processed and dispensed, the milk bank may be unable to cover their expenses. Mothers who are interested in more specific information can contact the Human Milk Banking Association of North America Inc. (HMBANA) or an area milk bank directly.

Procedure for Donating Milk

Mothers who have expressed and saved milk for another person's baby have found great emotional gratification and reward in knowing that they are helping a baby in need. You can facilitate the use of milk banks for both donors and recipients by providing a free breast pump and collection bottles, and by arranging for the transfer of milk to the nearest milk bank. Learn the location of milk banks as well as their policies regarding milk collection and distribution. HMBANA provides such information for professionals. When a mother expresses a desire to become a donor, you can provide her with guidelines and put her in contact with the nearest milk bank.

HMBANA provides donor education in both verbal and written form. Donors are instructed about situations that require disqualification from donating milk. Milk banks will not accept milk from mothers who are ill or who are taking any medication other than replacement hormones. Donors are taught clean technique for milk expression. That includes handwashing, breast cleansing, washing and sterilizing of pump parts, handling of sterilized equipment, labeling of the milk, proper milk storage, and proper technique for transportation of milk to the bank.

If the milk bank requires that the milk be frozen, the label should be attached to the jar before being placed in the freezer to ensure that the label will adhere. When milk is transported to the milk bank, it must be well insulated to prevent any thawing. The milk must stay frozen until it arrives at the milk bank. Milk banks that collect fresh human milk must see that it is refrigerated immediately after being collected and used within 24 hours. Some milk banks may require that milk be collected in a sterile container and marked with the mother's name, date of collection, number of ounces, and the name and dosage of any drugs taken by the mother. Others may accept excess stockpiled milk in a one-time donation. The individual milk bank will provide its own collection and storage guidelines, which may vary slightly from those described here.

Screening of Donated Milk

Potential milk donors are screened before their milk is accepted by the milk bank. After milk is received at the bank, according to HMBANA's protocols, frozen milk is thawed in a refrigerator and pooled under sterile conditions. It is then heat-treated to ensure the absence of HIV, hepatitis, and other viruses and bacteria for which the milk bank did not test. This also ensures that the mother was not in the window period between infection and antibody expression. Routine antigen testing similar to that of blood banks is also conducted to further rule out the presence of HIV in the milk. Fortunately heat-treated milk retains most of the immunologic and nutritional properties. Heat-treating at either 56°C or 62.5°C (**Holder pasteurization**) is carried out for 30 minutes. Then the milk is rapidly cooled and refrozen. Each batch is thoroughly cultured. If there is any bacterial growth, the milk is excluded from infant use.

When a need arises for raw human milk, the decision is made in consultation with all parties involved, with potential risks outlined carefully. The raw pool of milk is screened for bacteria and must have an acceptably low level of bacteria colonies of normal skin flora. This is true of all milk, whether or not it is raw. When colonies are unacceptably high, or if any bacteria other than normal skin flora is present, that milk is excluded from both raw and pasteurized use.

Donor milk should always be obtained through a milk bank. The informal sharing of human milk is not recommended. Home pasteurization is not controlled by a protocol that ensures the safety of the milk. There are serious liability issues for health care providers who arrange for one mother to supply milk informally to another mother's baby. The absence of a pasteurization safeguard makes this practice unsafe, even if they go through a screening process.

ALTERNATE FEEDING METHODS

Approach the issue of alternate feeding methods gently and with a lot of support. When they are needed, the mother's idealized view of breastfeeding has not materialized, and she must be allowed to verbalize her concerns and fears about her situation and her baby. The options and their risks and benefits to breastfeeding management need to be explained. Allowing the mother the freedom to make such a choice about what will fit best in her life gives her some control over an otherwise tenuous situation. The options available for a breast alternative include a cup or spoon, tube-feeding device for use at the breast, tube device used for finger feeding, and an artificial nipple and bottle. The appropriateness of each method to the mother's situation, including the risks, must be presented. She also needs to know the cost and the care and cleaning of each device. When the mother makes her decision, she will need thorough instructions, both verbal and written, with demonstration and close follow-up until the baby is breastfeeding again.

Cup Feeding

For the baby who is unable to breastfeed, cup feeding offers a baby-led alternative that does not invade the baby's oral cavity (Fig. 19.15). The cup provides an initial sensory stimulus of the lips, olfactory senses, and the tongue. The younger baby will lap the milk, which promotes appropriate tongue movement used during breastfeeding. The baby can pace his own intake, and because he is in control, respiration is easier and swallowing occurs when he is ready. Babies as young as 30 weeks' gestation are capable of maintaining their heart rates, respirations, and oxygenation while cup feeding (Lang, 1994). At 30 to 34 weeks, babies lap by protruding their tongues into the milk to obtain small boluses of milk. The milk often is held in the baby's mouth for some time before swallowing. As the baby matures, a sipping action begins to develop. Lang noted a correlation with cup feeding the preterm baby to the establishment of breastfeeding.

The method for cup feeding is easy for the mother and baby to learn. It is well worth the investment in avoiding the risk of the baby forming a preference for an artificial nipple. It may take the baby four or five feeds to catch onto the technique. A small cup with rounded edges works best, such as a shot glass, medicine cup, or a hollow-handed medicine spoon or even a conventional table spoon (Fig. 19.16). The small plastic cups used by fast food restaurants for catsup are a convenient choice. "Sippy" cups should be avoided because the spout does not allow the baby to trough his tongue correctly.

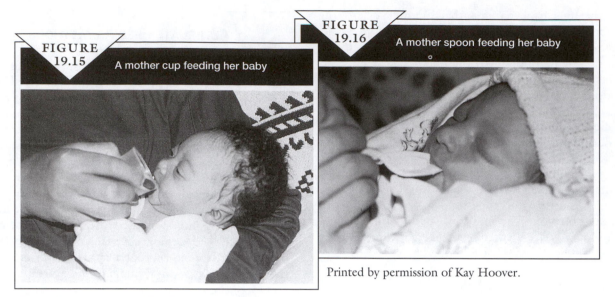

FIGURE 19.15 A mother cup feeding her baby

FIGURE 19.16 A mother spoon feeding her baby

Printed by permission of Kay Hoover.

Printed by permission of Kay Hoover.

Procedure for Cup Feeding

The cup should be filled about half way with approximately one-half to one-third an ounce of milk. Tucking a cloth under the baby's chin will catch any spills. The baby can be held in the mother's arms or in a semisitting position on her lap. Bring the cup to the baby's lips and rest the rim of the cup on his lower lip so that it touches the corners of his mouth. Tip the cup so that the milk just touches his lips. The baby will begin to lap the milk from the cup, and his tongue will form a trough to bring the milk to the back of his throat so that he can swallow it.

The milk must never be poured into the baby's mouth, because that will increase the risk of aspiration. The baby must be allowed to lead this activity and to rest between swallows. If he resists, it is best to stop, comfort him, and try again later when he is calmed. This method provides a low level of intervention that is much less invasive to the baby's oral cavity than finger feeding or the use of artificial nipples. Cup feeding is helpful in assisting the baby in learning to extend his tongue to and over the alveolar ridge.

▼ Tube-Feeding Device

A tube feeding device is intended to be used during a breastfeed to provide supplemental nutrition while the baby suckles at the breast. A commercial nursing supplementer consists of a plastic bag or bottle designed to hold expressed milk or an artificial baby milk. It is suspended by a cord around the mother's neck, or clipped to her clothing at shoulder level, so that it rests between her breasts. Thin, flexible tubing leads from the container to the end of the mother's nipple (Figs. 19.17 and 19.18). A less expensive noncommercial supple-

menter can be constructed with the use of a number 5, 6, or 8 French oral gastric tube on the end of a syringe or placed in a bottle (Fig. 19.19).

A tube-feeding device encourages nutritive suckling. It can be adjusted to deliver more supplement when the mother's milk production is low and less supplement as her production increases. A mother who is relactating or inducing lactation may find the use of this device to be helpful for supplementing her baby's intake while she in-

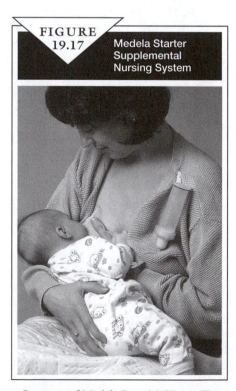

FIGURE 19.17 Medela Starter Supplemental Nursing System

Courtesy of Medela Inc., McHenry, IL.

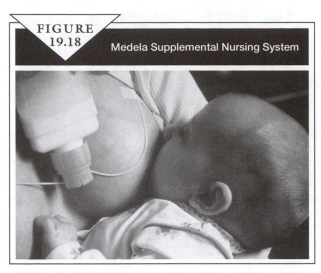

FIGURE 19.18 Medela Supplemental Nursing System

Courtesy of Medela Inc., McHenry, IL.

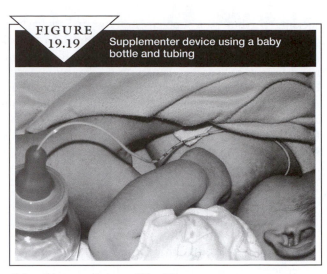

FIGURE 19.19 Supplementer device using a baby bottle and tubing

Printed by permission of Kay Hoover.

creases production. A baby who refuses to nurse at the breast can be encouraged by the flow of milk from the supplementer. A mother who has been expressing milk for an ill baby may need to use a supplementer during the transition from the milk expression to nursing. If the baby has been receiving the mother's milk from a bottle, the mother can replace use of the bottle with tube feeding. In any instance in which the baby will latch, a tube-feeding device is the least invasive and preferred method. It avoids the possibility of nipple preference from a bottle nipple and provides the mother with the breast stimulation she needs (Edgehouse, 1990).

Procedure for Tube Feeding

The container of milk is placed even with, above, or below the baby's head, depending on the desired rate of flow. Adjust the level of the container so that the baby has about one suck per swallow. As his suck becomes stronger, and milk flow increases, the container can be lowered. Tilt the feeding container so that it is easy to view bubbles rising to the top. Bubbles indicate that the baby is sucking and receiving milk effectively. The tube should extend about one-fourth of an inch beyond the end of the nipple. It can be taped to the mother's breast to keep it in place. The tape needs to be long enough to prevent it from coming loose in the baby's mouth. Paper tape is the least irritating to the mother's skin.

The baby suckles at the breast and the tip of the tube simultaneously. The flow of supplement from the container encourages him to continue suckling. In this way, the baby receives nourishment and stimulation of his oral reflexes. At the same time, the mother receives natural stimulation of her breasts to encourage milk production. Some babies may initially object to having the tube in their mouths and require time and patience in

getting accustomed to it. Others become so conditioned to nursing with the tubing that they may refuse to nurse without it. Advise the mother to check her baby's mouth daily to make sure that the tube is not irritating the roof of his mouth. After every use, the tubing should be flushed out with cold water, then washed with hot soapy water and rinsed with clear water.

Some styles of nursing supplementers have a flow-control valve that responds to the baby's sucking. Some, too, have various sizes of tubing to determine flow rate. It is unnecessary to compress the tube manually in order to control milk flow. In fact, doing so may damage the device or place the baby at risk by causing him to expend energy on non-nutritive sucking. Infants who are not at risk may be encouraged to start a feed without the supplementer and then make use of it when the need for additional supplement is indicated. Performing alternate breast massage during the feeding is helpful.

The substance used in tube feeding can be either expressed human milk or an artificial baby milk. Some infant formulas are thick and do not flow well through the narrow tubing. When powdered formula is used, it must be shaken well to avoid clogging the tubing. Some sources suggest avoiding the use of powdered formulas in a tube-feeding device because of the potential for clogging and the infant receiving insufficient supplementation. Human milk fortifiers can also clog tubing.

When it is evident that the baby is receiving increasing amounts of his mother's milk, the mother can reduce the supplement she offers at each feed. Such clues will be the presence of more milk in the breasts or increased amounts of milk left in the supplementer accompanied by good weight gain. Daily milk production is highest at morning feeds, and the amount of supplement can be reduced accordingly. Mothers need to note changes in suckling rhythm and supplement flow during feeds in order to switch breasts for optimum stimulation of milk production. The mother can watch for signs of sufficient nourishment, such as wet diapers, good skin turgor, and a consistent pattern of eating and sleeping. When she and her baby's physician are confident that milk production is adequate, the supplements can be decreased slowly—based on clinical evidence such as the baby's output and mother's milk production—and finally discontinued.

▼ Finger Feeding

Finger feeding is another means of getting needed nourishment to the baby (Fig. 19.20). In tube feeding, the tubing is placed on the end of the mother's nipple. In finger feeding, the tubing is placed on the end of the caregiver's or parent's finger. Finger feeding is more invasive than a tube-feeding device, and if it is used too long, finger feeding can become as addictive as an artificial nipple because the infant will imprint to it. Occasional finger feeding may be beneficial for a baby who needs help in organizing his suck. Although caregivers need to use a glove when demonstrating finger feeding, parents may finger feed without gloves. Because of the potential for allergy, latex is not recommended.

Procedure for Finger Feeding

As with tube feeding, you may use either a commercial nursing supplementer or a number 5, 6, or 8 French oral gastric tube on the end of a syringe that has the plunger removed. Removing the plunger allows for the infant to be in more control of his feeding rather than the adult who is feeding him. Another alternative is placing a long tube in a bottle on a table. Place the appropriate amount of expressed milk or substitute in the container that is attached to the tubing. Prime the tubing with the milk or substitute, then crimp it to stop the flow until it is in position. The baby should be held in an upright or semiupright position. Place the container of milk even with, above, or below the baby's head, depending on the desired rate of flow. The syringe or supplementer can be raised or lowered to achieve the appropriate flow. Position it so that it will be easy to view bubbles rising to the top. Bubbling indicates that the baby is sucking and swallowing effectively.

Lay the tubing along the fat pad of the finger, extending it about 1/4 inch beyond the finger tip. If you wish, you can tape the tube to your finger. Gently tickle the baby's lips so that he will open his mouth for your finger. Never push your finger into his mouth; wait until you are invited in by the baby. Place the fat pad of your finger with the tube on it into the baby's mouth against the soft palate (the finger nail will be against the baby's tongue).

The number of times the baby is finger fed and the amount of milk he is to be given will be determined by the baby's condition and the reason that finger feeding is required. If possible, hold the baby with his face skin to skin with the breast. Be sure that he is at a 45-degree angle to avoid milk getting into his ears. The mother's goal is for her baby to have one suck per swallow, as with breastfeeding. More than four sucks per swallow may be tiring to the baby. Advise the mother to check her baby's mouth several times each day to make sure that the tubing is not irritating the roof of his mouth. After every use, she needs to flush out the tubing first with cold water and then with hot soapy water, and finally to rinse it with clear water.

▼ Syringe Feeding

Some lactation consultants use a periodontal syringe either with finger feeding or at the breast (Fig. 19.21). Be

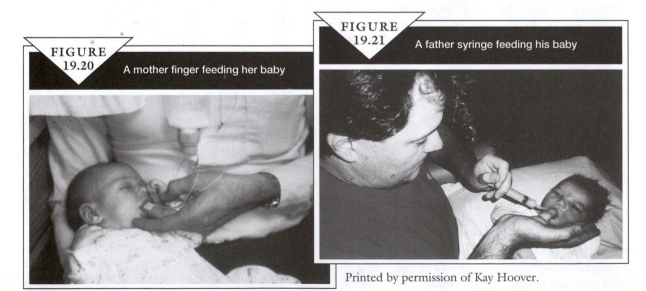

FIGURE 19.20   A mother finger feeding her baby

Printed by permission of Pat Bull.

FIGURE 19.21   A father syringe feeding his baby

Printed by permission of Kay Hoover.

extremely cautious about using this method of feeding because it can have potentially harmful consequences. Using a syringe with a plunger places the caregiver in control and not the baby. The fluid is pushed into the baby's mouth when he sucks, thus creating a potential of giving a greater bolus of milk than the baby can handle. This could cause aspiration, especially when done by someone who is inexperienced with the use of a syringe. Second, the periodontal syringe has a sharp point, presenting the possibility of scratching or gouging the baby's tongue, gums, or palate. For all of these reasons, syringe feeding is not recommended.

▼ Bottle Feeding

The lactation profession advocates for a method of alternate feeding that is least likely to interfere with breastfeeding. However, in reality, bottles and artificial nipples still remain a choice for mothers. They carry the powerful influence of cultural acceptance and encouragement, often to the point of excluding breastfeeding. Some mothers may find themselves in a situation that lacks support for the use of any alternative feeding device other than a bottle. A mother may decide that she herself is only comfortable with the use of the bottle. She may work with another alternative feeding method for some time and decide to switch to the bottle, because of lack of progress or pressure from her support network. Likewise, a baby may need to stay with a caregiver who is not comfortable with feeding methods other than a bottle. Parents deserve to know the risks involved with such choices. They need to understand that artificial nipples weaken a baby's suck and can contribute to malocclusion. Should they opt for the use of bottles and artificial nipples, they need to know the safest ways to implement their use.

In order to understand the concerns related to bottle and artificial nipple use, it is important to recognize the difference between the breast and an artificial nipple within the baby's oral cavity. When a baby is breastfeeding, his entire oral cavity is virtually filled with breast tissue, not just the nipple. There is no artificial nipple on the market that conforms to the individual shape of the baby's mouth in the way a human breast does.

The difference in the baby's mouth action on the breast and with the bottle must also be considered. On the breast, the baby is in charge. For the most part, when he suckles, the breast responds to his action with varying milk flows. When he stops suckling, the flow also stops. With a bottle, his action changes to one of protecting his airway. The bottle will provide a continuous drip of fluid and the baby must clamp the teat in order to get a break from the flow. No bottle and teat currently available is able to mimic the baby-led feeding at the breast.

Bottles and Nipples

Mothers who combine breastfeeding and bottle feeding will want to avoid any bottle nipple that has a small base. When the baby sucks on this type of nipple he tends to purse his lips, an action he may then use when he is put to breast (Fig. 19.22). A nipple with a wide base forces the baby to open his mouth wide, as he does with breastfeeding (Fig. 19.23). It is hoped that the wide base will help minimize latch-on difficulties when he switches back and forth between breast and bottle. If there is smacking or clicking when the baby drinks from the bottle, the base of the nipple probably is not large enough. No nipple that encourages the infant to purse his lips should be used unless there is no plan to resume breastfeeding.

Another issue related to artificial nipples is the choice between latex and silicone. Latex nipples are cheaper and are available in more shapes than those made of silicone. They do not last as long, however. Latex nipples may become rather gummy after use, particularly after boiling. There is also concern that boiling latex can release nitrates, which may have a cancer-causing effect. Additionally, increasing numbers of people are developing allergies to latex. Using latex teats

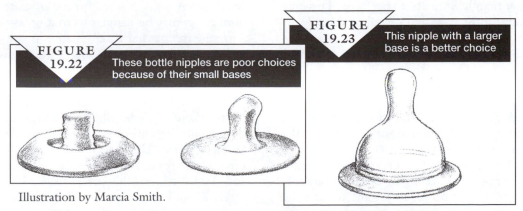

FIGURE 19.22 These bottle nipples are poor choices because of their small bases

Illustration by Marcia Smith.

FIGURE 19.23 This nipple with a larger base is a better choice

Illustration by Marcia Smith.

and pacifiers could precipitate this reaction in a susceptible infant. Although silicone nipples are firmer and more expensive, they withstand boiling better than the latex ones, thus lasting considerably longer. Silicone nipples are a potential source of silicone ingestion.

Selecting a Feeding Bottle

It probably does not much matter what type of bottle the mother chooses. However, because there are no antibacterial agents in formula, it is imperative that the bottle is able to be cleaned thoroughly with a bottle brush that can reach into every crevice. The elongated "O" shaped bottles designed for easy holding by the baby probably can not be cleaned as well as a plain bottle.

Teaching Bottle Feeding to Parents

The advantages of breastfeeding for the mother and baby extend far beyond the nutritional and immunologic benefits. When a mother chooses to breastfeed, she is making a health choice. She is choosing a method of communicating to her infant that is unique to the breastfeeding relationship. This lifestyle and relationship is the natural and normal one for new mothers. Certain adaptations can be made so that the bottle-fed baby and his mother receive some of the benefits of a breastfeeding relationship. It is the caregiver's responsibility to teach women the best and safest way to formula feed their infants when this mode of feeding is chosen.

Breastfed babies are held in several different positions for feeds. They breastfeed on both sides, which gives babies a different visual perspective when they change breasts. Bottle-fed babies also need that advantage. Mothers can be taught to cuddle their babies in the right arm for one feed, and in the left arm for the next feed. Likewise, breastfeeding always involves skin-to-skin contact between the mother and baby, contact that is continuous throughout the feed. Bottle feeding mothers need to be encouraged to provide frequent skin-to-skin contact with their babies. Additionally, there may be a temptation with bottle feeding to prop the bottle rather than hold the baby for feeds. This practice is dangerous for the baby and therefore strongly discouraged.

Breastfeeding mothers instinctively "groom" their babies while nursing. That is, they stroke, pat, and otherwise touch their babies with their free hand. This is a bit more difficult to do while bottle feeding. Bottle-feeding mothers can be encouraged to snuggle and hold the baby for at least 15 to 20 minutes after a feed so that he can benefit from this mothering.

Breastfed babies enjoy periods of non-nutritive sucking at the breast. This occurs usually at the end of a feed. A bottle-feeding mother may want to give her baby a pacifier at this time. Bottle-fed infants are unable to suck non-nutritively on the bottle because any movement of his mouth will cause formula to be expressed. Breastfed babies often have the opportunity to cuddle in bed with the mother during feeds, with both of them napping while the baby suckles. The bottle-fed infant does not generally have this opportunity. Encourage the formula-feeding mother to take her baby to bed with her after he is finished eating so he does not miss out on this special time with her.

▼

ARTIFICIAL BABY MILK

If a mother is unable to provide her own milk for all or a portion of her baby's feedings, and banked milk is not available to her, an artificial baby milk will need to be used rather than cow's milk until her baby is 1 year of age. Ideally, the infant formula choice is made carefully in conjunction with her baby's health care provider, with consideration given to her family's life circumstances and health history. It should be the choice of last resort, when all other options to provide human milk have been exhausted. Sadly, this is often not the case.

▼

Acceptable Medical Reasons for Foods Other Than Human Milk

There are rare instances in which a mother may not be able to breastfeed her baby. Perhaps she has a physical condition such as Sheehan's syndrome, long-term drug therapy, or severe congestive heart failure. If a mother is infected with HIV prior to the birth of her baby, and if she has access to a sanitary water supply, she should not breastfeed her baby. If the mother becomes infected with HIV after birth, she should not breastfeed because her baby was not exposed to the HIV in utero. The presence of HIV does not mean, however, that the baby cannot receive human milk. The mother's milk can be heat-treated, or banked human milk can be used. Because tuberculosis is spread through close contact with mothers, it may be dangerous to a breastfeeding infant. After the mother has received appropriate treatment for at least 1 week and is no longer infectious, she can return to breastfeeding. See Chapter 23 for more discussion of these conditions.

A mother who has an active herpes lesion on her breast where the baby will come in contact with the lesion cannot breastfeed on the affected breast until the lesion is healed. The baby may continue to nurse on the unaffected breast, and the mother can express her milk and discard it from the affected side. If a mother is severely ill with a condition such as psychosis, eclampsia, or shock, she may be unable to breastfeed for a period of time until her healing is sufficient to begin or resume breastfeeding. Mothers who must take certain medications, such as cytotoxic or radioactive drugs, may need to stop breastfeeding while the drug is present and active. Finally, if a mother specifically refuses to breastfeed, she will need instructions in the use of an alternative feeding method.

Medical reasons for artificial baby milk also may be due to the baby's condition. Use of human milk by any means is not possible for a baby with galactosemia because he cannot metabolize lactose—the main carbohydrate in human milk. This is an extremely rare condition that requires the use of a special formula. Although other inborn errors of metabolism, such as phenylketonuria (PKU) or maple syrup urine disease, require the use of milk substitutes, they also allow for intake of the mother's milk when it is carefully monitored. Human milk supplementation is required in situations such as hypoglycemia or dehydration, when the condition has not improved through increased breastfeeding or increased intake of human milk. Babies with very low birth weight or who are born preterm, less than 1000 g or 32 weeks' gestation, may require supplementation for a period of time (Akre, 1989). If it is determined that the baby needs supplementation, an alternative feeding method must be chosen that will interfere least with the return to breastfeeding and fit most comfortably into the family's lifestyle.

Choosing an Infant Formula

The decision to feed an artificial baby milk should not be made in haste and should be discussed with the infant's primary caregiver. Parents' choice of artificial baby milk is often based on which company left a case on the their doorstep, which discharge pack was given to them at hospital discharge, and which cents-off coupon is available. The physician's choice is often based on which formula company sales representative is the best salesperson. Consideration is not always given to which brand will agree best with the particular baby.

Sometimes the physician will rotate formulas. For example, babies who are born within a certain 4-month period may get one type of formula. The choice in the next 4 months is rotated to the next formula and so on. All artificial formulas are slightly different. Individual companies advertise that their brand contains more of one element than that of another manufacturer. Theirs, they argue, is "closest to mother's milk" in that particular element. These pronouncements can be confusing to parents, who may worry that they must select one element over another.

The next issue to consider is whether to purchase powdered, concentrate, or ready-to-feed formula. The cost may be a determining factor for parents. Powdered formula is the least expensive of the three types. In 1998 dollars, cost in the United States Midwest averaged about $146 per month to feed a baby powdered formula. This is the least expensive form, is probably the most portable, and has the longest shelf life. However, it is the most prone to mixing errors. Parents may not follow package directions or use the specific scoop provided with the can. Each company has their own particular set of instructions and the size of the scoop is not uniform from one manufacturer to another. Mothers need to be cautioned to read the instructions carefully and to use the scoop that came with that particular brand of formula. Additionally, caregivers should ask the mother to prepare the formula in the hospital as a return demonstration to ensure that she understands the correct procedure.

Concentrate is the next least expensive form of formula and is easier to mix than the powdered form. However, it is easy for parents to confuse concentrate with ready-to-feed. Even the most educated parents run the risk of misreading the label and feeding their infants with straight concentrate. Ready-to-feed formula is the most convenient of the three. It is also the most expensive, at an average of $206 per month in the United States Midwest. One of the advantages of ready-to-feed formula is that the mother does not need to make decisions about whether to use tap water or bottled water. Nor would there be changes to the baby's system when traveling, as there might be when various water supplies are used. However, ready-to-feed formula is the most expensive of the three types and must be discarded if an entire can is not used within the specified period of time.

Safety Tips from the American Academy of Pediatrics

Parents will need to ensure the safety of their infant's formula. The American Academy of Pediatrics (AAP) cautions mothers to check their water supply and make sure that it is safe for the baby to drink. Families with well water should have it tested. If there is any concern that their water supply is unsafe, they can purchase bottled water. To prevent lead poisoning, the water used for formula should be obtained from the cold water tap only. In older homes and in some newer ones, the water pipes are held together with lead solder. The AAP recommends that parents run the cold water for at least 1 minute before collecting it and longer if the water has not been used for several hours.

When traveling, parents will want to consider the safety of the water en route. If the mother is unsure about its bacteria level, she can use bottled water or boil the tap water for 5 minutes (boiling longer tends to cause the lead to concentrate). Bacteria can multiply rapidly in formula that is left at room temperature. Therefore, the formula must be refrigerated or chilled if it is stored in the diaper bag. A clean bottle will need to be used for each feeding, and utensils should be sterile. The can opener and top of the can should both be washed well with hot soapy water before opening the can. The expiration date on each can of formula must be carefully checked before using it to ensure that the date has not expired. Because there have been product recalls of infant formula, parents may be wise to record the lot numbers of each can in the event of a manufacturer's recall.

When parents choose to use artificial baby milk and bottles for feeding, it is the role of the health care professional to provide them with appropriate feeding guidelines in order to minimize the risk to their baby. In prenatal contacts with mothers, this information may be presented to assist the mothers as they make their infant feeding choice. Lactation consultants who provide education to maternity staff need to advocate that teaching of postpartum patients include complete and correct information for those who choose to bottle feed. Often, much information regarding proper bottle feeding and use of an artificial baby milk is glossed over or not discussed at all. This does a disservice to mothers and to their babies and does not provide true informed consent for their decision-making process. Parents need complete and accurate information in order to make responsible decisions.

▼

SUMMARY

There are appropriate uses for the various breastfeeding devices and techniques available to mothers, and they should be used only when a clear need has been demonstrated. If they are used inappropriately, some breastfeeding aids can impact negatively on breastfeeding. Begin with the least invasive methods for dealing with a problem in order to minimize interference. Provide guidance, support, and follow-up to ensure that the mother has a clear understanding of the proper use of the device. When mothers must be separated from their babies, help them select a method of milk expression that will best suit their needs. Learning hand expression may be all the mother requires. Make sure mothers know the proper collection and storage techniques for preserving the nutritional quality of their milk. Help them learn alternate feeding methods that work best for them. Above all, serve as an advocate for the mother and baby remaining together with minimal interventions. Incorporate special aids into care plans only when necessary.

▼

REFERENCES

Akre J. Infant feeding: The physiological basis. *WHO Bulletin Supplement* 67; 1989.

Arnold L. How to order banked donor milk in the United States: What the health care provider needs to know. *J Hum Lact* 14: 65–67; 1998.

Auerbach K. Sequential and simultaneous breast pumping: A comparison. *Int J Nurs Stud* 27:257–265; 1990a.

Auerbach KA. The effect of nipple shields on maternal milk volume. *JOGNN* 19:419–427; 1990b.

Balmer SE and Wharton BA. Human milk banking at Sorrento Maternity Hospital, Birmingham. *Arch Dis Child* 67:556–559; 1992.

Barger J. Lactation Management Course, Breastfeeding Support Consultants, Chalfont PA; 1998.

Barros FC. Use of pacifiers associated with decreased breastfeeding duration. *Pediatrics* 95:497–499; 1995.

Bernbaum JC, et al. Non-nutritive sucking during gavage feeding enhances growth and maturation in premature infants. *Pediatrics* 71:41–45; 1983.

Bornmann PG. Legal considerations and the lactation consultant—USA. *Lactation Consultant Series.* New York: Avery Publishing Group; 1986.

DeNicola M. One case of nipple shield addiction. *J Hum Lact* 2:28–29; 1986.

Drosten F. Pacifiers in the NICU: A lactation consultant's view. *Neonatal Network* 16:47–50; 1997.

Edgehouse L and Radzyminski SG. A device for supplementing breastfeeding. *MCN* 15:34–35; 1990.

Goldblum RM et al. Human milk banking. I. Effects of container upon immunologic factors in mature milk. *Nutr Res* 1:449–459; 1981.

Hamosh M et al. Breastfeeding and the working mother: Effect of time and temperature of short-term storage on proteolysis, lipolysis, and bacterial growth in milk. *Pediatrics* 97:492–498; 1996.

Hopkinson J et al. Glass is container of choice. Letter to Editor. *J Hum Lact* 6:104–105; 1990.

Howard C et al. The effects of early pacifier use on breastfeeding duration. *Pediatrics* 103(3):E33; 1999.

Hunziker UA and Barr RG. Increased carrying reduces infant crying: A randomized controlled trial. *Pediatrics* 77:641–648; 1986.

Kesaree N et al. Treatment of inverted nipples using a disposable syringe. *J Hum Lact* 9:27–29; 1993.

Lang S et al. Cup feeding: an alternative method of infant feeding. *Arch Dis Child* 71:365–369; 1994.

Nemethy M and Clore ER. Microwave heating of formula and breastmilk. *J Pediatr Health Care* 4:131–135; 1990.

Newman J. Breastfeeding problems associated with the early introduction of bottles and pacifiers. *J Hum Lact* 6:59–63; 1990.

Pierce K and Tully MR. Mother's own milk: Guidelines for storage and handling. *J Hum Lact* 8:159–160; 1992.

Pittard W et al. Bacteriostatic qualities of human milk. *J Pediatr* 107:240–243; 1985.

Pittard W. Bacterial contamination of human milk: Container type and method of expression. *Am J Perinatol* 8:25–27; 1991.

Quan R et al. Effects of microwave radiation on anti-infective factors in human milk. *Pediatrics* 89:667–669; 1992.

Righard L and Alade M. Breastfeeding and the use of pacifiers. *Birth* 24:116–120; 1997.

Sosa R and Barness L. Bacterial growth in refrigerated human milk. *Am J Dis Child* 141:111–112; 1987.

Victoria CG. Use of pacifiers and breastfeeding duration. *Lancet* 341:404–406; 1993.

Walker M. Management of selected early breastfeeding problems seen in clinical practice. *Birth* 16:148–158; 1989.

Wellstart. Expert work group meeting. Washington, D.C.; 1996. (Personal communication from Lois Arnold.)

Wilson-Clay B. Clinical use of silicon nipple shields. *J Hum Lact* 12:279–285; 1996.

Yokoyama Y et al. Release of oxytocin and prolactin during breast massage and suckling in puerperal women. *Eur J Obstet Gynecol Reprod Biol* 53:17–20; 1994.

BIBLIOGRAPHY

Arnold L and Larson E. Immunologic benefits of breastmilk in relation to human milk banking. *Am J Infect Control* 21:235–242; 1993.

Henderson T et al. Effect of pasteurization on long-chain polyunsaturated fatty acid levels and enzyme activities of human milk. *J Pediatr* 132:876–878; 1998.

Righard L. Are breastfeeding problems related to incorrect breastfeeding technique and the use of pacifiers and bottles? *Birth* 25.40–44; 1998.

20

TEMPORARY BREASTFEEDING SITUATIONS

When the mother of a breastfed baby faces a temporary dilemma in her breastfeeding experience, you can provide encouragement and suggestions to help preserve breastfeeding. Often, such situations involve a period of time when breastfeeding is interrupted. Understanding the influence that the mother's breastfeeding management has in respect to jaundice will help parents avoid its incidence or an unnecessay interruption in breastfeeding. Some babies will seem to lose interest in breastfeeding or to prefer one breast over another. Finally, parents who experience a delay in the initiation of breastfeeding, or who wish to relactate after having stopped, will need advice and support to work through such a time. These issues are all explored in this chapter.

HYPERBILIRUBINEMIA (JAUNDICE)

Clinically, hyperbilirubinemia (jaundice) is one of the most commonly treated medical conditions in the healthy newborn. It is apparent in up to 50 percent of full term infants in their first week of life (Woodall, 1992). Jaundice is characterized by a progressive yellow coloring of the skin and the whites of the eyes. In advanced cases, weakness and loss of appetite occur. Most jaundice is physiologic and will clear up spontaneously within a few days with no intervention and no ill effects. Physiologic jaundice needs to be distinguished from high bilirubin levels in the infant that are caused by mismanagement of breastfeeding, a rare factor in the mother's milk, or pathology.

Types of Jaundice

At birth, the healthy newborn's bilirubin level is 1.5 mg/dl or less. Over the next 3 to 4 days, it rises to a peak level of approximately 6.5 mg/dl. The bilirubin level then returns to a normal level of less than 1.5 mg/dl by around the tenth day of life (deSteuben, 1992). This natural rise and fall of the newborn's bilirubin is known as physiologic jaundice. In infants with mild jaundice, the yellow coloring may be difficult to detect visually under artificial light. When the bilirubin level rises above 12 mg/dl, it is considered to be exaggerated, or non-physiologic jaundice, if it has no identifiable cause. The term pathologic jaundice is applied when the elevated bilirubin is caused by a disease process.

Physiologic Jaundice

In utero, the fetus produces large amounts of red blood cells, which carry needed oxygen to him from his mother's blood via the placenta. This is his only source of oxygen until he leaves his mother's womb and is able to draw in oxygen through his lungs. Oxygen is carried by the hemoglobin portion of these red blood cells. Newborn infants have more hemoglobin than adults. The healthy full-term infant is born with both fetal and adult hemoglobin. Although fetal hemoglobin is efficient in handling oxygen in utero, adult hemoglobin is only efficient after birth. Because the fetal hemoglobin is not needed after birth, it is broken down and separated, and the globin portion is reused by the body. The heme portion undergoes many changes, the final byproduct of which is bilirubin.

Every newborn infant has an increased concentration of bilirubin. However, not all infants will have the high concentrations that result in the visible yellow coloring associated with jaundice. Many infants are able to dispose of bilirubin through normal physiologic processes. Under normal conditions, the bilirubin becomes bound chemically to proteins, such as albumin, which transport it to the liver. The liver converts the bilirubin through a process known as **conjugation** into a form that can be passed through the bile to the intestine. In the intestine, it undergoes further changes that enable it to be excreted in the baby's stools and, to a much lesser extent, in the urine.

Physiologic jaundice occurs when, because of the infant's immature system, bilirubin is produced faster than the liver can process it. Frequently in the newborn, red blood cells break down more quickly than the immature body can handle them, resulting in a temporary buildup of bilirubin. Maturing of the liver, bacterial colonization of the intestine, and the completion of the transition

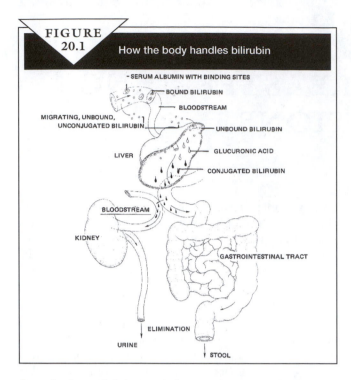

FIGURE 20.1 How the body handles bilirubin

from fetal to adult hemoglobin result in a gradual reduction of the bilirubin level. Bruising or blood incompatibilities can cause a rapid rise in bilirubin levels.

In physiologic jaundice there is a decreased rate of bilirubin conjugation. In conditions such as hepatitis, galactosemia, biliary atresia, or sepsis there is an abnormality of excretion or reabsorption of bilirubin. This unconjugated bilirubin is left to circulate freely in the bloodstream. If the bilirubin is bound (attached to albumin), it is not in itself harmful to the baby, because it will remain within the bloodstream. If it is unbound, however, it can migrate to other parts of the body, such as the brain, skin, muscle tissue, and mucous membranes where it deposits (Fig. 20.1).

Breastfeeding-Associated Jaundice

Breastfeeding-associated jaundice is generally a result of such iatrogenic causes as rigid hospital schedules, routine mother-infant separation, unnecessary supplementation of breastfeeding, and pacifier use. This may be coupled with a lack of education on the part of both the mother and the hospital staff regarding what is typical with breastfeeding. Additionally, the use of labor medications often results in sleepy babies who then become poor nursers. The end result of one or more of these conditions is inadequate intake of the mother's milk. The resultant elevated bilirubin levels are caused, not by dehydration, but rather by caloric deprivation and decreased stooling. Bilirubin levels may range from 9 to 19 mg/dl.

Breastfeeding-associated jaundice can be prevented through appropriate breastfeeding management. Establishing policies of obstetrical care that are based on the

WHO/UNICEF's *Ten Steps to Successful Breastfeeding* will eliminate interference with breastfeeding that perpetuates this type of jaundice. The lactation consultant who functions within a hospital can work toward instituting such policies.

Rates of breastfeeding-associated jaundice are the highest in health care settings where optimal breastfeeding care is not routine. Treatment should be aimed at increasing the number and quality of feeds. Attachment and positioning at the breast must be investigated, and the baby will need to be observed at feeds for swallowing. Rooming in is suggested in order to provide an increase in the number of feeds. The mother can be encouraged to provide frequent skin-to-skin contact at the breast to further increase feeding opportunities.

If the baby's suck is weak and ineffective, the mother may perform breast compression (alternate massage) to increase the flow of milk. If this does not increase the baby's swallowing, a tube-feeding device may be used at the breast. If the need for tube feeding arises, the mother can express her milk to increase milk production and provide milk in the supplementer. She will want to allow her baby unlimited access to the breast, with no limitations placed on frequency or duration. If phototherapy is prescribed, you can advocate for a trial period of increased feeds to promote increased stooling and lowering of the bilirubin before resorting to the use of phototherapy.

Late-Onset Jaundice

In very rare instances, jaundice is believed to be caused by a factor present in the mother's milk. This type of jaundice is frequently referred to as **breastmilk jaundice**. It occurs in less than one percent of infants (Drew, 1978). Arias (1963) observed that milk from some mothers caused jaundice in their infants by inhibiting the bilirubin conjugating enzyme in the liver. However, later studies led researchers to believe this was not the case (Murphy, 1981). Other studies have linked late onset jaundice to free fatty acids in the milk (Yung, 1977) but this, too, has been questioned (Constantopoulos, 1980). Although many possible causes have been investigated, experts cannot agree on the mechanism for this type of persistent jaundice.

Late-onset jaundice is different from other forms of jaundice. It develops extremely slowly and may not become apparent until between the fourth and seventh days of life, after mature milk has begun to replace colostrum. Bilirubin reaches a maximum concentration by the second or third week and may persist through the sixth week of life. The baby is lively and does not appear to be sick even when the bilirubin levels reach their peak of 15 to 20 mg/dl.

Late-onset jaundice is a self-limiting and benign condition (deSteuben, 1992; Wilkerson, 1988). Breastfeeding need not be discontinued in most cases of late-onset jaundice (Poland, 1981). The same treatment for physiologic jaundice can be applied, that is, increased feeds along with exposure to sunlight. If necessary, arrangements can be made to place the baby in a fiberoptic blanket for phototherapy at home, as long as the baby is otherwise healthy. There are no reports in the literature of kernicterus caused by late onset jaundice. Temporary cessation of breastfeeding is sometimes suggested as a treatment. However, although an interruption in breastfeeding may confirm the diagnosis of late onset jaundice, this has no reported benefits to the baby.

With this type of jaundice, parents need the reassurance that nothing is wrong with either the mother's milk or the baby. Also, prepare them for a long period of resolution. A familial tendency for this type of jaundice was noted by Grunebaum and colleagues (1991). When counseling a mother who previously experienced late-onset jaundice, it is important to keep this factor in mind.

Pathologic Jaundice

Pathologic jaundice can result from conditions such as infections in the blood or liver, diseases of the liver, obstructions in the gastrointestinal system, and interference with the binding of the bilirubin in the bloodstream. Many of these are circumstances that would also be associated with jaundice in an adult. Clinical evaluations and various tests are performed to pinpoint specific diseases. Treatment of the disease, as well as treatment of the jaundice, is necessary in these situations. Because of its diverse nature, it is possible for pathologic jaundice to appear any time after birth. The baby could have any combination of jaundice types, thereby making diagnosis relatively difficult. Blood incompatibility and certain drugs can also result in pathologic jaundice.

▼ ### Risks and Treatment of High Bilirubin

Unconjugated, unbound bilirubin is attracted particularly to tissues with a high-fat content, including the brain and nervous system. Under certain conditions that disrupt the blood-brain barrier—such as prematurity, asphyxia, and hemolytic disease—the bilirubin can pass the blood-brain barrier and deposit in nerve cells in the brain. Bilirubin has a toxic effect on brain and nerve cells, and can result in neurologic damage known as **kernicterus**. In extreme cases, it can cause death. The bilirubin level at which kernicterus occurs varies with the gestational and postnatal age of the infant, his birth weight, the presence of other disease, and the availability of albumin-binding sites. Generally, a healthy full-term infant will not develop kernicterus when his bilirubin level is below 20 mg/dl of blood (Newman and Maisels, 1990).

All jaundice warrants investigation of some sort, along with appropriate follow up. Jaundice becomes clinically significant when it develops within the first 24 hours of the baby's life, when levels become exaggerated, or when it is prolonged beyond 2 weeks in term babies and beyond 3 weeks in preterm babies (Dodd, 1993).

Detection of Jaundice

Jaundice is visible when the bilirubin level reaches 5 to 7 mg/dl. Of those babies with visible jaundice, 15 percent will have a bilirubin level of 10 mg/dl or higher. It is further estimated that 3 percent of these babies will have exaggerated or sustained bilirubin levels as a result of a normal development process in their ability to conjugate and excrete bilirubin (Steuben, 1992). If the infant is ill or premature, the safe level is lower, and the jaundice must be treated quickly and monitored closely. DeCarvalho and colleagues (1982) state that bilirubin levels are three points lower in babies who nurse more than eight times per day compared with those who nurse less. The researchers tentatively conclude that this may be due to increased suckling that stimulates the baby's gastrointestinal tract to eliminate bilirubin and prevent its recirculation.

As jaundice increases, the yellowing progresses from the head down to the chest, on to the knees, lower legs and arms, and finally to the hands and feet. Bilirubin levels correspond to the visual jaundicing of the baby's body. When jaundice reaches the level of the baby's shoulders, this correlates to a bilirubin level of 5 to 7 mg/dl. A bilirubin of 7 to 10 mg/dl will show jaundice to the level of the umbilicus. If the jaundice is present below the umbilicus, the bilirubin is 10 to 12 mg/dl. Jaundice below the knees corresponds to a bilirubin level greater than 15 mg/dl (Kramer, 1969).

When jaundice is suspected or detected visually, a blood test is performed to check the bilirubin level. Some hospitals routinely check the bilirubin levels of all newborns on the third postpartum day. Schmucher (1990) notes that the decision to draw a serum bilirubin level is most often made on the basis of the level of jaundice on assessment. The test usually consists of pricking the infant's heel in order to fill a very thin tube with blood for analysis. In addition, the infant is evaluated clinically to rule out disease and infection. Blood types of both the mother and baby are evaluated to rule out blood incompatibilities. A Coombs' test, which was performed at birth, is assessed in coordination with these other tests to check for antiglobulins in the baby's blood.

Treatment of Jaundice

When a significant bilirubin level is detected, the physician may rely on several types of treatment, depending on the baby's condition. For less severe jaundice, regular visual observation of the infant and periodic testing of the bilirubin level may be sufficient. Physiologic jaundice is usually very mild and causes no known lasting effects in the healthy full-term infant. In most cases, the bilirubin values rise slowly (less than 5 mg/dl increase in 24 hours). The bilirubin reaches a noticeable level by the third day of life. It remains slightly elevated for several days and falls by the end of the first week. Active treatment is rarely required as long as the bilirubin levels remain within a safe range.

Increased Feeds

Increasing the frequency of feeds in the early days often helps to reduce bilirubin levels. Increased feeds provide greater stimulation of the gastrocolic reflex, which increases gut motility and thereby reduces intestinal reabsorption of bilirubin through increased stooling (DeCarvalho, 1982; Varimo, 1985). It has been shown that when meconium, which is laden with bilirubin, is passed in the stool within the first 6 hours of life, the incidence of jaundice is decreased. Because colostrum has a laxative effect on the baby, it follows that early breastfeeds will help prevent jaundice by aiding in the efficient elimination of bilirubin. Frequent feeds provide the infant with more calories to prevent reabsorption of bilirubin. They also increase the movement and frequency of stools which helps minimize the recirculation of bilirubin. Additionally, frequent feeds help the mother establish milk production, which provides her baby with more fluids and better weight gain in the early weeks.

It is recommended that the practice of water supplementation be avoided, because it shows no significance in reducing the serum bilirubin levels (DeCarvalho, 1981). Placing the baby in his crib near a sunny window may help decrease jaundice, because bilirubin breaks down when it is exposed to sunlight or its equivalent. Any drugs that may contribute to the buildup of bilirubin should be discontinued for both the breastfeeding mother and her baby. The mother can use a tube-feeding device at the breast to encourage him to nurse and supply the fluids and nutrition he needs. The mother may begin expressing her breasts to provide her own milk in the supplementer. If she is initially unable to obtain adequate amounts from milk expression, an artificial baby milk can be used in the supplementer.

Phototherapy

When the bilirubin approaches a level that the physician has determined requires more active treatment, the baby may be placed under a special fluorescent light called a **bili light**. This treatment is termed **phototherapy**. It works in the same way as sunlight to break down bilirubin, forming products that are colorless and able to be excreted without conjugation. Phototherapy is recommended in the full term newborn if it appears that the bilirubin levels will reach 20 mg/dl. Often the treatment is begun when the level exceeds 15 mg/dl.

Newman and Maisels (1992) recommend the use of phototherapy in healthy full term newborns when the bilirubin level reaches 17.5 to 22 mg/dl. Dodds (1993) recommends phototherapy with levels reaching 15–20 mg/dl. Oski (1992) advocates waiting until the bilirubin level approaches 25 mg/dl. He asserts that the belief that a bilirubin level of 20 mg/dl is dangerous is based on observations made in the 1950s of newborns with Rh incompatibilities.

The American Academy of Pediatrics (1994) recommends phototherapy with a bilirubin level at 15mg/dl or above at 25 to 48 hours of life, with a bilirubin level of 18 mg/dl or above at 49 to 72 hours of life, and with a bilirubin level of 20 or above at 72 or more hours of life. There continues to be much discussion of what is a safe bilirubin level. It is important to keep informed of current practice recommendations.

Types of Phototherapy. For the traditional phototherapy conducted in the hospital, the baby usually has as much of his skin exposed as possible to maximize the effect. He is placed in an isolette to keep him warm, with his eyes covered to protect them from the light. He is usually left under the bili light continuously except for brief feeding periods. Some hospitals allow parents to hold their babies while they are under the lights, to provide skin contact and additional opportunities for bonding.

Although phototherapy results in lowered bilirubin levels, it does have side effects for the infant. He may have an increased **insensible** (not perceptible) water loss that could lead to dehydration. He may have loose stools, develop riboflavin (vitamin B$_2$) deficiency, experience temperature instability, or develop skin breakdown or rashes. The potential also exists for eye damage due to the lights and **apnea** (failure to breathe) may develop due to displaced eye patches (deSteuben, 1992). The infant may also become sluggish in his responses and have a noticeably weak sucking reflex. More frequent short feeds and additional fluids are usually indicated.

Traditional phototherapy increases mother-infant separation and thus has been shown to have an impact on breastfeeding. Elander and Lindberg (1984) report that the short period of separation associated with phototherapy can decrease the duration of breastfeeding. Home phototherapy using a fiberoptic blanket provides several advantages in the treatment of jaundice in the full term newborn (Fig. 20.2). It allows for more mother-infant interaction, the baby is clothed for better temperature regulation, and eye patches are not needed (Woodall, 1992).

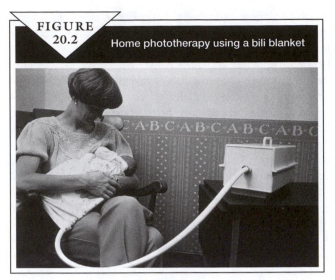

FIGURE 20.2   Home phototherapy using a bili blanket

Courtesy of Medela Inc., Mc Henry, IL.

When Woodall compared home phototherapy with traditional hospital phototherapy, she found no difference in the decrease of bilirubin levels over time. Nor was there a difference in the number of phototherapy hours required for treatment. James (1993) noted that with home phototherapy, breastfeeding continued at a higher rate among mothers as compared with the mothers whose infants were treated in the hospital. James also reported that the cost of hospital phototherapy was five times that of home treatment. Further, the home treatment group had no readmissions or complications, and Woodall noted increased parental satisfaction. Parents with babies receiving traditional hospital phototherapy showed concern regarding the inability to hold their babies and the need for the babies to wear eye patches.

You need to be aware of the local availability of home phototherapy. When counseling parents who face a possible extended hospital stay for their newborn due to jaundice, you can suggest that they explore the option of home phototherapy with the baby's physician. It is helpful to point out the differences of these therapies to the parents, who may be feeling overwhelmed with the thought of their baby needing to stay in the hospital.

Dodd further recommends the consideration of using intermittent phototherapy, which is performed 1 hour out of every 4. She notes that it has been shown to be as effective as continuous phototherapy. Additionally, as in the use of the fiberoptic blanket, it allows for greater mother-infant interaction and is less of an economic drain in health care costs.

Treatment of Jaundice in the Premature Infant

In premature infants, jaundice that is not truly physiologic occurs more frequently and may last for up to 3 or 4 weeks. Phototherapy is often used to lower biliru-

bin levels because the premature infant's brain is especially sensitive to bilirubin. His digestive system takes longer to mature to the point at which it can detoxify and eliminate bilirubin. The bilirubin levels that are permissible in the premature infant are inversely related to the degree of prematurity. Neonatologists treat physiologic jaundice in all infants aggressively. Experience with premature infants has demonstrated that neurologic impairment can occur with this type of jaundice (Guthrie, 1978). As the infant's liver matures and works more efficiently, physiologic jaundice decreases without treatment. However, exposure to sunlight and more frequent feeds will help reduce bilirubin levels more quickly. Discontinuing breastfeeding will not help treat this type of jaundice and will unnecessarily disrupt the establishment of milk production in the early days.

Parental Concerns Associated with Jaundice

Because newborn jaundice occurs so frequently, it is helpful for all prospective parents to learn about this condition so that they will be prepared in the event that their baby develops jaundice. It appears to occur more frequently among Asians, Native Americans, and Eskimos. Babies who are born at higher altitudes also have higher bilirubin levels.

The lactation consultant involved in prenatal education is in a key position to educate parents. Let them know that jaundice is a common newborn condition that can be resolved with great success. Reinforcing information for parents after their baby is born will help them integrate the facts and encourage them to focus on ways that they can ensure continued close contact with their baby during treatment.

When parents are informed about the causes of jaundice, they can take action to minimize its occurrence. The mother can avoid the use of drugs during pregnancy and minimize medications taken during labor and delivery. She can make arrangements ahead of time to nurse her baby shortly after delivery and very frequently in the first days after birth. By working with their baby's physician, parents can ensure that their infant is not given drugs that contribute to jaundice.

Parents can reduce emotional stress by arranging to be close to their baby whenever possible. They can request treatment at the mother's bedside and intervals of interaction where eye and skin contact are possible. Better yet, they can request home phototherapy rather than an extended hospital stay in order to eliminate separation from their infant. Encourage parents to keep themselves well informed of their baby's condition and treatment plans, and to discuss any concerns with their baby's physician. They may wish to discuss with the physician the questions that are presented in the next section.

Questions to Ask the Physician

◆ What is the cause of the jaundice?

◆ What tests have been done or need to be done? What are the results? What do the results mean?

◆ How long is it estimated the jaundice will last?

◆ What are the criteria for home phototherapy?

◆ If the baby is under the bili light or under observation, when can he be breastfed?

◆ If phototherapy is performed in the hospital, when can the parents have social contact with their baby?

◆ If breastfeeding has been interrupted, what is the rationale for this decision, how long will it be, or what must the bilirubin count be before breastfeeding can be resumed?

Using these guidelines, parents can work with their physician to develop a care plan that allows frequent feeding and access to their baby. If the baby remains hospitalized after the mother is discharged, encourage parents to inquire about parental rooming in. If this option is not available or the parents do not choose to room in, suggest that they plan frequent visiting times. If the baby is unresponsive as a result of phototherapy, visits may be discouraging, especially if the staff is also too busy to give parents their attention. Although his eyes are covered, the baby will benefit from parental voice and touch stimulation. You can reassure parents that the long-range outcome is excellent. Most jaundice resolves completely within a few days or weeks. See Table 20.1 for the counseling summary on jaundice.

TABLE 20.1
Counseling Summary—Jaundiced Baby

Mother's Concern	Suggestions for Mother
Parents bewildered by procedures and other aspects of baby care	◆ Discuss questions with the baby's physician and other care providers. ◆ Read available literature.
Separation of mother and baby	◆ Arrange for bedside treatment of baby, either from sunlight or portable bili blanket or lights. ◆ Arrange for regular intervals of interaction for eye and skin contact.
Treatment interfering with breastfeeding	◆ Arrange for fiberoptic blanket phototherapy. ◆ Arrange for regular contact with baby and frequent feeds. ◆ Use relaxation techniques to ensure letdown. ◆ Arrange for uninterrupted feeds.
Baby sluggish in his responses with weak sucking reflex	◆ Begin more frequent feeds. ◆ Use breast compression while nursing to encourage suckling. ◆ Use a tube feeding device. ◆ Use cup feeds if latch is poor.
Physician considering interruption in breastfeeding	◆ Ask for delay in treatment while baby is breastfed frequently to increase his intake of fluids. ◆ Ask for frequent checks of bilirubin level.
Breastfeeding must be interrupted	◆ Begin expressing milk as soon as possible to keep building and maintaining milk production.
Prevention of jaundice	◆ Avoid exposure to chemicals during pregnancy. ◆ Avoid jaundice-producing drugs during labor and delivery. ◆ Nurse within 1 hour after birth and frequently thereafter. ◆ Expose baby's skin to sufficient sunlight daily.

DELAYED ONSET OF BREASTFEEDING

At times, circumstances do not permit a new mother to begin breastfeeding immediately after her baby's birth. A delay may preclude breastfeeding for anywhere from a few hours to several months. A short-term delay (a delay of a few hours up to a couple of days) may result from the baby being born with a low body temperature, having aspirated meconium at birth, or having been born after a prolonged rupture of the mother's membranes. These conditions may necessitate that the baby and mother be separated until the condition is stabilized. In the case of prolonged ruptured membranes, some hospitals isolate the mother and baby together to avoid a separation. Prematurity, **respiratory distress syndrome**, and other birth complications may require several weeks or months of hospitalization. Although breastfeeding may be permitted at some point during the hospitalization, it usually is not possible in the early days.

Many women who plan to breastfeed give up this thought when they are separated from their infant or when breastfeeding is delayed for other reasons. The caregivers who are involved in the care of these mothers and babies must stress that a temporary situation does not preclude breastfeeding. Women who understand that breastfeeding is still possible will need a great deal of encouragement, support, and correct information on how to establish and maintain their milk production until breastfeeding is possible. Babies who are born with health problems need the benefits of their mother's milk to aid in their recovery. Mothers are usually encouraged by their physicians to express milk for their babies or to nurse them when it is permitted.

Expressing Milk to Maintain Lactation

When breastfeeding is delayed, it is important that the mother begin milk expression as soon as possible. She will need to continue to express on a regular basis in order to establish and maintain milk production. Even if the baby's prognosis and chances for survival are not optimistic, the mother may be comforted knowing that she is providing milk for her baby. If the baby is not allowed to be fed the mother's milk, the mother at least has the opportunity to be involved in a parenting role.

Advise that the mother express her milk for a total of eight times every 24 hours. If the baby is not able to nurse for an extended period of time, expressing milk during the night is not as crucial. If it is a short-term separation or close to the baby's return to breast, the mother may want to express during the night. If she drinks fluids before bedtime, she is likely to wake during the night to urinate and can take advantage of this night waking by expressing milk. Traveling to and from the hospital to visit her baby, expressing her milk throughout the day, and trying to recover physically from childbirth can create anxiety and exhaustion for the mother. Sleep and rest will be important to her.

Establishing letdown may be difficult for a mother who is worried about her sick baby and must turn to a breast pump in place of her baby for establishing and maintaining milk production. Suggest that she tape a picture of her baby to the breast pump and that she record her baby's sounds and play the tape while she is expressing. She may also find that expressing her milk is more successful following a visit to the hospital where she has spent time with her baby. Some mothers find that their milk production corresponds to the baby's condition, experiencing a decrease if the baby's condition worsens. The type of breast pump that is used will directly affect the mother's milk production. High-quality, hospital-grade, electric double pumps show the best yield. Despite the best efforts, the mother's milk production will decrease with time. It can usually increase again after the baby begins nursing.

The mother may find it useful to combine the use of both an electric and hand pump for expressing her milk. An electric pump requires less effort on the mother's part and is convenient for maintaining milk production on a long-term basis. She can arrange to rent one for use at home where it will be convenient for pumping. If she must travel a long distance to visit her baby and does not have access to an electric pump at the hospital, she can purchase a manual breast pump to use when she is away from home. Some women have been successful expressing milk manually or with a hand pump, without the use of an electric pump.

Transportation and Storage of the Expressed Milk

The mother will also be concerned with transportation and storage of her milk. The hospital may provide sterile bottles, along with instructions regarding how they want the milk handled. They may request fresh milk, in which case it is to be refrigerated but not frozen, because freezing destroys some live cells and other protective factors. To avoid waste, the amount of milk in each bottle should be only slightly more than the infant is currently taking. If the baby has not begun receiving the mother's milk, she will want to put only small amounts in each container (no more than one ounce) until she learns how much he takes at a feed. Advise the mother not to use soft plastic bottle liner bags to store her milk. She can inquire with the hospital staff about the use of special storage containers as well as other preferences and procedures. She may also want to specify, in writing, that her milk be given only to her baby until such time that her baby no longer needs it.

Transition from Milk Expression to Breastfeeding

When her baby is able to begin nursing, the mother may need help in making a smooth transition from milk expression to breastfeeding. Although ideally, the first breastfeed will occur in the hospital as the baby's condition improves, it may be delayed until after he is discharged. If the mother returns to the hospital for feeds, she can request a private, quiet place in which to nurse her baby. Perhaps a separate nursery or vacant patient room will be available. She can also request a comfortable chair and ample pillows for support.

The mother may find the first feed to be stressful, feeling unsure of how to breastfeed and doubting the adequacy of her milk production. Her baby may be confused about how to suckle at the breast and may have a poor sucking reflex, or he initially may appear disinterested in breastfeeding. The mother may need to increase her milk production and condition her letdown reflex. These are all issues that can be worked through with varying degrees of success. She will benefit from your support and advice until the transition is completed.

When the mother learns that her baby will soon be allowed to nurse, she can begin expressing her milk more frequently throughout the day and night in order to increase milk production. If she is unable to nurse every 2 or 3 hours, she will need to continue expressing to maintain production. If she is nursing frequently and finds that her baby is not satisfied, she may need to supplement with some of her own stored milk or infant formula until her milk production increases. It may take several days or even months to reach the goal of exclusive breastfeeding. Encourage the mother to concentrate on enjoying her baby and to take things one day at a time. The following guidelines may help the mother in making the transition from expressing to breastfeeding.

Guidelines for Conditioning the Baby to Breastfeed

◆ Express milk onto a breast pad, and place it near the baby.

◆ Place a picture of the mother in the baby's view.

◆ Insert a gavage tube through a bottle nipple.

◆ Provide frequent skin contact.

◆ Conduct practice sessions at the breast.

◆ Shape and hold the breast for the baby, using the Dancer hand position.

◆ Express milk into the baby's mouth.

◆ Use a tube-feeding device for feeds.

Mothers Who Return to Bottle Feeding

Because of the health benefits of human milk, physicians strongly urge mothers to breastfeed their ill babies. Some of these mothers may not have planned to breastfeed. A mother may provide her milk through expressing or nursing only as long as the physician indicates that it is essential to her baby's recovery. When the baby is out of danger, these women will switch to bottle feeding. Even a short-term commitment to breastfeeding can be the turning point toward an intimate bond between mother and baby. Remember that your role is to support the mother in her choices, which may mean guiding her through the weaning process when it is her wish. See Table 20.2 for a summary of counseling issues for a delayed onset of breastfeeding.

RELACTATION

Relactation is defined as re-establishing milk production in a mother who has greatly reduced milk production or has stopped breastfeeding. It may follow untimely weaning or separation of the mother and baby, as with the birth of a low-birth-weight infant or the hospitalization of the mother or infant. One of the most common motives for relactation is a baby's allergic reaction to artificial baby milk.

When a mother approaches you to begin the relactation process, it is important that you consider the reasons why the mother did not initially begin or continue with breastfeeding. Possibly breastfeeding was without

---

TABLE 20.2

Counseling Summary— Delayed Onset of Breastfeeding

◆ Begin pumping breasts soon after birth and continue regularly until baby can nurse.

◆ Tape picture of baby to breast pump.

◆ Play recording of baby's sounds.

◆ Express milk directly after visiting baby.

◆ Hand express or pump breasts when away from home.

◆ Place milk in clean container and keep chilled during transport.

◆ Express milk more frequently to increase production.

◆ Continue expressing milk until transition to breastfeeding is complete.

◆ Offer supplement if milk production is low.

problems and the mother weaned due to misinformation. The mother's milk production may not have been up to full potential, or the baby may have rejected the breast or suckled poorly. Along with these considerations, it is important to look at how much time has passed since her baby was at the breast and how he has been fed during that time. It may also be helpful to learn about the mother's breastfeeding management before her decision to wean. These underlying concerns must be investigated and the education and suggestions appropriate to her individual situation need to be incorporated into her plan of care for relactating.

Maternal Motivation

Further investigation into the mother's situation focuses on her primary reason for wanting to relactate. When she is highly motivated and enthusiastic about the process, as well as tempered by realistic goals, relactation is likely to be more successful for her. If her decision to relactate is at another person's urging, she may lack the motivation to persevere. Learn how the mother defines successful relactation and how she will react if her milk production does not meet the full needs of her baby. How will she react if relactation does not work? The mother needs to assess honestly her expectations and possible responses to these possibilities. You can discuss these issues with her, and provide a realistic and supportive picture that invites her thoughtfulness and aids in her decision.

You will need to determine what the mother knows about the process of relactation. Possibly she has little or no information about the suggested plan of care. The mother's decision to relactate must be based on knowledge of what to expect, and you need to be sure she has the appropriate information. You also need to consider the mother's sources of support. Who is supporting her in this endeavor? How do those in her immediate household feel about the process? If she is meeting opposition and plans to relactate, how will she deal with the lack of support? You can be available to consult with the family or friends of the mother, whether they are supportive or not. You may in fact be the mother's only source of support initially. Clearly, the success of relactation has many factors that come into play before the baby and the breast are reintroduced. After it is determined that the mother is motivated to carry through with relactation, you can address issues of milk production and encouraging the baby to take the breast.

The Process of Relactation

The mother's breasts are prepared for lactation through the physiologic changes that accompany pregnancy and birth. Estrogen concentrations fall rapidly immediately following birth. Prolactin levels drop to normal by about 3 weeks in a woman who is not breastfeeding (Lawrence, 1999). The degree of postpartum breast involution is also a determinant of success (Bose, 1981). It appears that a woman has a greater chance of success if she initiates lactation during the first 3 weeks postpartum. However, it is possible to establish lactation beyond that time as well.

Relactation success depends on the woman's determination and the amount of breast stimulation she receives. Her baby's willingness to suckle at the breast is another factor. To help a mother re-establish milk production, there are a number of suggestions you can pass along to her. Frequent suckling is by far the easiest way to accomplish the increase in milk production. If the baby is willing, suckling along with the use of a tube-feeding device at the breast will provide both stimulation for the mother's breasts and nourishment for the baby. During a breastfeed, **switch nursing** and breast massage will help increase milk production. With switch nursing the mother alternates between both breasts several times during a feed. If the baby is reluctant to suckle, the mother may initiate a pumping routine using a double electric breast pump. Pumping frequency should match her baby's feeding patterns. She can also incorporate breast massage into the routine. Once the baby is willing to suckle, it may be beneficial to the mother's milk production for her to express milk between feeds to provide further stimulation.

In addition to breast stimulation, the mother will want to give attention to her lifestyle throughout this period of relactation. Although the ideal situation would be one of total attention by the mother to the process of relactation, this may not always be possible. You can help the mother find practical ways to manage her life during this period in order to optimize her efforts. If it is available and accessible, the mother may wish to have a doula service help her with household routines. Family and friends may also provide invaluable support by doing simple errands, caring for siblings, or preparing meals. The mother will need adequate nutrition and rest in her daily routine. She specifically will want to examine possible milk-reducing influences in her life, such as oral contraceptives, nicotine, or herbal teas like peppermint and sage. You can help her find ways to reduce or eliminate such influences.

Until the mother's milk production is established well enough to serve as her baby's sole form of nourishment, she will need to supplement him with donor human milk or an infant formula. An effective means of offering supplements is the use of a nursing supplementer or other tube-feeding device (see Chapter 19). This approach avoids the baby developing a preference for a bottle nipple and provides maximum suckling at the breast. As the mother's milk production increases, her baby will take increasingly less supplement. The mother must work closely with her baby's physician, making sure that she decreases the supplement in relation to her milk production. She can keep a close check on the baby's weight as his supplement is decreased.

If her baby is undernourished, his suck may be weak, making it difficult for him to stimulate the mother's breast enough to build her milk production. An infant's willingness to suck corresponds to his age and to the length of time that elapses before he is first put to breast (Auerbach, 1985). Frequent and continuous skin-to-skin contact in a relaxed atmosphere without pressure may entice the baby to latch. A drowsy baby or a baby in a light sleep state may be encouraged to latch with skin-to-skin contact and some expressed milk or formula on the end of the nipple.

▼ Increasing the Mother's Success

Some success has been noted with recreating the birth experience (Shinskie, 1998). **Rebirthing**, or remedial co-bathing, is described as simulating the birth experience. The baby is placed on the mother's abdomen in a bath of warm water and allowed to find the breast on his own. With this technique, the baby and mother spend some gentle, calming time together in the bath water. After a period of time, the mother reclines and places the baby on her abdomen. The baby is allowed, without assistance, to crawl up to the breast, and to root and latch on. The mother may be encouraged to carry out the rebirthing technique when it seems to fit into her routine, as a means of calming both her baby and herself, and as a means of achieving a latch. The mother whose baby is reluctant to latch needs gentle reminders to work toward a correct latch rather than settle for a painful, inappropriate latch. See Chapter 16 and Chapter 13 for more suggestions on increasing milk production and encouraging the baby to nurse.

Because of the emotional and physical demands of relactation, the topic should be approached with caution. Ideally, the mother will inquire about relactation. If she does not, it would be advisable to suggest relactation only if the mother seems determined to breastfeed. The time-consuming task of combining supplementing with nursing and the stressful nature of such an endeavor may cause the mother to doubt her motives or the advisability of continuing her attempts. You can encourage her to view breastfeeding as a means of nurturing her baby and not one of feeding alone. Help her measure success in terms of her relationship with her baby rather than the amount of milk she produces or the length of time she nurses. A support system is essential to successful relactation, so arrange for her to receive frequent contact during this period.

▼ NURSING AN ADOPTED BABY

Nursing an adopted baby can provide emotional satisfaction for both the mother and infant as long as the mother has realistic motives for breastfeeding. The mother will need to **induce lactation** in order to breastfeed her adopted baby. It is doubtful that she will ever be able to nourish her adopted baby entirely on her milk alone. If she begins breastfeeding with this goal in mind, she may feel that her attempts are unsuccessful and disappointing. If, however, she views breastfeeding as an emotionally gratifying experience for herself and her baby, and as an opportunity to develop a warm and loving bond with her baby, she will find great satisfaction in her nursing experience.

As in relactation, you would not want to initiate the concept of breastfeeding an adopted infant. However, you can respond to a mother who is highly motivated and indicates an interest. It is extremely time consuming and difficult to induce lactation in the absence of a pregnancy. Without the estrogen concentrations of pregnancy that prepare a woman's breasts for lactation, prolactin may not have a sufficiently potent stimulative effect on milk secretion (Bose, 1981). Women who have lactated previously are three times as likely to have milky secretions while attempting to induce lactation as women who have never lactated (Auerbach, 1985). If the mother's inability to give birth resulted from a hormonal imbalance, that same imbalance could affect her chances of inducing lactation. Success also depends greatly on the woman's desire to nurse and the motherly feelings she develops that stimulate the letdown reflex.

In a study at Massachusetts General Hospital, involving five women who had adopted infants, all of the women achieved some degree of lactation within 11 days of first putting the infant to breast (Kleinman, 1980). Kramer (1995) published a report about women who had never been pregnant, for whom estrogens and either metoclopramide or chlorpromazine were used to begin milk production, along with frequent suckling. Women who had breastfed previously did not need the estrogen. Three of these women had never been pregnant or breastfed before. Although they may not have produced the same amount of milk as the other mothers, they were able to establish a rewarding nursing relationship with their babies.

▼ The Process of Inducing Lactation

The relactation techniques discussed earlier apply to the process of inducing lactation for adoptive mothers as well. An adoptive mother can use all the same measures for nipple preparation as biologic mothers. They will want to avoid soap and other drying agents, and check for inverted nipples. Breast massage and back rubs will help increase blood circulation to and within the breast; nerves in the breast radiate from the area between the shoulder blades. Suggest that she massage her breasts from five to eight times each day over a period of 3 to 6 months. The adoptive mother may also benefit from attending a support group for breastfeeding women while she waits for placement.

One of the most important preparations for a woman who is attempting to induce lactation is that of pumping her breasts to stimulate milk production. A hospital-grade electric breast pump with a double setup is recommended because it provides the most effective nipple stimulation. It may be some time before the woman sees any results from her pumping, and she can be encouraged by even the smallest amount of milk she produces.

If the woman knows when the baby's birth is expected, she can begin pumping for up to 1 month before placement. Often, parents receive only a few days' warning, which does not allow much time for breast preparation. If she does have prior notice, the adoptive mother can begin pumping several times a day for 10-minute sessions. By the time placement occurs, she should be pumping every 2 to 3 hours throughout the day. Many adoption agencies cooperate with the adoptive parents' plans to breastfeed. They may arrange to have the baby fed with an alternative feeding method in order to minimize nipple preference. They may also provide for breastfeeding sessions if placement does not occur soon after birth.

The length of time it takes for the woman's milk to appear and the amount of milk produced will vary with each individual mother and baby. Certainly, milk production will increase more rapidly after the baby begins suckling at the breast. The baby's age will also be a factor. Babies younger than 3 months are more likely to suckle when they are placed at the breast. In one Australian study, milk output nearly doubled when the mother massaged and expressed milk before and after feeds (Nursing Mothers' Association of Australia, 1985). Having the baby sleep in bed with the mother, so that he can suckle sleepily for comfort throughout the night, will enhance milk production as well. Jelliffe (1976) noted that breast stimulation is important for continued milk production. More recent work by Daly and Hartmann (1995) demonstrates that regular milk removal is necessary to ensure continued milk production.

The Massachusetts study cited earlier suggests that the milk of an adoptive mother will not be adequate for totally nourishing her baby. She most likely will need to supplement her baby with donor human milk or an appropriate infant formula to ensure optimal nourishment. You can encourage her to view her breastfeeding primarily as a means of bonding with her baby. The

mother's milk production will not be great enough to sustain her baby's growth, and the quantity will increase much more slowly than that of a biologic mother. She can use a tube-feeding device at most breastfeeding sessions to provide her baby with adequate nourishment and reduce the amount of time she needs to spend supplementing. She also can save time and reduce anxiety by preparing an entire day's feeding equipment and formula at one time.

When inducing lactation, the baby's health and well-being must always be the first priority. As the mother replaces the supplement with her own milk at the breast, she will need to proceed slowly with any decrease in the supplement. The supplement should be decreased in amount, not diluted. As a general guide, you can suggest to her that the decrease not exceed 25 ml per feed. Her baby's growth and output will need to be monitored for 4 to 7 days before another decrease in supplement takes place. A diary of supplemental feedings and nursing sessions—with attention to frequency, duration, and the baby's disposition—will help her monitor his intake. Frequent visits to the baby's physician are advised for weight checks and the monitoring of other signs of growth.

The best stimulation for establishing and maintaining milk production is the baby's suckling. His willingness to nurse will improve over time. An adopted baby's nursing schedule is similar in frequency and duration to that of a baby who is nursed by his biologic mother. The age at which he begins solid foods and initiates weaning is also similar to biologic babies. Because the adoptive mother will probably not be able to produce enough milk for her baby's total nourishment, she will need extra support and encouragement. You can help her educate the case workers and other caregivers who are responsible for her baby's welfare, emphasizing the beneficial nature of the nurturing relationship between mother and baby. See Table 20.3 for a counseling summary on relactation and adoption.

BABY LOSING INTEREST IN BREASTFEEDING

After 3 months or more of breastfeeding, and most commonly around 7 months of age, some babies seem to become disinterested in nursing. The baby may be happy to be put to breast, mouth the nipple, and then act disinterested or cry. This could happen suddenly or he may gradually decrease the number of feeds. Most often, such disinterest in breastfeeding lasts from only a few days to a week. However, some periods of nursing abstinence have been known to continue for 3 or 4 weeks. The mother may become very uncomfortable from overfull breasts and may be emotionally drained

TABLE 20.3

Counseling Summary on Relactation and Adoption

Mother's Concern	Suggestions for Mother
Inadequate letdown	Use relaxation techniques.
Building milk production	Begin nursing as early as possible.
	Use regular supplement and decrease amount as milk production increases.
	Use breast massage.
	Use frequent feedings.
	Get sufficient rest.
	Eat a nutritious diet.
	Keep a diary of breastfeeds and formula feeds.
Baby reluctant to nurse	Use soothing techniques for baby and increased skin-to-skin contact.
	Apply mother's milk or sweet substance to nipple.
	Slowly drop mother's milk into side of baby's mouth before placing baby on breast.
	Use nursing supplementer.
Preparation for breastfeeding	Massage mother's back and breasts.
	Stimulate nipples manually.
	Stimulate milk production by using breast pump.
	Avoid soap and other drying agents on breasts.
Low milk supply	Supplement baby with formula; do not dilute.
	View breastfeeding primarily as a means of nurturing baby's emotional health.
	Have baby checked frequently for weight gain.
	Monitor baby's weight while replacing formula with breastfeeding.
Nipple perference in baby	Use nursing supplementer, cup, spoon, or dropper.
Mother frustrated with part-time breastfeeding	Simplify bottle preparation techniques or use nursing supplementer.
	Learn to appreciate breastfeeding for nurturing relationship with baby.

from trying to satisfy her baby. Encourage her to relax and to be patient as she learns to cope with the change in her breastfeeding pattern. She can maintain milk production through expressing her milk regularly and putting her baby to breast frequently without pressuring him to nurse.

▼ Possible Causes of the Baby's Disinterest

It is sometimes difficult to pinpoint the cause of a baby discontinuing breastfeeding. You can help the mother understand her baby's changing needs as he develops.

Many times, the disinterest is a result of a developmental stage that will subside as the baby matures. He may simply have become a more efficient nurser and is able to obtain more milk in a shorter period of time. He may become interested in new objects and people. As a baby becomes more interested in his surroundings, he can easily be distracted from nursing.

The mother can respond in a variety of ways. She can either move away from the distraction or end the feed and resume when the baby is more interested. She might shift her position so that the baby faces the activity and has the best of both worlds as he nurses. She can also let him play and nurse intermittently at the breast for the feed. Babies enjoy and benefit from mother-infant interaction such as looking, touching, verbalizing, and smiling.

Extra evening or late night feeds, when all is quiet and the baby is too sleepy to be distracted, may make up for missed daytime feeds. Sometimes the baby needs his mother's undivided attention while nursing. She can refrain from activities such as talking, reading, or watching television during feeds. Retiring to a quiet darkened room for these brief periods of breastfeeding also helps. Some babies may show disinterest in breastfeeding after being subjected to parenting programs that aim to make the baby sleep through the night. These babies cannot differentiate between when breastfeeding is and is not allowed.

When a baby has an ear infection or a head cold, it is difficult for him to nurse if he must breathe through his mouth. If he has a cold or earache, the mother can consult her baby's physician about medications for decreasing the production of mucus or mechanical methods for removing it before nursing. Nursing in an upright position or with the clutch hold will take pressure off his ears and facilitate drainage in his nose. The mother can massage her breasts and express milk before nursing to promote letdown. She can also perform breast compression during the feed, so that her baby will not need to suck as hard to obtain milk. Teething pain may make it uncomfortable for the baby to nurse as well. Because of the pain, a teething baby may nurse sporadically, and may fuss and pull away from the breast. Comfort measures to ease the pain in his gums, such as rubbing them with a cool washcloth or allowing him to gum a cooled teether, will usually renew his interest in nursing.

The mother may have unknowingly rebuffed her baby with an overwhelming reaction to being bitten, and he may feel rejected. He may associate nursing with his mother becoming upset because of the biting and may not want to risk trying it again. Skin-to-skin contact between the mother and baby will help to re-establish trust between them. Suggest that the mother undress and take the baby to bed or into the bath with her. She can hold him close to her body with her breasts exposed so that he recalls what it feels like to be next to her skin and will hopefully be encouraged to nurse. Use of a baby sling also provides increased intimacy to build the baby's trust.

The baby may reject nursing because he is satisfying his sucking needs in some other way, such as sucking on his thumb or other object. The mother can put her baby to breast whenever he begins to do this. Sometimes solid foods or supplemental bottles cause the baby to become less interested in breastfeeding. If the mother is giving her baby supplements, she may want to cut back on them temporarily to rekindle his interest in the breast.

The mother may be experiencing overexertion, tension, poor eating habits, or fatigue. The baby may respond to the mother's emotions by decreasing his feeds. If the mother is aware of such a reaction in her baby, she may look at her own situation and resolve to care for herself with adequate rest, nutrition, and exercise, as well as finding ways to decrease her stress. During menstruation, the taste of the milk and the scent of the secretions on the mother's skin may change slightly, making feeds seem less familiar and therefore less desirable to the baby. When the mother's body returns to normal after several days, the baby will renew his interest in breastfeeding.

▼ What the Mother Can Do

Until her baby nurses again, the mother will need to express her milk after attempting to nurse in order to maintain milk production and prevent engorgement. She also needs to work out an alternate method of feeding her baby while she helps him through this phase. Use of a bottle and artificial nipple may cause nipple preference because of the different methods of sucking required between the breast and a bottle nipple. Choosing an alternative feeding method such as cup feeding will avoid this problem. Your objectivity can help the mother establish priorities and work toward resuming breastfeeding with her baby. Other measures the mother can use to encourage her baby to breastfeed are given in the following section.

Advise the Mother to

- Use relaxation techniques and massage before feeds.
- Increase skin contact with the baby before feeds.
- If the baby's gums are sore, rub them with ice or a finger before the feed.
- Nurse in a quiet, dark room without distractions.
- Attempt to nurse when the baby is almost asleep.
- Increase evening and nighttime feeds.
- Use breast compression while the baby is at the breast to increase milk flow.
- Hold the baby in an upright position for easier breathing during feeds.
- Express a little milk onto the nipple or the baby's lips to encourage him to feed.
- Get plenty of rest, add extra protein and fresh vegetables to her diet, and drink sufficient fluids to promote a feeling of well-being.
- If the baby prefers one breast, transfer him to the other breast by gently sliding him over rather than turning him around.

- Feed the baby in the presence of other breastfeeding babies.

- Put the baby to breast when he begins sucking on his thumb or other object.

- Discontinue the use of pacifiers.

- Nurse before offering any dietary supplements.

- Reduce the amount of supplements being given to the baby.

- Offer liquids by cup or other method that avoids an artificial nipple.

- Hand express or pump between feeds to maintain milk production.

- Check for illness or teething pain in the baby and contact his physician if necessary.

- Cleanse the breasts with clear water before feeds to remove deodorant, lotions, or other substances.

- Discontinue the use of any new brand of deodorant or lotion.

▼ BABY WHO PREFERS ONE BREAST

A baby's preference for one breast over another is a common occurrence. It is often difficult to determine a cause. One factor may be the hand preference of the mother. If a woman is right-handed, her baby may prefer her right breast. Or she may put him to breast on the left side more often while she uses her right hand for other tasks, unconsciously encouraging a preference. The mother might try evaluating her breastfeeding patterns and adjust positions so that her baby will nurse equally on both breasts.

The baby may dislike the appearance or feel of one of the breasts. Perhaps the breast has a mole, hair, or other difference that may cause him to prefer the other breast. He may dislike the smell of the skin on one side due to deodorant or perfume. You can suggest that the mother temporarily eliminate these products and wash with clear water before nursing. In rare cases, the baby seems to dislike the taste of the milk in one breast. Feeding the milk with the use of an alternative method such as a cup will help rule this out. Refusal may result from a plug of thick milk that has broken loose and is transported through the ducts and out of the nipple. As soon as the plug is cleared, usually after one pumping session, regular nursing resumes.

Perhaps the breast the baby refuses is more engorged, with firmer tissue in the areolar area that does not allow for a comfortable and productive suckle. In this instance, hand expressing or pumping to soften the breast tissue may encourage the baby to nurse on that breast. The baby's birth experience may have involved trauma to one side of his face, chin, neck, or shoulder, and he may be in pain when he is held in certain positions. A cold or ear infection can produce a degree of discomfort in the baby that leads to breast refusal. Careful attention to positioning may entice the baby to nurse. After the discomfort is relieved, the baby usually returns to the refused breast. At times, a baby's preference has led a woman to see her physician for an examination and a malignant growth has been found in the breast tissue (Saber, 1996). You can keep this rare possibility in mind without frightening the mother. Suggest that she have her breasts examined by a physician if all other measures fail.

▼ Encouraging the Baby to Feed at Both Breasts

There are some methods the mother can use to get her baby back on both breasts. She can begin the feed on the preferred breast first and express a little milk from the other breast to start the baby on it. Alternatively, the mother can begin with the less preferred breast, after first having obtained letdown by pre-expressing her milk. She might try doing this at times when the baby is drowsy and is less aware of which breast he is suckling. She can also try to entice the baby with expressed milk on her nipple. Using the clutch hold will sometimes fool him into thinking he is on the preferred breast, especially if he has an earache or a sensitive ear condition. Simply putting the baby to breast in any new position may also do the trick.

The mother will need to express milk from the less preferred breast regularly to relieve discomfort and maintain milk production in that breast. Some women may be content nursing primarily or totally on one breast. One breast can produce more than enough milk for the baby. Although it may be slightly larger for a time, the mother can conceal this difference in size with loose-fitting clothing.

▼ SUMMARY

Temporary breastfeeding situations often present a challenge to the mother. Preserving the breastfeeding relationship may involve altering the breastfeeding routine, as with jaundice. It may mean supplementing the baby at the breast while the mother increases her milk production. Alternatively, it may require maintaining lactation with the use of a breast pump, as with a nursing strike. With your support and suggestions, these types of situations can be navigated successfully, leading to a satisfying outcome for the mother and baby.

REFERENCES

American Academy of Pediatrics. Practice parameter: Management of hyperbilirubinemia in the healthy term newborn. *Pediatr* 49:558–565; 1994.

Arias IM et al. Neonatal unconjugated hyperbilirubinemia with breastfeeding and a factor in milk that inhibits glucuronide formation in utero. *J Clin Invest* 42:913; 1963.

Auerbach KG and A Sutherland. *Relactation and induced lactation.* Garden City Park, NY: Avery Publishing; 1985.

Bose CL et al. Relactation by mothers of sick and premature infants. *Pediatrics* 67(4):565–569; 1981.

Check WA. Hospital headway: Fighting fatal jaundice. *Family Health* 13:46–49; 1981.

Constantopoulos A et al. Breastmilk jaundice: The role of lipoprotein lipase and the fatty acids. *Eur J Pediat* 134(1): 35–8; 1980.

Daly S and Hartmann P. Infant demand and milk supply, Part 2: The short-term control of milk synthesis in lactating women. *J Hum Lact* 11:27–37; 1995.

DeCarvalho M et al. Frequency of breastfeeding and serum bilirubin. *Am J Dis Child* 136:737–738; 1982.

DeCarvalho M. Effects of water supplementation on physiological jaundice in breastfed babies. *Arch Dis Child* 56:568–569; 1981.

deSteuben C. Breastfeeding and jaundice: A review. *J Nurse Midwife* 37:59s–65s; 1992.

Dodd KL. Neonatal jaundice—a lighter touch. *Arch Dis Child* 68:529–533; 1993.

Drew JH. DIALOGUE: Breastfeeding and Jaundice, Part I. Breast Milk and Jaundice. *Keeping Abreast: Journal of Human Nurturing* 3:49–52; 1978.

Drew JH and Kitchen WH. The effect of maternally administered drugs on bilirubin concentrations in the newborn infant. *J Pediatr* 89:657; 1976.

Elander G and Lindberg T. Short mother-infant separation during first week of life influences the duration of breastfeeding. *Acta Paediatr Scand* 73:237–240; 1984.

Grunebaum E et al. Breastmilk jaundice: natural history, familial incidence and late neruodevelopmental outcome of the infant, *Eur J Pediatr* 150:267–270; 1991.

Guthrie, RA. DIALOGUE: Breastfeeding and Jaundice, Part I, Breast Milk and Jaundice, *Keeping Abreast: Journal of Human Nurturing* 3:49–52; 1978.

Jelliffe D. Hormonal control of lactation. In Schams D (ed). *Ciba Foundation Symposium, No. 45, Breastfeeding and the Mother.* Amsterdam: Elsevier Scientific Publishing; 1976.

Kleinman R et al. Protein values of milk samples from mothers without biologic pregnancies. *Pediatr* 97:612–615; 1980.

Kramer P. Breast feeding of adopted infants. *Br Med J* 311: 188–189; 1995.

Murphy H et al. Pregnanediols and breast milk jaundice. *Arch Dis Child* 56(6):474–476; 1981.

Poland RL. Breast-milk jaundice. *J Pediatr* 99(1):86; July, 1981.

Saber A et al. The milk rejection sign: A natural tumor marker. *Am Surg* 62:998–999; 1996.

Schumacher RE. Noninvasive measurements of bilirubin in the newborn. *Clin Perinatol* 17:417–435; 1990.

Shinskie D. Use of rebirthing to facilitate latch in neurologically impaired baby. *Clinical Issues,* 3(1):4–5; 1998.

Varimo P et al. Frequency of breastfeeding and hyperbilirubinemia. *Clin Pediatr* 25:112; 1985.

Wilkerson N. A comprehensive look at hyperbilirubinemia. *MCN* 13:360–364; 1988.

Woodall J et al. A new light on jaundice. *Clin Pediatr* 353–356; 1992.

Yung FC and Cheah SS. Breastmilk jaundice: An in vitro study of the effect of free fatty acids on the bilirubin-serum albumin complex. *Res Commun Mol Pathol Pharmacol* 17(4):679–88; 1977.

BIBLIOGRAPHY

Auerbach KG and Gartner L. Breastfeeding and human milk. Their association with jaundice in the neonate. *Clin Perinatol* 14(1):89–107; 1987.

Auerbach KG. When treatment for jaundice undermines breastfeeding. *Contemp Pediatr:*105–106; 1992.

Auerbach KG. Sequential and simultaneous breast pumping: A comparison. *Int J Nurs Stud* 27:257–265; 1990.

Banapurmath C et al. Initiation of relactation. *Indian Pediatr* 30:1329–1332; 1993.

Berkow R (ed). *Merck Manual,* 13th ed. Rahway, NJ: Merck, Sharp and Dohme; p. 984; 1977.

Gartner L. Disorders of bilirubin metabolism in Nathan and Oski (eds). *Hematology of Infancy and Childhood,* 4th ed. Philadelphia, W.B. Saunders; p. 90; 1993.

Hale T. *Medications and Mother's Milk.* Amarillo TX, Pharmasoft Publishing; 1999.

J Rosta et al. Delayed meconium passage and hyperbilirubinemia. *Lancet:* 2:1138; 1968.

James JM et al. Discontinuation of breastfeeding infrequent among jaundiced neonates treated at home. *Pediatrics* 92: 153–155; 1993.

Kramer LI. Advancement of dermal icterus in the jaundiced newborn. *Am J Dis Child* 118:454–458; 1969.

LaTorre A. et al. Beta-glucuronidase and hyperbilirubinemia in breast-fed babies. *Biol Neonate* 75:82–84; 1999.

Lawrence RA. *Breastfeeding: A guide for the medical profession.* St. Louis, MO, Mosby Inc.; 1999.

Madlon-Kay D. Evaluation and management of newborn jaundice by Midwest family physicians. *J Fam Pract* 47:461–464; 1998.

Maisels M et al. The effect of breast-feeding frequency on serum bilirubin levels. *Am J Obstet Gynecol* 170:880–883; 1994.

Martinez J et al. Control of severe hyperbilirubinemia in full-term newborns with the inhibitor of bilirubin production Sn-Mesoporphyrin. *Pediatrics* 103:1–5; 1999.

American Academy of Pediatrics. Practice parameter: Management of hyperbilirubinemia in the healthy term newborn. *Pediatrics* 49:558–565; 1994.

McCrae WM, Kernicterus in the newborn, *Nursing Times* 72:1088; 1976.

Mennella JA and Beauchamp GK. Maternal diet alters the sensory qualities of human milk and the nursling's behavior. *Pediatrics* 88(4):737–44; 1991.

Newman T and Maisels M. Does hyperbilirubinemia damage the brain of healthy full-term infants. *Clin Perinatol* 17:331–356; 1990.

Newman TB and Maisels MJ. Evaluation and treatment of jaundice in the term newborn: A kinder, gentler approach. *Pediatrics* 89:809–818; 1992.

Nursing Mothers' Association of Australia. *Adoptive Breastfeeding and Relactation.* Nursing Mothers' Association of Australia, Nunawading, Victoria; 1985.

Oski FA. Hyperbilirubinemia in the term infant: An unjaundiced approach. *Contemp Pediatr* 9:148–154; April, 1992.

Salariya E and Robertson C. Relationships between baby feeding types and patterns, gut transit time of meconium and the incidence of neonatal jaundice. *Midwifery* 9:235–242; 1994.

Scanlon JW (ed). Hand-held screening device for neonatal jaundice. *Perinatal Press* 6(5):66; 1982.

Seldman D et al. Hospital readmission due to neonatal hyperbilirubinemia. *Pediatrics* 96:727–734; 1995.

Simkin P and Edwards M. *When Your Baby Has Jaundice.* Seattle, WA: Pennypress; 1979.

Tay C et al. Twenty-four hour patterns of prolactin secretion during lactation and the relationship to suckling and the resumption of fertility in breast-feeding women. *Hum Reprod* 11:950–955; 1996.

Wilde C et al. Breast-feeding: Matching supply with demand in human lactation. *Proc Nutr Soc* 54:401–406; 1995.

CHAPTER

21

HIGH-RISK INFANTS

Ideally, the breastfeeding experience for both the mother and infant involves only the normal adjustments in the postpartum period. However, this is not always the case. The infant may experience a medical condition that will require altering the mother's breastfeeding routine. This may be due to the limitations of his illness and possibly to separation from his mother. The mother may require increased support in order to persevere and continue providing her milk to her baby. Fortunately, it is becoming more accepted that providing human milk is worth the effort when the baby is ill, particularly in the case of prematurity.

PROLONGED HOSPITALIZATION OF THE HIGH-RISK INFANT

When a couple plans for the birth of their baby, they anxiously anticipate bringing him home and settling in as a family. Sometimes, however, parents must return home alone, leaving their baby in the special care of medical personnel. All parents will react differently to such an untimely separation, and their need for support will be just as individual. Hospitalization of the **high-risk infant** creates anxiety and uncertainty for parents. The transition from hospital to home after he is discharged will be another trying time. It may help for you to familiarize parents with typical reactions and ways of coping, and to offer suggestions for interacting with their baby and planning for his homecoming. It will also help you to understand what these parents are experiencing, so that you can fashion your counseling to meet their needs.

Parents' Reactions

Except for a brief glimpse of their baby at birth, the parents of a high-risk infant have little opportunity to interact with him in the first hours after birth. Depending on the baby's condition, it may be several days or weeks before they can even hold him. When they see their baby in the nursery he most likely will be lying in an isolette or **stablelet**, with a myriad of tubes and monitors connected to his unclothed body. This can be a frightening scene if parents have not been prepared to expect it and given an explanation for all of the life-sustaining devices. The parents may be overwhelmed by the equipment and its correlation to their baby's chances for survival, and find it difficult to focus on their baby as an individual. Even with a favorable prognosis, parents may wonder silently if their baby will survive. They will want to know what can be done to help him, how soon he will be out of danger and disconnected from tubes and monitors, and when he can breastfeed and go home. They will feel helpless, wanting to do something for their baby and not knowing what or how.

You can help parents formulate questions for their baby's caregivers. Stress to them the importance of asking for explanations and clarification of anything they do not fully understand. They may have difficulty absorbing and processing all the information they receive from you and other caregivers. You may need to continually repeat, review, and clarify important points for the mother in regard to breastfeeding her high-risk infant.

Many parents of high-risk infants experience feelings of guilt, loneliness, and anxiety. They pass through the same type of grief process as parents whose baby has died, and they may avoid contact with other parents who have healthy babies. Mothers in the hospital may detach themselves from the other mothers and babies. Parents may even try to avoid involvement with their own baby in an instinctive effort to protect themselves from becoming attached to a baby they may lose. This is a very common and natural reaction, and such feelings usually subside after the parents are able to accept their baby's condition. They will have grieved for and mourned the healthy baby they had expected and are now able to accept the baby they have.

Parents may become overtired and anxious, putting a strain on their relationship. They can be encouraged to seek out sources of support, both within the hospital environment and within their community. Talking with other parents who have experienced similar situations may help them realize that their reactions are typical, and may give them techniques for coping.

Support groups for parents of high-risk infants are available in many communities. Attending one of the group's discussions can provide parents the opportunity to share their own feelings and concerns and to learn to put them into perspective. Mothers of high-risk infants who have sources of support are found to be more likely to continue breastfeeding (Kaufman, 1989). You can become aware of available support and make appropriate referrals. It is equally important that you inquire about the mother's own family and friends as support systems.

Because a high-risk infant requires a great deal of attention and care, parents' needs often go unrecognized or unmet. You can take an interest in the mother and draw her out by encouraging her to talk about her labor and delivery experience. Focus on her rather than on the baby. She may need to share her feelings about the birth, her baby, and her ability or inability to cope. Ask her how she is sleeping, how her appetite is, and whether she is taking her pain medication. In other words, show concern for her! Your most important role in relation to the mother is that of a supportive listener. She will be receiving information and advice from many sources and may need someone who will listen to her in an accepting, objective, and interested manner. Sincere and honest concern is natural. Let her know that you care and that you are there for her.

Another important aspect of counseling the mother with a high-risk infant is that of advising her about breastfeeding. It may be several weeks or months before she is able to put her baby to breast. She will need to learn how to build and maintain milk production during that period, and how to facilitate letdown by artificial means (i.e., expressing her milk instead of receiving the suckling stimulation from her baby). She also must cope emotionally with the delay in her breastfeeding. More information on this topic appears later in Chapter 22.

Baby's Care

Tremendous advances have been made in improving the morbidity and mortality rates of high-risk infants. This is due, in large part, to the care that is available to these infants in special care facilities. Such pediatric **tertiary** care centers have the necessary equipment and specially trained staff to care for seriously ill infants. Many times babies can be cared for at the hospital where they were born. This can be a comfort to the parents when the hospital is near their home. In some instances, a high-risk pregnancy is detected early enough so that the woman can deliver in a tertiary care facility that has the means to care for both the mother and baby.

When the infant must be transported from one facility to another, parents go through a very real grief experience. Their infant is being placed in the care of medical personnel who, although very competent, are complete strangers to the parents. They may be separated from their baby by a distance that will make visitation difficult. The very fact that their baby is transferred to a special care facility underscores the seriousness of his condition. Many times, as the baby improves, he can be transported back to the hospital in the parents' community until he is ready for discharge.

The Neonatal Intensive Care Unit

The neonatal intensive care unit (NICU) itself is a very overwhelming place for both the parents and their baby (Fig. 21.1). In his intrauterine environment he was exposed to his mother's rhythmic body sounds and her voice. There was no sharp variation in light. He was continuously bathed in warm amniotic fluid and rocked by his mother's movements. In contrast, the NICU is a very noisy environment with continuous white noise and harsh mechanical sounds occurring at varying times. Voices are not often distinct. The lighting is continuously bright, with no daily rhythmicity. Touch in the NICU is often anything but gentle and soothing. Most contacts with the high-risk infant are either technical or medical in nature. Thus, the baby may associate touch with unpleasant events. There is often debate among health care professionals regarding how much stimulation is appropriate for the high-risk infant. (See the discussion of **kangaroo care** later in this chapter.) As the lactation consultant working with parents of high-risk infants, you can become aware of current research in NICU care. Advocate for a more baby-friendly environment that encompasses the best of high-tech developmental care. Share with the mother ways she can nurture her infant through gentle, warm, and loving touch.

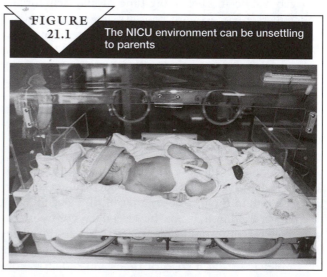

FIGURE 21.1 The NICU environment can be unsettling to parents

Printed by permission of Kay Hoover.

Human Milk for the Baby in the Neonatal Intensive Care Unit

Human milk may be vital to the progress of a high-risk infant who is at risk for developing a variety of infections (Hylander, 1998). The ingestion of human milk can help protect these babies through its immunologic properties. Emphasize the importance of human milk for a high-risk infant and encourage the mother to provide her own milk to her baby.

Interaction between Parents and Baby

The impact of early separation on parents' relationships with their high-risk infant can be minimized if the parents initiate as much meaningful interaction as possible. The overwhelming nature of the experience may make parents hesitant or fearful to participate. You can help bridge this gap by inquiring about and addressing their concerns. Encourage their participation and provide explanations in simple and concrete terms. Often, parents are not aware of what is normal and expected in the NICU or even with their own baby. It is helpful to point out what to expect of their baby based on his condition and gestational age. Culp (1989) found that parents feel less anxiety and more realistic expectations when the baby's behavioral capabilities are pointed out. They can visit their baby in the nursery, touching and fondling him as much as is permitted for his condition. Babies have better weight gains and quicker recoveries when they are held and cared for by their mothers during hospitalization (Hurst, 1997; Sloan, 1994).

Eye-to-eye contact between the parents and their infant is important as well. Parents can ask that eye patches be removed temporarily during their visit. They will benefit by having some time alone with their baby, without the hovering presence of hospital staff, so that they can interact together as a family. Parents can be encouraged to take part in caring for their baby in such areas as feeding, bathing, and diapering. This is especially important in the days preceding the baby's discharge, so that they can gradually begin assuming their roles as caretakers.

Nyqvist (1993) looked at the concerns of former NICU mothers and their advice to other mothers with babies in the NICU. Mothers were often concerned about the lack of privacy and the ability to simply sit and hold their babies and get to know them. You can help the mother adapt by arranging for privacy screens or for her to room in when the baby is able. Encourage the mother to have private time whenever the baby's condition permits.

Mothers in the Nyqvist study also revealed concerns regarding feeds. They preferred that they, not the nurses, feed their babies whenever possible and wanted breastfeeding to be given preference over the use of gavage feeding or bottles. You can advocate for feeding practices that protect breastfeeding such as not using artificial nipples and not requiring successful bottle feeds before time at the breast. These experienced mothers also advocated close physical contact and breastfeeding as soon as possible, both of which enhance the baby's well-being. Finally, they advised that mothers ask questions. You can encourage these behaviors in the mothers in your care. You can also advocate for change in NICU policies whenever necessary.

In discussing these forms of interaction with parents, keep in mind that many times there will be logistical problems such as caring for siblings, and transportation to and from the hospital. Time commitments also present challenges for the mother in terms of rest, expressing her milk, and spending time with other family members. Although they will want to spend as much time as possible with their baby, parents will also be pressured by these other demands. They should not be made to feel guilty or negligent if they cannot visit the hospital as often as you or others think appropriate.

▼ Taking the Baby Home

Many parents of hospitalized infants perceive their baby as needing special care. They are often anxious at the time of discharge and overwhelmed with the thought of caring for him full time. Discharge may be anticipated or may come as a complete surprise. Parents' emotions will be a mixture of elation, anxiety, caution, and insecurity in their roles as full-time caretakers. Before the baby can be discharged, he must be physically stable and able to tolerate feeds by mouth. He must also maintain his body temperature and have a good sucking reflex. Small infants are discharged today much sooner than in the past. There is no longer a "magic" weight that must be obtained. Today, it is common for a 3½ pound infant to be discharged, as long as he can meet three criteria. He must be able to maintain his temperature in an open crib, take the prescribed amount of fluid by any means, and be in a stable medical condition.

The mother can prepare for her baby's homecoming by arranging for household help, freezing meals for later use, stocking up on grocery items, and any other aids that will allow her time with her infant. She will want to discuss a feeding plan with her baby's physician before discharge. If supplements are required, she will need to know how often they are to be given, as well as any special care procedures or restrictions. Scheduling a visit with the local physician she has chosen to care for her baby will provide continuity of care and ensure that her baby's physician is familiar with him after he is discharged from the care of hospital personnel.

After the baby is home, encourage that the parents limit visitors. The baby will still be recovering physically. Additionally, the mother will most likely be drained both physically and emotionally. Both parents need to have quiet time together with other family members, re-establishing relationships and integrating the baby into the family. Many parents experience an initial phase of excitement, followed by exhaustion, until the transition is completed and enjoyment and self-confidence return (Klaus, 1995). See Table 21.1 for a counseling summary on prolonged hospitalization.

You can assist the mother through this time of transition by increasing your contact with her before her baby's discharge from the hospital. Inquire about the mother's most pressing concerns, and address them or refer the mother to appropriate assistance. McKim (1993) found that mothers of high-risk infants are concerned about issues such as crying, breathing noises, spitting up, and infant behavior, all of which relate to feeding. It is important that these issues be addressed with parents. Point out typical infant behaviors and breathing noises, explain how to burp, and describe normal "spit up." Mothers are often unaware of the cues given by their babies in the early days. It is helpful to point out cues such as rooting that indicate readiness to feed. Also teach infant responses that show signs of overstimulation, such as the baby's breathing changes, frowning, arching his back, waving his arms, hiccoughing, and loss of eye contact (Burns, 1995; Farran, 1989). These cues are all described in Chapter 11.

The crying behavior of a preterm high risk infant will vary according to his gestational age. His cries may be more high pitched and uneven than those of a full-term baby, and they seem to occur more frequently as well. Boukydis (1989) noted that a greater number of preterm babies develop colic-like symptoms than do full-term babies. This can be very trying for parents as they adjust and attempt to know and console their child. You can provide anticipatory guidance regarding what to expect and how to cope with crying. Additionally, ongoing support through postdischarge follow-up can assist these mothers through their transition to home. McKim (1993) reported that mothers who believed that they did not receive enough information regarding their babies' care and expected behavior were more anxious and less confident in caring for their babies. You can ease this anxiety and help build maternal confidence.

BABIES NOT BORN AT TERM

The average gestation time for a fetus ranges from 37 to 42 weeks. When a baby is born before or after that time, he will very likely require specialized care for a period of time. The length of hospitalization and degree of care needed will depend on the baby's condition and the number of weeks before or after term when he was born. An explanation of prematurity and postmaturity will help you understand these birth outcomes, enabling you to pass on appropriate information to parents. You can familiarize them with the typical characteristics of these babies as well as implications for breastfeeding.

Small for Gestational Age Infants

If, according to infant growth charts, intrauterine growth was slowed when birth took place, the infant will be considered small for gestational age (SGA). This is also referred to as intrauterine growth retardation (IUGR). Because of limited amounts of **adipose tissue**, these infants often have problems regulating their blood sugars and temperatures. They frequently have early feeding problems, and may breastfeed poorly and require supplementation with their mother's expressed milk or with an artificial baby milk until their condition has stabilized and they begin to gain weight. After their condition has stabilized, these infants seem to demand very frequent feeds, as if they are trying to gain the weight they should have gained in utero. Mothers need to be informed that these infants "love to nurse" and will breastfeed frequently and for long periods of time. Such a pattern is expected and is a normal outcome in this condition.

TABLE 21.1	
Counseling Summary—Prolonged Hospitalization	
Mother's Concern	**Suggestions for Mother**
Mother's emotional needs unrecognized	Discuss birth experience and adjustment factors with supportive person.
Early separation from baby	Provide quality interaction through touching, eye contact, and time alone with baby.
Exhaustion from traveling to and from hospital and caring for baby at home	Arrange household help. Prepare and freeze meals before homecoming. Stock grocery supplies before homecoming.

◀ Prematurity

An infant is considered premature when he is born before 37 weeks of gestation. A complete assessment of the infant is made at birth. The assessment includes gestational age, intrauterine growth, and such physical characteristics as skin, posture, reflexes, and fat deposits. Birth weight is also a consideration. Most premature infants weigh less than 5½ pounds (2500 g). There are two general classifications for premature infants. A premature infant is considered **appropriate for gestational age (AGA)** if his rate of intrauterine growth was normal. As described earlier, when intrauterine growth was slowed, he is considered SGA.

The Premature Infant's Appearance and Status

A premature infant's skin has a gelatinous appearance, and is loose and wrinkled. Blood vessels and bony structures are visible because there is very little subcutaneous fat. Fine downy hairs may be present on the infant's forehead, sides of the face, back, and extremities. Hair on his head is scanty, and he usually has no visible eyebrows. Because the cartilage needed to support his ears is not yet fully developed, his ears can be folded in many positions. His head will appear large in proportion to the rest of his body because skull growth is completed before other body growth.

The heart of a premature infant is well developed. However, his lungs and rib cage may not function efficiently at birth due to muscular weakness. Heat regulation is poorly developed, and care must be taken to stabilize and monitor his body temperature. Premature infants tend to have a higher rate of physiologic jaundice than do full-term infants. This is due to their immature liver and digestive systems and low levels of **glucuronic acid**. (See the jaundice discussion in Chapter 20.) Because iron stores are laid down during the last 6 weeks of pregnancy, babies who are born before that time will probably need to receive iron supplements. All premature infants do not automatically require iron supplements however. Each baby needs to be tested to determine if there is an iron deficiency.

Taking the Infant Home

Within certain parameters, premature infants are usually discharged when they have reached 35 weeks of gestational age. They must demonstrate a good sucking reflex and few respiratory problems. There must be no signs of disease or complications and the infant must exhibit a good weight gain. Some hospitals will discharge an infant as small as 3½ pounds (1600 g) if he is doing well. Babies who are born with extremely low birth weight (less than 3 pounds or 1350 g) who also have serious respiratory, heart, or brain problems, or other medical complications will most likely be hospitalized for a more extended period.

After the baby is home, he will require special care. He cannot be treated like the average baby simply because he was discharged from the hospital. He will need to be protected from infectious illness and any other conditions that could compromise his health. Parents will want to continue to have their baby's physician closely supervise his progress, particularly when medical problems are evident. Caution them against expecting their baby to catch up very quickly developmentally. It may take as long as 2 years for a premature infant to reach the developmental state of a full-term baby of the same age. However, their overall outlook is excellent, with most premature infants reaching their full physical and mental potential.

Breastfeeding the Premature Infant

Breastfeeding a premature infant poses some challenges in the early days and weeks. However, when one considers what human milk has to offer any infant, premature or full term, the challenges seem less imposing. In light of the health concerns that accompany prematurity, mother's milk becomes all the more important.

Human milk is the preferred way to feed a premature infant. It helps establish **enteral** (through the digestive system) tolerance and allows for an earlier discontinuation of **parenteral** (intravenous) nutrition. Human milk has a positive effect on both direct and indirect bilirubin levels. Studies also show long-term improved neurodevelopment in premature infants who are fed human milk (Gross, 1993).

Human milk offers the preterm infant the advantages of having physiologic **amino acids** and fat. It provides greater **bioavailability** of nutrients, a lower **renal solute load,** enzymes to aid digestion, and anti-infective properties. Human milk feeds greatly diminish the incidence of necrotizing enterocolitis. In fact, because of these health benefits, human milk is often prescribed even when the mother does not intend to breastfeed.

This is not without controversy, however. Much debate exists as to whether or not the preterm infant needs human milk fortifier added to the human milk he receives, particularly in the case of very low birth weight infants. Concern is expressed over the total volume of protein and minerals such as calcium and phosphorous found in human milk (Hall, 1989; Wheeler, 1990). The focus is often on weight gain rather than brain growth (Ebrahim, 1993). This ignores the fact that human milk is clearly the feeding of choice to promote neurodevelopment.

Lucas (1994) points out that preterm infants who are fed human milk, when compared with their formula-fed counterparts, showed no negative differences on Bayley psychomotor and mental developmental tests at 18 months. This calls into question the claim that human milk is deficient in meeting the preterm's needs. Further research shows that preterm infants can catch up to their expected intrauterine growth at 38 to 42 weeks postconception when they are exclusively breastfed (Ramasethu, 1993). Clearly more research is needed in this area.

Another area of controversy revolves around the preterm's physical ability to breastfeed. Often, breastfeeding is withheld until the infant "proves" that he is able to bottle feed well. This is based on the premise that breastfeeding is more "stressful" for the premature infant when, in fact, the opposite is true. Breastfeeding infants have less oxygen desaturation during a feed than their bottle-feeding counterparts (Blaymore, 1993). They also have fewer episodes of apnea and **bradycardia** (slow heart rate).

Size is an issue as well. Preterm infants often are not allowed to breastfeed until they reach a certain weight. Size, however, is not intimately related to the infant's ability to coordinate his sucking, swallowing, and breathing. Sucking motions and swallowing of amniotic fluid occur early in gestation. Each preterm infant needs to be assessed on an individual basis for his readiness to go to breast—irrelevant of his ability to suck on a bottle. Premature infants are ready to breastfeed when they are able to coordinate sucking and swallowing. They will put their fists to their mouths, and feed with only occasional disruptions in breathing and heart rate.

Deciding to Breastfeed a Premature Infant

The personnel encountered by the mother while her baby is in the NICU can be very influential in promoting breastfeeding for her baby. Having a specific protocol that covers education, non-nutritive time at breast, non-nutritive sucking, and then the transition to breastfeeding was shown to increase the rate of breastfeeding in one NICU (Bell, 1995). This influence is particularly true of the baby's physician.

The lactation consultant working with families and staff in the NICU must strive to keep up-to-date on breastfeeding matters that relate to preterm infants. In turn, they need to update the staff as appropriate. Caregivers who work with NICU families must give up-to-date, correct, and referenced information, not information that is based on personal experiences. Presenting the facts to mothers does not allow for a "neutral" position regarding infant feeding. Breastfeeding is clearly the optimal way to feed a baby. Withholding the facts in order to avoid guilt fails to provide valuable information. The mother deserves to hear all the facts and make her own decisions based on current, accurate information.

When a baby is born prematurely, breastfeeding education often focuses on the significant advantages that a mother's milk offers to her baby. It is also helpful to point out the benefits to the mother. Only her milk is the same age as her baby, and it will change to meet her baby's needs as her baby's needs change. At a time when she can do little else for her baby, expressing her milk is something she can do. And what a valuable gift her milk is! The mother deserves to hear what a unique and important contribution she makes to her baby's health and development.

Establishing and Maintaining Lactation

In order to provide her valuable milk for her baby, it is recommended that the mother begin to express milk from her breasts within 6 hours of her baby's birth. (See Chapter 19 for a discussion on pumping for a hospitalized baby.) The mother may be overwhelmed by the birth of her premature baby, and will undoubtedly need help getting started with breastfeeding. The nursing staff on the postpartum unit will need to instruct the mother in establishing lactation with hands-on and written instructions. The goal is to help her develop a plan for milk expression that will meet her and her baby's needs until the baby can be put to breast for feeds.

It is advisable that the mother express at least eight times every 24 hours. One expressing session should occur during the late evening or early morning hours. She will want to allow for at least 10 minutes of expressing time for each breast, using a hospital-grade electric breast pump (Auerbach, 1994; Stern, 1990; Stine, 1990). If she pumps both breasts at the same time, she can initially pump for 12 minutes total time. It is very important that the mother pump as frequently as she can in the first few days after the birth. This frequent pumping in the first 2 weeks will determine the amount of milk she is able to produce during the rest of her breastfeeding experience. A pumping diary can help the mother keep track of her efforts.

Initially, the mother will express only a few drops of colostrum. The amount will increase gradually over the course of her first days of pumping. Reassure her that her colostrum is valuable and that the amount is normal. Those few precious drops may be sent to the nursery and spoon fed to her baby if he is able to tolerate oral feeds. Or they may be placed on a breast pad and placed in the isolette with her baby in order to familiarize him with his mother's scent.

The mother may find that breast massage before and during pumping sessions leads to faster expression of her milk and possibly increased amounts. It will help the mother to know that longer pumping sessions do not increase milk yield. Her greatest volume of milk pumped will be in the first 10 to 12 minutes (Auerbach, 1990). To increase volume, she can increase the frequency of pumping sessions throughout the 24 hours. When double pumping, she can be encouraged to pump at least for 12 minutes.

Her yield may also be assisted by means to help her milk ejection reflex. This includes sensory stimulation through a picture of her baby or the smell of his clothing. The use of auditory and visual relaxation are other methods (Feher, 1989). Massaging the mother's back while she is pumping can assist milk ejection. If these less invasive measures fail to increase the mother's yield, she may wish to discuss the use of galactogogues—such as fenugreek or blessed thistle—or prescription medications such as metoclopramide (Ehrenkranz, 1997).

It will help the mother to know that her milk production may fluctuate depending on her baby's condition. Changes in her own lifestyle may also affect it. If her baby experiences a setback, the mother may notice a drop in milk volume. If she returns to work while her baby remains in the NICU, she may notice a decrease in supply. Over time, in spite of a favorable prognosis for her baby, the mother may notice an unexplainable decrease in milk production or an increased time required for her milk ejection reflex. Sometimes the opposite is true, and the mother will have much more milk expressed than her baby is able to use. This milk can be stored for later use or donated to a milk bank. Keep the follow-up of these mothers a high priority in order to provide support to them through these rough periods. Without your support, most mothers of premature infants will encounter problems with milk production.

Preserving the Safety of the Milk

With consideration to the more fragile state of the premature infant, a mother who is pumping for her preterm infant needs to practice good hygiene in order to ensure the safety of her milk. Encourage her to shower daily and to wash her hands before each pumping session. After a pumping session, the pump parts that come in contact with her milk should first be rinsed clean of milk with cold water and then washed in hot soapy water. Additionally, the pump parts must be boiled daily. The milk for her premature baby should be stored in sterile hard plastic or glass containers that maintain the integrity of the milk composition.

Unlike milk that is expressed for full-term infants, the milk for a premature infant should not be layered with milk from other pumping sessions. Milk from each pumping session needs to be stored separately and labeled according to the NICU's specifications. The mother also will want to inquire with her baby's nurses regarding how the milk is to be received, whether it should be fresh or frozen. She should be encouraged to provide fresh milk whenever possible. If the baby is unable to tolerate oral feeds, or if the mother is unable to deliver the milk to her baby within 24 hours after it is expressed, the hospital may request that she freeze her milk. When transporting frozen milk, the mother needs to be aware that melting ice gives off heat and may thaw some of her milk. The frozen milk can be wrapped in newspaper or a towel and kept in a cold insulated container for transport. Provide the mother with written instructions for pumping hygiene and care of her milk for her easy reference through this difficult time.

Feeding the Preterm Infant Expressed Human Milk

Initial feeds of the preterm infant are often via gavage tubing. A gavage tube may be **nasogastric**, passing through the nose into the stomach, or **orogastric**, passing from the mouth to the stomach. Occasionally, a **gastrostomy** tube is placed through the skin directly into the stomach.

Freshly expressed milk is preferred for feeds when the baby is not yet able to go to breast, because its composition is most suitable for the baby. Frozen milk will have lost a small portion of its protective properties. However, it is still preferable to an artificial substitute in terms of nutrition and the protection that is afforded the premature infant. As the baby is able to tolerate these enteral feeds and as he grows more clinically stable, he will be able to progress to oral feeds, including feeding at the breast. In the mother's absence, he can receive feeds via an alternative feeding method, such as cup, spoon, or dropper. As previously discussed, the use of artificial nipples and bottles to provide supplements is not recommended for premature infants. Bottle feeding is associated with physiologic and biochemical changes in the infant such as **hypoxemia, hypercapnia** (high carbon dioxide levels), apnea, bradycardia, and **cyanosis.** Babies as young as 30 weeks gestation and as small as 1100 g are capable of effectively handling feeds at the breast. Research demonstrates that it is physiologically easier for a preterm infant to suckle on the human breast than with an artificial nipple (Anderson, 1993, 1989; Meier 1988). Mead (1992) showed that the preterm infant can suckle well enough at the breast to maintain good weight gain.

Kangaroo Care

Readiness to breastfeed begins when the baby is stable. The NICU staff and the baby's parents can assist the baby in making the transition from gavage feeds to breastfeeds in a variety of ways. The mother can continue to place drops of her milk on a breast pad and leave it in her baby's isolette to increase his familiarity with her scent. During gavage feeds, she can put her baby to breast to build his association with sucking and eating. Teach the mother ways to assist her baby and the normal expectations of the experience. As the baby's condition permits, **kangaroo care** can also be initiated (Anderson, 1993, 1989; Hamelin, 1993; Ludington-Hoe, 1992; Weibley, 1989; Whitelaw, 1990). Stable infants, even when they are still on a ventilator, may begin kangaroo care.

Kangaroo care provides the baby a chance to be placed skin to skin with his mother in close proximity to her breasts. It allows him the opportunity to become gently familiar with his new feeding environment and explore his new feeding method. The baby is held skin to skin upright and prone between his mother's breasts, wearing only a diaper. He and his mother are then wrapped together to maintain his temperature appropriately (Fig. 21.2). The mother can wear a button-down shirt and no bra for ease of kangarooing. In order not to overstimulate her baby, she needs to sit quietly at first, with minimal or no talking, singing, stroking, or rocking. As her baby's condition improves she will notice an interest on his part to maintain eye contact. Often during this kangarooing, her baby will be in a quiet alert state initially, and then settle down to sleep. Fathers are encouraged to kangaroo their baby as well.

Kangaroo care offers many advantages to the preterm baby and his parents. The skin-to-skin contact has a soothing effect on the baby. Less crying is noted, his heart rate and respirations are more regular, and he has better sleep periods. The baby also is better oxygenated and is able to maintain his temperature. Babies who receive kangaroo care tend to gain weight faster and to be discharged from the hospital earlier. The effects are long term as well, with less crying noted at 6 months of age and a decreased rate of serious infection in the 6 months following kangaroo care (Sloan, 1994). The mother receives benefits from kangarooing as well. It has been reported that mothers feel more attached to their babies and more confident in caring for them when they use kangaroo care (Hurst, 1997).

Kangaroo care has been shown to increase the success of breastfeeding for the preterm infant. Time spent lying quietly by the breast—becoming familiar with the scent, sight and sensations—gradually develops into rooting, licking, and tasting. You and the NICU personnel can encourage the mother that this is a very important step in her baby's progress toward exclusive breastfeeding. As he becomes stronger and more alert, these kangaroo care times will lead to the baby latching onto the breast with active suckles. A small study showed greater improvement in milk production in mothers who practiced kangaroo care for about 4 hours per week than in mothers who did not practice this skin-to-skin contact (Hurst, 1997).

Feedings at the Breast in the Hospital

When the baby shows readiness to feed at the breast, the mother can gently be guided to promote his attachment and suckling. Initial feeds will involve only minimal "feeding" time, interspersed with much resting time. Assure the mother that this is normal and expected. It is a time when she and her baby are getting to know one another, and it will involve much practice at first. Ideally the location should be quiet and private, and near any needed equipment.

Instruct the mother to hold her baby at the level of the breast, supporting his entire body. Holding her baby in the clutch position will enable her to see and handle him. The mother will want to support her breast with the C-hold to compel her baby to root and open his mouth. Modifying this hold into the Dancer hand position will support her baby's jaw at the same time she is minimizing the weight of her breast in his mouth. This jaw and cheek support may help increase her baby's milk intake (Einarsson-Backes, 1994). To encourage her baby to nurse, the mother may use breast massage before and during the feed. Some mothers use a breast pump to initiate milk flow.

Encourage the mother to approach the feed in a relaxed and unhurried manner. Her baby will need frequent rests during feeds at the breast. If he experiences gulping and choking, the mother can be taught to adjust her position and that of her baby to accommodate milk flow. She can hold her baby so that the back of his throat is somewhat higher than the breast, or she may sit in a semireclined position. Another option for the mother is to express her milk before the feed and allow her baby to nurse with a less intense milk flow. This allows him to "practice" his sucks without being overwhelmed by milk (Naranayan, 1991).

If possible, during feeds, the mother will want to avoid any unnecessary stimulation from bright lights, loud noises, stroking, rocking, or talking to her baby. Learning his new skill of feeding at the breast will require a great deal of his attention. Too much outside stimulation can overwhelm him. If at any time during the feed her baby seems irritated or fussy, the mother

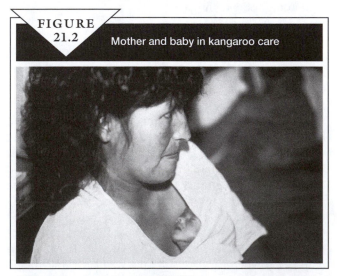

FIGURE 21.2 Mother and baby in kangaroo care

Printed by permission of UNICEF.

can kangaroo him by her breast and allow him the comfort of simply being there.

Your support during these early feeds is quite valuable to the mother. She may feel overwhelmed by this new experience (Gunn, 1991). Concerns frequently cited by mothers are what to expect of their preterm baby and how to know that he is getting enough milk (Hill, 1994). The mother needs to know how to tell when her baby is in a pattern of nutritive, or high-flow, sucks and swallows. She may also need to become familiar with the gadgets that are used during her baby's transition to the breast. A tube-feeding device may be used to encourage more effective sucking at the breast. Some breastfeeds may need to be followed with a sup-

TABLE 21.2
Counseling Summary—Preterm Infant

Mother's Concern	Suggestions for Mother
Anxiety about taking small baby home	◆ Continue close medical supervision of baby.
Anxiety about beginning breastfeeding	◆ Keep realistic expectations. ◆ Allow transition period.
Baby tires easily at breast	◆ Wake baby frequently during feed. ◆ Stimulate baby to nurse. ◆ Nurse frequently for short periods as long as baby is suckling and swallowing.
Weak rooting reflex	◆ Provide skin-to-skin contact. ◆ Turn baby's head toward breast. ◆ Help baby open his mouth. ◆ Form nipple and bring baby to breast.
Weak sucking mechanism	◆ Use Dancer hand position to increase intraoral negative pressure.
Intermittent sucking and resting during feeds	◆ Plan to allow lengthy time for each feed.
Nipple preference	◆ Express milk until letdown occurs. ◆ Avoid artificial nipples. ◆ Cup feed when the mother is not present for feeds.
Difficulty interesting baby in breast	◆ Provide frequent skin contact and nuzzling. ◆ Familiarize baby with smell of mother's milk.
Difficulty positioning baby at breast	◆ Use pillows to bring baby to breast level. ◆ Use clutch hold for positioning and Dancer hand position under baby's chin.
Difficulty determining whether baby is getting enough milk	◆ Determine with NICU staff the number of wet diapers and stools to expect each day ◆ Determine follow-up visit schedule with pediatrician. ◆ Determine minimum feeding frequency to expect and what to do if baby does not meet that goal. ◆ Consider renting electronic scale for daily weights at home. Plan with pediatrician what weight gain to expect. Learn from nursing staff how to determine accurate weights.

plementary feed. For increased calorie supplement, the creamy portion of expressed milk that rises to the top can be used. Alternatively, the mother can express hindmilk after a breastfeed (Valentine, 1994). In some instances, the neonatologist may recommend test weights to determine milk intake at the breast in order to calculate supplement needs. The electronic scale has been shown to provide an accurate estimate of the preterm's milk intake at the breast (Meier, 1990). Many mothers find the use of such a scale to be very reassuring. You can provide her with encouragement about her progress with pumping and, eventually, breastfeeding.

Going Home with a Premature Infant

When her baby is nearing his discharge from the hospital, the mother may experience quite a range of emotions, from excitement and anticipation to apprehension and dread. The day she has been waiting for is finally approaching, and yet her baby still seems so fragile. To ease this transition for the mother, she can be encouraged to room in with her baby in the hospital 2 or 3 days before discharge. This allows her to function in an independent mode with help available when she needs it. It is especially important that 24-hour rooming in is provided for her, if possible. Nighttime care of the infant seems especially threatening to new parents.

After she is home, the mother may continue using the hospital routines for the first few days to ease the transition for both her and the baby. During this time, she needs to keep expressing her milk. As her baby gradually begins to breastfeed more frequently and more efficiently, she can decrease her pumping time. If her baby was sent home being supplemented or needing special devices, she will be able to discontinue these gradually as well. Many practitioners advise mothers that some degree of pumping will be necessary until the infant reaches his expected due date.

Your follow-up will ease the mother's worries as she initiates these changes. Her baby's weight can be assessed periodically as the feeding routines change. The mother may need to be reminded of her baby's feeding cues and expectations because those that are taught by caregivers for full-term infants do not always work for preterm infants. The biggest worry of mothers who take their preterm infant home is how to tell if the baby is getting enough milk. Kavanaugh (1995, 1997) and Meier (1990) recommend the use of electronic balance scales at home to help mothers recognize that their babies are consuming adequate milk. They believe that doing this will enable many mothers to continue who would have quit breastfeeding because the anxiety over milk transfer outweighed their desire to nurse.

The mother can be encouraged to regard her baby's gestational age, rather than his age from birth, as an indicator of what to expect. Through this time, the breast can provide him a safe and reassuring place that has remained constant as he moved into his new environment. You can reassure the mother that she has overcome many obstacles—from pumping, to first feeds, and finally her baby's discharge from the hospital. She has provided her preterm baby with a unique and valuable gift that will benefit him for a lifetime. See Table 21.2 for a counseling summary on the preterm infant.

▼ Postmaturity

A postmature baby is one who is born after 42 weeks of gestation. Delivery may be facilitated by inducing labor or by performing cesarean birth. The danger of postmaturity involves deterioration of the placenta, which progressively becomes less efficient after the normal gestation period of 37 to 42 weeks. Postmature infants may be appropriate for gestational age in body length but are often **small-for-date** because of the progressive increase in placental dysfunction. Fetal oxygenation will be marginal or depressed before labor, and meconium may be released during labor. The stresses of labor are poorly tolerated following birth. The baby may have difficulty maintaining respiration, blood sugar levels, and nervous functioning. These are all situations that generally are manageable.

Some postmature infants have skin that is dry and cracked, with a texture similar to parchment paper. The infant's skin is sagging and loose, with an absence of vernix. He may have profuse scalp hair, as well as long nails on his fingers and toes. If meconium was released, there can be a yellow-green staining of the baby's skin and nails. A postmature baby may be sluggish during his initial attempts at breastfeeding. He may need to be coaxed and prodded in much the same way as the premature baby. Basically, however, breastfeeding a postmature infant progresses in much the same way as that of a full term infant.

▼ COUNSELING A MOTHER WHOSE BABY HAS DIED

Probably one of the most distressing situations you will encounter will be caring for a mother whose baby has died. At such a time it seems difficult to find just the right words, to avoid any painful remarks, and perhaps most important, to be supportive. With appropriate counseling techniques, some insight into the mother's emotions, and a feeling of empathy, you can be confident in your ability to handle the encounter and comfort the mother in her grief.

After listening to the mother relate what has happened, you can let her know how shocked and saddened you feel. Avoid telling her "I know how you must feel," or "I can imagine what you are going through." You cannot begin to know what the mother is feeling unless you have experienced a similar loss. Instead, you can reflect back to the mother how she must feel. Appropriate statements may be, "You must be devastated," or "I can't imagine the loss you feel."

To encourage the mother to talk, you can tell her that other mothers who have suffered similar losses have found it helpful to talk through their feelings. Let her know that you will be glad to listen. At the same time, assure her that you do not want to invade her privacy. Unless her feelings are shared and worked through, her grief will continue without resolution. People close to the mother may feel uncomfortable listening to her relate her birth experience and the circumstances surrounding her baby's death. She may appreciate being able to turn to you, knowing that you will be concerned and interested in listening to her.

Having an insight into the mother's feelings will help you in your counseling. For many mothers, the bonding process began on the day they learned they were pregnant or when they first heard the baby's heartbeat. The parents need others to acknowledge that their baby, even though very young, stillborn, or never cared for by them, was loved even before birth and was a person who meant a lot in their lives. Avoid comments such as, "At least you can have more children" or "It was for the best." The mother may feel she would rather care for an imperfect baby than no baby at all. She cannot be consoled by the thought of replacing her dead baby with a new one. She is grieving for the baby she has just lost. You can acknowledge the infant's importance by asking his name and using it during your discussion.

Parents need to pass through a grief process before their loss can be totally resolved. There are many different terms used for this process. Essentially, it begins with a stage of denial and ends in acceptance of the loss. The range of emotions they experience between these two stages are presented in Figure 21.3. The time it takes parents to pass from the denial phase to that of acceptance will vary greatly, and could take as long as 18 to 24 months.

Acceptance of their loss will depend on many factors, among them the amount of support and understanding that the parents receive from friends and family. The mother may need to talk about her baby long after most people have tired of hearing it. You may be the one person she feels will be receptive, especially if you have built a close relationship with her. Try to key into the mother's needs and sense how often she would like to hear from you. It will be much easier for her to receive a call than to pick up the phone and feel she is bothering you with more rambling about her baby. In choosing your comments carefully, perhaps the list in Table 21.3 will be helpful.

▼ Breastfeeding Concerns

The mother may have concerns specific to breastfeeding, especially if she and her baby had begun nursing. Even if she had not begun to breastfeed, the mother's breasts may fill up with milk a few days after delivery and can become engorged and painful. Offer the mother suggestions for relieving the fullness without stimulating her breasts to the extent that more milk is produced. Advise her to express her milk just enough for comfort. All other comfort measures for engorgement can be used as well (see Chapter 14).

Continuous application of cabbage leaves to the breasts will encourage the milk to dry up and offer the mother relief. Remind her to change the cabbage leaves about every 2 to 3 hours. A mother who had been pumping her breasts to maintain her milk production for a premature or ill baby will have more difficulty stopping lactation. She may need to continue pumping and decreasing slowly in a weaning pattern so as to avoid problems associated with abrupt wean-

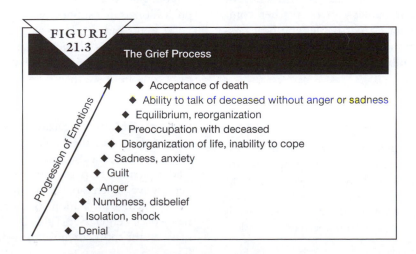

FIGURE 21.3

The Grief Process

Progression of Emotions

◆ Acceptance of death
◆ Ability to talk of deceased without anger or sadness
◆ Equilibrium, reorganization
◆ Preoccupation with deceased
◆ Disorganization of life, inability to cope
◆ Sadness, anxiety
◆ Guilt
◆ Anger
◆ Numbness, disbelief
◆ Isolation, shock
◆ Denial

TABLE 21.3
Do's and Don'ts for Counseling Grieving Parents

DO show your genuine concern and caring.

DO be available to listen and empathize.

DO say you are sorry about what happened.

DO allow the mother to express as much grief as she feels.

DO encourage parents to be patient with themselves.

DO allow the mother to talk about her baby.

DO talk about the special qualities of the baby she lost.

DO acknowledge the impact of the baby's death.

DO reassure the parents that they did everything possible for their baby.

DO refer to the baby by name.

DO show your sadness and disappointment.

DON'T let your own sense of helplessness keep you from reaching out to the mother.

DON'T avoid the mother because you are uncomfortable with her situation.

DON'T say you know how the mother feels.

DON'T suggest that the mother should be feeling better by a certain time.

DON'T tell parents what they should feel or do.

DON'T change the subject when the baby is mentioned.

DON'T try to find something positive about the baby's death.

DON'T point out that they can always have other children or suggest that they should be grateful for any other children they already have.

DON'T suggest that the baby's care by the parents or medical personnel was inadequate.

DON'T avoid using the baby's name for fear of causing pain for the mother.

DON'T be overly cheerful or casual.

Adapted with permission from a list compiled by the Compassionate Friends.

ing. A mother who had begun nursing her baby may also need to express her milk to decrease her milk production gradually. Mothers who had been nursing or expressing milk for their babies can be further comforted in knowing they gave their babies the best possible care, both nutritionally and emotionally. Some mothers donate their milk to a milk bank for a period of time.

 Support Systems for Parents

Parents who have lost a child may benefit from professional counseling available through local clergy and social service organizations. Talking with other parents who have had similar experiences can also help their perspectives and encourage them to share feelings. This is especially vital to parents who have experienced the loss of a baby. As time passes, they may have a continuing need to talk about their loss, and will benefit from the ongoing support they receive from other parents and professionals in a support group.

Parents can also learn their rights and options, questions to ask their physicians, and helpful suggestions for arrangements following their baby's death. They have the right to hold or see their baby after he has died, a practice particularly helpful for parents of a stillborn infant. Some hospitals take pictures of the deceased infant for parents to keep. This is especially important to parents who choose not to see their infant because many have the desire to see their baby months later when it is too late. These pictures help parents put their baby's death into perspective. There are many support groups for grieving parents across the nation, often affiliated with a hospital or medical center. See Table 21.4 for a counseling summary on the mother whose baby has died.

TABLE 21.4

Counseling Summary—Mother Whose Baby Has Died

◆ Listen to the mother's feelings.

◆ Reflect back her feelings through the use of counseling skills.

◆ Express your concern and sorrow.

◆ Help her acknowledge that her baby was a person who meant a great deal to her.

◆ Support her as she passes through the grief process by being patient and receptive, and by choosing your comments carefully.

◆ Help the mother gradually reduce her milk production.

◆ Direct the mother to support groups, social service organizations, and professional counseling, as applicable.

▼

SUMMARY

The lactation consultant is a valuable resource for the high-risk infant and his mother. This support includes counseling the mother regarding how to fit breastfeeding into her baby's situation. You may also be needed to support the mother as she works through her feelings surrounding this unexpected outcome, feelings that go beyond breastfeeding. You are there to help her develop a realistic picture in the beginning and to plan for her baby's nutrition. This may occur long before her baby is able to go to the breast. You can guide the mother through the initiation of pumping and caring for her stored milk. Be available to her to support the early breastfeeds and to guide her through the transition of bringing her baby home from the hospital. Sadly, sometimes, you may need to support a mother whose baby has died. Your participation in the mother's health care team will be critical in these types of circumstances.

▼

REFERENCES

Anderson G. Skin to skin: Kangaroo care in Western Europe. *Am J Nurs* 89:662–666; 1989.

Anderson G. Current knowledge about skin to skin (Kangaroo) care for preterm infants. *Breastfeeding Review* 8:364–373; 1993.

Auerbach K. Sequential and simultaneous breast pumping: A comparison. *Int J Nurs Stud* 27:257–265; 1990.

Bell E et al. A structured intervention improves breastfeeding success for ill or preterm infants. *MCN* 20:309–314; 1995.

Blaymore J. Breastfeeding of very low birth weight infants. *J Pediatr* 123:773–778; 1993.

Boukydis Z. Crying and preterm babies. *Intensive Caring Unlimited* 7:7; 1989.

Culp R et al. A tool for educating parents about their premature infants. *Birth* 16:23–26; 1989.

Ebrahim G. Feeding the preterm brain. *J Trop Pediatr* 39:1430–1431; 1993.

Ehrenkranz R and Ackerman B. Metoclopramide effect of faltering milk production by mothers of premature infants. *Pediatr* 78:614–620; 1986.

Einarsson-Backes L. The effect of oral support on sucking efficiency in preterm infants. *Am J Occup Ther* 48:490–498; 1994.

Feher S et al. Increasing breast milk production for premature infants with a relaxation/imagery audiotape. *Pediatrics* 83:57–60; 1989.

Gross S and Slagle T. Feeding the low birth weight infant. *Clin Perinatol* 20:193–209; 1993.

Gunn T. Breastfeeding preterm infants. *N Z Med J* 104:188–189; 1991.

Hall R et al. Hypophosphatemia in breastfed low birth weight infants following initial hospital discharge. *Am J Child Dis* 143:1191–1195; 1989.

Hamelin K and Ramachandran C. Kangaroo care. *Can Nurse* 89:15–17; 1993.

Hill P et al. Mothers of low birthweight infants: Breastfeeding patterns and problems. *J Hum Lact* 10:169–176; 1994.

Hurst N et al. Skin-to-skin holding in the neonatal intensive care unit. *J Perinatol* 17:213–217; 1997.

Hylander MA et al. Human milk feedings and infection among very low birth weight infants. *Pediatrics* 102(3); p. e38; 1998.

Kaufman K and Hall L. Influences of the social network on choice and duration of breastfeeding in mothers of preterm infants. *Res Nurs Health* 12:149–159; 1989.

Kavanaugh K et al. Getting enough: mothers' concerns about breastfeeding a preterm infant after discharge. *JOGNN* 24:23–32; 1995.

Kavanaugh K et al. The rewards outweigh the efforts: Breast-feeding outcomes for mothers of preterm infants. *J Hum Lact* 13:15–21; 1997.

Klaus MH et al. *Bonding: Building the foundations of secure attachment and independence.* Addison Wesley; New York; 1995.

Ludington-Hoe S et al. Selected physiologic measures and behavior during paternal skin contact with Colombian preterm infants. *J Dev Psych-01* 18:223–232; 1992.

McKim E. The information and support needs of mothers of premature infants. *J Pediatr Nurs* 8:233–244; 1993.

Mead L et al. Breastfeeding success with preterm quadruplets. *JOGNN* 21:221–227; 1992.

Meier P. Bottle and breastfeeding: Effects on transcutaneous oxygen pressure and temperature in preterm infants. *Nurs Res* 37:36–41; 1988.

Naranayan I et al. Sucking on the 'emptied' breast: Non-nutritive sucking with a difference. *Arch Dis Child* 66:241–244; 1991.

Nyqvist K and Sjoden P. Advice concerning breastfeeding from mothers of infants admitted to a neonatal intensive care unit: The Roy adaptation model as a conceptual structure. *J Adv Nurs* 18:54–63; 1993.

Ramasethu J et al. Weight gain in exclusively breastfed preterm infants. *J Trop Pediatr* 39:152–159; 1993.

Sloan N et al. Kangaroo mother method: Randomised controlled trial of an alternative method of care for stabilised low-birthweight infants. *Lancet* 344:782–785; 1994.

Stern J and Reichlin S. Prolactin circadian rhythm persists throughout lactation in women. *Neuroendocrinology* 51:31–37; 1990.

Stine M. Breastfeeding and the premature newborn: A protocol without bottles. *J Hum Lact* 6:167–170; 1990.

Valentine C et al. Hindmilk improves weight gain in low-birth-weight infants fed human milk. *J Pediatr Gastroenterol Nutr* 18:474–477; 1994.

Weibley T. Inside the incubator. *MCN* 14:96–100; 1989.

Wheeler R et al. Calcium and phosphorous supplementation following initial hospital discharge in <1800 gm birthweight breastfed infants. *Am J Perinatol* 7:389–390; 1990.

Whitelaw A. Kangaroo baby care: Just a nice experience or an important advance for preterm infants. *Pediatrics* 85:604; 1990.

BIBLIOGRAPHY

Auerbach K and Walker M. When the mother of a premature infant breastfeeds: What every NICU nurse needs to know. *Neonatal Network* 13:23–29; 1994.

Belec L et al. Antibodies to human immunodeficiency virus in the breast milk of healthy, seropositive women. *Pediatrics* 85:1022–1026; 1990.

Bobat R et al. Breastfeeding by HIV-1-infected women and outcome in their infants: A cohort study from Durban, South Africa. *AIDS* 11:1627–1633; 1997.

Bose CL et al. Relactation by mothers of sick and premature infants. *Pediatrics* 67(4):565–569; 1981.

Bradshaw J. Breastfeeding twin, triplets and quads: Making the impossible easy. *Newsletter: National Capital Lactation Center* 16; Summer, 1996.

Bu'Lock F et al: Development of coordination of sucking, swallowing and breathing: Ultrasound study of term and preterm infants. *Dev. Med Child Neurol* 32:669–678; 1990.

Burns K et al. Infant stimulation: Modification of an intervention based on physiologic and behavioral cues. *JOGNN* 23:581–589; 1995.

Croxson M et al. Vertical transmission of hepatitis C virus in New Zealand. *N Z Med J* 110:165–167; 1997.

Curtin G. The infant with cleft lip or palate: More than a surgical problem. *J Perinat Neonatal Nurs* 3:80–89; 1990.

Cutting W. Breastfeeding and HIV infection. *Br Med J* 305:788; 1992.

Datta P. et al. Mother-to-child transmission of human immunodeficiency virus Type I: Report from the Nairobi study. *J Infect Dis* 170:1134–1140; 1994.

Dunn D and Newell M. Quantifying the risk of HIV-I transmission via breastmilk. *AIDS* 7:134–135; 1993.

Dunne W and Jevon M. Examination of human breast milk for evidence of human Herpesvirus 6 by polymerase chain reaction. *J Infect Dis* 168:250; 1993.

Farran A et al. Infant stimulation in the NICU. *Intensive Caring Unlimited* 7:13; 1989.

Furman L et al. Breastfeeding of very low birth weight infants. *J Hum Lact* 14:29–34; 1998.

Greve L et al. Breastfeeding in the management of the newborn with phenylketonuria: A practical approach to dietary therapy. *J Am Diet Assoc* 94:305–309; 1994.

Gross SJ et al. Nutritional composition of milk produced by mothers delivering preterm. *Journal of Pediatrics* 96(4):641–44; 1980.

Hira S et al. Apparent vertical transmission of human immunodeficiency virus type I by breastfeeding in Zambia. *J Pediatr* 117:421–424; 1990.

Hurst N et al. Skin-to-skin holding in the neonatal intensive care unit influences maternal milk volume. *J Perinatol* 17:213–217; 1997.

International Lactation Consultants' Association. ILCA's position paper on the issue of HIV and infant feeding. *J Hum Lact* 13:269; 1997.

Kampinga G et al. Primary infections with HIV-1 of women and their offspring in Rwanda: Findings of heterogeneity at seroconversion, coinfection and recombinants of HIV-1 subtypes A and C. *Virology* 227:63–76; 1997.

Klaus MH and Kennell JH. *Maternal-Infant Bonding.* St. Louis: C.V. Mosby Co.; 1976.

Kriess, J. Breastfeeding and vertical transmission of HIV-1. *Acta Paediatr* 421(Suppl):113–117; 1997.

Lambert J and Watters N. Breastfeeding the infant/child with cardiac defect: An informal survey. *J Hum Lact* 14: 151–155; 1998.

Lucas A and Cole TJ. Breast milk and neonatal necrotising enterocolitis. *Lancet* 386; 1519–1523; 1990.

Lucas A et al. A randomized multicenter study of human milk versus formula and later development in preterm infants. *Arch Child Dis* 70:F141–F146; 1994.

Lucas A et al: Breast milk and subsequent intelligence quotient in children born preterm. *Lancet* 339; 261–264; 1992.

Mathew OP and Bhathia J. Sucking and breathing patterns during breast and bottle feedings in term neonates. *Am J Dis Child* 143:588–592; 1989.

Measel CP and Anderson GC. Nonnutritive sucking during tube feedings: Effect on clinical course in premature infants. *JOGGN* 8(5):265–272; 1979.

Meier P and EJ Pugh. Breastfeeding behavior of small preterm infants. *MCN* 10:396–401; 1985.

Meier P et al. The accuracy of test weighing for preterm infants. *J Pediatr Gastroenterol Nutr* 10:62–65; 1990.

Neifert M and Thrope J. Twins: Family adjustment, parenting, and infant feeding in the fourth trimester. *Clin Obstet Gynecol* 33:102–112; 1990.

Newberg D et al. A human milk factor inhibits binding of immunodeficiency virus to the CD4 receptor. *Pediatr Res* 31: 22–28; 1992.

Nommsen-Rivers L and Heinig M. HIV transmission via breastfeeding: Reflections on the issues. *J Hum Lact* 13:179–181; 1997.

Orloff S et al. Inactivation of human immunodeficiency virus type I in human milk: Effects of intrinsic factors in human milk and of pasteurization. *J Hum Lact* 9:13–17; 1993.

Oxtoby M. Human immunodeficiency virus and other viruses in human milk. Placing the issues in broader perspective. *Pediatr Infec Dis J* 7:825–835; 1988.

Palasanthiran P et al. Breastfeeding during primary maternal human immunodeficiency virus infection and risk of transmission from mother to infant. *J Infect Dis* 167:441–444; 1993.

Polywka S et al. Hepatitis C virus infection in pregnancy and the risk of mother-to-child transmission. *Eur J Clin Microbiol Infect Dis* 16:121–124; 1997.

Raiha N. Protein fortification on human milk for feeding preterm infants. *Acta Paediatr* Suppl 405(Suppl):93–97; 1994.

Ruff A et al. Breastfeeding and maternal-infant transmission of human immunodeficiency virus type I. *J Pediatr* 121: 325–329; 1992.

Schanler R. Suitability of human milk for the low-birthweight infant. *Clin Perinatol* 22:207–222; 1995.

Schanler R and Abrams S. Postnatal attainment of intrauterine macromineral accretion rates in low birth weight infants fed fortified human milk. *J Pediatr* 126:441–447; 1995.

Sollid D et al. Breastfeeding multiples. *J Pernat Neonat Nurs* 3:46–65; 1989.

Stiehm E and Vink P. Transmission of human immunodeficiency virus infection by breastfeeding. *J Pediatr* 118:410–411; 1991.

Van de Perre P et al. Mother-to-infant transmission of human immunodeficiency virus by breast milk: Presumed innocent or presumed guilty? *Clin Infect Dis* 15:502–507; 1992.

WHO Press. HIV and breastfeeding. *Central African J Med* 38:314–315; 1992.

Williams R and Medalie J. Twins: Double pleasure or double trouble? *Am Fam Phys* 49:869–873; 1994.

Woerner J. The joy of multiples. *Int J Childbirth Education* 8:35–36; 1993.

22

WHEN BREASTFEEDING IS INTERRUPTED

Ideally, a breastfeeding mother and her baby are together during feeding times with no interruptions in feeds. However, in today's world, this is often not realistic, nor in many cases desired by the mother. There are many different occasions that may result in a separation of the mother and baby. Some of these situations will be temporary, whereas others will require regular long-term periods of separation. The separation may be for a few hours or a few days, or the mother may be away for regular daily separations because of returning to work or school. She may also be away from her baby over a long period of time because of illness and hospitalization. Some of these separations may not involve missed breastfeeds. Others will require the use of an alternative feeding method during the absence. Mothers who experience such separations will have special needs in terms of managing feeds and maintaining milk production. They will benefit from emotional support and encouragement as well.

finding time to spend with each family member. She also needs to know that her baby will accept nourishment by an alternative feeding method during her absence. This requires planning well in advance to allow time to work out possible problems of her baby not accepting the feeding method. The mother's comfort is an issue as well. She will need to express milk regularly in order to relieve any overfullness and to maintain milk production. She may experience conflicting emotions about the separation and about planning to continue breastfeeding in spite of obstacles. Effective use of counseling skills will help you listen and respond to the mother's concerns about the cause of the separation, especially if her baby is hospitalized. This can be a trying time for her family. Your support and encouragement will be especially appreciated.

MANAGING BREASTFEEDING THROUGH A SEPARATION

Being separated from her baby can create stress and anxiety for a new mother. This is especially true when the separation is a result of illness. You can help relieve some of the mother's anxieties by accepting and supporting her decisions concerning breastfeeding. If she chooses to combine breastfeeding with a daily or prolonged separation, she will need advice about milk expression and maintaining milk production. You can help her in obtaining a pump and offer her practical suggestions for its use. The mother will need to be strongly motivated to overcome any potential difficulties and pressures that may confront her. This discussion focuses on how you can help a mother whose separation from her baby affects her breastfeeding management.

The Mother's Needs

When a mother is separated from her baby during usual nursing times, she may face challenges regarding attitudes of family members, child care arrangements, and

Considerations for Timing of the Separation

Often mothers have no control over the timing of a separation. A working mother may have a limited maternity leave, or hospitalization may be necessary for either mother or baby. For those who do have a choice, however, there are some factors to be considered. An important breastfeeding consideration for the mother is that she delay missed breastfeeds until her milk production is well established. Barring any interference, most mothers will have breastfeeding well established by the time the baby is 2 months old and can likely manage a separation by that time. The transition is even smoother if a separation can be delayed until the baby is old enough to begin eating solid foods, at around 6 months of age. At that time, there will be less need for supplemental feedings while the mother and baby are apart. There are also many other factors unrelated to breastfeeding such as the emotional needs of both the mother and baby, and separation anxiety that occurs at around 9 months. The mother can assess her particular situation to determine when the separation will be least disruptive.

Maintaining Milk Production

A mother's milk production will naturally diminish to some extent if she experiences a substantial separation from her baby. She cannot remove milk from her breasts as efficiently as her baby does when he nurses. In order to maintain the ability to produce sufficient milk for her baby, a mother must remove milk from her breasts regularly. You can provide her with instructions on how to hand express or use a breast pump. Many mothers who are away from their babies on a regular basis find it convenient to express milk routinely. Others, depending on the length of absence, may prefer to not express and save their milk. Instead, they express only enough to relieve discomfort during the separation and allow their milk production to diminish slightly. Their babies will receive infant formula during the absence rather than human milk. This choice will depend on each mother's preference and the circumstances of her separation. Your role is to support her decision.

Nourishing the Baby during the Absence

When a breastfeeding mother is away from her baby during nursing times, she must make arrangements for some form of nourishment until she returns. The feeding method and type of food are factors to be considered. Although a bottle may be convenient, it can cause the young baby to develop a nipple preference that will interfere with breastfeeding. Although a cup or medicine spoon will eliminate nipple preference, it may require more time for feeding. If a bottle is used, those with nipples that encourage the baby to open his mouth wide seem to make the transition from breast to bottle easier for the very young baby. Therefore, the mother will want to use a nipple with a large base (see Chapter 19).

The mother may choose to provide her own milk or may prefer that her baby be given infant formula. Depending on the length of her absence and the baby's age, he may receive juice, water, or solid foods. Experimenting with feeding methods for at least 2 weeks before the separation takes place will help the baby learn to accept nourishment by some means other than breastfeeding.

Motivation to Continue Nursing

Motivation and determination are critical factors for a mother in continuing to breastfeed despite a separation from her baby. Some mothers may assume that they must wean their babies when a separation occurs. You can assure the mother that breastfeeding is perfectly compatible with both short-term and long-term separations. If weaning does become inevitable, you can reassure the mother that the quality of her breastfeeding experience is the important factor in determining success, not its duration. If the separation has prompted the mother to compromise her initial goals for breastfeeding, she can still work toward a satisfying experience if she remains flexible and positive.

If a mother is not totally committed to breastfeeding, she may choose to deal with the separation by weaning her baby. Some mothers may want to continue nursing despite feeling very discouraged. By assessing each mother's motives you can help her achieve the outcome she truly wants. Mothers who deal with a separation will benefit from a great deal of support and practical suggestions, whether the decision is to wean or to continue nursing.

Coping with Difficulties

A separation between mother and baby can create physical problems related to breastfeeding, as well as emotional tension and anxiety. The mother must remove milk from her breasts regularly in order to avoid such problems as leaking, plugged ducts, engorgement, and mastitis. Despite her diligence in expressing her milk, she may still experience problems because of not being able to remove milk from her breasts as efficiently as her baby does when he nurses.

The mother will be taxing her energy reserves, whether it be from working or traveling back and forth to the hospital. Therefore, she will want to pay close attention to adequate rest and nutrition. If the separation is due to the mother's illness, she will have an even greater need for rest and good nutrition to aid in her recovery, as well as to build or maintain her milk production.

The mother needs to be mindful that when she skimps on her nutrition, it may affect her sense of well-being and her ability to function efficiently. She can eat and drink to thirst, choosing healthy foods and beverages. Drinking something directly before or during the times she expresses will help her remember to supply herself with adequate fluids. Sufficient rest is also important to the mother's well-being.

At times, a baby may demonstrate a strong desire to remain with his mother when he is with her. Other times, he may appear to reject her and seem to be more attached to the person who cares for him. This can be either a source of comfort to the mother or a source of jealousy and anxiety. Many mothers experience a sense of guilt about a separation, regardless of whether it was planned or unplanned, or optional or unavoidable. This feeling of guilt may be related to the mothers' absence from her baby or to her original goals for breastfeeding. Sometimes the guilt may motivate the mother to reconsider her options and alter her situation.

You can play a key role in helping mothers cope with the anxieties caused by a separation from their babies.

They will need constant support, both throughout the separation and when they are reunited with their babies and resume breastfeeding. Practical suggestions will also be important in giving mothers correct information and special hints that will make the separation easier for them.

▼ Following the Separation

When the period of separation has ended and breast-feeding can be resumed, the mother may benefit from knowing a few tricks to get her baby back onto the breast. If milk production has declined, she can hand express or pump to rebuild it. She may be able to entice her baby to nurse by feeding her milk from a tube-feeding device or medicine dropper while putting him on the breast. The mother may need to supplement feeds for up to 1 week after her baby resumes breastfeeding until milk production increases to meet her baby's requirements. Encourage her to arrange for assistance with household chores so that she can spend the week renewing her breastfeeding relationship with her baby.

Other suggestions for getting the baby back on the breast are presented in Chapter 20.

▼ SHORT-TERM SEPARATIONS

Most breastfeeding mothers find that they are away from their babies for a usual feeding time at some point during their breastfeeding experience. Such short-term absences sometimes helps a woman adjust to her new role as mother and caretaker of a small baby. They offer a break from the routine of baby care and help her maintain a positive perspective. A brief time away can help a mother strike a compromise between mothering and outside interests such as volunteer work, sports activities, crafts, or exercise classes. A mother may have responsibilities that necessitate a short absence, such as doctors' appointments or attending functions for other family members. She may wish to simply plan an evening out with her partner, go to the hairdresser, or shop with a friend.

TABLE 22.1
Counseling Summary—Separation of Mother and Baby

Mother's Concern	Suggestions for Mother
Overfullness, leaking	◆ Express milk during absence.
	◆ Wear breast pads.
	◆ Nurse directly before and after separation.
Low milk production	◆ Express regularly during missed feeds.
	◆ Drink to thirst.
	◆ Nurse frequently when with baby.
Nourishment for baby	◆ Feed mother's milk or artificial baby milk.
Nipple preference	◆ Use cup or medicine spoon.
Baby not accepting alternative feeding method	◆ Have another person feed the baby with alternative feeding method before separation occurs.
	◆ Suggest more than one alternative feeding method.
Baby's behavior	◆ Recognize baby's reaction to separation from his mother.
Ability to express milk	◆ Practice milk expression before separation.
Timing of separation	◆ Delay separation until milk production is established (at around 2 months).
Difficulty obtaining milk	◆ Establish routine to condition letdown.
	◆ Improve milk expression technique (i.e., practice hand expression or acquire more efficient breast pump).
Avoiding missed feeds	◆ Arrange for mother and baby to be together for feeds by baby being brought to mother or mother going to baby.

These events may be planned at times that will avoid missed feedings. Many times the baby can accompany the mother, depending on the event. For those occasions when the baby is left at home, expressed mother's milk can be provided through an alternative feeding method. The mother can express milk in the morning and throughout the day for a few days before the planned separation. She can then store her milk in the freezer. If she becomes uncomfortably full or experiences leaking during the separation, she can express milk for her own comfort as well as to avoid breast problems. She may choose to use manual expression or to carry a hand-held pump for that purpose. See Table 22.1 for a counseling summary on separation of the mother and baby.

![marker] **Hospitalization of Mother or Baby**

Hospitalization can occur at any time during a mother's breastfeeding experience. Whether planned or unexpected, any separation causes emotional stress. Stress is intensified when it is because of an illness or injury. The mother will be dealing with the anxieties caused by the separation as well and will need support for more than breastfeeding. Special situations that may necessitate a baby's prolonged hospitalization following birth are discussed in Chapter 23. Here we focus on more general aspects of hospitalization and offer guidelines to assist the mother.

There are a few factors that apply regardless of whether it is the mother or baby who is hospitalized. The mother can explore the possibility of remaining with her baby continually or arrange for them to be together at feeding times. If rooming in is available, she can inquire about the cost and whether or not she must provide for the additional bed or meals. If the mother needs to pump to maintain milk production, she can ask about using a hospital breast pump while she is there. She will need to remove milk from her breasts regularly throughout the day. If the baby is not allowed to consume the mother's milk, pumping is still important for her to maintain her milk production. Table 22.2 will help a mother who must plan for a hospitalization.

TABLE 22.2	
Preparation for Hospitalization	
Points to Consider	**Suggestions for Mother**
Explore your options	◆ Learn if hospitalization is necessary.
	◆ Request a second opinion.
	◆ Learn if hospitalization can be delayed until the baby is older and milk production is established.
	◆ Learn whether early discharge is possible if home nursing care is arranged. Contact local Visiting Nurses Association for home care.
Be assertive regarding your wishes	◆ Discuss all concerns and wishes with your physician to avoid separation or to work toward minimizing missed feeds.
	◆ Examine hospital policies concerning rooming in and use of hospital breast pump.
Become well informed	◆ Learn about hospital procedures and factors surrounding hospitalization.
	◆ Review informed consent as discussed in Chapter 3.
	◆ Inquire with local Chamber of Commerce about support groups available.
	◆ Contact resource groups.
	◆ Contact United States Department of Health and Human Services for literature about hospitalization of children, including review of books available commercially.
Keep clear, well-organized records	◆ Record expenses for income tax deductions, i.e., child care, travel, and breast pump rental, as these may be paid by insurance.
	◆ Write down all details of your care plan, and provide copies for yourself, your physician, and hospital.
Prepare for transportation to and from the hospital	◆ Arrange for your mate or a friend or other relative to take time off from work to drive you to and from the hospital if this is acceptable to your care provider.

▼ When the Mother Is Ill

Whenever a mother contracts an infection—whether it be a cold, fever, or more serious illness—her body responds by producing antibodies in her milk that help to protect her breastfeeding baby. Although some viruses may be transmitted through human milk, in most cases, the presence of antibodies to counteract them offsets the potential harm to the baby. Often, a more likely mechanism of disease transmission from the mother to her baby is through close contact such as touching and close mouth and nose contact, not through the mother's milk. When the mother becomes ill, her baby has probably been exposed already through contact with her during her most contagious period. The most effective treatment for the baby would then be to continue breastfeeding while the mother receives any necessary medication. The mother could also decrease the baby's exposure to the disease by careful handwashing before contact with her baby. In extreme cases, she can wear a mask over her nose and mouth.

Therefore, a breastfeeding mother who develops a cold or fever need not worry about infecting her baby through her milk. She will want to practice good hygiene and limit facial contact with her baby during the infectious period. She also needs to rest and follow the treatment prescribed by her physician in order to return to good health quickly and not compromise her milk production.

Hospitalization of the Mother

In most cases, a mother who is hospitalized due to illness or injury can continue to breastfeed, provided that she is not consuming medication that could be harmful to her baby. If rooming in is permitted, she may ask to be assigned to a floor that will accommodate a young baby. Depending on the mother's condition, she may need to have another adult in the room to help her care for her baby. If her condition does not permit rooming in or it is not available, perhaps she can arrange for someone to bring her baby to the hospital during the day and stay to care for the baby and help the mother during feedings if necessary. Another alternative is for the baby to be brought to the hospital intermittently throughout the day in order to breastfeed.

Continuing to nurse through a complicated medical situation may not be the best choice for every woman. If her medical condition would be compromised by her breastfeeding or if she finds it difficult to deal with the situation, weaning may be a better alternative. Many mothers, however, have continued to breastfeed throughout a hospitalization. One mother underwent a breast biopsy on an outpatient basis without ever missing a feed. While a mother's medical condition may make nursing or caring for her baby challenging, her determination and advance planning will ease these difficulties. She will benefit from help in planning for the hospitalization, managing breastfeeding during the time she is hospitalized and returning to a regular routine after she has returned home.

▼ When the Baby Is Ill

For a variety of reasons, a baby may remain hospitalized for a prolonged period after birth. Also, he may return to the hospital due to complications, a contagious illness, or injury. Many mothers will want to remain with their babies and can inquire about rooming-in policies for mothers of sick babies. If a mother is not able to stay with her baby, she can perhaps visit him regularly each day and, if permitted, nurse him during her visits. Traveling back and forth to the hospital can be very tiring to a mother, especially if it occurs directly after the birth at a time when the mother needs to give attention to her own recovery. If the baby is hospitalized in a high-risk center, the mother can ask about having him transferred to a facility closer to her home after his condition has stabilized, where she can visit him more easily. Occasionally, a baby contracts a contagious illness that requires that he be isolated from other babies in a special isolation room. Most often, the mother would be safe rooming in with her baby and she can inquire about this option.

A baby who must undergo surgery will benefit from his mother's presence immediately before and after the procedure. Physicians generally request that a patient consume nothing within 8 hours preceding surgery. However, human milk is digested so easily that a baby's stomach would be empty much sooner and he would be considerably hungry by the time he underwent surgery if he were not permitted a later feeding. Realizing this, physicians may permit breastfeeding closer to the time of surgery. The mother can ask her baby's physician about when the last feeding is permitted before surgery. It is suggested that an infant can nurse up to 3 hours before surgery (Litman, 1994; Tomomasa, 1987). The mother will also want to know how soon she will be allowed to see her baby and nurse him following surgery, and whether she can be with him in the recovery room.

After the Hospitalization

After the mother and baby are together at home, they will both benefit from frequent contact and support. If breastfeeding was interrupted during the hospitalization, the mother may need help increasing milk production. If the separation was for an extended period, she may need to relactate if she wishes to continue breastfeeding. Even if the mother and baby were able to nurse during the hospitalization, they may still need some help in re-establishing their breastfeeding routine. The anxiety and worry about the situation that precipitated the hospitalization will not necessarily subside just because they are settled at home. The mother may need to talk out her feelings and will appreciate having a compassionate and concerned listener.

SUPPORTING THE WORKING MOTHER

Mothers are often faced with a choice that will require regular separations from their baby. This most often involves a return to work or school. The lactation consulting profession is doing an exemplary job of influencing women to initiate breastfeeding. However, many of society's attitudes, particularly those that involve a woman's return to work or school, do not support an atmosphere that is conducive to the mother continuing to breastfeed. This is evident in both attitude and action. Breastfeeding is often viewed as an interruption in the woman's "real" life, with careers and lifestyles touted as a priority over the child's needs. Today's women are expected to place their career or economic base ahead of child-rearing. You will frequently find yourself in a position to help mothers work through the sometimes conflicting goals of motherhood and career.

Ideally, the mother who is considering a return to work or school will seek assistance and information in the prenatal period in order to explore her options adequately in an unhurried manner. This is an excellent time for the mother to begin looking at her options, as well as her needs and desires. When a mother chooses to combine breastfeeding with a work situation that involves a separation from her baby, many factors will affect her success in combining the two roles. Research has demonstrated that the women who are most likely to continue breastfeeding while working are older and more educated. They work less hours per week and in more professional jobs (Hills-Bonczyk, 1993; Ryan, 1989). Timing of the mother's return to work also has an impact on the length of time the mother breastfeeds. Employment within 2 months postpartum appears to shorten the mother's breastfeeding duration (Gielen, 1991).

In the United States, employment seems to be viewed as a socially acceptable reason for mothers to wean (Van Esterik, 1981). Mothers themselves may feel there are very few occupations that will allow them to combine breastfeeding with employment. Chalmers (1990) noted that only 1 percent of the women in her study believed that combining the two was workable, despite the fact that 87 percent of her study participants believed it was desirable to work and breastfeed. Based on the research, it would appear helpful for you to focus your education on the feasibility of combining maternal employment with breastfeeding. Greater effort with outreach will also benefit younger and less educated mothers who must work full time and who have shorter maternity leaves.

Making the Decision to Return to Work

Often, a mother has assumed that her circumstances can lead only in one direction. She may, in fact, have many more creative solutions for incorporating motherhood into her life. When the mother begins an honest investigation of her circumstances, she can begin to piece together a plan. Help her recognize, though, that after she is home with her new baby, new goals may alter that plan.

Prenatally, she can discuss her feelings and concerns with her partner and other support persons in her life. She can also seek input from her employer. She will want to become familiar with her employer's policies regarding maternity leave, as well as issues involved with her return to work as they relate to her child's needs—such as breastfeeding. Some questions a mother may want to consider as she plans her return to work are listed in the next section.

Questions Regarding a Return to Work

◆ What resources are available to her?

◆ How long will she be able to stay on maternity leave?

◆ Can her working hours be altered, reduced, or eliminated?

◆ Does her employment provide any measure of flexible working options such as job sharing, on-site child care, telecommuting from home, flex hours, or part-time hours?

◆ Does her work require separation from her baby, or is an alternative available that will keep the mother and child together?

◆ Can the mother begin a home-based business that does not require her to leave her baby?

After the mother has gathered specific information pertaining to her own situation, she will want to consider the impact of long-term separation on her child. Information and classes on breastfeeding and working offer practical advice for the mother who wishes to combine her career and breastfeeding. There are some aspects missing from this information, however. Maternal employment options should encourage the mother's productivity while keeping her with her baby and enabling her to meet her baby's needs (Chalmers, 1990; Furman, 1992; Greiner, 1993; Walker, 1992). The simple fact is that babies need their mothers, not just their mothers' milk. Just as the baby's nutrition while the mother is absent is important, so is the quality of substitute care that often accompanies maternal employment. Research has demonstrated that although most employed parents express high satisfaction with their substitute care arrangements, more than 70 percent of substitute care facilities provide "barely adequate" child care. And 15 percent of these facilities provide "abysmal" care (Brownlee, 1997). You need to address these issues honestly with mothers in order to help them make more informed choices.

◄ Before Returning to Work

During the woman's pregnancy, you can look for appropriate moments to encourage her to plan her postpartum goals and explore employment options. As part of her investigation, the mother can be encouraged to take a closer look at her current employer. Is her supervisor knowledgeable about and supportive of breastfeeding? Are her co-workers supportive? Is there an appropriate location and time allotment for lactation breaks? You can assist the mother in communicating with her employer and co-workers about breastfeeding by providing the mother with literature. She can point out to them that breastfeeding affords the baby health benefits, thereby reducing the number of illnesses and lost time from work to care for an ill child.

Feeding Options

You can help the mother explore feeding options for her baby. These options may include breastfeeding on breaks throughout the day if there is substitute care on-site or nearby. She might reverse her child's nursing cycle by providing most or all of his feeds at times when she is with him, referred to as **reverse cycle nursing**. A mother will most likely need information on a breast pump so that she can remove milk from her breasts if feedings are missed. Before she returns to work, she can begin collecting milk for later separations. Some women choose to wean to an artificial baby milk for feedings during the separation and continue to breastfeed when together with their baby. Still others will choose complete weaning.

Child Care Options

As the mother is exploring her choices for substitute child care, she will want to add the handling of her milk to her list of inquiries of the care provider. Is the care provider familiar with breastfeeding and the use of mother's milk? The mother will need to meet with the child care provider to discuss the needs of a breastfeeding baby. Is the provider familiar with alternative feeding methods? Is she aware of the positive aspects of breastfeeding to the care provider—less fussiness, less spitting, no staining of clothing, less illness, less diaper odor, and less waste? Ultimately, both the mother and her substitute child care provider will need to feel comfortable in the arrangement. You can provide information that is useful for both of them, particularly facts related to milk storage and handling. Mothers also need to be aware of the increased risk of illness in the baby if they put the child in day care and stop breastfeeding at the same time.

Breastfeeding Management Before Returning to Work

After the baby is born, the mother can be encouraged to initiate good breastfeeding practices while in the hospital and to use her support systems for both information and encouragement. As she settles in at home, spending time just enjoying her new baby and their precious relationship will benefit both the mother and baby. At approximately 2 to 3 weeks before her return to work, she can begin the hands-on planning for her baby's needs during the separation. As she familiarizes herself with the techniques for manual expression and the use of a breast pump, your assistance will help her learn these techniques and increase her self-confidence. The mother can begin expressing on the unused breast at the end of a feed or express between feeds. In addition to practicing her technique, this will enable her to begin storing her milk for her baby.

As the mother is building a supply of frozen milk, she can also be encouraged to plan for her baby's use of an alternative feeding method. She can enlist the help of another person close to the baby to feed him the expressed milk. Her own milk at a comfortable temperature may encourage her baby to accept the new method of feeding. If a bottle with an artificial nipple is used, the nipple itself can be warmed. Occasionally, a baby will outright refuse any alternative method while his mother is nearby, and she may need to leave the immediate area. The baby often is more receptive when the person feeding him is someone who is very familiar. It is also best not to try a new feeding method when the baby is too hungry to deal with something unfamiliar.

During this time, as she becomes more proficient with expressing her milk and her baby is more accepting of his new feeding method, the mother can do several trial runs with the baby's substitute care provider. She may also begin easing into a feeding routine that mimics her work schedule. As she finds herself in the midst of these intense changes, she can be encouraged to keep open communications with those closest to her. When one's life is so full of caring for a young baby and combining it with employment, adjustments will be needed in other areas. Housework and errands will become less of a priority as the mother considers what must be done, what can wait, what can be streamlined for greater efficiency, and who is able to do it best.

Combining employment with a young baby presents challenges, regardless of how the baby is fed. The breastfeeding mother can be reassured that the special bond afforded by breastfeeding will provide her and her baby with a unique way to reconnect before and after the day's work. The first feeding at the end of the work day provides special time for the mother and baby to be alone with one another and enables the mother to get some much needed relaxation. The baby also has a chance to become reacquainted with his mother after having been away from her. Additionally, breastfeeding's health benefits that reduce the risks of many illnesses will, in turn, reduce the working mother's stress. Breastfeeding mothers have an opportunity for rest during their nighttime hours, because breastfeeding only minimally interrupts their sleep. Mothers who encourage their babies to switch to reverse cycle nursing will find less of a need to express milk during working hours.

▼ Returning to Work

When the time comes that the mother returns to work, several suggestions may make the transition a bit smoother for both her and her baby. If possible, she might start out part time, either in terms of days per week or hours per day. Based on a traditional workweek, returning to work on a Thursday or Friday will allow the mother to feel less overwhelmed in the transition. If the return to work was a bit rocky, she and the baby will have the weekend to recoup and get ready for a full workweek. The night before work, the mother can pack a bag for her baby and herself in order to avoid a harried morning start. She can set her alarm to allow extra time in order to snuggle and feed her baby before beginning the workday.

Child Care Provider

By the time the mother returns to work, she and her substitute care provider will have decided on issues related to feeding. Suggest that the mother provide a written list of instructions related to the care of her milk, as well as her baby's special preferences. The mother's milk may be offered in a cup, medicine spoon, or bottle. The caregiver will want to watch for signs of hunger so that the baby does not become overly hungry. The mother can ask that the baby be held in the same position as he is held for breastfeeding. It is important that he be allowed to draw the milk or bottle nipple into his mouth rather than it being forced by the caregiver.

Both the mother and substitute care provider need to discuss the amount the baby takes at feedings. They can discuss how he handles an artificial nipple and how he is doing in general. The care provider will want to avoid feeding the baby too close to the time the mother is to arrive, because the mother will want a hungry baby to relieve her full breasts. If the baby is very hungry just before the mother's return, the caregiver can provide only a partial feed. Together, the mother and care provider can help make the transition as smooth as possible.

Expressing Milk While at Work

When the mother is at work, she will gradually learn to blend the expressing strategy she refined at home with her new work routine. She will benefit from your support as she prepares to return to work and after she has implemented her plans. Part of this support can include information about the importance of expressing her milk. When the mother understands its importance, she is more likely to feel committed to do it. You can help her recognize that regularly removing her milk will maintain her milk production and help her avoid engorgement, mastitis, plugged ducts, and excessive leaking.

She will be reassured in knowing that she is providing her baby with health and nutrition that cannot be duplicated. Furthermore, she is saving money for her family by avoiding the cost of infant formula, the various feeding devices, and medical costs incurred due to more frequent illnesses. Knowing how beneficial her milk is to her baby will be comforting to the mother at times when she is feeling discouraged.

The mother's previous expressing routine may not have been precisely what it will be after she is actually at work. She will need encouragement and reassurance that it will take time to figure out the best strategy for expressing her milk. Ideally, she will be able to match her lactation breaks to her baby's feeding needs. At the very least, she will want to respond to fullness in her breasts. If her baby is still quite young, she may find it best to express milk every 3 hours. A double breast pump will decrease the mother's pumping time, requiring only about 10 minutes to stimulate her milk production adequately and remove the available milk. If she is single pumping or hand expressing, her time will increase to 20 minutes. As her baby grows older, the time between pumpings will naturally decrease. The mother will know best how to combine the needs of her baby, her body, and her job. You can provide support and information to help the mother form solutions.

The mother's letdown reflex may noticeably be affected by her return to work. She is learning a new routine and integrating her maternal role with her workplace role. She is also experiencing a degree of separation from her child, with its accompanying worries and doubts about how her child will fare. She will benefit from ideas to enhance her letdown and make her expression times more efficient. First, she will want to express her milk in an area that is comfortable for her, with attention to privacy, her chair, the room temperature, and options for passing the time while expressing her milk. Massaging her breasts and, if possible, using moist heat will provide a degree of relaxation. Stimulating her senses in a way that reminds her of her baby will also help. She may play an audiotape of his sounds, keep a picture of him close by, or even have an article of his clothing with her.

As the mother is collecting her milk at work, she can store it in quantities her baby will generally take at one feeding. Initially this may be uncertain. As she and her baby settle into a routine, this will become more clear. It is helpful for her to know that her freshly expressed milk may remain at room temperature safely for up to 8 hours. If the mother does cool her milk, she needs to take care to not allow it to warm on her commute home. See Chapter 19 for more discussion of collecting and storing human milk.

Mother's Comfort and Adjustment

As the mother adjusts physically to her new routine, she may notice changes within her body. Her milk production may fluctuate as she experiences emotional ups and downs. You can reassure her that this is a common event that can be resolved. If she has times when expressing is delayed, her breasts can become quite full. She may also experience some leaking during this time of adjustment. Some mothers keep a complete change of clothes at their workplace in case it is needed. Prints rather than solid colors will help to conceal breast fullness, leaks, or lopsidedness. A jacket or sweater can also be kept handy and wearing breast pads will absorb leaked milk. The mother will need easy breast access for ease of pumping at work, as well as for her baby to nurse just before leaving for work and on reuniting with her after work.

The mother's planning of her time after work hours is equally as important as her plans during work. You can help her view breastfeeding as an opportunity to relax with her baby after work, rather than another chore that needs to be completed. Placing quiet time with her baby as a priority over other demands may help the mother deal with her afterwork pressures. Often babies react to the separation from their working mothers by increasing their breastfeeding. This is helpful to both the mother's milk production and her need for rest. If it leads to reverse cycle nursing, the mother can be encouraged to take her baby to bed with her to meet her need for sleep.

▼ The Baby-Friendly Workplace

There is a trend in the workplace to create a more family-friendly environment for working parents. Many breastfeeding women return to work soon after the birth of their baby. Consequently, employers can significantly influence a woman's ability to continue breastfeeding. Many businesses and large corporations are putting programs in place that support breastfeeding mothers. *Working Woman Magazine* published a list of the top 100 corporations for women. Over 80 percent of these corporations had some type of lactation program (Working Woman, 1998). The benefits of support for the breastfeeding mother extend beyond the individual mother and child. Employers find that employee morale and loyalty increase, with less time lost from work. The lower incidence of days off also results from less illness in the baby because of the protection he receives from breastfeeding (Cohen, 1997), which could decrease health care costs for the company. Accommodating breastfeeding can be considered as part of the company's overall health awareness program. When employers take an active interest in the families of their employees, they improve cohesiveness and productivity within the company.

Approaching the Employer for a Lactation Station

You can be instrumental in helping your clients achieve support at work by giving them suggestions for approaching their employer. One recent research study found that employers were more supportive of breastfeeding if they had previous experience with a breastfeeding mother (Bridges, 1997). The mother may also want to garner support from others before approaching her employer. A fellow employee is usually the most effective person for this purpose. Other possibilities are another breastfeeding mother or breastfeeding advocate, the corporation's nurse, a wellness program director, or a health educator. This person can help the mother determine the best way to approach the employer, as well as the appropriate preparations to make beforehand.

It is best that the idea of a lactation station be presented to the employer in a written proposal. The proposal should identify the necessary time, space, and environment that the program will require. Additionally, it will help to know the potential costs and whether the company's budget can support these costs. Pointing out the cost-benefit ratio will illustrate in the long run how the company can save money in health care benefits. Research on the health savings of breastfeeding will lend further credence to the proposal. Offering more than one option may increase the mother's chances for success with the employer, and she should be prepared to discuss alternative solutions and make compromises in her original plan.

The mother can survey other employees to find out how many are pregnant, those who plan to breastfeed, and those who would make use of a lactation station. This will help garner support for the program as well as provide concrete data to present to the employer. The mother can demonstrate to the employer that the cost of the program will be less than the cost of training or replacing a new employee.

Elements of an Employer Breastfeeding-friendly Program

There are many measures employers can take to support breastfeeding mothers. They can provide extended paid maternity leave to allow the mother to remain at home with her baby for as long as possible. Breastfeeding breaks can be incorporated into the mother's work schedule. Information about child care can be provided by the employer. Better yet, the company can provide child care at or near the work site. Mothers can be given the option to bring their baby to work so that they can breastfeed rather than express their milk. Some companies even provide prenatal and postpartum programs for parents. The physical arrangements and environment at work are discussed in the following section, as well as the mother's time away from work responsibilities.

Physical Arrangements

The biggest challenge to establishing a lactation station may be finding available space that is private. The room will need a door that can be locked to prevent embarrassing interruptions. A screen inside the door could offer additional privacy. The room will need to have comfortable chairs with arm support, and a table or desk on which the mother can place her breast pump, baby's picture, beverage, and other items that she may need. Employees who go on maternity leave can receive a single page describing the pumping station so they will know their employer supports breastfeeding. This information can also be used to show employees the importance of the program.

Several employers have found it helpful to have a sign-in book at the pumping station or room. This enables them to track and report the number of employees from different departments who use the space and the breast pump. Employees are encouraged to provide feedback on how they found the conditions of the station and additional items that may be useful. Usually, the employees express gratitude and praise.

Time to Express Milk or Breastfeed

The time allotted for mothers to express their milk needs to be valued and respected. This is not just a typical coffee break. It is a health practice for both the mother and her baby, grounded in a significant amount of research. Employers are encouraged to allow the mother freedom to leave her work space when she determines the need. She requires enough time to reach the room, sufficient time for unhurried pumping, and time to return. The understanding should be that no questions will be asked and no one will complain. The employer can establish this policy with the co-workers, recognizing that the mother is doing this for her baby's health. Allowing time for cigarette breaks seems to be standard in many companies. A break for breastfeeding—a healthy choice—certainly warrants the same accommodation!

Positive Environment

The support of management will be crucial to the mothers' ability to balance work with breastfeeding. Some employees, especially females, may make negative comments about the mother's efforts. Ironically, male co-workers often seem to be more supportive of her breastfeeding than are other women. A positive climate established by management will encourage co-workers to support the mother in a meaningful way. Company policy needs to incorporate protection of the mother's right to pumping time and intolerance of nonsupport from other employees.

The climate in the pumping area should be nonstressful and soothing. The mother could relax to a tape player playing soothing music, and with books and pamphlets to read while she is pumping. Providing a refrigerator for the mother's milk is another gesture that shows a commitment to her efforts. It would also be helpful to have a mirror so that she can check to be sure that her clothes are back in place before leaving the room. Another service provided by some employers is having a lactation consultant on call for any concerns or special situations that arise.

Employers are a significant contributor to mothers reaching their breastfeeding goals. You can be instrumental in helping employers in your own community establish policies that will support their breastfeeding employees. Stressing the financial and health benefits will strengthen your efforts in this regard. A useful resource is *Support for the Breastfeeding Employee*, National Maternal and Child Health Clearinghouse, 8201 Greensboro Drive, Suite 600, McLean, Virginia. 22107. Phone 703–821–8955, Ext 254.

▼

SUMMARY

In our industrialized culture, the acceptance of mother-baby separation, coupled with the fact that illness may also necessitate a separation, requires that the lactation consultant become knowledgeable about ways to help mothers continue breastfeeding in spite of time away from their babies. The mother who is ill or whose baby is ill will need practical ideas to deal with the illness, her milk production, and the baby's feeding needs. Your support will be a valuable resource to the mother throughout the stress of a hospitalization. Often, separations are due to social or economic needs and may allow for more planning on the part of the mother. You can help the mother recognize her options and arrange to provide her milk to her baby. Continued assistance after she has implemented her plans will help her to find ways to fine tune her course of action with pumping, milk storage, use of alternative feeding methods, and routine changes. In some cases, you may be actively involved in a corporate lactation program, providing mothers within the company support before and during their breastfeeding experiences.

▼

REFERENCES

Bridges C et al. Employer attitudes toward breastfeeding in the workplace. *J Hum Lact* 13:215–219; 1997.

Brownlee S and Miller M. Five lies parents tell themselves about why they work. *US News and World Report*; May 12, 1997.

Chalmers B et al. Working while breastfeeding among coloured women. *Psychol Rep* 67:1123–1128; 1990.

Furman L. A second look at breastfeeding and full time maternal employment. *Am J Dis Child* 146:540; 1992.

Gielen AC et al. Maternal employment during the early post partum period: Effects on initiation and continuation of breastfeeding. *Pediatrics* 87:298–305; 1991.

Greiner T. Breastfeeding and maternal employment: Another perspective. *J Hum Lact* 9:214–215; 1993.

Hills-Bonczyk S et al. Women's experiences with combining breastfeeding and employment. *J Nurs Midwife* 38:257–266; 1993.

Litman R et al. Gastric volume and pH in infants fed clear liquids and breast milk prior to surgery. *Anesth Analg* 79:482–485; 1994.

Ryan A and Martinez G. Breastfeeding and the working mother: A profile. *Pediatrics* 83:524–531; 1989.

Tomomasa T et al. Gastrointestinal motility in neonates: Response to human milk compared with cow's milk formula. *Pediatrics* 80:434–438; 1987.

Van Esterik P and Greiner T. Breastfeeding and women's work: Constraints and opportunities. *Stud Fam Plann* 12:184–197; 1981.

Walker M. Why aren't more mothers breastfeeding? *Childbirth Instr* 19–24; Winter, 1992.

▼

BIBLIOGRAPHY

Ajusi AD et al. Bacteriology of unheated expressed breast milk stored at room temperature. *East Afr Med J* 66(6):381–387; 1989.

American Academy of Pediatrics. Breastfeeding and the use of human milk. *Pediatrics* 100(6):1035–1039; 1997.

Arnold L. Storage containers for human milk: An issue revisited. *J Hum Lact* 11(4):325–328; 1995.

Auerbach K. Assisting the employed breastfeeding mother. *J Nurs Midwife* 35:26–34; 1990.

Barger J and Bull P. A comparison of the bacterial composition of breast milk stored at room temperature and stored in the refrigerator. *Int J Childbirth Education* 2(3):29–30; 1987.

Barker J. Family Ties. *Performance* 18–23, 1995; Baker J. Mothers in the corporate world. *Rental Roundup* 7:1–2; 1990.

Bocar D. Combining breastfeeding and employment: increasing success. *J Perinat Neonat* Nurs 11:23–43; 1997.

Cohen R and Mrtek MB. The impact of two corporate lactation programs on the incidence and duration of breastfeeding by employed mothers. *Am J Health Promotion* 8:1–6; 1997.

Corbett-Dick P and Bezek S. Breastfeeding promotion for the employed mother. *J Pediatr Health Care* 11:12–19; 1997.

Dimico G. Teaching breastfeeding to working mothers. *Int J Childbirth Education* 20–21; 1991.

Duckett L. Maternal employment and breastfeeding, Clinical issues in perinatal and women's health nursing: Breastfeeding *NAACOG*, 3(4):701–712; 1992.

Freed GL et al. Pediatrician involvement in breastfeeding promotion: A national study of residents and practioners. *Pediatrics* 96:490–494; 1995.

Freed GL et al. National assessment of physician's breastfeeding knowledge, altitudes, training, and experience. *JAMA* 273:472–476; 1995.

Haider R and Syeeda B. Working women, maternity entitlements, and breastfeeding: A report from bangladesh, *J Hum Lact* 11(4):273–278; 1995.

Healthy Mothers, Healthy Babies. *What Gives These Companies a Competitive Edge? Worksite Support for Breastfeeding Employees.*; Washington DC; July, 1993.

Kavanaugh K et al. Getting enough: Mothers' concerns about breastfeeding a preterm infant after discharge. *JOGNN* 24:23–32; 1995.

Kavanaugh K et al. The rewards outweigh the efforts: Breastfeeding outcomes for mothers of preterm infants. *J Hum Lact* 13:15–21; 1997.

Lawrence RA. Breastfeeding: A guide for the medical profession. St. Louis, MO: Mosby Inc.; 1999.

Medela Sanvita soars in Scottsdale. *Rental Roundup* 10:1–2; 1993.

Morse J et al. Patterns of breastfeeding and working: The Canadian experience. *Can J Public Health* 80:182–188; 1989.

Riordan J and Auerbach KG. *Breastfeeding and Human Lactation*. Boston, MA; Jones and Bartlett; 1993.

Rogers B and Banchy P. Establishing an employee breast pumping facility. *J Hum Lact* 10(2):119–120; 1994.

Saunders SE Carroll J. Post partum breastfeeding support: Impact on duration. *J Am Diet Assoc* 88:213–215; 1988.

Slusser W and Powers NG, Breastfeeding Update I: Immunology, Nutrition and Advocacy. *Pediatri Rev.* 18(4):111–119; 1997.

USDA. *Breastfeeding Babies Welcome Here!* USDA Food and Nutrition Service; Division Food and Nutrition Service, Alexandria, VA; October, 1993.

Weibley T. Inside the incubator. *MCN* 14:96–100; 1989.

Working Woman. Special Issue, Annual survey of family-friendly companies, One hundred best companies for mothers. p 14–94; October, 1998.

23

MOTHERS AND BABIES WITH LONG-TERM SPECIAL NEEDS

The typical breastfeeding experience revolves around a mother and her baby who begin nursing shortly after birth and continue relatively problem free. For some mothers, there will be circumstances that require special assistance in their management of feeds. Mothers who give birth to more than one baby require some ingenuity and resourcefulness in managing breastfeeding. You will encounter mothers who have a nursing child at home when they give birth to a new infant and can assist these mothers as they balance the needs of both children. A variety of health conditions—both in the health of the mother and infant—have the potential to impact a mother's management of breastfeeding. All of these special circumstances are addressed here, with suggestions for you and the mother.

MULTIPLE BIRTH

A mother who delivers more than one baby at a time can breastfeed just as successfully as the mother of a single baby. Although she may have more demands on her time and she may experience some special challenges, she will also find that breastfeeding brings a calming element to an otherwise hectic life. Breastfeeding will be emotionally gratifying for both the mother and her babies. It is certainly a more pleasurable expenditure of time than preparing formula and heating bottles while listening to the cries of hungry babies! It also saves parents the expense of buying double the amount of infant formula.

Breastfeeding encourages the mother to regard each of her babies' needs individually. The mother of multiples may need to pay closer attention to her breastfeeding schedule than the mother of a single baby. With creative planning and flexibility she will find a routine that works best for her. Breastfeeding encourages the mother to spend more time in close physical contact with her babies, enabling her to provide a maximum amount of skin contact with each one. Encourage her to breastfeed her babies separately at least one time every day, and to spend other time alone with each

baby as well. Bonding is important to the emergence of individuality in each baby. Breastfeeding enhances this attachment.

Breastfeeding Management

A mother who is breastfeeding more than one baby will benefit from special help in managing feeds. While in the hospital, it is important that she have all of her babies together for feeds. Some hospitals keep twins together in the same bassinet or isolette. This is referred to as co-bedding and is beneficial to the babies. The mother then will master the practical aspects of feeding them. If one of her babies must remain in a special care nursery, she can nurse the baby who is able to be with her and express her milk for the other one. The mother will need plenty of pillows to help her position more than one baby at her breasts during a feed. She may require the help of another person who can hold the head of one baby after he is positioned at the breast, while the mother helps the second baby latch onto the other breast. If she has more than two babies, the remaining baby can be fed with an alternative method while two are nursing. The mother can rotate babies at each feed so that all of them receive equal time on the breast.

There are a variety of methods a mother may choose to nurse her babies. She may nurse both babies simultaneously and reverse breasts for each baby at the next feed. She may confine each baby to one breast only and always reserve the same one for the same baby. The possible drawback to this technique is that one baby may have a stronger suck than the other, and the mother may develop a larger breast on that side because of greater stimulation and milk production. She might then confine each baby to one breast and alternate breasts each day. Figure 23.1 illustrates three positions for nursing both babies simultaneously.

Many mothers prefer to nurse their twins simultaneously rather than separately. The mother can enjoy nursing times more if she does not hear the hunger cries of her other baby. Otherwise, she may rush

**FIGURE
23.1**

**FIGURE
23.1**   Positions for nursing twins

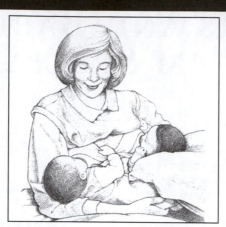
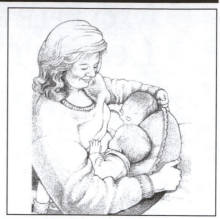

Babies are crisscrossed, with each one in the cradle hold, with support from the mother's hands under their buttocks and pillows placed under the mothers' elbows.

Babies are placed with one in the cradle position and one in the clutch position, with pillows supporting the mother's arms. A pillow on her lap may also help.

Both babies are placed on a pillow in the clutch position. A footstool can add to the mother's comfort.

Illustrations by Marcia Smith.

through the feed and find it less relaxing. She may also have less opportunity to interact in a meaningful way with her babies. Occasionally, though, one baby may be hungry at a time when the other baby is not interested in nursing. The mother might delay feeding the hungry baby until the other one is willing to nurse so that she can economize on the time she spends with feeds. It is important that you not add to the mother's dilemma by causing her to feel guilty about doing this. Each mother must work out her own way of managing feeds and will appreciate your support in her decision. At another time you can discuss with her each baby's individual needs and the importance of responding to them.

More than two multiples require even more creative scheduling than twins. It is not possible for a mother to nurse all babies at one time, and it would be very time-consuming for the mother to nurse each baby separately. She would literally be nursing around the clock! She can, however, nurse two babies at one time while she or someone else offers an alternative feeding method to the third baby or babies. Alternatively, she can nurse the first two babies simultaneously and the other or others on both breasts afterward. In the early days, she will most likely need the help of another person to help at feedings. The mother should be sure to offer the breast to all three babies throughout the day so that they all receive milk from the breast. When she becomes adept at this routine, the mother will be able to manage on her own. As with twins, she will want to be sure that all babies receive the same amount of time at the breast and that both of

her breasts receive equal stimulation. It may be helpful for her to keep a log for each baby's diapers and feeds. Table 23.1 presents a counseling summary for multiple births.

◆ Parenting Challenges with Multiples

Initial bonding may be difficult with multiples, and even more so when one baby remains hospitalized longer than the other one. The mother may have had the opportunity to cuddle and nurture one baby and develops a closeness that appears to be threatened when the second baby comes home. She may need to work harder to develop a close relationship with the second baby. Sometimes this dilemma is never totally resolved. When the second (or more) baby arrives home, she can elicit help to care for the first baby in order to spend more time getting to know the new arrival.

The mother's feelings about giving birth to multiples can range from delight to dismay. These emotions will fluctuate depending on how each day goes for her. She may feel stressed by the constant demands on her time and energy. Household priorities will need to accommodate the demands of more than one baby, and the mother will need to incorporate time-saving techniques into her daily routine. Preparing simple nutritious meals can be emphasized for her own health and sense of well being.

A mother of multiples may be pressured by well-meaning friends and family to begin supplemental foods earlier than usual or to wean at an earlier date. Help her recognize that her babies are individuals and will grow at

TABLE 23.1

Counseling Summary—Multiple Births

Mother's Concern	Suggestions for Mother
Lack of time for all tasks	◆ Plan nursing schedule.
	◆ Carefully evaluate priorities.
	◆ Use time-saving methods for household chores.
	◆ Prepare simple nutritious meals.
	◆ Enlist help from others.
Bonding with more than one baby	◆ Breastfeed separately at least one time every day and spend time alone with each baby every day during the first few weeks.
Bonding with baby who has a delayed homecoming	◆ Regard babies as individuals and meet their separate needs.
	◆ Obtain help with babies who are already settled in and spend more time with new arrival.
Nursing two babies at the same time	◆ Let each baby nurse exclusively on one breast, *or*
	◆ Put babies on alternate breasts at each feed, *or*
	◆ Let each baby nurse on one breast for the entire day and alternate breasts daily.
Spending too much time nursing babies separately	◆ Whenever one baby is hungry, nurse both.
Nursing three or more babies	◆ Nurse two at a time and get help from another person to feed the other baby with alternative feeding method.
	◆ Alternate babies so that a different one is fed with alternate means at each feed.
	◆ Nurse the first two babies simultaneously and the other baby on both breasts afterward.
Greater susceptibility to mastitis	◆ Avoid long periods away from the babies.
	◆ Remove milk from the breasts when feeds are missed.

varying rates. Although growth spurts may occur simultaneously, it is more likely that they will come at slightly different times for each baby. The babies may be ready for solid foods and weaning at different times as well. Mothers who nurse multiples are more likely to supplement their babies earlier than the mother of a single baby. Some may breastfeed exclusively for several months, whereas others may elect to supplement regularly every day. Occasional supplements given by another person will allow the mother to have some time alone for a few hours if she wishes. This will help her keep a perspective on her mothering. Some mothers find this to be a workable compromise and the only way they are able to manage breastfeeding with multiples. Your support as her lactation consultant will be important in helping the mother learn how to manage her breastfeeding.

Family and friends may be unsupportive of the mother's breastfeeding. Mothers of Twins clubs, which offer excellent support and advice about caring for multiples, are available in many communities. However, Mothers of Twins clubs are not intended to provide breastfeeding support. Help in this area should be incorporated simultaneously with support from a lactation consultant or breastfeeding support group.

Mastitis may be more common for mothers of multiples, partially because of fatigue, and also due to the mother's abundant milk supply. A missed feeding by one or all babies can result in engorged breasts more quickly than in the case of a mother with one baby. Because of this, the mother with multiples will need to be more accessible to her babies for feeds. When she is away, she must be sure to express milk from her breasts to avoid engorgement and the possibility of plugged ducts.

Breastfeeding is a rewarding and comforting element in the lives of babies whose individual personalities are emerging and who can enjoy close personal bonding with their mother. Multiples tend to be regarded as a single entity, a group. It is reassuring to each individual baby to be nurtured at the breast and feel the close special attention of his mother.

TANDEM NURSING

Tandem nursing describes the breastfeeding of two or more children of different ages. A mother may still be breastfeeding one baby when she becomes pregnant with another. Her baby may continue nursing throughout the pregnancy and remain nursing after the new baby arrives. Or, a child who had previously weaned may show a renewed interest in breastfeeding when he sees the new baby at his mother's breast. A very warm relationship can develop between nursing siblings and their mother. Breastfeeding can provide a good lesson in sharing and touching, and encourages affection and close friendship between siblings.

Breastfeeding during Pregnancy

When a mother becomes pregnant while she is still nursing a previous child, she may be reluctant to give up the special relationship she and her nursing child enjoy. Her child too may be reluctant to give up nursing and may resist any attempts at weaning by the mother. There is no proven danger to the mother or the developing fetus in allowing a child to nurse while the mother is pregnant. The exception is a woman who has experienced or is at risk for premature labor. She may need to wean her child to avoid the possibility of miscarriage.

The pregnant woman may experience some discomfort that could discourage her from continuing to nurse. Nipple tenderness is a common condition in early pregnancy, and the mother may also experience discomfort when the child touches her breasts. Some women report feeling nauseated whenever the older child nursed during their pregnancy. When colostrum production begins, the child may discontinue nursing due to the changing composition and taste of the mother's milk. When a woman nurses throughout her pregnancy, colostrum will return briefly. Anecdotal evidence suggests that the composition of the milk appears to change. Some women may experience a decrease in milk yield during pregnancy, which may cause the child to lose interest in breastfeeding (Moscone, 1993).

If the mother continues to nurse during her pregnancy, she will want to be sure that she is eating nutritiously. Encourage her to consume enough nutrients to meet her own nutritional needs as well as those of her fetus and her nursing child. Although her child will receive additional nourishment from supplemental foods, he will still be depleting the mother's own nutritional stores.

Breastfeeding Siblings

In deciding whether to nurse more than one baby at the same time, the question of adequate milk production is not an issue. The increased suckling will continue to increase the mother's milk production, enabling her to sustain both her older child and her infant. The important issues, then, are the emotional needs of her older child and her own comfort and physical well-being. If she believes that her older child will benefit from the emotional nurturing of breastfeeding, she may choose to continue nursing. If she is uncomfortable with her child nursing and believes that it is too demanding, she may want to wean the older child rather than transmit her resentment to him whenever he nurses.

If the mother elects to wean her older child from the breast, she will want to do so gradually as in any other weaning situation. It can be more difficult when she is still nursing her young baby because the older one may want to nurse whenever he sees the baby at the breast. The mother can remedy this by nursing her baby at times when the older child is not around, or when he is happily occupied with other things. Substituting other special activities and snacks to take the place of breastfeeding will help her older child move easily from breastfeeding to total weaning.

Simultaneous feeds are much easier when one of the babies is a toddler, because the toddler can position himself at the breast. He may also be old enough to understand the need to wait to nurse and the concept of taking turns, which may make separate feeds manageable. Each child will indicate a preference for feeds at a particular time of day, and the mother may want to nurse each of them separately at this special time in order to give them both close individual attention. Because the older child is receiving additional nutrients from other foods, the mother needs to put her younger baby to breast first, when milk production and release is greatest. The older child can then nurse on the less full breast, thereby obtaining less milk.

Another option is to reserve a particular breast for each child and to alternate breasts daily to equalize nipple stimulation. Because the toddler is a more efficient nurser and will increase the mother's milk production, the mother may find that she produces so much milk that her younger baby receives too strong a flow of milk and chokes when attempting to nurse. In this event, she can allow her older child to remove some of the milk before putting her baby to breast. See Table 23.2 for a counseling summary on tandem nursing.

TABLE 23.2

Counseling Summary—Tandem Nursing

Mother's Concern	Suggestions for Mother
Nursing during pregnancy	◆ Give special attention to diet to ensure adequate nutrients. ◆ Discontinue breastfeeding if contractions occur frequently.
Mother resents nursing older child	◆ Wean the older child gradually. ◆ Nurse the baby when the older child is otherwise occupied. ◆ Substitute other activities for breastfeeding.
Ensuring baby gets enough milk	◆ Let the baby nurse first, *or* ◆ Reserve a particular breast for each child and alternate daily.
Baby overwhelmed by abundant milk supply	◆ Let the older child nurse first for a short time to reduce flow, then put the baby to breast.

▼ SPECIAL MATERNAL HEALTH CONDITIONS

There are a variety of medical conditions that may have an impact on a mother's breastfeeding. Any condition that requires the mother to take medication should be studied carefully in terms of breastfeeding safety. Conditions discussed in this chapter include diabetes, hypothyroidism, cystic fibrosis, and phenylketonuria.

▼ Diabetes

Women with diabetes can breastfeed safely regardless of the type of diabetes they have. The three classifications of diabetes mellitus are insulin-dependent, noninsulin-dependent, and gestational diabetes. Because gestational diabetes virtually disappears following delivery, there are no special breastfeeding guidelines for these women. Diet-controlled diabetic women have no breastfeeding restrictions. Most diabetic women who control their condition through the use of oral hypoglycemic agents are switched to insulin therapy during pregnancy for the safety of the fetus. Insulin is not excreted in human milk, so insulin-dependent women may breastfeed safely, with insulin therapy continued throughout lactation if necessary.

It is helpful for you to acquire a working knowledge of how diabetes affects the body, so that appropriate advice can be given. Diabetes occurs as a result of insufficient insulin production or inefficient use of insulin by the body's cells. The body is unable to metabolize carbohydrates for energy and thus burns fat as its energy source. When the fat is metabolized, there is an increase in the amount of ketones excreted into the urine. When the kidneys are unable to keep up with the input of ketones, the blood sugar level is affected. Uncontrolled blood sugar levels can cause coma.

The Diabetic Breastfeeding Mother

The diabetic mother is an integral part of her health care team. She is responsible for monitoring her blood glucose levels, following a restricted diet, and administering her own insulin. A woman's insulin needs will drop dramatically after the delivery of the placenta. Therefore, the insulin-dependent woman must conduct frequent blood glucose tests in the first few days postpartum to determine her requirements. Insulin levels will fluctuate erratically until lactation is established and again when weaning is initiated. Therefore, careful monitoring is imperative.

Though diabetes is not detrimental to breastfeeding, there is evidence that lactogenesis is delayed in insulin-dependent diabetics as compared to nondiabetics by up to 2 to 3 days. This phenomenon has not been proven to interfere with the mother's overall lactation outcome. However it is important that you be aware of the possibility and counsel mothers appropriately. Breastfeeding early and regularly postpartum is especially important for diabetic mothers to assist stage II lactogenesis (Arthur, 1994; Ferris, 1993; Hutt, 1989; Jackson, 1994; Ostrum, 1993).

Because of an altered hormone balance, the diabetic woman may actually experience a remission throughout lactation. Sugar is absorbed from the mother's system to produce the energy needed for milk production, and lactose is used for the mother's milk. Additionally, breastfeeding expends several hundred calories daily. These factors often allow a higher caloric intake and lower insulin dosage.

Diabetes treatment is highly individual. Some women may need to increase, rather than decrease, their dosage of insulin. Many diabetic women feel their healthiest and have better control over their diabetes during lactation than at any other time in their lives. In a study reported by Whichelow and Doddridge (1983), a breastfeeding mother's insulin requirement was 40 units at 3 months postpartum as compared with 45 units before pregnancy. This was true despite a daily increase of 50 g of carbohydrates.

During lactation, diabetic women generally require an increase in calories, carbohydrates, and protein. Again, this varies with every woman. Dietary guidelines need to be part of the new regimen she plans with her physician. If her blood sugar gets too high, acetone is released and transmitted to her baby through her milk. After several days of exposure to high acetone, the baby may develop an enlarged liver. An increase of carbohydrates and perhaps an increase of insulin dosage will control the risk of acetone migrating into the mother's milk. If blood sugar is too low, the woman may experience diabetic shock. Epinephrine could then be released into her system, thereby inhibiting letdown and milk production. Tight control of blood sugar levels is extremely important.

Diabetic women are prone to yeast infection that can affect both the mother's vaginal area and nipples. Moisture provides a breeding ground for fungus and can cause nipple soreness. Keeping the nipples dry between feeds will help to avoid this complication. If sore nipples fail to respond to the usual treatment, a yeast infection may be the cause. A topical fungicidal cream can be obtained from the mother's physician and applied to the nipples between feeds. The baby's physician must also be consulted in order to treat the baby's mouth at the same time. See Chapter 14 for a discussion of thrush.

The diabetic woman's delicate balance of diet, insulin, and exercise can be disturbed by an infection or by a digestive or emotional upset. During lactation, she will need to minimize stress and remove milk from her breasts regularly to avoid plugged ducts and mastitis. If mastitis occurs, the mother must monitor her blood sugar closely and make necessary adjustments in her treatment regimen. During any interruption in breastfeeding, and especially during weaning, adjustments will be needed in caloric intake and insulin dosage in order to compensate for the decrease in utilization of sugar for lactation. Whenever she finds sugar present in her urine, the mother must increase her insulin dosage gradually and reduce caloric intake to respond to her nursing schedule. If the interruption is short lived, a simple reduction in food intake may be sufficient, with no change in insulin dosage.

With modern monitoring techniques, both in the hospital and at home, many diabetic women are able to carry their babies to term and to breastfeed with few complications. Diabetic women are often highly motivated to breastfeed and have a good working knowledge of nutrition as a result of their condition. By carefully monitoring her blood sugar level, working closely with her physicians—which may include an obstetrician, a pediatrician, and an endocrine specialist—and managing her breastfeeding appropriately, a diabetic woman can breastfeed without compromising her health or that of her baby. In Australia, one study found that mothers who were diabetic breastfed for a longer time than nondiabetics, even though they did not initiate lactation as early and even though the babies received more supplements (Webster, 1995). See Table 23.3 for a counseling summary on diabetes.

TABLE 23.3

Counseling Summary—Diabetes

Mother's Concern	Suggestions for Mother
Effect of breastfeeding on diabetes	◆ Monitor the condition carefully and adjust caloric intake accordingly.
	◆ Consume enough carbohydrates to avoid acetone being released in the mother's milk.
Monilial infection of nipples	◆ Keep the nipples dry between feeds to prevent occurrence.
	◆ Monitor nipple condition closely and request topical fungicide from the physician.
Breast infection	◆ Regularly remove milk from the breasts to avoid infection which may upset insulin balance.
Weaning	◆ Make any changes in insulin and food *gradually*.

Hypothyroidism

Hypothyroidism is a condition caused by a deficiency of thyroid secretion. Symptoms are sluggishness, low blood pressure, dry skin, possible obesity, and sensitivity to cold. Replacement therapy with natural or synthetic hormone preparations can totally eliminate these characteristics. A mother who is properly managed while she is receiving thyroid supplementation can breastfeed with no risk to her baby's health. The supplementation she receives merely brings the mother's own thyroid to a normal level. Therefore, the amount of thyroid secretion the baby receives through her milk is equal to that of any other breastfeeding mother.

There is one word of caution for the mother who is severely hypothyroid and receiving unusually high dosages of thyroid supplement. The additional thyroid that passes to her baby through her milk may mask latent hypothyroidism while he is being breastfed. After weaning begins and the level of thyroid intake decreases, the baby with latent hypothyroidism could suffer brain damage. Many hospitals routinely screen for hypothyroidism in newborns in conjunction with screening for phenylketonuria (PKU) and other disorders. It is also worthwhile to note that many severely hypothyroid women are unable to become pregnant, so the likelihood of your encountering such a mother is rare. Untreated hypothyroidism can adversely affect a mother's milk production. If a mother consults you regarding low milk production and has a history of thyroid problems, you might recommend thyroid testing. Thyroid testing may also be in order when a mother presents with low milk production that has no identifiable cause.

Cystic Fibrosis

Cystic fibrosis is an inherited disease with symptoms that usually manifest themselves in infancy. It is characterized by chronic respiratory infection, pancreatic insufficiency, and heat intolerance. Although cystic fibrosis has no known cure, the use of antibiotics has prolonged the life span of those with the disease. Breastfeeding by a mother with cystic fibrosis is possible. The ailment may compromise the mother nutritionally, and the caloric requirements of breastfeeding may further compromise her nutritional status. Therefore, the breastfeeding mother with cystic fibrosis must give careful attention to her nutritional requirements.

Some researchers question the amount of bacterial exposure to the breastfeeding infant of a mother with cystic fibrosis. Others believe that breastfeeding does not expose the infant to any more bacteria than he would receive otherwise. Concern about possible exposure arises from the fact that women with cystic fibrosis are usually chronic carriers of *Staphylococcus aureus*, a potential pathogen (Welch, 1981). However, the infection would not be transmitted via the milk but rather by the close contact between the mother and infant. Consequently, exposure is also true of formula-fed babies of cystic fibrosis mothers. The infection risk is not limited to the breastfed baby.

The lymphocytes in the mother's milk are sensitized to pathogens and provide protection to the baby. It is suggested that the milk of these mothers be analyzed periodically. Their babies must be monitored for bacterial exposure and the mothers monitored for nutritional status. This is especially true during exacerbations of the mother's respiratory symptoms (Michel, 1994; Shiffman, 1989). More studies need to be conducted before a definitive recommendation can be made about the safety of a cystic fibrosis mother breastfeeding her baby.

Maternal Phenylketonuria

Phenylketonuria, commonly known as PKU, is a rare inherited disease that can cause brain damage if it is not detected and treated immediately after birth. The success of newborn screening for PKU has led to many female PKU babies growing to maturity normally and having children of their own. This has led to a new problem of maternal PKU, a situation that has potential dangers for a developing fetus. A woman who had PKU as an infant will need to return to a special PKU diet during her pregnancy. The **phenylalanine** overload in her body, resulting from having been on a regular diet, will affect the growing brain of her fetus. The brain damage is done before the infant is born and regardless of whether or not the fetus has inherited PKU. A woman may not even be aware that she had PKU as an infant. The phenylalanine overload during infancy may not have been high enough to cause the disease in the woman, although it could be high enough to cause brain damage in her developing fetus. The woman simply may not remember that she had PKU because she would probably have been on a regular diet from the age of 5 years.

When a woman becomes pregnant, or better yet when she is contemplating beginning a family, she can ask her parents whether she had PKU as an infant. She might also request that her physician perform a simple test for PKU. After delivery, the woman with PKU will want to consult her physician about breastfeeding management. There is no data to suggest that breastfeeding would be contraindicated. A recent article presents the case of twin sisters with PKU who were placed on special diets before conception and during pregnancy. They both then breastfed their infants for several months. Although the phenylalanine in both mothers' milk was higher than in that of non-PKU women, their breastfed babies maintained normal phenylalanine levels (Fox-Bacon, 1997).

▼ Tuberculosis

When a mother has active tuberculosis, if maternal disease is discovered before birth and treatment is initiated immediately, breastfeeding can be permitted as long as maternal therapy is continued and infant **prophylaxis** is initiated. However, when active maternal disease is discovered after the infant is born, all contact between the mother and infant will need to be suspended until appropriate therapy is initiated and continued for at least 2 weeks. This contact includes breastfeeding. During the interruption in breastfeeding, mothers can express and discard their milk every 2 to 4 hours to establish their milk production (Freed, 1996; Lawrence, 1997).

▼ Hepatitis C

The risk of mothers transmitting hepatitis C to their infants through breastfeeding appears to be quite low. Lawrence (1997) states that breastfeeding is acceptable. Other sources state that if mothers of newborns are known to have hepatitis C, they should not breastfeed. That recommendation is based on the fact that the risk is unknown, not because transmission of the infection has been established (AAP, 1994; Freed, 1996). There is also contrary evidence to suggest that human milk, even if it contains the virus, does not cause infection in newborns (Lin, 1995).

▼ Herpes

Herpes can pose a significant health hazard to an infant. There are several diseases in the herpes family, and the degree of danger varies among them. These infections are grouped together because all share a common structure, have similar biologic behavior, are transmitted by a virus, and are highly contagious. Several of the herpes infections manifest themselves as skin lesions that begin as small red pimples. They develop into fluid-filled blisters, and then dry up and heal.

Varicella zoster and the herpes simplex viruses fall into this group. During the active phase, the blisters cause a burning, tingling, and itching sensation, often accompanied by fever and enlarged lymph nodes. Exposure to active herpes lesions can be fatal to the neonate, so all active lesions must be covered to prevent exposure. In its 1997 statement, the American Academy of Pediatrics does not include herpes in their list of conditions that contraindicate breastfeeding. Avoiding possible transmission by covering lesions on the breast seems a wise precaution. They state that "breastfeeding is acceptable if there are no herpetic lesions in the area and exposed, active lesions are covered" (AAP, 1997a, 1997b; Lawrence, 1997). Sexual contact should be avoided when the lesions are active.

Epstein-Barr

The Epstein-Barr virus (infectious mononucleosis) afflicts mostly young adults. It is rarely contracted beyond the age of 35. Although little is known about how it is transmitted, Epstein-Barr poses no threat to the breastfeeding infant.

Varicella Zoster

The two zoster viruses are shingles and chickenpox. Chickenpox affects mainly young children whereas shingles is generally an adult affliction. Both zoster infections are contracted through direct contact or through droplets from the nose or mouth. If the mother is infected at the time of delivery, she must be isolated from her infant until the lesions heal completely. Her milk can be given to her infant (Frederick, 1986; Lawrence, 1997).

Herpes Simplex

Both of the herpes simplex viruses are contracted through direct exposure to the lesions. Most herpes simplex infections tend to rest in the skin or tissues of the nervous system. The infection remains there without symptoms until it is activated. Common activating agents are fever, physical or emotional stress, exposure to sunlight, and certain foods or drugs. The infection can be present in the infant without any maternal history. It can be identified in the infant by upper and lower respiratory symptoms, a hoarse cry, and fever.

Herpes simplex I (cold sore) usually appears on the mouth and nose areas. Herpes simplex II (genitalis) is usually transmitted through sexual contact. It produces painful blisters on the skin and the moist lining of the sex organs. In addition to the other herpes simplex symptoms, herpes genitalis causes painful intercourse, urinary problems, and swelling in the groin area. Neonates who contract the disease usually do so through direct contact with the infected tissue. Mortality rates are extremely high for infants who are exposed to herpes genitalis during vaginal birth. If a woman has had active lesions within three weeks of delivery, a cesarean birth is usually performed before she goes into labor.

Cytomegalovirus

The fifth member of the herpes family is cytomegalovirus (CMV). Although nearly all adults are infected with CMV by the age of 50 years, the infection rarely causes symptoms. Symptoms may include fatigue, fever, swollen lymph glands, pneumonia, and liver or spleen defects. When contracted in early infancy, the usual source is the infant's mother. The most frequent site of CMV reactivation in postpartum women is the breast. Excretion of CMV in human milk seems to peak after 2 to 12 weeks (Ahlfors, 1985). The virus is not usually active during the first 8 days following birth, and few positive samples are found after 2 months. The benefits of human milk outweigh the minimal risk of transmission through the mother's milk (Stagno, 1980). Lawrence (1997) states that, because of the passive antibodies, term infants can be breastfed even when the mother is shedding the virus in her milk.

Infants acquire immunity to CMV through **transplacental** antibodies. The greatest danger of CMV to breastfeeding infants is the event of an infant of a seronegative mother receiving donor milk from a **seropositive** mother (Dworsky, 1982). Because the infant has not received transplacental antibodies, the infection is life threatening. This is especially dangerous for premature infants or infants who are immunologically impaired. CMV in human milk can be destroyed through pasteurization at 62°C for 8 minutes. However, this procedure also destroys many of the milk's immunologic properties.

▼ Human Immunodeficiency Virus

Mothers who test positive for the human immunodeficiency virus (HIV) run the risk of exposing their babies to the virus and thus to the danger of acquired immunodeficiency syndrome (AIDS). AIDS is a terminal condition that destroys the immune system. HIV is transmitted through the blood and through other body fluids. It occurs predominantly among homosexual men and intravenous drug users. The occurrence of HIV among heterosexuals is on the rise, however, including incidences among women.

Most HIV-infected women are intravenous drug users or sexual partners of men in the high-risk group. Women in this group would place their infants at risk for HIV if they were to breastfeed. At the present time, based on the limited available research, any woman who tests seropositive for HIV should not breastfeed a seronegative infant. If the mother lives in conditions that do not allow for safe use of human milk substitutes, the risk of her infant's death is increased by *not* breastfeeding. Therefore, breastfeeding may be the preferred alternative. If the mother and baby are both HIV positive, it is doubtful that breastfeeding would do further harm. These babies rarely live long, and the benefits of breastfeeding would outweigh any additional exposure, especially when formula feeding is not a safe alternative.

Vertical transmission of HIV from the mother to the infant may occur prenatally, during birth, or postpartum. In most cases, the timing of the infection cannot be determined. There have been reports in the literature of mother-to-child transmission that suggest breastfeeding as the route. However, not all children of breastfeeding mothers who test positive for HIV become HIV positive. This leads researchers to wonder whether breastfeeding is dangerous or protective when a mother is HIV positive. It is quite possible that a factor, or factors, present in the mother's milk may decrease the risk of transmission. Many unknown variables exist in the instances of transmission that are attributed to breastfeeding. Further research is warranted. Figure 23.2 contains the official position of the American Academy of Pediatrics regarding breastfeeding for HIV positive mothers.

With the increasing prevalence of HIV infection around the world, more and more women of childbearing age are becoming infected and hence are capable of passing the infection onto their babies through pregnancy, birth, or breastfeeding. According to the World Health Organization (1993), roughly one-third of babies who are born to HIV-infected mothers become infected. Much of this mother-to-baby transmission occurs during pregnancy and delivery, although recent data confirm that some of it occurs through breastfeeding.

The WHO has concluded that in communities where infectious disease and malnutrition are the main cause of infant deaths and the infant mortality rate is high, the usual advice given to mothers should be that they breastfeed their babies. This is because their baby's risk of HIV infection through their milk is likely to be lower than the risk of death from other causes if the baby is not breastfed. Women in these circumstances should seek advice from their health care providers in making their decision on how to feed their infants with the safest method.

On the other hand, in communities where the main cause of death during infancy is not infectious disease and the infant mortality rate is low, the WHO consultation concluded that the usual advice to pregnant women known to be infected with HIV should be to use a safe feeding alternative for their baby rather than to breastfeed. Women infected with HIV also have the option of expressing their milk and heat treating it before feeding their babies or choosing to use donor milk. Voluntary and confidential HIV testing, including pre- and post-testing counseling, should be available to the women, and they should be encouraged to seek testing before delivery (WHO, 1998).

FIGURE 23.2 Statement by the American Academy of Pediatrics on HIV and breastfeeding

The World Health Organization has developed recommendations for breastfeeding in the developing world (AAP, 1995). The following recommendations are made by the American Academy of Pediatrics for the United States, where infectious diseases and malnutrition are not major causes of infant mortality and where safe alternatives to breastfeeding are available.

1. Women and their health care providers need to be aware of the potential risk of transmission of HIV infection to infants during pregnancy and in the **peripartum** period, as well as through human milk.
2. The AAP recommends documented, routine HIV education, and routine testing with consent of all women seeking prenatal care so that each woman will know her HIV status and the methods available both to prevent the acquisition and transmission of HIV and to determine whether it is appropriate to breastfeed.
3. At the time of delivery, provision of education about HIV and testing with consent of all women whose HIV status during this pregnancy is unknown are recommended. Knowledge of the woman's HIV status assists in counseling on breastfeeding and helps each woman understand the benefits to herself and her infant of knowing her sero status and the behaviors that would decrease the likelihood of acquisition and transmission of HIV.
4. Women who are known to be HIV-infected must be counseled not to breastfeed or provide their milk for the nutrition of their own or other infants.
5. In general, women who are known to be HIV-**seronegative** should be encouraged to breastfeed. However, women who are HIV-seronegative but at particularly high risk of **seroconversion** (injection drug users and sexual partners of known HIV-positive persons or active drug users) should be provided education about HIV with an individualized recommendation concerning the appropriateness of breastfeeding. In addition, during the perinatal period, information should be provided on the potential risk of transmitting HIV through human milk and about methods to reduce the risk of acquiring HIV infection.
6. Each woman whose HIV status is unknown should be informed of the potential for HIV-infected women to transmit HIV during the peripartum period and through human milk and the potential benefits to her and her infant of knowing her HIV status and how HIV is acquired and transmitted. The health care provider needs to make an individualized recommendation to assist the woman in deciding whether to breastfeed.
7. Neonatal intensive care units should develop policies that are consistent with the above recommendations for the use of expressed human milk for the nutrition of neonates. Current **OSHA** standards do not require gloves for the routine handling of expressed human milk. However, gloves should be worn by health care workers in situations where exposure to human milk might be frequent or prolonged, for example, in milk banking.
8. Human milk banks should follow the guidelines developed by the United States public health service, which includes screening all donors for HIV infection and assessing risk factors that predispose to infection, as well as pasteurization of all milk specimens.

SPECIAL INFANT HEALTH CONDITIONS

Occasionally, you may encounter an infant whose physical condition presents special breastfeeding considerations. Babies can be born with a variety of birth defects, some of which affect their ability to breastfeed. In addition to the nutritional benefits derived from breastfeeding, it may be easier to accept a special situation if the mother knows she is doing everything possible to comfort and nurture her baby and when she recognizes that her baby depends on her. Bonding between parent and child can be enhanced by breastfeeding, lessening emotional stress, and helping the family through this difficult time. Conditions presented here include PKU, cleft lip, cleft palate, and neurologic impairment.

Infant with Phenylketonuria

PKU results when an infant lacks an enzyme needed to change phenylalanine, an amino acid that is found in food protein, into a form the body can use. If it is left untreated, the body becomes overloaded with phenylalanine. Skin rashes, convulsions, mental impairment, and other problems may result. An infant with PKU appears healthy at birth. He can avoid permanent damage if diagnosis and treatment are initiated promptly during the first weeks of life. Diagnosis can be done with a simple blood test and is required by law, with exceptions made for religious beliefs.

A PKU infant must immediately be put on a diet that restricts the level of phenylalanine intake while providing sufficient amounts of it to allow the infant to grow appropriately. The amounts of phenylalanine intake must be strictly monitored. This diet regulation is suggested to continue throughout the person's lifetime in order to maintain normal cognitive function.

Traditionally, a PKU infant was weaned from his mother's milk and put on a diet of milk-based formula and a special phenylalanine-free formula. The exact level of phenylalanine in human milk is difficult to determine without the aid of technical equipment. It is low (approximately 40 mg/dl) when compared to cow's milk and other artificial baby milk, which range from 73 to 159 mg/dl. The infant's diet is adjusted for phenylalanine on the basis of weekly blood tests. After control has been established, the infant may be able to consume up to 20 ounces of human milk daily, along with a supplement of phenylalanine-free formula, to meet his requirements of phenylalanine. Continuing to breastfeed will maintain the mother-infant bond and ensure adequate milk production. It also will help reduce the emotional stress for parents when they learn that their baby has a chronic illness. Additionally, it has been shown that the PKU babies fed human milk initially had higher IQs (Riva, 1996).

Breastfeeding may be interrupted while physicians are stabilizing phenylalanine levels and determining the infant's diet prescription. The mother can express her milk during this time in order to maintain production. After control is established (with the level of phenylalanine below 10 mg/dl) and the amount of phenylalanine-free formula needed has been determined, the mother's milk can be added to the diet. Some physicians may recommend an alternative that would allow the mother to continue breastfeeding without interruption, using one of two procedures. One method is to allow the infant to continue nursing and offer a phenylalanine-free formula at each feed, while maintaining a consistent daily intake of a prescribed volume of human milk and phenylalanine-free formula. The other method is to substitute a phenylalanine-free formula for one or two breastfeeds per day, with the mother expressing her milk at the missed feeds. The primary disadvantage of these two methods is the infant's prolonged exposure to potentially toxic levels of phenylalanine. However, this can be monitored closely with frequent analysis of the infant's serum (Duncan, 1997).

Low-phenylalanine or phenylalanine-free formula was designed to be supplemented with cow's milk or a cow's milk-based formula. Consequently, vitamin and mineral supplements may be needed to augment the nutrients present in the mother's milk. If not, the addition of phenylalanine-free formula to the infant's diet may result in a decrease of nutrient absorption. Also, fluid requirements may be minimal because of the lower solute load of human milk.

Between 3 and 12 months of age, it is recommended that the baby's diet be challenged with a phenylalanine load to reconfirm the diagnosis. The baby is given a natural protein load that has been calculated to provide a specific amount of phenylalanine for 3 days. This is usually in the form of cow's milk or an evaporated milk formula. If the mother does not wish to interrupt breastfeeding during that time, she will need to have the phenylalanine content of her milk measured to minimize error.

Managing Feeds

When such unique circumstances place restrictions on a mother's nursing pattern, she will need a great deal of support, as well as advice on how to manage feeds

and monitor her baby's intake. She may have difficulty maintaining milk production, and the additional worry about her baby may affect her letdown reflex. She may also be prone to plugged ducts or mastitis because of restricted feeds. She will want to remove milk from her breasts through manual expression or pumping whenever necessary after feeds. Periodic test weighing will need to be done in order to track the amount of mother's milk the baby has consumed. Amounts of phenylalanine-free formula can be premeasured. However, the only way to measure average intake of the mother's milk is through daily weight checks using an electronic scale.

To ensure efficient utilization of amino acids, phenylalanine-free formula should be given to the baby within 15 minutes of supplemental food containing protein, such as human milk. Feeding the prescribed amount of phenylalanine-free formula through a tube-feeding device at the breast will save the mother time. Powdered formula may clog the tubing. However this can be avoided by mixing the formula with warm water and reblending it just before pouring it into the container. The use of a tube-feeding device at the breast seems to be the most effective way of preserving the quality of the breastfeeding relationship.

There are some disadvantages to offering the phenylalanine formula separate from the breast. Absorption of nutrients in the mother's milk may be less efficient. The baby may fill up on the first substance, either the formula or mother's milk, and not take the second one well. If he falls asleep at the breast at the end of a feed, he will need to be disturbed to be supplemented. You can help the mother find a routine that best fits her own situation.

If levels of phenylalanine are high during the initial prescription phase, the baby could be breastfed once or twice a day after pumping. Although he will not get much milk, he is still stimulating milk production and receiving the emotional benefits of being at the breast. After pumping, the mother can put her baby to breast, after the phenylalanine-free formula. This will avoid the baby becoming frustrated from hunger. She might also use a tube-feeding device while the baby nurses on a breast that has just been pumped. If the volume of the mother's milk increases too rapidly, she can reduce feeds on a just-pumped breast or use only one breast at a feed. If the mother's milk volume is inadequate, she can nurse more frequently to increase milk production.

Dietary Changes

As the infant with PKU grows, his dietary requirements will change. The mother may find that her baby refuses present amounts of formula or her milk, that his phenylalanine levels are within the desired range, and that growth is adequate. She can then ask that the energy content of her milk be evaluated to determine if a dietary change is required. Guidelines for introducing solid foods are the same as for any other breastfeeding infant, except that high-phenylalanine foods such as eggs, meat, cheese, and milk are not recommended.

Weaning a PKU infant from the breast will, of necessity, be more structured than that of other breastfeeding babies. The mother must monitor phenylalanine intake closely by replacing each dropped feeding with the correct amount of phenylalanine-free or low-phenylalanine formula or solid foods in order to maintain a balance. Weaning may need to be done earlier than usual if physicians have difficulty controlling phenylalanine levels in the baby. When considering weaning, the mother will want to designate a target date and estimate what her baby's weight will be in order to determine his requirements for phenylalanine, protein, and energy at that time. She can then, in consultation with a PKU nutritionist, calculate the amounts of phenylalanine-free or low-phenylalanine formula and other supplements needed to provide the necessary levels.

Although breastfeeding a PKU infant entails a great deal of close monitoring and added inconvenience, it can be accomplished. It will require a special motivation by the mother, access to daily or weekly blood checks for the baby, a support system such as a nursing mothers' support group or La Leche League, and a cooperative medical team. Many medical professionals are learning more about breastfeeding as it relates to PKU and will work with the mother toward a positive outcome. A counseling summary on the infant with PKU is presented in Table 23.4.

Galactosemia

Galactosemia is an inherited disease in which the liver enzyme that changes **galactose** to glucose is absent. Galactose is a simple sugar found in lactose, referred to as milk sugar. The infant with galactosemia is unable to metabolize lactose. Without treatment, the infant would progress from lethargy, to cerebral impairment, and ultimately, to mental retardation. Galactosemia requires immediate and total weaning from all milk—including human milk—as well as other foods that contain galactose. The infant is placed on a special formula that is free of galactose, such as Nutramigen. Occasionally, babies with galactosemia may be breastfed; however, such cases are rare (Forbes, 1988).

Cleft Lip and Cleft Palate Infant

When an infant is born with a physical defect, the effect on family members and their relationships will depend on the type of defect and its severity. The medical expertise and emotional support available to parents will also be a factor. A cleft lip or cleft palate is of particular concern when parents plan to breastfeed their baby, because a cleft can affect the infant's ability to generate suction and thereby his ability to obtain adequate nourishment. However, many feeding problems are overcome when parents understand the sucking mechanism and learn how to help their baby to adapt to breastfeeding in other ways. In order to help their baby, parents first need to understand what a cleft lip and a cleft palate involve in terms of physical structure of the mouth.

TABLE 23.4	
Counseling Summary—PKU Baby	
Mother's Concern	**Suggestions for Mother**
Maintaining proper pheny- lalanine intake for baby	◆ Offer recommended amounts of phenylalanine-free formula and limit breastfeeding as prescribed by the physician.
Nursing restricted	◆ Maintain milk production through regular pumping or manual expression.
	◆ Have the baby nurse on the just-expressed breast.
	◆ Use an electronic scale to determine the amount of the mother's milk consumed.
Managing feeds	◆ Use only one breast per feed.
	◆ Offer phenylalanine-free formula and the mother's milk at the same feed, either by using a tube-feeding device or offering first one and then the other.
Weaning	◆ Carefully plan weaning and substitute nourishment according to the baby's present weight and projected weight for the date weaning will be completed.
	◆ Closely monitor phenylalanine intake by replacing a dropped feed with the correct amount of phenylalanine-free or low PHE formula and solid foods.

A cleft is an opening in the upper lip or palate, or both, that develops when these oral structures fail to fuse during the first trimester of pregnancy. A cleft in the palate means that there is an opening to the nasal cavity in the roof of the mouth. Clefts can occur on one side of the mouth (unilateral) or both sides (bilateral). They can be a cleft of the lip only, a cleft of the palate only, or most commonly, a cleft of both the lip and palate (Figs. 23.3 and 23.4). This discussion relates to an isolated cleft, not a cleft that occurs as part of a more generalized malady. Such a major malady would require specialized medical care and would often preclude breastfeeding. The mother would need referral to a physician who could make the final determination as to the severity of the condition.

Approximately one in 700 children is born with a cleft, ranking it as about the second most common birth defect. The child born with a cleft usually faces continuous treatment until adulthood, involving plastic surgery, orthodontics, management of ear fluid, and sometimes speech therapy. Each child's condition is unique and the treatment plan will vary. Cleft palate treatment centers specialize in treating clefts and offer a comprehensive team approach to each child's needs. The child's prognosis and outcome, as well as his future potential, are generally excellent.

Parents' Reactions to a Cleft

The reactions that parents experience after having a child with a cleft can vary greatly. Most parents respond with shock and some degree of guilt. They may ask themselves, "What did we do to cause this?" Others may go through some of the other feelings associated with grief, such as denial, anger, rejection, and mourning for the "perfect" child. There is no set pattern or time progression for these emotions. You can be most helpful by listening and taking cues from the parents.

Allow the mother to freely work through whatever stages her feelings take until she reaches a point of acceptance. You can provide encouragement by commenting on how well she is doing with aspects of her mothering and on her baby's positive attributes. It is not constructive to mention that the child could have been afflicted with a worse problem. This denies the mother's feelings and can hamper communication. It is unrealistic, and therefore ill advised, to tell parents that surgery performs such miracles that afterward no one will ever know their child had a cleft. Although surgery has made tremendous advances and produces remarkable results, traces of the cleft will exist.

The type of cleft can have some impact on the parents' reactions. Facial visibility of an unrepaired cleft lip, with or without cleft palate, leads to an immediate emotional response. A cleft palate is visible only when the infant cries. Generally, surgery to repair a cleft lip is performed much sooner (at about 3 months of age) than that of a cleft palate (at about 1 year). Thus, parents of an infant with a cleft lip have a more immediate need to deal with the condition on several levels.

FIGURE 23.3 Cleft lip and palate, single cleft lip and palate (unilateral), and double cleft lip and palate (bilateral)

Cleft may extend through soft palate and uvula

Uvula

Single cleft lip and palate (unilateral)

Double cleft lip and palate (bilateral)

Source: *The Mosby Medical Encyclopedia*. New York; The C.V. Mosby Company 1985; p. 170. Printed with permission.

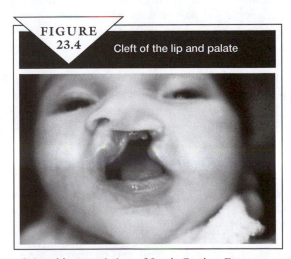

FIGURE 23.4 Cleft of the lip and palate

Printed by permission of Sarah Coulter Danner.

In any case, it is often helpful to give parents information in gradual doses during the newborn period. They may benefit from the repetition of facts as they progress through the range of emotional reactions and become more receptive to explanations and suggestions. Support is extremely valuable and crucial.

Breastfeeding According to Type of Cleft

Understandably, parents may be apprehensive about feeding a child with a cleft. Methods of feeding infants with clefts are often difficult and time consuming, especially in the early weeks. Unfortunately, many caregivers still do little to help parents overcome their fears or give them the support they need to overcome obstacles. Mothers are often discouraged from attempting to breastfeed cleft infants despite the fact that breastfeeding can be a positive technique for these children. Children with cleft palate are apt to have fluid in the middle ear and thus are prone to ear infections. Therefore, the immunologic properties of human milk can be particularly valuable (Paradise, 1994). Additionally, breastfeeding offers these children improved speech development and aids in their visual development.

The birth order of the infant can have some effect on breastfeeding outcome. The milk production of multipara women will probably be better established initially than that of primiparas. These women may, therefore, have an easier time lactating. In terms of providing the mother with the most effective help to accomplish breastfeeding, it is first important to determine the type of cleft with which the infant is afflicted.

Cleft Lip

An isolated cleft lip presents no physiologic impediment to breastfeeding. The infant can nurse at the breast as well as his noncleft peers, and he can mold his open cleft around a breast perhaps more easily than a small rubber nipple. It may help for the mother to place her thumb over the cleft lip while her baby nurses in order to improve the seal that forms around the breast by the lips. In many cases, the breast tissue will fill the cleft to seal it off. Breastfeeding position is not an issue as it is with a baby who has a cleft of the palate. The mother will still benefit greatly from support and encouragement, despite the relative ease with which breastfeeding can be accomplished.

Cleft Palate

A cleft palate poses a different picture altogether. In breastfeeding, the tongue draws the nipple into the mouth while the tongue and palate create a vacuum which holds the breast in the baby's mouth. His gums compress the breast behind the lactiferous sinuses so that he can strip the milk from the breast. With a cleft palate, because of the hole between the infant's mouth

and nose, the infant is unable to create a vacuum and hold the breast in his mouth. To compensate for this inability, the mother can cup her breast as she brings her baby toward her to latch on. She will need to continue holding her breast in the baby's mouth throughout the feed. The mother can massage her breasts before and during the feed so that the lactiferous sinuses will be filled with milk. This will also make it easier for her baby to transfer milk.

In a unilateral cleft, the breast needs to enter the infant's mouth on the side of the cleft in such a way that the infant's cheek on the side of the defect touches the breast. When the cleft is bilateral, the breast should enter the infant's mouth at midline. The infant can straddle the mother's body while being held upright, or he can be held in a clutch (football) position. Regardless of the position in which the baby is held, he will need to be held upright so that his nose and throat are higher than the breast. This will prevent milk from leaking into his nasal cavity.

Often the child finds the beginning of a feed easiest, when the breast is firmer. Extracting the hindmilk is sometimes difficult. In any case, the infant should be put to breast on cue and with great frequency—at least every 2 hours—in the newborn period. Despite a cleft palate, the infant will suckle on the breast. The mother may not feel that the sucking sensation is particularly strong, especially if she has had the experience of breastfeeding other children.

Encourage the mother to be very attentive to the weight pattern of an infant with a cleft palate. Weight checks should be performed every week to determine that the baby is gaining weight adequately. Anticipatory pumping, or pumping in the early days, will help create a copious milk supply. If the baby does not remove milk from his mother's breast sufficiently, she will need to pump her breasts after the feed. The expressed milk can be given to the infant either with or after the next feed. If possible, it is best to avoid the use of bottles so that the infant does not develop a preference for the artificial nipple. The expressed milk can be given with a tube-feeding device at the breast while the infant is nursing. Otherwise a cup or medicine dropper can be used to provide the supplement after the infant has finished each feed.

Some infants with cleft palate will choke quite often during feeding. Choking and milk leaking through the nose occur frequently with cleft palate babies, regardless of feeding method. Although feeding can be a time-consuming, frustrating process in general, it often becomes easier after the first month. The mother can use special techniques that will aid her in her attempts to breastfeed. Breast pumping will help to maintain milk production and make milk readily available at the beginning of a feed. If the infant tires easily during feeds, short and frequent feeds are advised. If the baby is reluctant to nurse, skin-to-skin contact with the mother is suggested. The mother also can initiate a feed before the infant is completely awake.

Cleft Lip and Palate

If the infant has both a cleft lip and palate, the techniques discussed relative to cleft palate will apply. Long-term use of a breast pump for expressing hindmilk is more likely to be necessary than when the infant has a cleft palate only. The more extensive the cleft, the more difficult the feeding will be. Some mothers in this situation will pump exclusively and provide their milk with an alternative feeding method. It is recommended that the mother continue to put her infant to breast as often as possible, however, to enhance bonding and nipple stimulation for milk production. It also provides a nice time for "comfort" nursing.

Surgical Repair

Infants with a cleft lip, with or without a cleft of the palate, will usually have lip repair surgery performed at about three months of age. Some hospitals permit infants to resume breastfeeding immediately following surgery. If the mother is not able to breastfeed during this time, she can be encouraged to express her milk for the infant and feed it through an alternative method. She can also store and freeze some milk in preparation for the event, in case her milk production decreases due to the emotional stress of surgery.

When an infant with a cleft lip and palate has his lip repaired, it will probably not improve his nursing ability significantly because the breastfeeding difficulties lie with the palate, and not the lip. However, lip repair will provide an important psychological lift to the mother. Some cleft palate centers fit feeding plates, called **obturators**, over part of the cleft palate, theoretically to assist in feeding (Fig. 23.5). Although its effectiveness for this purpose is disputed by some experts, the obturator does sometimes have psychological benefits for parents. In Japan, a modified plate was reported to help partially breastfed babies gain weight at a similar rate to that of formula-fed babies. One such baby breastfed to 14 months (Kogo, 1997).

Pierre Robin Syndrome

Pierre Robin is a syndrome in which there is a receding lower jaw and displacement at the back of the tongue, combined with a cleft palate and an absence of the gag reflex (Fig. 23.6). Pierre Robin syndrome, not to be confused with a simple cleft palate, is not very common. The infant with Pierre Robin syndrome, can suffer severe respiratory distress and have difficulty maintaining an airway, particularly during the newborn period. He can also have difficulty thriving. The possible severity of this situation and concerns over survival usually require that feeding at the breast be avoided.

Pierre Robin syndrome occurs in many different degrees. An infant with a very slight case may be able to breastfeed. For the infant who cannot breastfeed initially, expressing and providing the milk to the infant can be recommended. After the infant with Pierre Robin syndrome gets through the crucial early stages of his life and has developed sufficiently so that he can maintain an airway without difficulty, the outcome is positive for him. At this time, the mother may be able to put the infant to breast, depending on the recommendations of the infant's physician.

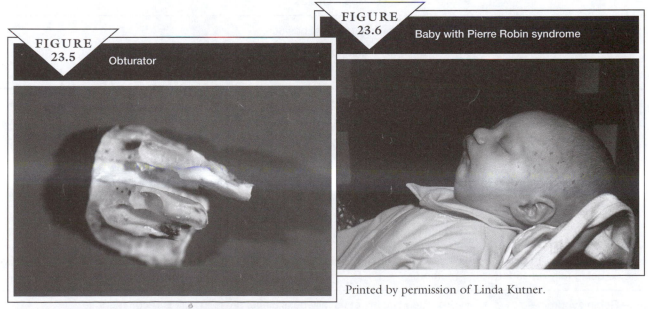

FIGURE 23.5 Obturator

Printed by permission of Sarah Coulter Danner.

FIGURE 23.6 Baby with Pierre Robin syndrome

Printed by permission of Linda Kutner.

Support for the Parents

Many new parents, especially those of first-born children with clefts, tend to attribute all behavior and problems of the infant to the cleft rather than realizing that much of it is part of the usual newborn pattern. You can help parents put the cleft into proper perspective and to view the child as normal in other respects. Encourage the mother to become an advocate for her child and to become comfortable with questioning and understanding all aspects of her child's treatment. It is very important that you avoid evaluating or judging their breastfeeding along the lines of one that does not involve a cleft. As mentioned before, the cleft palate feeding regimen can be trying, frustrating, and extremely time consuming. Help the mother recognize success in every effort.

Some mothers find themselves emotionally or physically unable to continue breastfeeding for as long as they might have wished. If it becomes necessary for the

TABLE 23.5	
Counseling Summary—Cleft Lip and Cleft Palate	
Mother's Concern	**Suggestions for Mother**
Nursing with a cleft palate	◆ Lip will usually mold around the breast.
	◆ If necessary, cover the cleft with the finger to ensure good suction.
Ensuring adequate nourishment	◆ Massage the breasts before nursing to fill the lactiferous sinuses.
	◆ Hold the breast in the baby's mouth.
	◆ With a unilateral cleft, the breast enters on the side of defect. The baby's cheek on the side of the defect should touch the breast.
	◆ With a bilateral cleft, the breast enters at the midline. The baby's body straddles the mother.
	◆ Use a feeding plate (obturator) to partially cover the cleft.
Maintaining milk production	◆ Closely monitor weight gain, wet diapers, and frequency of feeds.
	◆ Express milk after feeds and feed milk to the baby in a tube-feeding device or medicine dropper.
	◆ Pump or hand express after feeds to adequately remove milk from the breast and stimulate milk production.
	◆ Use breast shells between feeds to stimulate milk production.
	◆ Avoid the use of nipple shields.
Choking and milk leaking out nose during feed	◆ Feed the baby in an upright position.
	◆ Push the baby's chin to his chest to stop choking, then resume feed.
	◆ Acceptance of these conditions and patience during feeds can overcome problems.
Baby reluctant to nurse	◆ Use short frequent feeds.
	◆ Nurse while the baby is still sleepy.
	◆ Use a tube-feeding device at the breast.
	◆ After feeds, express milk and feed it in a bottle with premie nipple.
Interrupting breastfeeding for surgical repair	◆ Express to remove milk from the breast and maintain milk production.
	◆ Feed expressed milk to the baby with an alternative feeding method that avoids nipple preference.
Disappointment due to baby never being fully breastfed	◆ Realize that breastfeeding is worthwhile as a nurturing technique, as well as a feeding method.
Pierre Robin syndrome	◆ Breastfeeding is not usually possible; expressed milk is recommended.

mother to wean, her disappointment over losing the nursing relationship may require special counseling. You can assist the mother by providing support and information about weaning. Remind her that her infant benefitted from the breastfeeding relationship and the human milk he received. For additional support, cleft palate parent support groups exist in many parts of the country. They can give parents a unique, useful opportunity to relate to others who have dealt positively with the experience. Both the mother and lactation consultant will want to keep an open mind, and be flexible and creative in meeting the challenges which this particular situation brings forth. A counseling summary on cleft lip and palate is presented in Table 23.5.

▼ Neurologically Impaired Infant

A healthy, full-term infant has a mature suck and swallow reflex, which is essential for suckling at the breast. A neurologically impaired infant rarely has a fully developed or strong suck and swallow reflex. This condition will cause the beginning days of breastfeeding to be more challenging, and feeds will take more time as breastfeeding continues. Such difficulty will depend on the severity of the impairment and the mother's ability to cope with the emotional stress and practical management of breastfeeding. Babies who are born with a neurologic impairment have a higher percentage of premature births and therefore may be hospitalized longer than most babies. The mother may need to deal with separation from her baby as well as possible nipple preference because of bottle feeding. General techniques for breastfeeding babies with neurologic impairments will involve providing support to compensate for low muscle tone and patience while the baby learns and relearns how to suckle.

Infant with Down Syndrome

Down syndrome is a congenital **anomaly** that afflicts one out of every one thousand infants. Its cause is the presence of an extra chromosome, resulting in an infant with oval eyes that slant slightly upward, a protruding tongue that seems too large for his small mouth, small ears, a wide flattened nose, muscular weakness, hypotonicity (low muscle tone), and a short stature (Fig. 23.7). His growth and development, although slower than that of the uncompromised child, will allow him to do most things other children can do. Physically, he may have incomplete heart and gastrointestinal development, respiratory infection, digestive upset, and obesity. An infant with Down syndrome is especially benefitted by breastfeeding because of the many immunologic factors in human milk and its easy digestibility. The infant's tendency toward obesity may also be reduced by nourishing him with human milk in his infancy.

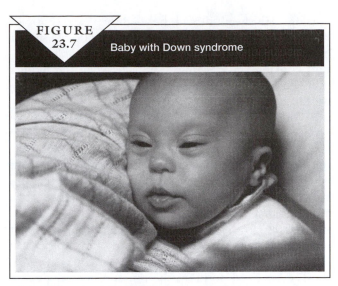

FIGURE 23.7 Baby with Down syndrome

Printed by permission of Sarah Coulter Danner.

Breastfeeding an infant with Down syndrome does present special challenges. Cardiac complications may be present, most likely in a mild form that will allow breastfeeding to take place with little difficulty. At the other extreme, a cardiac condition may be so severe that the activity required for breastfeeding is too stressful and is contraindicated. Most babies with Down syndrome are able to breastfeed. The mother will need to minimize the effort required by careful attention to positioning and supporting the baby, and by watching for signs of fatigue.

The infant's hypotonia will cause his head, arms, and legs to be loose and floppy. He may also have difficulty rooting and sucking because of weak reflexes. He may be sluggish in his nursing and become easily fatigued at the breast, making it difficult for him to remove milk from the breast sufficiently. During his learning period at the breast, he will require extra assistance and patience. As he learns to nurse and exercises and stretches his muscles, his muscle tone will improve. Encourage the mother to view early breastfeeds as practice sessions. She and her baby can get to know one another, and the mother can learn how to hold and rouse her baby. She may need to work for several minutes to stimulate her baby to an alert state for nursing. The rousing techniques presented in Chapter 12 will all be helpful.

Any of the conventional breastfeeding positions may be used for an infant with Down syndrome. The mother will need to support her baby's body so that he is required to exert only minimal effort to hold up his head and body. The side-lying position, with the infant supported by several pillows and his head propped higher than the rest of his body, seems to work well for many of these infants. When his body is well supported, the baby can then reserve as much energy as possible for nursing. His head should be slightly flexed but not drooped too far forward. It should be positioned so that his throat is slightly above the level of the nipple to prevent choking and gagging, especially when the mother leans backward slightly to allow her nipple to tilt upward.

To initiate feeding, advise the mother to press down on her baby's chin to help him open his mouth. She can check to make sure that his bottom lip is turned outward and not inward over the alveolar ridge. The infant with Down syndrome has a flaccid, flat tongue that initially may be unable to cup around the nipple and form a trough that carries the milk to the back of his throat. By pressing down on the center of the tongue with her finger several times before each feed, the mother can help her baby learn to shape his tongue correctly. With the Dancer hand position, she can cup her baby's chin and hold his cheeks lightly with her thumb and index finger. Her other three fingers can support her breast during the feed.

To help her baby obtain her milk with ease, the mother can massage and express milk to initiate letdown before putting him to breast. Her goal is to nurse for 10 to 12 minutes on each breast every 2 to 3 hours. If her baby does not suckle well, she will need to express milk after the feed and feed it to her baby in a cup or spoon at that feed or the next. A tube-feeding device may also be used to feed the mother's expressed milk or formula to the baby. Because her baby will be somewhat passive, the mother will need to initiate feeds frequently. She can learn to observe her baby for subtle signs of wakefulness, such as lip and eye movements, that will cue her to pick him up for feeds.

Regardless of whether the infant with Down syndrome is bottle fed or breastfed, he will gain weight and grow in length more slowly than the average infant. Slow weight gain by itself is not an indication that breastfeeding is providing insufficient nourishment. If the mother expresses milk after every feed to ensure adequate stimulation for good milk production, and if she feeds her baby the thick hindmilk, she will probably be able to meet her baby's nutritional needs through her milk.

Parents of babies with Down syndrome may experience shock and grief at the birth of their "less than perfect baby." Although breastfeeding will present more challenges, the bond developed through breastfeeding will help the parents love their baby as they work through their emotions. You need to provide extra support and encouragement to these mothers. Praise them for their efforts and remind them of all the beneficial aspects of breastfeeding for an infant with Down syndrome. Refer the parents to a Down syndrome support group to help them deal with their grief in the company of other parents who are in the same situation.

Hydrocephalus

Hydrocephalus is an excessive accumulation of cerebrospinal fluid in the intracranial cavity. It is caused by an interference in the flow or absorption of fluid through the brain and the spinal canal. The infant's head will enlarge as the fluid increases. In most cases, he will have a high-pitched cry, muscle weakness, and severe neurologic defects. Breastfeeding is possible with adjustments in positioning. The infant's head needs to be positioned slightly higher than the breast and he needs to be fed frequently to avoid reflux.

Spina Bifida

Spina bifida is a nerve defect present at birth that results in a gap in the bone that surrounds the spinal cord. It is relatively common, occurring about 20 times for every 1000 births. Surgical repair is unnecessary if the gap is very small. If it is large enough to allow parts of the spinal cord to protrude, surgery may be required. Most of these infants will have weakness or paralysis of the lower extremities. Surgery to repair the defect usually is performed as soon as possible—within 24 to 48 hours after birth. The infant will be in the neonatal intensive care unit following the surgery. Therefore, the criteria for expressing and transporting milk will need to be described to the parents.

The baby can be brought to the breast as soon as it is allowable. His body will need a great deal of support with pillows. The mother, once she is positioned comfortably and surrounded by pillows, will need someone to carefully lift the baby and bring him to her for feeds. The mother's position will need to be altered slightly to avoid pressure on the baby's spinal column. Feedings will need to be brief until the baby has recovered. Longer feedings can be implemented after the baby grows stronger. The recovery process may take several weeks. During this time, you can support the mother as she pumps to provide milk for her baby. Then you can be available to help her adjust her position after the baby arrives home.

Infant with Brain Damage

Infants with brain damage can have varying degrees of mental deficiency and learning ability. A severely brain damaged infant will be unable to maintain concentration because of an extremely poor attention span. Reflexes that are instinctive at birth will soon be forgotten and will require reteaching. Learned abilities will also be forgotten and will require constant and continual reinforcement. Thus, infants with brain damage may require ongoing techniques to aid in the development of the sucking reflex. This will call for great patience and perseverance on the part of the parents.

The severity of brain damage will determine the degree to which an infant is able to breastfeed. In many cases, the infant's brain mechanism does not pick up the impetus to perform specific functions. Although reflexes may be present, he may not have the ability to coordinate them with the stimulus. Although the reflexes for rooting and sucking are satisfactory in an uncompromised infant, they may be insufficient for enabling the brain damaged infant to breastfeed. In the early months, he may be able to respond to these reflexes. As the months pass, the reflexes regress from instinct to a learned ability. The mother must be prepared to constantly coax her baby to nurse because he may continually forget how to nurse. Additionally, the baby may have difficulty swallowing, resulting in gagging and choking. This can be remedied by nursing the baby in an upright position and stroking downward under the chin to aid his swallowing.

Because a brain-damaged infant cannot maintain his level of concentration, he may lose interest in nursing before he removes milk adequately from the breast. The mother can try nursing for brief 5-minute periods and nurse more frequently. Because her infant may become very frustrated waiting for letdown, the mother can express her milk to initiate letdown before putting him to breast. A tube-feeding device may also be useful for nourishing the baby while he suckles at the breast.

Support for the Parents

Parents of neurologically impaired infants will need an extensive network of support, and you will be an important part of this network. Because breastfeeding a challenged infant will be accompanied by a myriad of difficulties, you will need to have frequent contact with the mother. Reinforce her commitment to breastfeed, and praise her for her diligence in coping with difficulties. Encourage parents to draw on each other for strength and support and put them in touch with special support groups for parents of challenged children.

The mother frequently may feel like giving up with breastfeeding and wonder if bottle feeding would be more convenient. You can assure her that mothers who bottle feed their babies experience the same challenges as breastfeeding mothers. The mother will undoubtedly pass through periods when she has extremely negative feelings about her baby. She needs to deal with the "death" of her normal healthy baby and accept a new, imperfect baby. This mother's depression can be much more severe than simple postpartum depression and she needs a great deal of support. You may be the only person with whom she can express her true feelings. She needs to know you are there for her and that you genuinely care. It may be difficult for you to deal with a special situation like this, and you will need support yourself from those close to you to enable you to cope. A counseling summary on the neurologically impaired infant is presented in Table 23.6

TABLE 23.6	
Counseling Summary—Neurologically Impaired Infant	
Mother's Concern	**Suggestions for Mother**
Baby has difficulty grasping breast	◆ Position the baby close to the breast and adequately support his body.
	◆ Position the baby's lower lip outward from his gum.
	◆ Press the baby's tongue down to create a groove for the nipple.
	◆ Use the Dancer hand position to support the breast and the baby's chin.
Baby has difficulty sucking	◆ Feed milk by a cup, dropper, or spoon.
Maintaining milk production	◆ Pump or express to remove milk from the breasts after feeds.
Baby gags or chokes during feeds	◆ Position the baby's head so his throat is slightly above the nipple.
	◆ Stroke downward under the chin to aid swallowing.
Baby loses interest after several minutes of nursing	◆ Pre-express milk to initiate letdown.
	◆ Express milk onto the nipple or into the corner of the baby's mouth.
	◆ Nurse more frequently for five-minute periods at a time.
	◆ Use a tube-feeding device to maintain milk flow.
Mother overwhelmed with caring for baby	◆ Talk with other parents of handicapped babies.

SUMMARY

Mothers with a variety of special circumstances are able to reach their breastfeeding goals. Your assistance will be valuable to them as they learn to manage feeds and meet the needs of their babies. Mothers of multiples find tremendous enjoyment and fulfillment in nurturing their infants at the breast. Those who nurse an infant and older child at the same time experience the bonding of their children with one another as well as with the mother, as she responds to the needs of both. Despite certain health conditions, mothers are able to establish sound breastfeeding management that does not compromise the health of either the mother or her infant. Breastfeeding helps normalize the relationship between a mother and her compromised infant, as well as protect the infant's health through human milk. As a lactation consultant, you need to be prepared to assist mothers in all of the special circumstances presented in this chapter.

REFERENCES

Ahlfors K and Ivarsson S. Cytomegalovirus in breast milk of swedish milk donors. *Scand J Infect Dis* 17:11–13; 1985.

American Academy of Pediatrics. Perinatal herpes simplex virus infections. *Pediatrics* 66:147–149; 1980.

American Academy of Pediatrics. *Statement on Breastfeeding*, 1997b.

American Academy of Pediatrics. *1997 Redbook: Report of the Committee on Infectious Diseases.* Elk Grove Village, IL: AAP; 1997a.

American Academy of Pediatrics. *Committee on Pediatric AIDS. Pediatrics* 96:977–979; 1995.

Arthur P et al. Metabolites of lactose synthesis in milk from diabetic and nondiabetic women during lactogenesis II. *J Pediatr Gastroenterol Nutr* 19:100–108; 1994.

Duncan LD and Elder S. Breastfeeding the infant with PKU. *J Hum Lact* 13(3):231–235; 1997.

Dworsky M et al. Persistence of cytomegalovirus in human milk after storage. *J Pediatr* 101:440–443; 1982.

Ferris A et al. Perinatal lactation protocol and outcome in mothers with and without insulin-dependent diabetes mellitus. *Am J Clin Nutr* 58:43–48; 1993.

Forbes A et al. Composition of milk produced by a mother of galactosemia. *J Pediatr* 113:90–91; 1988.

Fox-Bacon C et al. Maternal PKU and breastfeeding: Case report of identical twin mothers. *Clin Pediatr* 36:539–542; 1997.

Frederick I et al. Excretion of varicella–herpes zoster virus in breast milk. *Am J Obstet Gynecol* 154:1116–1117; 1986.

Freed G and Clark S. Breastfeeding and maternal illness. *Contemporary Pediatrics* 57; 1996.

Jackson M et al. Total lipid and fatty acid composition of milk from women with and without insulin-dependent diabetes. *Am J Clin Nutr* 60:353–361; 1994.

Kogo M et al. Breast feeding for cleft lip and palate patients, using the Hotz-type plate. *Cleft Palate-Craniofac J* 34:351–353; 1997.

Kriess J. Breastfeeding and vertical transmission of HIV-1. *Acta Paediatr* 421(Suppl):113–117; 1997.

Lawrence R. *A Review of the Medical Contraindications to Breastfeeding.* Technical Information Bulletin. Washington, D.C.: National Center for Education in Maternal Child Health, USDHHS; October, 1997.

Lin H et al. Absence of Infection in breast-fed infants born to hepatitis C virus–infected mothers. *J Pediatr* 126:589–591; 1995.

McBride M and Danner S. Sucking disorders in neurologically impaired infants: Assessment and facilitation of breastfeeding. *Clin Perinatol* 14:1:109–130; 1987.

Michel S and Mueller D. Impact of lactation on women with cystic fibrosis and their infants: A review of five cases. *J Am Diet Assoc* 94:159–165; 1994.

Morris S. Developmental implications for the management of feeding problems in neurologically impaired infants. *Sem in Speech Lang* 6:293–315; 1985.

Moscone S and Moore MJ. Breastfeeding during pregnancy. *J Hum Lact* 9(2) 83–88; 1993.

Ostrum K and Ferris A. Prolactin concentrations in serum and milk of mothers with and without insulin-dependent diabetes. *Am J Clin Nutr* 58:49–53; 1993.

Paradise J et al. Evidence in infants with cleft palate that breastmilk protects against otitis media. *Pediatrics* 94(6):853–860; 1994.

Riva E et al. Early breastfeeding is linked to higher intelligence quotient scores in dietary treated phenylketonuric children. *Acta Paediatr* 85:56–58; 1996.

Shiffman M et al. Breastmilk composition in women with cystic fibrosis: Report of two cases and a review of the literature. *Am J Clin Nutr* 49:612–617; 1989.

Stagno S et al. Breast milk and the risk of cytomegalovirus infection, *N Engl J Med* 302:1073–1076; 1980.

Webster J et al. Breastfeeding outcomes for women with insulin dependent diabetes. *J Hum Lact* 11:195–200; 1995.

Welch M. et al. "Breast-feeding by a mother with cystic fibrosis. *Pediatrics* 67:664–666; 1981.

Whichelow M and Doddridge M. Lactation in Diabetic Women. *Br Med J* 287:649–650; 1983.

WHO/UNICEF, Consensus Statement from the WHO/UNICEF Consultation on HIV Transmission and Breastfeeding, Geneva, Switzerland, April 30 to May 1, 1992. *Weekly Epidemiological Record* 67:177–184; 1992.

WHO. *Breastfeeding and Human Immunodeficiency Virus (HIV).* World Health Organization, EB93/17 10 November; 1993.

WHO. *HIV and Infant Feeding.* World Health Organization; 1998.

▼

BIBLIOGRAPHY

Beck Breastfeeding the baby with a cleft lip. *Keeping Abreast Journal* 3:122; 1978.

Belec L et al. Antibodies to human immunodeficiency virus in the breast milk of healthy, seropositive women. *Pediatr* 85: 1022–1026; 1990.

Bobat R et al. Breastfeeding by HIV-1 infected women and outcome in their infants: A cohort study from Durban, South Africa. *AIDS* 11:1627–1633; 1997.

Braun and Palmer (eds): *Early Detection and Treatment of the Infant and Young Child with Neuromuscular Disorders.* New York: Therapeutic Media; 1992.

Campbell AN and Tremouth MJ. A new feeder for infants with cleft palates. *Arch Dis Child* 62:1292–1293; 1987.

Centerwall WR et al. *Cleft Lip and/or Cleft Palate.* Light for the Way, Inc; 1984.

Crossman K. Breastfeeding a baby with a cleft palate. A case report. *J Hum Lact* 14:47–50; 1998.

Curtin G. The infant with cleft lip or palate: More than a surgical problem. *J Perinat Neonatal Nurs* 3:80–89; 1990.

Cutting W. Breastfeeding and HIV infection. *Br Med J* 305: 788; 1992.

Danner S and Cerutti E. *Nursing Your Neurologically Impaired Baby,* Rochester, NY: Childbirth Graphics; 1984.

Danner S and Wilson-Clay. *Breastfeeding the Infant with a Cleft lip/Palate.* Lactation Consultant Series, LLL, Unit 10. Avery Publishing, New York; 1986.

Datta P et al. Mother-to-child transmission of human immunodeficiency virus Type I: Report from the Nairobi study. *J Infect Dis* 170:1134–1140; 1994.

Dunn D and Newell M. Quantifying the risk of HIV-I transmission via breastmilk. *AIDS* 7:134–135; 1993.

Dunne W and Jevon M. Examination of human breast milk for evidence of human Herpesvirus 6 by polymerase chain reaction. *J Infect Dis* 168:250; 1993.

Edwards M and Watson ACH (eds). *Advances in the Management of the Cleft Palate.* Edinburgh: Churchill Livingstone; 1980.

Ehrenkranz R and Ackerman B. Metoclopramide effect on faltering milk production by mothers of premature infants. *Pediatr ICS* 78:614–20; 1986.

Ernest KE et al. *Guide to Breastfeeding the Infant with PKU* U.S. Dept. of Health & Human Services, Pub No. (HSA)79–5110 U.S. Washington, DC: Government Printing Office; 1980.

Fernhoff P and Lammer E. Craniofacial features of isotretinoin embryopathy. *J Pediatr* (4) 105:595–597; Oct 1984.

Grady E. "Breastfeeding the baby with a cleft of the soft palate." *Clin Pediatr* 16(11):978–981; 1977.

Greve L et al. Breastfeeding in the management of the newborn with phenylketonuria: A practical approach to dietary therapy. *J Am Diet Assoc* 94:305–309; 1994.

Hira S et al. Apparent vertical transmission of human immunodeficiency virus type I by breastfeeding in Zambia. *J Pediatr* 117:421–424; 1990.

Hutt P. The effects of diabetes on lactation. *Breastfeed Rev* 14:21–25; 1989.

International Lactation Consultants' Association. ILCA's position paper on the issue of HIV and infant feeding. *J Hum Lact* 13:269; 1997.

Jacobson S et al. Incidence and correlates of breast-feeding in socioeconomically disadvantaged women. *Pediatrics* 88 (4):728–736; 1991.

Jain L et al: Energetics and mechanics of nutritive sucking in the preterm and term neonate. *J Pediatr* 111(6):894–898; 1988.

Kampinga G et al. Primary infections with HIV-1 of women and their offspring in Rwanda: Findings of heterogeneity at seroconversion, coinfection and recombinants of HIV-1 subtypes A and C. *Virology* 227:63–76; 1997.

Kovalenko AF and Zhuchenko LV. Nursing of children with congenital cleft upper lip and palate in the first year of life, Surgical Stomatology Faculty N. 1. Pirogov Odessa Medical Institute, Facial and Jaw Surgery Clinic, Odessa Scientific Research Institute of Stomatology; February 27, 1973.

Lewis MB and Pashayan HM: Management of infants with Robin anomaly. *Clin Pediatr* 19(8): 519–528; 1980.

Neifert M and Thorpe J. Twins: Family adjustment, parenting, and infant feeding in the fourth trimester. *Clin Obstet Gynecol* 33:102–112; 1990.

Newberg D et al. A human milk factor inhibits binding of immunodeficiency virus to the CD4 receptor. *Pediatr Res* 31:22–28; 1992.

Nommsen-Rivers L and Heinig M. HIV transmission via breastfeeding: Reflections on the issues. *J Hum Lact* 13:179–181; 1997.

Orloff S et al. Inactivation of human immunodeficiency virus type I in human milk: Effects of intrinsic factors in human milk and of pastuerization. *J Hum Lact* 9:13–17; 1993.

Oxtoby M. Human immunodeficiency virus and other viruses in human milk: Placing the issues in broader perspective. *Pediatr Infec Dis J* 7:825–835; 1988.

Palasanthiran P et al. Breastfeeding during primary maternal human immunodeficiency virus infection and risk of transmission from mother to infant. *J Infect Dis* 167:441–444; 1993.

Palmer S and Horn S. Feeding problems in children. In Palmer S, and Evkall S (eds). *Pediatric Nutrition and Developmental Disorders.* Springfield IL: Charles C Thomas; pp. 107–121; 1978.

Ruff A et al. Breastfeeding and maternal-infant transmission of human immunodeficiency virus type I. *J Pediatr* 121:325–329; 1992.

Smale SD and Onyx PH. *Survey of Breastfeeding Mothers 1976–1980.* Presented at American Cleft Palate Association Conference. Lancaster, Pennsylvania; 1980.

Smale SD and Onyx PH. *Techniques and Aids for Breastfeeding the Infant with Cleft Lip and/or Palate.* Paper presented at the Fourth International Congress on Cleft Palate, Acapulco, Mexico; May, 1981.

Sollid D et al. Breastfeeding multiples. *J Pernat Neonat Nurs* 3:46–65; 1989.

Stiehm E and Vink P. Transmission of human immunodeficiency virus infection by breastfeeding. *J Pediatr* 118:410–411; 1991.

Townsend D: Nursing after cleft lip surgery. *New Beginnings* 6:147–148; 1989.

Van de Perre P et al. Mother-to-infant transmission of human immunodeficiency virus by breast milk: Presumed innocent or presumed guilty? *Clin Infect Dis* 15:502–507; 1992.

Weatherly-White RCA et al: Early repair and breast-feeding for infants with cleft lip. *Plast Reconstr Surg* 879–885; 1987.

Williams R and Medalie J. Twins: Double pleasure or double trouble? *Am Fam Phys* 49:869–873; 1994.

Woerner J. The joy of multiples. *Int J Childbirth Education* 8:35–36; 1993.

24

PROFESSIONAL CONSIDERATIONS

Contributing Authors: Jan Barger, Linda Kutner, and Carole Peterson

As a lactation consultant, you are an integral member of the breastfeeding mother's health care team. This position carries with it tremendous responsibilities. It is important that you give serious consideration to your professional growth in order to deliver optimal care. This growth process will take you through a progression of stages as you acquire the role of lactation consultant. The process is similar to the acquisition of the parental role described in Chapter 17. As you navigate through this journey, you will learn to appreciate the importance of formal lactation education and extensive clinical experience. This chapter explores networking with colleagues and participation in your professional association, which will form an essential part of your own support system. Safeguards for providing appropriate care to mothers and babies are discussed in terms of professional certification and standards of practice. Additionally, you will learn to recognize your own limitations and times when you need assistance. This awareness will help you maintain a positive perspective that enables you to give the best of yourself to mothers and infants.

ACQUIRING THE ROLE OF LACTATION CONSULTANT

Moving into a new role, whether it is a new career or motherhood, is a dynamic process. The process of becoming a parent is described in *Acquiring the Parental Role*, by Bocar and Moore (1987). They discuss four stages in the process—the Anticipatory Stage, the Formal stage, the Informal Stage, and the Personal Stage. This process from novice to expert was later adapted in the context of a person entering the lactation profession (Barger, 1998). Examining the lactation consultant's role within this framework will help you understand the challenges and dilemmas that are involved in assuming this new role.

Anticipatory Stage

In the Anticipatory Stage, the aspiring lactation consultant collects information about the role of lactation consultant from many sources. Contact with a lactation consultant during your own breastfeeding experience may have sparked in you an interest in the profession. You may be a health professional seeking to expand your role with women and children, or perhaps your interest arose from having breastfed your own children.

Whatever the source of your interest, you will gather information from other lactation consultants, the professional association, the certification board, providers of lactation education, and professional journals. Your perception of being a lactation consultant may be somewhat idealized at this stage. You may envision balancing work at home with family responsibilities. Perhaps you anticipate making a substantial salary doing something you love. Or you may seek the "perfect" job in a clinic or hospital setting. You will soon recognize how much there is to learn and the need for formal training. This will direct you to enroll in a lactation management training program. After completing your training, you will enter the Formal Stage as a lactation consultant **intern**. Interns are those who have completed the didactic segment of their lactation management education and are involved in acquiring the clinical experience necessary toward becoming certified.

Formal Stage

The Formal Stage begins when the lactation consultant intern begins to care for mothers and infants. The lactation consultant role is defined by formalized expectations that are stated in objective, written terms. The International Lactation Consultant Association (ILCA) has developed standards of practice for the lactation consultant. Additionally, the International Board of Lactation Consultant Examiners has a Code of Ethics that governs the lactation consultant's actions and ethics. Most institutions in which a lactation consultant would be employed will have a written job description to define the role within that particular institution.

During your internship you will begin the process of breaking down preconceived ideas and teachings. It will become clear that there is conflicting advice among the "experts" on many aspects of breastfeeding management. Wanting to do everything the "right" and "best" way, you must learn to choose from more than one method to determine your own practices. You may perform lactation management rigidly and formally according to your perceived "rules" as you try to do everything right. This can be a difficult time for you to make decisions based on the individual mothers' and babies' needs. You may still view things as black and white in your execution of a care plan. For example, if you have been taught that bottles contribute to a baby developing a preference for an artificial nipple, or that a 'good' lactation consultant never uses a nipple shield, you may be reluctant to use either, even when they might be appropriate.

Although you are eager to work independently, you will prefer the security of a mentor to guide you during this stage. Reactions and comments from the mentor will have a great impact on you, and you will need moral support and affirmation as you progress toward independence. You will be learning how to apply your knowledge in order to individualize your practices for each mother and baby. You will soon believe you are adequately performing the essential plans of care and begin to feel comfortable caring for new mothers. You will gain confidence in sharing your knowledge and skills with colleagues. You no longer think that you must know everything and will gain confidence to move on to the next stage of role acquisition which is the Informal Stage.

Informal Stage

As you enter the Informal Stage, you will begin to modify the rigid rules and directions you had sought out and used during the Formal Stage. You are comfortable considering all the different approaches to care and weighing various options. Networking with other lactation consultants will help you mature in your own role as you continue to learn that there may be many ways to approach various aspects of breastfeeding management. Your interactions with mothers and other lactation consultants become more spontaneous, and there is less fear of imperfection. You then enter the Personal Stage.

Personal Stage

Finally at the Personal Stage, you evolve further in your role to a style that is consistent with your own personality. You are better able to understand the motives and whims of new mothers. You recognize that mothers are responsible for their own choices, and you learn to not

feel guilty for undesirable outcomes. Consequently, you are more accepting of a mother who chooses a path that you regard as less than optimal. Although you seek other opinions, you are quick to discard them if they do not fit with your own approach. You are able to look critically at research and adapt it to your own practice. You are comfortable in your role as a lactation consultant and enjoy opportunities to teach others. If you have not already become certified previous to this stage, you will now sit for the certification exam provided by the International Board of Lactation Consultant Examiners. After passing the exam, you will be a qualified International Board Certified Lactation Consultant (IBCLC).

Facilitating the Role Acquisition

Each aspiring lactation consultant will progress through these stages at her own pace. The pace at which you progress will be determined by your comfort level at each stage. Other lactation consultants can be valuable as mentors during your Formal Stage. It is through such exposure to a variety of practicing lactation consultants that you will emerge with your own unique approach. During the Personal Stage you might model yourself after an experienced lactation consultant whom you have observed. The flexibility you learn to adopt in your approach will carry through to enable you to remain flexible in developing your plans of care for mothers and babies.

Recognizing this dynamic process of role acquisition illustrates that there are few hard and fast rules about working with mothers and babies. You will learn to adapt theoretic knowledge to each situation. Any lactation consultant who has not changed her practice substantially during the past 5 years has failed to remain current with new information that has surfaced during that time. As we continue to discover and understand what Mother Nature gave us, our practices will continue to change!

PREPARING FOR THE PROFESSION

Preparing for any new profession can be a daunting task. Chances are, since you are reading this text, you have already come a long way in the process. Much groundwork has been laid in the lactation profession in its short existence. It will continue to evolve as we define this young profession further. Fortunately, standards of practice and entry-level education and assessment are defined and provide a starting point for budding lactation consultants.

Educational Preparation

It is amazing how much there is to know about breast-feeding. Consider the size of this text alone if you have any doubt of that! New practices and recommendations appear continually, sometimes making it difficult to remain current. You need to be aware of controversies regarding new practices and consider them with respect to basic information and solid research. You will then be able to decide carefully whether the newer ideas are better than the old ones. Remaining current is essential to your growth and development as a lactation consultant. Anyone who wishes to work in a helping role with breastfeeding mothers has a professional responsibility to give optimal care.

The knowledge and skill base in the lactation field is broad and extensive. The information learned in this text can help you identify areas in which you need further instruction and experience. In the early years of the profession, many lactation consultants gained their knowledge through self-directed education. As the profession continues to evolve past its infancy, it recognizes the value of formal education in lactation management. The International Lactation Consultant Association can be contacted for a list of educational programs offered throughout the world. Even the experienced health professional will benefit from specialized instruction in lactation management.

Essential Elements of a Lactation Management Program

A lactation management program needs to include information and discussion specific to the practice of lactation consulting. Ideally, instruction would include documentation; developing private, hospital, clinic, or public health based practices; and review of the standards of practice as defined by the professional association. Emphasis should be placed on preparing the practitioner for practice as an IBCLC, with a focus on practical aspects of lactation management. Information on obtaining clinical experience should also be provided (Kutner, 1998a).

A lactation management course should address the subjects defined in the grid for the IBLCE exam, which are

- Maternal and infant anatomy, physiology, and endocrinology
- Maternal and infant nutrition, biochemistry, immunology, and infectious diseases
- Maternal and infant pathology, pharmacology, and toxicology
- Psychology, sociology, and anthropology

- Growth parameters and developmental milestones from preconception to beyond twelve months
- Reading and interpretation of research
- Ethical and legal issues related to the practice of lactation consulting
- Technology related to breastfeeding
- Public health issues surrounding lactation

Clinical Experience

Formal didactic education is only one of two important elements in your training. You also need to acquire extensive hands-on clinical experience. This, in fact, is a requirement for candidates of the certification exam offered by the International Board of Lactation Consultant Examiners (IBLCE). The greatest challenge to candidates for the exam (and therefore candidates for the profession) is acquiring the necessary number of practice hours. You may be able to make arrangements with a hospital-based lactation consultant to supervise you in providing services for mothers while you gain experience. Some hospitals have lactation clinics located within their facilities. Perhaps you can volunteer or be hired into a physician's office, WIC agency, or other clinic. A manual is available for those looking to obtain breastfeeding consultancy hours. It is entitled *Clinical Experience in Lactation: A Blueprint for Internship,* and it gives clear guidelines for finding broad-based clinical experiences. The text identifies the specific types of experiences needed to prepare one for the certification exam and for working as a professional lactation consultant (Kutner, 1997a).

Other Educational Experience

The lactation consultant and the public are best served when an individual entering the profession has previous education outside the field of lactation. Areas that help provide a basis for practice are the basic sciences, nutrition, child development, social sciences, and communication. If your educational preparation is in a non–health-related field, you will want to consider courses in the areas of anatomy, physiology, psychology, and sociology. A curriculum of basic college courses in a two-year program may include the courses identified in Table 24.1.

In addition to basic education, there are courses relative to the lactation field that are especially recommended for lactation consultants. Again, if you do not have a health-related degree, you will benefit from courses that will help to fill the gaps in your education. Table 24.2 identifies courses that would be helpful for lactation consultants.

TABLE 24.1

Basic College Courses in a Two-year Program*

Discipline	Semester credit hours
Communications	9 credit hours (English composition and speech)
Math and Science	20 credit hours
Humanities	6 credit hours (languages, fine arts, literature, and philosophy)
Social Sciences	6 credit hours (psychology, sociology, and anthropology)
Contemporary Studies and Life Skills	3 credit hours (art, music, and computer science)
Electives	18 credit hours

TABLE 24.2

Courses Helpful for Lactation Consultants*

Introduction to Anatomy and Physiology	4 credit hours
English Composition I	3 credit hours
English Composition II	3 credit hours
Fundamentals of Speech	3 credit hours
Microbiology	4 credit hours
Introduction to Psychology	3 credit hours
Child Psychology	3 credit hours
Introduction to Sociology	3 credit hours
Family in Society	3 credit hours
Computer Basics	3 credit hours
Medical Terminology	2 credit hours
Medical Law and Ethics	3 credit hours
Basic Nutrition	3 credit hours
Introduction to Human Disease	3 credit hours
Psychology of Human Development	3 credit hours
Child Development	3 credit hours
Marriage and the Family	3 credit hours
Counseling	3 credit hours
Pharmacology	4 credit hours
Chemistry	4 credit hours
Biology	4 credit hours

*These lists of courses (Tables 24.1 and 24.2) will assist the aspiring lactation consultant in identifying areas that will strengthen her knowledge and skills in the field. The lists are reprinted with permission from the text, *Clinical Experience in Lactation: A Blueprint for Internship*, by Kutner and Barger, Breastfeeding Support Consultants, Chalfont, PA; 1998.

Professional Networking

The individual lactation consultant is not alone in promoting, protecting, and supporting breastfeeding. The field of lactation consulting has grown tremendously since the first meeting of ILCA and the creation of IBLCE, both in 1985. Thousands of lactation consultants have been certified worldwide. Opportunities abound for networking with others for advice on a particular issue. It is important to make sure you have experienced lactation consultants with whom you can network. With the growth of the lactation consulting profession, there are increasing numbers of knowledgeable and skilled lactation consultants who may serve as a mentor for you until you feel confident in your own abilities. Even after becoming a qualified IBCLC, you will continue to benefit from mentoring and networking with other experienced lactation consultants.

Becoming a member of ILCA will bring you in contact with over 4000 lactation consultants worldwide. With your membership, you will receive the *Journal of Human Lactation* and the member newsletter, the *ILCA Globe*. These periodicals share new research and practical tips to help you in your own practice. Case studies are helpful for learning more about what does and does not work in practice. Reading the *Consultants' Corner* provides ideas for encountering the unexpected as well as innovative approaches to an old problem. Other newsletters and journals are also available and are listed in Appendix B.

Additional forms of networking include attending professional conferences for lactation consultants and other breastfeeding advocates. A listserv on the Internet is specifically designed for lactation consultants. Communicating through *Lactnet* provides much needed breastfeeding information as well as the opportunity to ask questions of a large number of people at the same time. To subscribe to *Lactnet*, simply address your e-mail to *listserv@library.ummed.edu*. In the body of your letter, type *subscribe Lactnet* followed by your name. You will immediately begin receiving up-to-date posts about breastfeeding issues.

Certification

Many health professionals who work in the maternal and infant health field incorporate their knowledge of breastfeeding into an existing practice. This may be, for instance, a pediatric nurse practitioner, physician, midwife, or hospital staff nurse. Others may wish to specialize in the care of breastfeeding mothers and infants. To help you prepare for taking the certification exam, it is suggested that you take a comprehensive course in lactation management. However, just completing a course will not provide certification that is recognized by the profession. Although some courses may bestow the title "certified" to their graduates, this title is not recognized by the profession. The only certification recognized by the professional association is that received by successfully completing the exam provided by the IBLCE. Candidates for the exam must meet minimal requirements regarding education in lactation management and number of hours in clinical experience. Successful completion of the exam allows you to use the title International Board Certified Lactation Consultant (IBCLC). Recertification is required every 5 years. See Appendix A for information to contact IBLCE.

STANDARDS OF PRACTICE FOR THE LACTATION CONSULTANT

Practicing as a lactation consultant means providing quality care to the public and accepting responsibility for that care. ILCA states that quality and service constitute the core of a profession's responsibility to the public (ILCA, 1995). To support that belief, ILCA developed the *Standards of Practice for Lactation Consultants*. ILCA believes that "all individuals representing themselves as lactation consultants, whether or not they are IBCLC, should adhere to these standards of practice in any and all interactions with the clients' families." Standards of practice have been defined as "stated measures or levels of quality" that serve as models for the conduct and evaluation of practice (AWHONN, 1991). Those who describe themselves as lactation consultants should provide the level and quality of care described in the ILCA *Standards of Practice*.

All lactation consultants work in concert with the infant's and mother's primary caregiver. You provide a level of care that facilitates continued health and wellness, particularly as it relates to breastfeeding management and early parenting issues. You focus on helping breastfeeding women and their families achieve their own breastfeeding goals. No matter what your practice setting, you will assess, plan, implement, and evaluate a variety of situations, both simple and complex. You are expected to individualize your approach and to prioritize practices to meet the physical and emotional needs of the breastfeeding mother and infant. Standards, as described in ILCA's *Standards of Practice*, are summarized below (Kutner, 1998b).

Standards of Practice for Plan of Care

In order to provide the best care possible to breastfeeding dyads in your practice, you must function within a set of standards. Standards of clinical practice were formalized by ILCA in 1995 and revised in 1999, to provide you with an appropriate guide in your clinical setting. You must assess the mother and child individually, evaluate the physical appearance and findings of the mother and child, and document the findings appropriately. This includes taking a formal history on both a general level and one specifically related to lactation. You then need to carefully consider the information you have gathered and develop a plan of care that is based on the mother's needs and goals. Part of this plan of care must include appropriate follow up, and it must be documented accordingly.

Implementation of the plan of care is the next step. You must provide appropriate guidance to the mother that includes discussion of the risks and benefits of any suggested interventions. Demonstrations should be given of all suggested techniques, along with written instructions for reinforcement. Any plan of care for the breastfeeding dyad must include provisions for safety, hygiene, infection control, and **universal precautions**. After you and the mother have worked out an agreeable plan, the primary caregiver of the mother or child, or both, must be made aware of the interaction and plan. This needs to be done in writing and may be carried out verbally as well, depending on the immediate needs of the mother or child. You also have a responsibility to make referrals to other care providers and support groups whenever appropriate. All steps involved in implementing the mother's plan of care must be included in your documentation. Chapter 10 explores the plan of care for breastfeeding further.

Finally, it is your responsibility to evaluate the outcome of any plan of care that has been implemented. If a planned intervention is not working, this will be discovered through evaluation, which will, in turn, lead to a modification of the plan. If the intervention is working, this knowledge will impact on future situations. Evaluation of the plan of care needs to be documented in the mother's record for consistency and future reference.

Standards of Practice for Education and Counseling

You will provide breastfeeding education in a variety of settings, and you will educate mothers and families to make informed decisions regarding infant feeding. You will provide anticipatory guidance that promotes optimal breastfeeding and minimizes breastfeeding difficulties. When difficulties arise, you will provide support and education that encourage the mother and her family to continue breastfeeding through resolution. Your role as an educator will extend to colleagues as well. You have the responsibility to educate other caregivers—professional and paraprofessional—in order to optimize breastfeeding care for mothers and their babies further.

▼ ## Standards of Practice for Professional Responsibilities

In addition to adhering to your profession's standards, you must also function within the broader standards of the health care industry. You have a responsibility to practice in an ethical manner, realizing that you are an advocate for the mother and child at all times. In that role, you are expected to be aware of any changes in your profession's standards as well as clinical research. You must be clinically competent and accountable for your professional actions, which include

◆ Respecting the privacy of the mother-child relationship

◆ Maintaining awareness of changing practices and of professional or ethical issues

◆ Recognizing limitations in your knowledge or skills

◆ Obtaining clients' written consent before providing care

◆ Communicating relevant information to the primary caregiver (or caregivers)

◆ Collaborating with and referring to other health care professionals as appropriate

◆ Participating in appropriate professional organizations

◆ Lending support to colleagues

▼ ## Standards of Practice for Legal Considerations

You must practice within the laws of the geopolitical region in which you live and respect the breastfeeding dyad's rights to privacy and issues that are confidential in nature. All records will be retained for the period of time that is acceptable for your geopolitical area. It is imperative that you obtain liability insurance before practicing as a lactation consultant. If you have a professional position within the health care field and are not doing anything beyond that scope of practice, your professional liability insurance will provide you with sufficient coverage. Non–health professionals are advised to secure some form of liability insurance. Contact ILCA for information on firms that provide insurance for lactation consultants.

Legal Issues Involving the Lactation Consultant–Client Relationship

When you accept a client, certain expectations and duties are created that are contractual in nature. Those duties exist whether or not you are being paid for your services. You will have a duty to render the appropriate level of care unless you are authorized to withdraw. You have a duty to refer the client to another caregiver if you are unable to render appropriate care and to not abandon the client.

This relationship is established whenever you and the mother have contact, whether in person or over the telephone. In some cases, a client relationship is created by the act of making an appointment. When a mother arrives by previous appointment, you are obligated to give her care or to make alternate arrangements by referring her to another competent practitioner. During an examination, if you should discover a problem that is beyond your competency, you must advise the mother of your concerns. Make sure she understands that she will need follow-up care and refer her to a competent practitioner when the problem is beyond your level of competency.

Telephone conversations may create a client relationship if you indicate acceptance or give comments in the nature of treatment. The content of the conversation will determine whether or not it constitutes a relationship. There are several things you can do to avoid creating this relationship. First, when receiving a call, identify yourself and obtain the name of the person who is calling. You may listen to the caller's complaints. If an appointment is made, make it clear that the appointment is being made for evaluation in order to determine whether you can accept the new client. If no appointment is made, you can inform the mother of her options. She may go to the local emergency room, or she can contact an appropriate physician or other lactation consultant. Remember that as soon as you give comments in the nature of advice, you have created a relationship with the client.

There are instances that do not create a client relationship. If a physician requests that you see a patient or review the patient's record, this does not constitute a relationship. However, if the physician relies on you for lactation advice and you are aware of this, a relationship between you and his patient is implied and you will want to see the patient as soon as possible. Another instance is when you have an affiliation with a hospital. Generally no relationship exists between you and mothers who were once in that hospital. However, this rule will not apply if you are contacted by the mother via a hospital hot line.

Duration of the Relationship

Whenever a relationship has been established with a client, you are legally required to continue care until the need for your services no longer exists, until the mother withdraws from your care, or until you withdraw in a manner that does not constitute "abandonment" of the mother. If you choose to withdraw from the relationship, you must give the mother appropriate notice of your intentions either by talking with her or by sending a certified letter with a return receipt requested. In the letter, you should state the mother's status, any need for follow-up care, and your intention to withdraw by a definite stated date—a date that will allow the mother to seek alternative care. You must indicate that until the stated date you will be available for emergencies. Also, you must state that the mother's physician can obtain a copy of all records with written permission of the mother. Be aware that a client's failure to pay will not justify your withdrawal without giving her sufficient opportunity to obtain alternative care. After notifying the mother of your intent, you must refer her to a competent replacement or to a specialist when her problem is outside the lactation consultant's competence.

You can avoid the worry of abandonment by performing services when they are needed. When you are asked by a physician to evaluate one of his patients, you can tell the patient verbally, "I have been contacted by Dr. ____ to evaluate you and your baby." Also, write this in the patient's chart. When you terminate the relationship, tell the patient, and write in the chart, "I am signing off this case and will no longer follow this patient. However, I will remain available if I am notified that additional consultations or assistance are required."

Substituting your services with those of another lactation consultant does not constitute abandonment. To avoid problems, you can notify the replacement of case details, both verbally and in writing. If possible, notify the client about the replacement as well. If a client fails to keep a follow-up appointment or to follow your advice, there are safeguards as well. Be sure that the client understands the nature of the condition and is informed of the risks of failing to seek medical attention. Provide her with an opportunity to visit you for counseling or care. While you will share all of this verbally with the client, you also will want to follow it up in writing with a certified letter.

Informed Consent

It is important that you obtain informed consent before providing care to mothers. Although informed consent may not be a legal requirement in some states, you are wise to discuss specific areas with mothers so that they may be fully informed. You will want to discuss the nature of the mother's problem, the nature of the proposed treatment, and reasonable alternative treatments. Inform the mother of the chance of success with the proposed treatment as well as any inherent risks. Also make sure that the mother understands any risks related to failing to undergo treatment. You can explore alternative treatments and risks with other lactation consultants to learn what they explain to their clients. Consult current medical literature as well to document frequency and severity of risks so that you can include this in your consent form.

Standard consent forms ordinarily do not provide sufficient information about the disclosures made to the patient or client to establish that consent was an adequately informed one. For lactation consultants in a busy practice, adequate legal protection may be obtained by writing up an information sheet for the courses of treatment. Both you and the mother will sign the form attesting to the fact that the mother acknowledges receipt of the information. One copy can be retained for your files and another copy given to the mother. Generally, in the United States, competent adults are capable of giving valid consent for infants. Therefore, the mother's signed consent covers both her care and that of her infant. See Figure 24.1 for a sample consent form for breastfeeding care.

Record Retention

Patient records need to be kept for a period of time for a variety of reasons. They will record details of the mother's and infant's health, and make it possible to give the mother her record to share with other care providers. Records will also help defend professional negligence suits, comply with state statutes and other regulations, and obtain third-party payment by substantiating fees.

If you work in a physician's office, the state's medical practice act or licensing statutes may dictate the type of information to be included in the patient's record. Typically, these require a written record of patient history, examination results and test results. To remain ac-

FIGURE 24.1 Consent form for breastfeeding care

I acknowledge that (your name) has explained to me that (I am/I may be/my baby is/my baby may be) affected by (condition) and has made the following treatment recommendation:

I acknowledge that the following information has been provide to me:

Purpose of the care/treatment: (purpose)

Alternative forms of care/treatment: (alternative care/treatment)

Risks of alternative care/treatment: (risks)

Risks of not undergoing care/treatment: (risks)

I further acknowledge that I have had full opportunity to discuss this information with (your name) and hereby consent to the following lactation consultant care or treatment (specify care or treatment)

_____   _____

Date   Patient/client or person authorized to
                          consent for patient/client

_____   _____

Date   (Your name and credentials)

Printed by permission of Breastfeeding Support Consultants.

credited, a hospital's records must contain identification data, patient medical history, reports of relevant physical examinations, diagnostic and therapeutic orders, evidence of appropriate informed consent, clinical observations, reports of procedures and tests, and conclusions at the termination of hospitalization or evaluation of treatment. You will want to keep a record of every telephone call; long distance telephone bills, if this applies; and appointment calendars. These will demonstrate that you followed up on a mother's care or responded in a timely fashion to a complaint. They will also demonstrate dates of appointments or the mother's failure to keep an appointment.

Avoiding Liability

There are several things you can do to avoid placing yourself at risk for liability. The monograph, *Legal Considerations and the Lactation Consultant—USA*, contains important reading on the topic of liability (Bornmann, 1986). Become familiar with your state's laws regulating the practice of medicine. Familiarize yourself with protocols in your practice setting. Obtain malpractice insurance, and keep it in force continuously. Build positive relationships with the mothers in your care. Be sure not to guarantee results or create unrealistic expectations for mothers. Empower them to make their own decisions and serve as their consultant, not their decision maker.

Recognize that there are times when you should not accept a case. Perhaps you get an uncomfortable or negative feeling about a particular situation. A case may be beyond your level of competence, or you may not have time to handle it. Document everything you do as well as what you chose not to do and why. Avoid making any negative notations in the mother's record that she may later read. Organize your work space with necessary paperwork accessible to make it convenient for documenting what you do. Keep a copy of everything you document. Finally, if you are in private practice, consider incorporating your practice to limit your personal liability.

▼
Standards of Practice for Ethical Issues

As a lactation consultant, you will work as a member of the health care team. It is important that you work with both the mother's and baby's physician, and that you send appropriate reports. Be careful not to undermine the physician's position, and try to work within the parameters of the physician's advice as much as possible. If you disagree, discuss the discrepancy with the physician. If a mother asks you for a referral to another physician, lactation consultant or other caregiver, try to suggest at least three names.

If you work in private practice, it is best to inform the client of your fees before you initiate an assessment. You may wish to post fees in your office. When asked over the telephone what the fees will be, you can respond, "As a lactation consultant in private practice, my fees are similar to those of the baby's physician. An office or home visit is $_____ and generally lasts about _____ hours. It includes. You may pay by cash or check at the end of the consultation." If you make breastfeeding equipment available as a service to mothers, you are expected to charge the standard fees for each item. Inform mothers of all fees at the beginning of the consultation so that there are no surprises later. Also, make sure that rental equipment such as breast pumps are scrupulously cleaned and in good working condition. Many lactation consultants will waive cleaning fees on rental equipment if the equipment is returned in clean condition.

Examples of Ethical Situations

A variety of situations may occur that require a lactation consultant to give even more careful consideration to the possible ethical ramifications of an action or practice. A few are presented here as examples (Barger, 1998). Food for thought is presented at the end of each scenario. The points are intended to identify issues that may be considered, and to serve as a stepping stone to determine how you would respond in each case.

Situation One

Tracy is referred to you by the pediatrician who cares for her son, Michael. Michael is 6 weeks old and is about 5.02 over birth weight. As you are taking a history and doing a breastfeeding assessment on this dyad, Tracy tells you that she is feeding Michael on a 3-hour schedule during the day. He is now sleeping about 8 hours at night, and feeds about 6 times in a 24-hour period. You suggest to her that she feed Michael more often, including waking him at night, as one of the goals to increase his weight and milk production. She tells you that it is important that he stay on the schedule. On further gentle questioning, you discover that Tracy is taking a church-related parenting class that condemns, among other things, the use of cue-related feeds. Babies are expected to sleep through the night at 6 to 8 weeks of age. She has been told that to increase the numbers of feeds would cause Michael's "metabolism to go into chaos." You probe a bit further and learn that for the first 4 or 5 weeks, Michael would cry for up to 40 minutes at a time. The program taught that babies would not eat well if they were fed more frequently than every 3 hours. Therefore, Tracy left Michael in his crib to "cry it out." She tells you, "It is important for the baby to learn that the parents are in control." She rejects your suggestion to use a supplemental feeding device. You recommend that she express her milk between feeds to increase milk production. However, Tracy feels that will throw her schedule off, and rejects this suggestion as well. You finally convince Tracy to agree to supplement Michael after each feed until he is gaining the appropriate amount of weight.

Issues to Consider:

◆ How much do you "push" to salvage the breastfeeding relationship?

◆ How much do you discuss her parenting methods with her?

◆ To whom, if anyone, do you report her parenting behavior, and why or why not?

Situation Two

You have started to do some lecturing about breastfeeding in your state. A hospital in a city about 4 hours from you has invited you to present a 1-day conference. As you begin to make plans to speak, you learn that the conference is sponsored by a major manufacturer of infant formula. Although there is nothing that specifically forbids you from taking money from the formula industry, you feel uncomfortable going ahead with the lecture. As you discuss it with one of your colleagues, she says to you, "You ought to go ahead with it. If you don't do it, there is no telling who they might get to give the conference—it might even be the formula representative herself. At least this way you know the nurses will receive appropriate information!"

Issues to Consider:

◆ If you go ahead with this plan, what underlying message does it give?

◆ Does the end justify the means? You know you would give good information but at what price to your own ethics?

◆ Is there any way to circumvent this problem and still get the message to the staff without taking formula money, and without forgoing compensation?

Situation Three

You are a new lactation consultant working in a hospital. On several occasions, you have been told by mothers that their pediatrician has given them information about breastfeeding that you find shockingly outdated. You are in a quandary. You cannot believe this prominent physician does not know the basics about breastfeeding, but it seems that he is woefully lacking in this area. You have also seen how he can sarcastically cut down nurses when they do not agree with him. You recognize that most physicians in your community are supportive of breastfeeding and have been receptive to learning more about breastfeeding management. However, you must help the mother within the context of her relationship with this particular physician.

Issues to Consider:

◆ If you decide to approach this physician, what tact will you take?

◆ How do you correct the misinformation the mothers have received?

◆ If the misinformation continues, what will you do, if anything, that will not jeopardize your new job?

▼

DEVELOPING RESOURCES

Frequently during your consulting career, you will find a need to seek assistance. It may be for an unusual breastfeeding situation, a medical question, or some other circumstance that you do not believe that you can address adequately with your existing information. In order to offer women the services and support that will aid them in breastfeeding, you will need to develop resources to help you deliver complete and correct information. Develop contacts with people in areas you believe will enhance your consulting. Establish an advisory relationship so that you may call on them when questions arise. Hospitals, physicians, dietitians, pharmacies, medical libraries, service organizations, and colleges can be valuable resources for you.

It is important to keep these resources in mind and to cultivate contacts with others in related fields so that the mothers in your care will have access to the information and services they need. Keep a list of referral resources such as a physical therapist, occupational therapist, speech and language therapist, physician who will clip a frenulum, craniosacral therapist, and accupuncturist. In addition to establishing personal resources, you need to develop a reference library with breastfeeding texts and periodicals. You can also keep an updated list of books and other materials that may be of interest to parents.

▼

PROMOTING YOUR SERVICES

Before promoting your services, you will want to conduct a needs assessment to determine the market for lactation consultants in your community. How many lactation consultants are already employed in local hospitals, physician's offices, and clinics? How many private practice lactation consultants are located within comfortable driving distance for parents? After you have determined the best potential settings for employment, decide which services you can offer that will fill the needs of your target market. Establish baseline data on breastfeeding statistics in order to demonstrate a need for your services. How many mothers initiate breastfeeding? For how long do they breastfeed? Identify current policies, practices, and attitudes. What breastfeeding resources are currently available for parents and caregivers?

Referral System

Maintaining a referral system is integral to the delivery of your assistance to breastfeeding women. This applies regardless of your work setting. Suggestions specific to individual settings are discussed in Chapter 2. They are predicated on the fact that if you want to help breastfeeding mothers, they need to know how to access your services. All areas of your community need to be aware of your services. This includes hospitals, birthing centers, physicians, childbirth educators, breastfeeding support groups, community groups, pharmacies, providers of breastfeeding devices, and anyone else who may encounter breastfeeding women. Studies show that women who receive breastfeeding education and support prenatally are more likely to achieve their goals. Therefore, if you work in a hospital setting, you want to ensure that mothers who are served by your hospital will receive this exposure before their delivery. Lactation consultants in private practice will depend on referrals for their entire practice.

Community Awareness

Another challenge is to make the community aware of your services. If you are in private practice, you can develop an attractive logo that identifies you easily to prospective clients and referral sources. Use the logo on printed brochures, business cards, letterhead, postcards, and all other materials that promote your services. A professional look to all printed material will speak well for you. Remember that your own personal appearance and demeanor will also have a great impact on the impressions you make.

There are a variety of ways in which you can obtain free exposure in the community. Consider providing outreach programs to educate the public about breastfeeding. You can offer to present breastfeeding information to classes in high schools as part of their health curriculum. Some newspapers will print an article about members of the community who have recently achieved special honors. Figure 24.2 shows a sample news release for a graduate of a lactation management program. It can be adapted and expanded to apply to individual circumstances. Participating in health fairs, trade shows, and charities will also advertise your services. World Breastfeeding Week

FIGURE 24.2 Sample news release

NEWS RELEASE
THROUGH: (Your name, title, address, phone number)
Date:

FOR IMMEDIATE RELEASE

(Your name) recently completed an intensive training program to give her the skills and information needed to practice as a Lactation Consultant. The training was conducted by the Center for Lactation Education, which is a division of Breastfeeding Support Consultants, Incorporated in Chalfont, Pennsylvania. The course covered all aspects of counseling skills, breastfeeding management, problems and special situations, working effectively with the medical community, nutrition, anatomy and physiology of the breast, and properties of human milk. Following completion of the program, (your name) became certified as a lactation consultant through the International Board of Lactation Consultant Examiners, the official certifying body for lactation consultants. (Your name) is also a member of the International Lactation Consultant Association.

Reprinted with permission of Breastfeeding Support Consultants.

offers an ideal time for you to sponsor a breastfeeding program in your community. A local radio or television station may be willing to conduct an interview.

Offer to speak for no charge in the community in order to become recognized as an authority on breastfeeding. Produce promotional items such as pens, note pads, magnets, and buttons that advertise your services. Provide inservice education at no cost to childbirth educators and other health professionals in your area. This will open doors for later referrals and relationships. Offer professional discounts or in-kind services to groups such as your local breastfeeding coalition, ILCA affiliate, or La Leche League. Something as simple as bringing refreshments when you visit other health care professionals may make an impression that will bring you to mind at a later time.

Writing a Resumé or Curriculum Vitae

A well-written resumé or curriculum vitae (referred to as a CV) will help you make a professional impression to a potential employer. Services are available for developing these documents through employment agencies and computer software programs. However, the task does not need to be daunting. Begin by taking a personal inventory of your background, work experience, and strengths to incorporate into a resumé or CV. The purpose of either of these documents is to showcase your talents. Send your resumé or CV with a cover letter that states the kind of position you are seeking and why you are applying to the particular facility. Follow up with a telephone call a short time later to request an interview.

There are distinct differences between a resumé and a curriculum vitae. The choice will depend on what you have learned about the facility and which format you feel will pique their interest. Below is a description of both documents.

Resumé

A resumé is a brief, one-page, promotional piece that identifies a specific job or interest. Applicable personal data to be included are name, address, telephone number, fax number, and e-mail address. Then state your objective or career goal and identify any skills and abilities that may be useful in the position you are seeking. This may include such things as knowledge of foreign languages, public speaking abilities, artistic talents, and computer capabilities. Follow this with a history of your education, employment, formal education, and other professional training. List dates of graduation, degrees

or certificates received, major and minor subjects, and any scholarships or honors. Your work history can be organized either by job or by function.

Work History by Job

List each job separately, even if more than one position was at the same facility. List dates of employment, name and address of the employer, nature of the business, the position that you held, specific job duties, any special assignments or use of special equipment, your scope of responsibility (e.g., how many people you supervised and the degree of supervision you received), and noteworthy accomplishments (backed up by concrete facts and figures).

Work History by Function

List functions (fields of specialization or types of work) you performed that are related to your present job objectives. Describe briefly the work you have done in each of these fields, without breaking it down by jobs.

FIGURE 24.3   Abbreviated curriculum vitae

Your Name, RN, MA, MSN, IBCLC
100 N. State Street
Anytown, PA 00000
Phone: 215-555-1234
Fax: 215-555-5678
E-Mail: yourname@aol.com
SSN-###-##-####

Education
Breastfeeding Support Consultants-Lactation Management-1992
University of Illinois, Chicago, IL-Masters in Nursing (MSN)-1990
Michigan State University, East Lansing MI-Counseling (MA)-1986
Wheaton College, Wheaton, IL-Psychology (BA)-1982
School of Nursing, Oak Park, IL-Nursing Diploma (RN)-1980
Parkside High School, Jackson, MI-1977

Licenses and Certifications
RN-Pennsylvania-1998 to present
RN-Illinois-1980 to present
RN-Michigan-1983 to 1990
IBLCE (International Board Certified Lactation Consultant)-1992 to present

Current Positions
Contributing Editor, ILCA Globe, 1996 to present
Member of Education Committee-ILCA-1997 to present
Lactation consultant-Anywhere Pediatrics, Anywhere, IL 1992 to present
Clinical Instructor, Mother-Baby Unit; Community Hospital, Anywhere IL, 1995 to present
Staff Nurse, Mother-Baby Unit; Community Hospital, Anywhere IL, 1991 to 1995
Staff Nurse, Labor and Delivery, University Hospital, Anycity, MI 1983 to 1988
Staff Nurse, Pediatrics; Community Hospital, Anywhere IL, 1980 to 1983

Previous Publications and Presentations
Lectures on various aspects of breastfeeding in workshops, seminars, conferences, and hospital inservices an average of 10 times per year since 1994. Published in the ILCA *Journal of Human Lactation* on breastfeeding topics and book reviews.

Complete CV available upon request

You may also list volunteer activities related to your present objectives, such as breastfeeding counseling.

Curriculum Vitae

A CV is an extensive, scholarly piece that reflects all of your professional activity. It will begin with the same personal data as a resumé: name, address, telephone number, fax number, and e-mail address. List your educational background, professional practice, academic appointments, memberships to professional associations, and any publications or articles you have written. Indicate outside professional interests and related community and consultant activities. Include all professional presentations and licensure.

Because some CVs may number several pages, a one-page abbreviated version can be developed with a note at the bottom that the complete CV is available on request. A sample of an abbreviated CV appears in Figure 24.3. This individual has demonstrated extensive experience in maternal-child health as well as participation in her professional association. She is relocating to a new city and is interested in obtaining a position as a full-time lactation consultant in the community hospital. This abbreviated CV will help her present a professional image and open the door to a possible position in the hospital.

▼ Developing a Lactation Consultant Job Description or Proposal

In addition to an impressive CV, you may want to approach a facility with a formal job proposal. Perhaps a prospective employer will be receptive if you request a position on a trial basis for a period of 6 months. During that time, you can train staff, establish breastfeeding protocols, and collect data to justify the continuation of your position.

Below is a list of possible elements to include in a job description or a proposal for a new position as a lactation consultant. In developing your proposal, you may select from these items. The list is based on proposals and job descriptions shared with Breastfeeding Support Consultants (BSC) over the years and is printed with permission of BSC. Thank you to all the lactation consultants who have generously shared their ideas to benefit others in the profession.

Items are categorized in such a way that you may consider the types of activities which may be included and the expertise required. Not all will apply to a particular position. Determine what the specific needs are of the facility so that you may design your proposal based on their needs. Also try to identify the appropriate person to receive the proposal. Often this will be the Director of Maternal-Child Nursing or a similarly titled position.

Cover Letter or Introductory Remarks

Begin with rationale for establishing a lactation consultant position. Give a brief description of your role in the mother's and infant's health care team, and describe how you see yourself functioning in their facility. Focus on the benefits to the hospital of having a lactation consultant on staff. You might also indicate the cost-benefit issues to the hospital for your services.

Objectives

Demonstrate that the establishment of a lactation consultant position will enhance the facility's reputation in the community as a concerned provider of health care to mothers and babies. Suggest that the position can be funded through an increased number of mothers who will choose to deliver there because of the facility's reputation. Cite that with a lactation consultant on staff the facility will:

◆ Provide a positive breastfeeding experience for both the mother and baby.

◆ Promote bonding between the mother and her baby.

◆ Promote healthier babies and mothers.

◆ Provide consistent breastfeeding teaching and support.

◆ Increase the incidence of mothers choosing to breastfeed.

◆ Increase the incidence of mothers continuing to breastfeed at 6 months.

◆ Decrease the incidence of unresolved breastfeeding problems.

Teaching Services

Indicate the educational programs you can provide to both parents and staff.

◆ Teach prenatal infant feeding classes.

◆ Teach in-hospital breastfeeding classes.

◆ Teach postpartum classes.

◆ Provide inservice education for staff.

◆ Assist with orientation of staff.

◆ Maintain a resource center for patient and staff materials.

◆ Conduct bedside teaching of staff through a mentorship or preceptor program.

Services to Mothers and Infants

Identify the services you can offer to mothers.

◆ Individual consultation during the hospital stay, which may include:
 Conduct daily rounds to breastfeeding mothers.

Give anticipatory guidance to mothers.
Revisit mothers who are experiencing problems.
Perform a breastfeeding assessment.
Develop a plan of care with the mother.
Provide problem-solving advice and support.
Document teaching and progress on the patient charts.

- Coordinate or provide home follow-up through telephone calls, postcards, or visits.
- Provide a 24-hour hot line where mothers can call and have their questions answered immediately. An alternative is to provide a 24-hour warm line where mothers leave a message on an answering machine or voice mail, and the call is returned at a later time.
- Refer mothers to a support group and other community resources.
- Coordinate counseling and support of mothers who wish to provide human milk for a high-risk infant.
- Coordinate dispensing of all breastfeeding devices.
- Provide an outpatient lactation clinic for weighing infants and discussing problems.

Working with Staff

Indicate the manner in which you will work with staff. This may include

- Initiate case conferences and confer with staff on patient needs.
- Serve as a resource for staff, physicians, and support group counselors.
- Consult with the mother's and baby's primary care providers.
- Discuss appropriate referrals with primary care providers.
- Provide on-call service for consultations with staff.
- Participate as a team member with staff and physicians to provide comprehensive care.
- Coordinate or participate in a breastfeeding committee.

Writing, Reviewing, and Revising Printed Materials

A lactation consultant needs the writing and editing skills necessary for development or revision of printed materials and protocols. Services you may wish to provide include

- Establish, review, and revise standards of care that support breastfeeding.
- Develop, review, and revise breastfeeding policies.

- Develop, review, and revise breastfeeding care plans.
- Develop and revise a charting system for documentation, teaching, and progress notes.
- Develop, review, and revise patient literature.
- Maintain statistics to assess the effectiveness of your services.
- Publish a monthly breastfeeding newsletter for staff.

Professional Requirements

Learn the preferences in the facility regarding credentials as well as experience that would be required for a lactation consultant practicing in that facility. Some facilities may require that the lactation consultant have a degree in another area of health care. Others will not. Be sure to include any education and experience that will complement the position you are seeking. This serves the purpose of a conventional resumé by identifying skills and abilities that will make you attractive for the position you are seeking.

- IBCLC certified through the International Board of Lactation Consultant Examiners.
- Membership in the International Lactation Consultant Association.
- Graduate from a lactation management course.
- Graduate from a school of nursing or other facility.
- Current licensure in the state in a related field.
- College degree in psychology, sociology, education, or other related field.
- Skills, knowledge, and attitude to promote breastfeeding.
- Communication skills for interactions with patients, families, and colleagues.
- Knowledge of cultural, psychological, psychosocial, nutritional, and pharmacological aspects of breastfeeding.
- Understanding of current breastfeeding practices and research findings.
- Participation in continuing education through seminars, workshops, and networking.
- Support for the facility's philosophy and policies.

Fee for Services

The reality in any business is that the bottom line is money, and this is no different in health care. You have identified in previous sections of the job proposal how your services will enhance the facility's delivery of care. You now need to demonstrate how the facility can cover the costs of your services. Better yet, you can show how your services will actually generate more revenue for the facility. One way to do this is to indicate areas where the facility can charge a fee for your services. Some insurance companies will reimburse for lactation services. Check the current status of the insurance carriers for women in your community and in the facility they use. Fee-for-service offerings may include

- In-hospital assistance
- Prenatal class
- Home or outpatient follow-up. This may include telephone counseling with an unlimited 24-hour hotline, an office visit, or a home visit
- Outpatient consultation services

Equipment and Other Resources

The facility will want to know what additional expenses your position will require. Therefore, in your proposal, indicate the initial investment that will be required in terms of equipment and other resources. This may include

- Office space
- Desk and chair
- File cabinets
- Computer and printer
- Telephone
- Answering machine or voice mail
- Internet access
- Beeper
- Comfortable cushioned armchair
- Electric breast pumps and other breastfeeding devices
- Infant scale
- Secretarial support
- Funds for reference books and continuing education
- Dictation services

▼

STAFF EDUCATION

As an ultimate goal, you want to achieve a continuum of supportive breastfeeding care for the mothers and babies you serve. If you are the breastfeeding expert in your facility and everyone saves all the breastfeeding problems for you to handle, then you are not doing your job! You need to train others to help you and to carry through with consistent care. By empowering others, you will be helping yourself. It will give you the ability to remain creative and energized, as well as minimize the number of problems.

In order for breastfeeding mothers to receive the best possible health care and advice, they must be cared for by health providers who are knowledgeable in lactation and who possess the necessary skills to facilitate learning. A knowledge deficit regarding breastfeeding has been found within all health care professions (Bagwell, 1993). Often, professional schooling includes little or no real breastfeeding education. Breastfeeding may be viewed as something that should just come naturally and is often neglected in continuing education. If staff members are consistently leaving the difficulties for you to resolve, then the mothers, infants and staff are losing out on valuable time. The longer a mother has a problem often results in a longer time to resolution of the problem.

Lactation consultants can provide other members of the health care team with necessary knowledge through inservice training and clinical supervision. Professional development can be accomplished through both scheduled group inservices and individualized clinical situations. If you are approached by a staff member with concerns regarding a specific mother and baby, you can accompany that staff member to the mother's room and involve the staff member in the consult (Fig. 24.4). Scheduled inservices need to meet the needs of both new staff and those with experience. You might consider including occasional seminars with more involved infor-

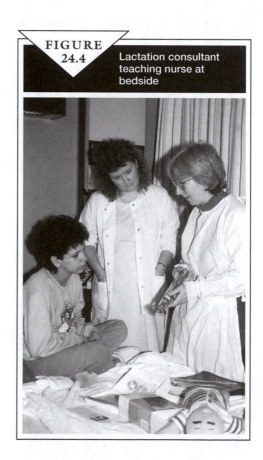

FIGURE 24.4 Lactation consultant teaching nurse at bedside

FIGURE 24.5   Pretest on breastfeeding

True   False

____ ____   1. Infant formula is just as healthy as human milk.
____ ____   2. Bottles and infant formula given to breastfeeding babies in the first 2 weeks do not interfere with breastfeeding.
____ ____   3. Breastfeeding is to human milk as bottles are to infant formula.
____ ____   4. Duration at the breast needs to be limited in the early days to prevent sore nipples.
____ ____   5. Even with time limits, most breastfeeding women will experience sore nipples.
____ ____   6. Breastfed babies typically will want to feed every 3 hours.
____ ____   7. Water supplementation will help prevent jaundice in breastfeeding infants.
____ ____   8. Formula supplementation is necessary when the mother has a low milk supply; when the supply has been re-established she can discontinue supplementing.
____ ____   9. Weaning is recommended when mothers are taking most medications.
____ ____ 10. Mothers who plan to return to work are advised to wean about 1 week before they return.
____ ____ 11. Breastfeeding mothers and babies take more of the physician's time than do those who are bottle feeding.
____ ____ 12. The best time to start breastfeeding is after the mother's milk comes in.
____ ____ 13. The best way to tell that a baby is getting enough milk is that he sleeps for at least 3 hours after each feed.
____ ____ 14. After the mother's milk supply is established, babies typically nurse for about 5 minutes on each breast at a feed.
____ ____ 15. Mothers need to feed from both breasts at every feed, limiting the time on the first side so the baby will take the second side.

(All answers are false)

Printed by permission of Breastfeeding Support Consultants.

mation and short breastfeeding bytes at unit meetings or on bulletin boards. You can also participate in the orientation of new staff members (Stokamer, 1993).

See the sample pretest in Figure 24.5 that can be used for staff education. This test can be used for hospital staff, physicians, residents, and others who will be attending educational offerings. It identifies misconceptions and areas of strength and weakness. Readers are welcome to use this test for their own teaching.

Creating Enthusiasm Among Staff

Staff education can take many forms. Consider launching a breastfeeding initiative with a motivational program for the staff. A workshop or conference will energize people and generate enthusiasm for learning more about breastfeeding. You could design a breastfeeding bulletin board with monthly updates and include highlights of particular staff members who have done something noteworthy related to breastfeeding. Post breastfeeding messages where people are likely to read them, such as in the locker room or on the back of the stall door in the restroom. Award staff with a small token of appreciation for attending a breastfeeding program. Some facilities give each staff member a badge that reads *Ask me about breastfeeding*. In addition to serving as a token of thanks, it also identifies that staff member to mothers and other staff as someone who can help them with their breastfeeding questions.

Your effectiveness in teaching other staff members about breastfeeding management will be enhanced when you create a receptive learning climate. In Chapter 3, you learned that one element of adult learning is the use of humor as a communication tool. In many ways, humor is simply allowing your humanness to shine forth. Be willing to make mistakes in front of colleagues. You are a role model to them. Let them see that in the real world we all make mistakes, and show them how we recover from our mistakes. Weave humor into your teaching. Humor is graphic and creates images in the learner's mind that help the learner remember better and longer. Modeling the use of humor is a first step to teaching staff how to use humor themselves as a communication tool with patients. Role playing situations in the classroom helps relieve anxiety and makes the anticipated situation in reality less awkward.

MATURING THROUGH CONSULTING EXPERIENCES

At times, lactation consulting may present experiences that are discouraging to you. There will be times when something unfavorable happens that you cannot correct. Whenever you experience discouraging consulting situations, it is helpful to talk with a colleague to express your frustrations or doubts. Some circumstances that may occur during your career are presented in the following sections.

Mothers Who Do Not Follow Your Advice

You will invariably encounter mothers who choose not to follow through on your advice. Some of these outcomes may result in what you consider to be inappropriate or ill-advised action by the mother. One mother may wean unexpectedly or earlier than you would advise. Another may supplement with formula or introduce solid foods at an early age. It is discouraging when a mother fails to follow through on your advice. It is equally frustrating to see a breastfeeding experience deteriorate because a mother has chosen not to follow through on the suggestions and advice that you have given her. However, you need to remember that what a mother does with your advice is her responsibility, and she will be the one who must live with the outcome. As long as you have given the appropriate support and information, you have fulfilled your obligation to the mother. You must then step back and respect her choice.

Medical Complications

It is discouraging for both the mother and lactation consultant when a mother is unable to breastfeed her baby for medical reasons. She may express her milk for a period of time and then have difficulty getting breastfeeding established. When a mother who is highly motivated and determined is unable to breastfeed, you may view it as failure on your part. Other times, more tragic events, such as a baby dying or the mother having radical breast surgery, may leave you feeling helpless. These tragedies can affect you deeply because you have learned to cultivate warmth and caring, and may find it difficult to remove yourself emotionally from the situation. You may need to work through the grief process just as the mother does.

External Interference

Some discouraging situations may involve people other than the mother in your care. Perhaps a mother's partner is unsupportive and resents your involvement. A member of the medical community may be unsupportive of your efforts or may consistently give incorrect breastfeeding information. These situations make it extremely difficult to provide necessary help and advice to a mother. Yet at the same time, they offer challenges. You can provide information to educate the partner or physician and try to determine the cause of the misinformation or lack of support. You can be open and frank with the mother about her partner's feelings and arrange follow-up contacts at times when he is not at home. You can work along with the mother in providing literature

to her physician and encourage the mother to share the positive aspects of her breastfeeding with her physician.

Professional Burnout

After having consulted with many mothers, your experiences may seem to become repetitive, boring, discouraging, or frustrating. You may find it a nuisance to deal with common problems such as sore nipples, fussy periods for the baby, sleeping through the night, and other events you have discussed endlessly with mothers. By considering the point of view of each mother and her needs and anxieties of first-time mothering, you can hopefully keep these in perspective. The term **burnout** is often used to describe this reaction. Burnout may occur any time that you become overly involved in your work. Although almost everyone gets burned out to some degree, idealists who have high standards and believe that they have to do all the work themselves tend to burn out more quickly in their efforts to achieve perfection.

Working in a caring profession carries a high risk of becoming stressed and burned out. When this happens, there is a lack of enthusiasm to perform tasks. Accompanying this problem may be a low tolerance level, and a loss of creativity and openness to change. The most stressful jobs seem to be those that combine big demands with a relative lack of autonomy. Emotional burnout can occur when you fail to achieve a balance, and it is a response to unrelieved stress. Lactation consultants and others who care for breastfeeding mothers are often available to clients 24 hours a day. The nurturing nature of the lactation profession impels many caregivers to provide constant access to mothers whenever a concern or problem arises. Lactation consultants often suffer from what one practitioner calls "compassion fatigue syndrome." We give and give and then give more to our clients. Failure to achieve a balance between professional responsibilities and personal needs places you in danger of professional burnout.

Mothers tend to wait until a problem seems unresolvable before they call for help. Therefore, many breastfeeding contacts for lactation consultants in private practice involve a mother in crisis. The mother is often in tears and needs her problem resolved immediately. Many times, there seems to be too much work and too little time for those who care for breastfeeding mothers. Because the lactation profession is still relatively new, there are not sufficient numbers of lactation consultants for the mothers who need them. Nationwide, in 1998 there was one lactation consultant for approximately every 1000 births. Add to that the fact that breastfeeding promoters often experience resistance from a medical system that is unwilling to accept newly researched breastfeeding policies and practices. These factors can intensify the tendency to become burned out. When burnout occurs, caregivers may distance themselves from the patient. By releasing feelings and tension, you can return to the mother and give compassionate care. Signs of emotional burnout appear below.

Signs of Emotional Burnout

◆ Tunnel vision

◆ Loss of coping skills

◆ Lack of focus and concentration

◆ Unexplained physical pain

◆ Fatigue

◆ Irrational behavior, a feeling of being on an "emotional roller coaster"

◆ Avoiding obligations and other avoidance behaviors

◆ Feeling that life is out of control

◆ Insomnia

◆ Irritation

◆ Depression

◆ Inability to manage time

Overcoming Burnout

In order to progress past emotional burnout, you first need to recognize that the problem is with the job, not with you. Accept your limitations and acknowledge that "this is too much for me today." It is often very difficult for us to admit to ourselves our own limitations. You need to establish personal boundaries. Trying to be everything for everybody does not work. This makes it especially important that you empower others to give breastfeeding mothers the help they need. Trained people can certainly help with the first levels of care, and this will help minimize the types of problems that cause stress.

Learn how to take a short time-out. Visualization and slow, deep breathing will help you relax and reclaim your strength and perspective. Physical exercise can also help rejuvenate you. Your sense of humor and your ability to find humor in situations will be especially important during times of stress. See Figure 24.6 for a relaxation exercise that may help you cope with stress before it leads to burnout. You can do this exercise while you are sitting at your desk, or in the car waiting for a traffic light (although you may want to leave your eyes open if you are at a traffic light!).

Making Time for Yourself and Your Family

One of the reasons why care giving professionals become burned out is that they never learn how to say no! This is especially true of women who take on more work because they believe their family, friends, and clients

FIGURE 24.6 Relaxation exercise

Sit up straight and place your feet flat on the floor. Close your eyes, and allow your arms to fall comfortably to your side. Take a long, deep cleansing breath and continue to breathe slowly and deeply. Visualize a peaceful scene: Perhaps a warm beach with waves rolling to the shore, or a field of wild flowers. Next, tighten the muscles in your legs, all the way down to your toes. Hold the tension for a few seconds, and then release. Tighten your stomach muscles, hold, and release. Remember to keep breathing slowly and deeply. Tighten the muscles in your arms. Make a fist with your hands and squeeze them tight, then release. Tighten the muscles in your face, clench your jaw, frown, and release. Rotate your head to the right . . . to the left . . . down to your chin . . . and back to the center. Raise your shoulders to your ears and back down. Take a deep cleansing breath, and open your eyes.

need them. Women, especially mothers, feel torn by all the demands on their time. They spend so much effort trying to please everyone, that they have no time or energy left for themselves.

Networking at conferences and affiliated meetings is a perfect time to get rejuvenated in the lactation field. Spending time with others in similar situations and learning new techniques can help breathe life into a job that is wearing you down. You also need to learn how to balance all that you do. Determine exactly what is important, and then prioritize your list. If you are attempting to do too many things, you will not be able to give your best to those things that are most important. Learn to delegate responsibilities so that you can put your valuable time and energy into the most important functions. Train others on the staff to take calls and answer basic breastfeeding questions. This gives ownership to others and enables everyone to focus on the priorities. When you multiply yourself by delegating and training staff, you will recognize that you do not shoulder the responsibility alone.

In order to overcome burnout, you also need to recapture some personal time to enjoy your family and friends. You need to plan quality time for yourself and your family. You have undoubtedly heard the question, "How many people on their death bed wish they had spent more time at the office?" Take the time to cultivate and nurture relationships with the important people in your life. You may actually need to schedule blocks of time into your calendar in order to assign this the priority it deserves.

You also need time for the most important person in your life—you! Make yourself take a vacation. Your vacation may simply entail time spent at home without work responsibilities. That means relaxing and pampering yourself. It does not mean painting your mother-in-law's house or cleaning the attic! You need special time just for yourself, engaging in activities that your busy schedule has not allowed. You might spend the entire time reading a favorite book or watching classic movies. The goal is to relax and rejuvenate yourself. You will be surprised how much clearer your thinking will be when you return to work after just a few days. You will then be able to give the best of yourself to others.

Renewing Enthusiasm

One lactation consultant reported that she knew she was burned out when she saw a new mother approaching her office to pick up a breast pump and her first reaction was, "Darn! Someone is here to pick up a pump and she has her baby with her!" She knew that she would be required to do more than simply provide a pump to the mother. When you are disturbed by the prospect of helping a mother and baby, you know you have reached a critical point. To prevent yourself from reaching that stage, take measures to help maintain your enthusiasm and perspective.

You cannot give the best of yourself when you are feeling stressed and stretched to the limit. Learn to say NO when others ask more of you than you have to give. Use an answering machine to screen telephone calls and take messages at times when you feel more prepared to answer the telephone. Limit the commitments you place on your time. And keep your sense of humor! People with a sense of humor are healthier, happier people.

Try to be aware of the times that make you feel uncomfortable and why. Learn how to work out these kinds of problems by discussing them with a colleague. If you have been losing interest in your work for some time, it may be appropriate for you to re-examine the goals you had hoped lactation consulting would help you fulfill. Perhaps you have reached your original goals and need to form new ones. If you examine what you would like to gain from your role, a new direction for your efforts may become obvious to you.

Do you still believe that educating mothers and helping them develop satisfying breastfeeding experiences are rewarding and worthwhile pursuits? If not, why do you feel this way? Do you still believe that promoting breastfeeding to physicians, nurses, students, and the general community is a worthwhile goal? Have you been stifled in this pursuit by nonlistening or uncooperative individuals? Perhaps it is time to take a new approach or to get outside help with community education. Have you considered visiting clinics, high school health classes, and local women's clubs for the purposes of educating the public? Perhaps you could write a weekly column on breastfeeding for your local newspaper or a newsletter. If the goal of educating others about breastfeeding is still important to you, then you might look for new ways to achieve it.

Have you stopped growing as a lactation consultant? You have gained a lot of knowledge, varied skills, and a more thorough understanding of yourself during your initial years of practice, but now you may feel you have become stagnant. For continued growth, you may need to be exposed to greater challenges, and new and more complex ideas and issues. Perhaps you can assist with the teaching of lay counselors in the community. Many seasoned lactation consultants, after years of clinical practice, may find it challenging to become clinical instructors for lactation consultant interns. Teaching others almost always leads to growth and increased self-understanding. Attending special presentations and conferences, and associating with others in the health care system can provide a means for personal education and growth. Perhaps new reading materials would offer stimulation to you. Deeper, more technical books and medical or counseling journals may interest you.

Do you see your lactation consulting as a means of bringing about social change? Do you want to encourage close, warm relationships between people? Do you want to promote the nuclear family as a lifestyle? Perhaps it is not clear to you just how your efforts can effect such changes. You can reflect on the specific actions you might take to bring about your goals. For example, it is well known that babies who are separated from their mothers for long periods after birth have a significantly greater chance of being abused. Perhaps you can work with your local hospital toward continued close contact of mothers and babies after birth. Do you believe that the father's participation in birth and infant care brings about a closer, more family-centered lifestyle? If so, then it may be worthwhile for you to find a means of encouraging a father's participation in events that are related to his child's birth and early life. When you can define your goals and relate them to your actions in this manner, you will be on your way toward developing a satisfying new role for yourself.

Lactation consulting does take time and practice. Most of all, it requires that you care about other people. Each experience is unique, and in each one you will learn and grow along with the mothers in your care. When your goals are clearly defined and you have directed your actions toward those goals, your role brings a sense of accomplishment and fulfillment. The reward and fulfillment comes from the knowledge that you are giving valuable help to others and that you are able to enjoy counseling breastfeeding mothers.

▼ Avoiding Pitfalls in Consulting

In the lactation consultant profession, remember that every consultant and every mother is unique. Therefore, consultations will vary from one dyad to the next. Your style of caring for mothers will also differ from another lactation consultant. This is no different than other arms of the health profession. As long as you help the mother feel better and reach her breastfeeding goals, you have done your job. Being aware of potential pitfalls will help you deliver an effective level of care. Perhaps the experiences of others, as described later, will help you avoid these pitfalls.

Not Accepting Your Own Limitations

Admit to the mother that you do not have all the answers and that you may need to get help from outside sources. Realize that your influence on the mother's behavior is limited. Encourage mothers to determine their own solutions.

Getting Overly Involved in a Mother's Private Life

If you find that a mother is relying on you too much, back off and encourage her to take charge of her own decisions. Build her confidence and offer her information with minimal guidance. If problems are serious and outside the realm of breastfeeding, encourage her to contact her minister, physician, or other agencies for advice and support. You are not a professional guidance counselor. Help mothers understand that your services are restricted to lactation consulting and related topics.

Discussing Your Own Breastfeeding Experience

Many times, a mother asks her lactation consultant how long she breastfed, or some other aspect of her own personal experience. It is important to maintain a professional relationship with clients. It is doubtful that she really wants to know about your breastfeeding experience. More likely, she has a question about her own breastfeeding. You can use counseling skills to determine the real purpose of the question. You might say, for example, "You're wondering how long to breastfeeding your baby." Discussing aspects of your own life diminishes the mother's experience. Keep the discussion focused on her.

Making Value Judgments

At times, it may be challenging to remain objective and to avoid your own value judgments from being relayed to mothers. Remember that your role with mothers is to help them become informed consumers. You are responsible for giving correct and appropriate information and advice. What the mother does with that advice is her choice. Encourage mothers to make the decisions that fit into their own lifestyle, and then support their choices. Always leave mothers with a graceful exit if they are not comfortable with your suggestions.

Interrupting

Becoming an effective listener is an essential skill for lactation consultants. Use counseling skills to draw out the mother and engage her in conversation, and resist the urge to jump into a conversation before the mother finishes her train of thought. Do not change the subject until you are sure the mother has explored it to her satisfaction. This is a pitfall that is common in many social and professional interactions. Avoiding it will come with practice, practice, practice!

Overwhelming the Mother with Facts or Suggestions

Many lactation consultants fall into the trap of overwhelming mothers with too much advice and information. Remember to restrict the amount of information you give to a mother at any one time. As a general rule, offer only three suggestions at one time. You can always follow up the contact with another one. Remember, less is more!

Being Too Solution-oriented

Being in a helping role within the health profession, there is always the risk of becoming too focused on solutions at the expense of other issues in the mother's life. You can avoid this by listening carefully for feelings and concerns the mother is expressing. Learn to read between the lines and to read her body language. Allow the mother time to define her situation and to work out her own answers. Enter into problem solving only after you have gathered sufficient information and impressions.

Failing to Provide Follow up to a Mother

We hope we have convinced you of the importance of following up with clients to learn if your advice has been helpful. Always follow through to learn whether the situation has improved and to give the mother support. Encourage her to contact you if she needs your further assistance. If there are times when you will not be available, make sure you have arranged backup. This is especially important if you will be away for an extended length of time. If your particular role does not allow you to contact her personally, you can put her in touch with another lactation consultant or a support group in the community so that she has a resource. The important issue is that the mother knows where to go for help.

▼

SUMMARY

As an integral member of the mother's health care team, it is important that you continue to grow and thrive in the profession. Appropriate education and clinical experience will prepare you to enter the profession. Understanding the stages of role acquisition will help you anticipate each new challenge. Availing yourself of the networking and support from colleagues and your professional association will enhance your effectiveness with mothers and babies. Becoming certified and adhering to the profession's standards of practice and ethics will ensure that you are providing appropriate care. Finally, you will give the best of yourself to mothers when you recognize your own limitations and seek assistance when appropriate.

▼

REFERENCES

Association of Women's Health, Obstetric and Neonatal Nursing (AWHONN). *Standards for the Nursing Care of Women and Newborns;* Washington DC; 1991.

Bagwell J et al. Knowledge and attitudes toward breast-feeding: Differences among dietitians, nurses, and physicians working with WIC clients. *J Am Diet Assoc* 93:801–804; 1993.

Barger J. *Acquiring the LC Role.* Lactation Management Course, BSC Center for Lactation Education; 1998.

Bocar DL and Moore K. *Acquiring the Parental Role.* Lactation Consultant Series #16. New York: Avery Publishing Group; 1987.

Bornmann PG. *Legal Considerations and the Lactation Consultant—USA.* Lactation Consultant Series New York: Avery Publishing Group; 1986.

International Lactation Consultant Association (ILCA). *Standards of Practice for Lactation Consultants* (1st ed). Raleigh, NC; 1995.

Kutner L and Barger J. *Clinical Experience in Lactation: A Blueprint for Internship.* Breastfeeding Support Consultants; Chalfont, PA: 1998a.

Kutner L. *Lactation Management* Course. BSC Center for Lactation Education; 1998b.

Stokamer C. In-Service breastfeeding program development: Needs assessment and planning. *J Hum Lact* 9:253–256; 1993.

▼

BIBLIOGRAPHY

Bocar DL. The lactation consultant: part of the health care team, Clinical issues in perinatal and women's health nursing: Breastfeeding. *NAACOG* 3(4):731–737; 1992.

Freudenberger HJ. *Burnout: The High cost of High Achievement.* New York: Bantam Books; 1980.

Hancock L et al. Breaking point. Newsweek; 56–62; March 6, 1995.

Nelson DS. Humor in the pediatric emergency department: A 2–year retrospective. *Pediatrics* 89:6, 1089–1090; 1992.

Schaef AW. *Meditations for Women Who Do Too Much.* San Francisco; Harper Collins; 1990.

Schaef AW. The Addictive Organization. San Francisco: Harper and Row; 1988.

25

CRITICAL READING AND REVIEW OF RESEARCH

Contributing Author: Sandra Breck

There are three kinds of truths: Lies, damn lies, and statistics.
Attributed to Benjamin Disraeli by Mark Twain

By studying this and other texts, you have learned a lot of state-of-the-art information and techniques to use in your practice as a lactation consultant. One more skill you need so that your practice remains current is the skill of critically reading the lactation science literature. To lactation consultants who are comfortable with helping breastfeeding mothers, this skill feels very different and, often, more difficult. Like all the other skills we learn, it improves with practice.

This chapter will give you background information on the processes of science as you will find them used in scientific journal articles. It will also explain the structure of the scientific article. Then, comes a "how-to" section on the critical reading of articles aimed at readers who have little previous experience. Two mock articles and commentary follow, so that you can practice the techniques presented in the chapter. Improving your critical abilities is a process of practice and feedback. You will have an opportunity to practice this process without criticism from others. Then you will be ready to tackle a real article and savor the satisfaction of knowing you are offering families the most carefully considered, evidence-based practice they can receive from a thoughtful lactation professional.

TYPES OF ARTICLES IN SCIENTIFIC JOURNALS

Scientific journals contain many types of articles. Commonly, the first prose to appear is an editorial, and some journals will print more than one. Editorials are very interesting and important to read. The editor is a prominent person in the field whose knowledge is broad and whose perspective on how the field is changing is often insightful. It is important to recognize, however, that editorials are not studies and do not report on a particular study. Therefore, they cannot be subjected to the kind of critical analysis to which this chapter is devoted.

Case Studies

Case studies are a type of article that is published by many biomedical journals. They report on one or more **cases** of a problem, diagnosis, or treatment. A case study often is published because there is a lot of interest in the topic. However, because the diagnosis is unusual or the treatment would be risky, it is unlikely that any experiments ever will be conducted. An example of this in lactation literature is a case study of mothers who need to use a medication that is not often prescribed during breastfeeding. Typically, the physician who treated the mother will describe her medical history and what led to the decision to try the medication. A description of the **outcome** for the mother and baby will follow. Such a case study has a **sample** of one mother and one baby. There can be no comparison subjects or comparison treatment. Thus, a case study cannot be subjected to critical analysis. It is still important information to retain because it may be the only information available on the use of that particular drug in breastfeeding. The information may help guide an especially difficult decision in **clinical practice**. However, because it is only one example of a given situation, it cannot be used to **generalize** to most breastfeeding mothers and babies.

Meta-Analysis

Meta-analysis is a technique that combines the data and results of several studies in order to improve the strength of the conclusions. Although meta-analyses are important studies, the analysis approach discussed in this chapter does not apply to them. If you read a meta-analysis, you may want some help from a researcher or statistician before you implement the recommendations made in the study. Scientific journals still publish a lot of debate questioning the validity of the criteria for a good meta-analysis. This type of study relies heavily on statistical **assumptions**, so many clinicians need help in judging their quality. Many such articles contain the words "meta-analysis" in their titles or abstracts, so you should be able to identify them.

Review Articles

Review articles are written by one or more experts in the field who summarize, and often critique, the best and worst studies published on a topic. They differ from a meta-analysis in that they do not combine the data and results the way a meta-analysis does. The opinions of the experts clearly play a role in their selection and the critical analysis of the articles to review. Little or no original data is presented in a review article. Therefore, critical reading of this type of article is not covered by this chapter. However, if you wish to learn about an area of clinical research that is new to you, reading a review article can be a very productive way to begin. You will discover some of the most recent information, some of the important scientists in the field, and some of the current controversies. Most of these articles will contain the word "review" in the title or abstract. If you want to find a review article, you can use the word "review" in your database search or in your request to the librarian.

Clinical Practice

Clinical practice articles often appear in many nursing, dietetic, physical therapy, and medical journals because these are applied sciences. These are written by authors who have experience in a particular diagnosis, problem, deficit, or preventive technique and want to share their accumulated wisdom with other clinicians. The *Journal of Human Lactation*, for example, usually has several of these articles in each issue, offering invaluable help from one lactation consultant to another. Because such articles have not tried to study a problem scientifically, there are usually no presentations of data in graphs, tables, or figures. There also are no **hypotheses** or research questions. There may be some summary information about how, for example, mothers who followed Protocol X coped with Problem Y, but there is no comparison group nor an attempt to show that Protocol X is better than some other protocol. Although these articles are helpful, there is no substantive test of the authors' ideas. Therefore, they do not constitute the same quality of evidence for changing care practices as does research.

Research

Research reports are the type of article addressed by this chapter. As discussed later, there are many types of research. Their strength is that they put to a scientific test a long-held belief or new idea. Researchers subject themselves and their work to the processes of scientific investigation and to the scrutiny of their peers. They take the risk that their colleagues may find their work wanting. Therefore, as lactation consultants, we must approach the work of our colleagues respectfully. Each article deserves careful attention for both the growth of our human understanding about lactation and for the benefit of the families in our care. You will recognize research articles after you have read this chapter because they follow the basic structure described in the following sections.

STRUCTURE OF A SCIENTIFIC ARTICLE

The purpose of this section is to make it easier for you to read a scientific article. Most scientific articles will follow a format that provides experienced readers with a maximum amount of information in a limited amount of journal space. Although this "condensed" feeling can be daunting to those who do not read such articles very often, the more you read, the easier it will become. You will learn to appreciate those well-written journal articles that condense effectively, and you will come away knowing exactly what the researchers did and why. They will have explained what they wish they had done differently, as well as what they believe they can justifiably conclude from their work. With practice, you will also come away with a pretty clear sense of whether or not you agree with their conclusions and will be able to give clear reasons for your decisions. The growth of the science of lactation depends on this clear communication and on feedback to researchers.

Identifying Information

At the very top of many scientific journals, especially the European ones, there is information identifying the journal using its standard abbreviated name. For example, *Acta Pediatr* is the abbreviation for the journal *Acta Paediatrica*, a Scandinavian journal. Although the format for the name, volume number, pages, and year of publication varies from one journal to another, the format used by *Acta Paediatrica* illustrates the commonalities.

Example: Acta Paediatr 22:120–125, 1970.

◆ Acta Paediatr is the journal's abbreviation.

◆ 22 is the volume of the journal. Most journals publish one volume every year, however some publish two volumes per year.

◆ 120–125 are the pages where the article is located. Most journals paginate continuously for 1 year. So, volume 22 starts with page 1. If the first issue for that year ends, say, at page 112, then the second issue begins at page 113, and so on. This continuous pagination is the reason that many journals do not include the issue number in the identifying information; it is not needed. However, some do include it, usually right after the volume number, like this: 22 (2):120–125, 1970. Many journals publish an issue every month but some (like the *Journal of Human Lactation*) publish quarterly, and others (like *Lancet*), publish weekly. When you look up an article or request one from a library, it is very important to carefully copy the numbers from the reference list you use.

◆ 1970 is the year of publication. In some journals, the year is listed directly after the name of the journal.

All of this information is very handy to have at the top of the first page of the article. Those journals that do not put it at the top usually put it at the end of the abstract or somewhere else on the first page.

Title of the Article

A well-chosen title will tell you a lot about an article. In some journals, the title explains the main finding and may be two sentences long. This helps busy readers choose which articles are highest priority for their reading.

Authors

As you read research regularly, you will begin to recognize the research interests of particular lactation scientists who will publish several articles on aspects of a limited scope of problems. Many times, you can acquire a good reference list on a single topic just by knowing a few researchers' names and noting the references in their articles. If you do not have a library to perform a computer search and do not have Internet access, you can build your own library of articles by authors' names. This will help when you are preparing a presentation or documenting the need for a practice change.

Abstract

Most journals ask authors to write a brief summary of (1) the reason the study was done, (2) a description of the main subjects and methods, (3) the findings, and (4) the conclusion. This **abstract** is often the best guide for deciding whether the entire article is worth reading. Although it will not answer all of your questions about the study, it will indicate what the authors thought was most important about their study. Abstracts vary in length and format, and from one journal to another. Each journal sets its own requirements.

Introduction

Usually, the authors will spend a few paragraphs explaining why they chose to study the problem cited in the article. Many studies are supported by funding from a particular source. The authors will need to justify their acceptance of funding from the source, and that kind of justification is often contained in the introduction. You may also find clues to why the authors made certain decisions, such as why they only studied infants under 6 weeks old, or collected data only during a particular season.

Review of the Literature

The purpose of this section of the article is to explain the issues surrounding the problem studied. It will review research that was conducted in the past. Many funding sources will not support a study on a question that previously has been addressed many times. Therefore, the researcher must identify some aspect of the problem that has not been covered or demonstrate that past research has not clarified an important aspect. The literature review narrows down the subject of interest. It cites previous studies and their findings, and shows how the current study is different or better. Authors sometimes will also explain weaknesses of past studies that are corrected in the current study.

In some journals, (the *New England Journal of Medicine*, for example), the review of the literature is combined with an introduction. There may not even be a heading to identify this first part of the article. Nearly all articles contain a discussion of the research problem and of past studies before they begin to explain the current research. Literature reviews could be very long, and journals usually want them to be limited to the most relevant studies. If you read such a review and do not find a study cited there that you know was published, space considerations could be the main reason.

Methods

The goal of the methods section is to tell the reader how the scientists **operationalized** the hypotheses and questions they studied. Subject recruitment is often described first. Subjects may have been asked to participate by a member of the research team who had certain criteria in mind (such as a previous preterm birth or giving birth to twins). Alternatively, subjects may have volunteered to be part of the study after hearing about it in childbirth class or a newspaper advertisement. Sometimes the study was based on charts or other records and the subjects were never aware that they were being studied. Usually, journals require that the authors tell that the study was approved by a **human subjects review group** and that the subjects gave informed consent.

Instruments

The methods section describes the **tools (instruments)** that were used to measure the outcome under study. The instrument may be a written questionnaire or survey, an electronic balance scale, a chemical test, biopsy, or ultrasound. The authors often explain a lot of detail about the methods, and the difference in results between two studies may be explained by differences in the measurement instruments. For example, a milk sample collected early in a feed will not have the same proportion of hindmilk as a sample from a breast that was drained more fully. One study takes early samples of milk and finds low vitamin A levels. The other study takes a sample after a complete feed and finds higher vitamin A content. The difference might be due to the greater fat content in the complete feed sample because vitamin A is fat soluble.

Definition of Terms

The methods section defines the terms that are used in the study. When the authors include "breastfeeding" dyads, they need to define what they mean by breastfeeding. Was it exclusive breastfeeding or partial breastfeeding, or both? Did they ask mothers about the amount of formula the baby consumed, or did they actually measure it?

Statistical Methods

Statistical methods used are usually outlined in the methods section. The authors will tell what methods they used and why they chose those particular ones. They may explain that they applied more than one statistical test to the data to strengthen the conclusions. This can be the least familiar part of the article to read. However, if you keep track of statistical terminology, you can develop a list of tests that you can look up in a text. Some texts that explain statistics without using calculus are listed in Appendix B.

Results

The most important study results are often displayed in graphs, tables, or charts. The title of the table or graph will explains its topic. Statistical significance of results will be explained in the key below the table. Another helpful use of tables is to summarize information about the subjects. Tables often compare the experimental group to the **control group** on relevant characteristics.

Most authors will phrase their results very carefully. Because their article has been through **peer review**, they usually cannot claim findings that are not fairly well supported by the work they present. However, reading only the results or the abstract of a study can limit the reader's understanding of both the general problem and this particular study's approach to it. Many clinicians are tempted to read just the results because it seems like so much work to wade through the methods. The effort to understand the methods, though, may prevent clinicians from inappropriately adopting a recommended change in practice that does not really fit their clinical practice well. The results of a study, in other words, need to be read in the context of the rest of the article so that the findings can be judged based on the specifics of that study.

Discussion

The discussion is the easiest part of the article to read. The authors review their reason for conducting the study, review more of the relevant literature, sum up their most important results and then suggest applications and further research. They also explain any weaknesses or problems with the project. Some of these explanations are in response to the comments of peer reviewers. These can be very helpful to the reader who is too unfamiliar with a particular area of research to think of alternative methods or interpretations. Although the earlier parts of the article are fairly standard and are prescribed by the journal itself, the discussion shows more of the authors' thinking and creativity. By the time a study is complete and ready for publication, the researchers have raised many questions in their own minds, and they often explore them in the discussion.

References, Literature Cited, and Bibliography

In this final section you will find the articles the authors cite in their review of the literature. It will also include any article that was cited in their methods section if they used a method described in a different article. Many journals also will permit the listing of additional articles related to the main topic.

CRITICAL READING OF A SCIENTIFIC ARTICLE

This discussion of critical reading will suggest an order in which to read the parts of an article. As you acquire more experience, you will create your own approach. For beginners, it might be helpful to use this standard approach with the first several articles you read. Using this method will also help you compare in a defined way the strengths and weakness of a study. This will improve your ability to determine why they differ in their findings and clarify why you find a particular study unsatisfying.

Critical reading is not a process that can be fully captured in a "recipe" format. If it were, you and another reader would come to the same conclusions every time. Rather, you will find that not only will you differ from other readers, but if you reread an article at a later time, you may assess its strengths and weaknesses differently than the first time you read it. This is where the fun lies in critical reading, in the challenge of the puzzles the science investigates.

Some readers will be frustrated that they cannot clearly label a given study as "good" or "bad" and either reject it entirely or apply every finding. Most studies are a mixture of well done science and things that could have been done better. Honest investigators admit this in the discussion section. These imperfections reveal the nature of science. Science is a process, not a body of facts written in a textbook. The evidence for or against "truth" accumulates over time, as the result of many imperfect studies. Clinicians who want to find the best science to use in their practice will find that they must keep reading because there is no final story. Following the development of our human understanding of a particular problem is fascinating and exciting once you are familiar with the tools scientists use to share their work with one another.

Following the discussion of critical reading, you will be guided through the reading of two mock articles. Using the format described, you will be asked to stop and answer each question for yourself as you progress through the article. You will get more out of this process if you actually try to be critical at each stage rather than just reading the answers the text provides (of which you should also be critical!). Finally, some general themes of critical reading will be presented. They are not the final words on the subject. Your own experiences are valuable, too. Expect to grow as a reader and a clinician from your continuing efforts to consider the science of lactation carefully. The steps to critical reading are discussed in the following sections.

◄ Step 1: Look at the Title

A well-written title will indicate the subject of the article. From reading the title, determine what you expect the article to present. Sometimes, a title may lead your thinking along one track and the article turns out to ac-

tually be about a different facet than you were expecting. If you are aware of what you were expecting, you can adjust more readily to what the authors really meant.

Next consider what you already know about this subject. Try to be specific in terms of the knowledge you have from other studies you have read or from textbooks, lectures, and experience. Do you know, for example, that sore nipples usually decrease by day 5 to 10 postpartum? Do you know that in the Hispanic community, support for breastfeeding from the mother's mother may be more important than support from her baby's father? Have other sources taught you that immunoglobulins are decreased by processing at high temperatures?

Taking time to review what you know will help you notice discrepancies between your knowledge and what the authors claim later in the article. There may be legitimate reasons for those discrepancies. The scientists have learned something new, for instance. Your reading will be more critical if you identify your own knowledge before you begin. Usually, this does not take very long. You may have chosen to read the article because of its importance for a problem that already interests you and that you have encountered several times in practice. What you already know about it will be fairly easy to recall. With new subject matter, your knowledge will be limited, so that review does not take very long either!

You then can conjecture how you would have studied the topic. If you are new to reading research, you may not have many ideas. But try this step anyway. If the topic is breastfeeding twins, where would you go to find subjects? Would you want any specific age of twins? Would gender of the babies be relevant? If the mothers had two other children, would that change the findings? If the twins had been born before 35 weeks, could that complicate the causes of problems you are studying? Do you really need to find twins who received very little food other than human milk? For the question you are asking, is it possible to do an experiment, or can you simply observe mothers and babies who have made their own choices? Will it be fairly easy to come up with 20 or more twin sets who meet the criteria? Or is the problem so unusual that the numbers of subjects will be small? Is this a problem that happens in one ethnic or cultural group more than others? If so, do you want to do a comparative study or focus more on just the one group? The more such questions you can ask yourself about how you would have done the study, the more readily you will grasp the significance of the choices the researchers made.

What should result from this brief review is a short list of aspects you expect to find in the study. For example, you may expect the study to include both first-time breastfeeders and experienced ones. Or, you may expect it to include only preterm infants weighing over 2500 g. If the result turns out to be different from your expectations, you will be very interested in the reasons. This may lead you to uncover a deficiency in the study.

Step 2: Read the Authors' Names

Noting author names is especially helpful if you have read a previous work by the author or authors and found the work to contain a problem. You will want to determine whether or not the authors corrected the problem in this study. If the authors have studied a related problem previously in a way that you thought was valuable, you will be alerted to any changes in their methods or focus. If you have never read work by these authors, noting their names will give you a reference point for future reading.

Step 3: Read the Abstract

Reading the abstract will be the first point at which your identified assumptions about what the study is about or who it includes may be supported or contradicted. The abstract should briefly tell you the main characteristics of the subjects and methods. If the study's colicky babies are older than 6 months of age, and you wanted help for 6-week-old infants, you may stop right then and look for a different article. If the title proclaims the article to be about treating engorgement but does not include cabbage leaves, you will want to read the introduction and literature review to determine why it was omitted.

The article may report a finding that contradicts what you know about the subject. It is hoped that this will not cause you to stop reading. Sometimes lactation consultants think an article that reports such results cannot possibly be correct. The assumption may be that the scientists must have done something wrong. The results alone cannot answer that question. It takes more reading to determine whether the contrary findings are justifiable or not. Reading the abstract will alert you to the importance of specific aspects of the study that may justify the unexpected findings.

The abstract may also give you your first hint of the recommendations that the investigators believe are warranted by their results. Knowing the direction in which they want to apply their findings prepares you to read for specific inclusions or exclusions in their work. For example, they may state in the abstract that they believe all new mothers should be given a videotape on positioning to take home with them. You may want to determine whether or not they included any low-income women in their study. They may suggest that all new mothers need a visit from a lactation consultant before discharge. You may question whether they measured the

lactation knowledge of the nursing staff or whether they included any mothers who had nursed several babies. Lactation consultants can learn as much from mothers as the other way around!

Reading the abstract will heighten your awareness of what the scientists believe is most important about their study. The abstract does not include much rationale for decisions made by the investigators. You must read the entire study for that. However, questioning while you read the abstract will help you get more out of the article itself.

Step 4: Study the Tables and Graphs

Make a quick overview of the tables and graphs to determine how many there are, their titles, and whether they are understandable. For each one, ask yourself why the authors chose to put this particular information in a summary form. Often, the reason is that it saves space. Sometimes, it is because they want to highlight an unusual aspect of their sample, method, or results. If a treatment produced a dramatic improvement in the patients' problems, for example, a graph may show that most clearly. Take special note of graphs or tables that display results you consider to be minor while ignoring results that seem to be more important. You may become aware of a **bias** in such a presentation. Also ask yourself if the table agrees with the text. This seems very basic. However, sometimes the text will portray one picture and the table another. If you cannot explain this in a plausible way, it may be a flaw in the article or an editorial error.

Step 5: Read the Results

Read the results to get firmly in your mind what the authors claim to find. You need to understand their claims in order to read about their methods effectively. Pay particular attention to the subjects in the study and the relationships between **variables**.

Subjects

Within the results, you want to identify the subjects who actually ended up in the study. Perhaps they intended to include half first-time breastfeeding mothers and half experienced breastfeeding mothers. This section of the article will tell you what their final sample was. You will then need to decide whether it was an appropriate sample for the question they were asking. You also need to decide whether the results they found are justified based on the kind of subjects they actually acquired. Most researchers try very hard to anticipate a certain number of study dropouts. However, they are sometimes unlucky (or they planned poorly) and more subjects drop out from one of their groups than from the others. Consider whether their results could have been different if their original plan had worked. Dropouts can affect the results. Some leave the study because their problem was solved quickly and they no longer needed the treatment. Some leave because there are side effects of the treatment that they cannot tolerate. Others drop out because the research process is a burden. Additionally, in our mobile society, some families move before they complete a study.

Consider the implications of each reason for dropping out of the study. If those dropouts had remained in the study, might the findings have been different? Suppose a study of women who returned to employment at 6 weeks postpartum was trying to determine what factors made it likely that they would continue breastfeeding to 12 weeks. One factor to study might be employer support. The researchers might enroll women in the hospital who were planning to return to work at 6 weeks and yet continue nursing until at least 12 weeks. If a few women dropped out because they expected lack of support from their employer, the remaining subjects would disproportionately include more mothers who expected support from their employers. It would then be likely that both those who continued and those who stopped expected support. This might lead the researchers to conclude that there was no difference between them in the support. In reality, a higher proportion of those who expected no support simply left the study. The dropouts caused the study to suffer from **homogeneity** with respect to employer support, so no difference in the "employer" factor could be detected.

Relationships

The investigators will usually tell you that their study found a relationship between two or more variables. For example, they may have found a relationship between giving discharge packs containing formula to new mothers and early discontinuation of breastfeeding. The discharge packs are the **independent variable** and the duration of breastfeeding is the **dependent variable**. Think about all the logical steps they need to have established to substantiate that finding.

The Data Needs to Be Consistent with the Claims

In the discharge pack example, this might be: More of the mothers who received packs need to have stopped breastfeeding earlier than did the mothers who did not receive packs. The number of mothers who stopped compared with those who continued needs to be significantly different in a statistical sense—**statistically significant**. It also needs to be convincingly different to you. Similarly, "early" weaning must be meaningfully different than "late" weaning.

There Must Be No Other Equal or Better Explanation

In the discharge pack example, this might be that the data ruled out the following possible competing explanations in the discharge pack group:

- More mothers with sore nipples
- A higher proportion of preterm infants
- More mothers who only intended to breastfeed 6 weeks or less

Ruling out these possible explanations makes it more likely that the discharge pack itself is the cause of the early weaning.

There Must Be a Plausible Mechanism That Links the Two Variables

In the discharge pack example, the mechanism for this causation might be that a discharge pack is a subtle signal to the mother that her health care professionals do not really believe she can make sufficient milk for her baby. Because she then doubts the adequacy of her milk supply, she weans early.

The first time you read the results section, you can try to say in your own words what these three steps are according to the article. Determine whether the results are what the authors expected based on their theories and hypotheses. Before you read the article any further, get the results clear in your mind, whether those results were predicted or not.

Step 6: Read the Methods (or Subjects and Methods)

The topics covered in this section are the most important to your critical reading because they determine whether or not the authors can justify their conclusions. The design of the study, the definitions of terms, the tools for measurement, and the statistical tests all contribute to your evaluation and are covered in the next section.

Design of the Study

There are several shorthand ways of describing the design of the study to a scientific audience. When you recognize these basic study designs, you are able to understand aspects of subject selection, data gathering, and comparisons that are drawn. You also will know the kinds of conclusions that are warranted by the study's design.

Retrospective Study

A **retrospective study** uses two comparison groups. The cases have the problem of interest and the **controls** do not. Designing a study by designating cases first results in a design based on **output variables**. Output variables describe the subjects after follow-up or treatment. For example, the cases might be babies readmitted to the hospital with weight loss in excess of that expected during the first week of life. The controls would be babies without such weight loss, possibly found by a search of the charts in a pediatric practice. The purpose of such a comparison might be to determine whether there were any differences in the number of feeds or stools in the first 4 days of life, or differences in the highest bilirubin level achieved that could be associated with the need for readmission. Such a retrospective study is also called a **case-control study**.

When the methods section declares that the design is retrospective, you would expect to read a description of the groups chosen for comparison. You then would want to decide whether the groups were appropriate. Retrospective studies depend a lot on records that were kept before the study was conducted. If a retrospective study concluded that babies who had stooled only once during their first 24 hours were at higher risk of readmission, you would want to know whether the record-keeping of stools passed was accurate. In a retrospective study, the use of existing records may be all that is possible. The evidence gained from such a study may not be as strong as when the record-keeping is more deliberate and planned.

Prospective Study

In a **prospective study,** subjects are sampled based on input variables that are believed to influence the outcomes. A prospective study might be one in which the authors had held staff education classes and designed new record-keeping tools before data collection began. From the starting date forward in time, the staff would be asked to keep especially careful count of the number—and, perhaps color and size—of the stools on a certain **cohort** of babies designated as infants born from January 1 to June 30, 2000. If the number of stools was found to be related to the risk of readmission for weight loss, there would be greater confidence in this prospective study than in the retrospective one. The researchers ensured the accuracy of data collection before the study. Prospective studies are also called **cohort studies**.

Cross-sectional Study

A **cross-sectional study** relies on record-keeping or memory much as a retrospective study does. However, an affected group is not identified first. Rather, data is gathered from everyone at the same time. Let's say we wanted to do the study about stooling and readmission rates in a cross-sectional design. Data collection might then be done at the time of all infants' two-month visits. After data is gathered, the affected group (those who had been re-admitted, in this example) are identified.

The information about their stools, feeds, and bilirubin is compared to the unaffected group. Cross-sectional studies are adequate for suggesting causative factors and relevant variables. Confidence in their findings is limited by the possibility that the data collection was too dependent on recall or missed too many possible subjects on the collection day or days.

Descriptive Study

A **descriptive study** will list many relevant variables of a defined sample rather than compare two groups. A family practice office might want to know the characteristics of its childbearing families before designing a preconception class. The study might describe how many families in the previous year had borne a first child, how many had had a second child, how many had breastfed and for how long, and so on. Even though the information was gathered from one particular sample, its findings might be published so that other family practices with similar types of families might benefit from the information. In descriptive studies, it is very important that the sample be described thoroughly and carefully, so that readers know the degrees of similarity and difference between their own groups of families and the one studied.

Qualitative Study

Another type of descriptive study is the **qualitative study**. Researchers in this type of study will observe subjects and events in a natural setting rather than establishing a control. These researchers are often looking for the meaning of an event or practice to the person experiencing it. Variables in a qualitative study usually are not measured in numbers, and differences between variables are not expressed numerically. Qualitative variables are often words that the researcher believes will change together, that is, category labels. For example, as "ethnic heritage" changes so does the "critical support person." The emphasis in qualitative research is on getting a sense of the whole or comprehending the emergent properties of an experience instead of breaking down a phenomenon or experience into parts. Qualitative studies in breastfeeding, for instance, have described the feelings of women who breastfed a child for several years as well as the empowerment of low-income women through breastfeeding. When you are evaluating such studies, you can use the more general ideas in this chapter. In addition, because qualitative work by itself does not claim that practice should change in a particular way, qualitative research critique is discussed separately later in the chapter.

Experiments and Trials

In research about breastfeeding, it is less common to find studies designed as **experiments**. Problems that involve humans are difficult to conduct as experiments.

However, comparisons of equipment or differences between animals might be studied experimentally. The best information about a problem that involves humans comes from studies called **randomized clinical trials**. They are similar to experiments. These trials attempt to avoid bias in the comparisons they draw. If the trial is also **blinded,** then knowledge of which treatment the patient received is kept secret until analysis of the data is begun. In that way, the patient's or lactation consultant's assessment of the effectiveness of treatment is not influenced by knowing to which treatment group the patient belonged. Also, the treatment groups are as similar as possible to one another at the beginning of the study. A big effort is made to identify any differences that do exist. Furthermore, in the randomized clinical trial, the treatment groups were treated the same in all ways except for the treatment itself.

Suppose there were a new drug to eliminate mastitis caused by yeast. To conduct a blinded study, the new and old drugs would be disguised, perhaps in identical capsules, and taken in the same manner. In that way, no one could tell which was which. Only a system of codes would be able to detect the difference for later analysis. Both groups are first time breastfeeders of babies 2 to 6 months old who are otherwise healthy. Therefore, the groups are as similar as possible. The mastitis is diagnosed and its severity graded by strict criteria and by the same two clinicians for all the subjects. Recommendations for other aspects of treatment (pain relief, treatment of baby, and so on) are the same for all subjects. In a tightly controlled study like this, differences in cure rates between the two drugs are more likely to be attributable to the drugs than in a case-control or other less controlled study.

There are several reasons why more studies are not blinded, randomized trials. First, ethical concerns preclude **random assignment** of people to potentially poorer treatments. Second, it is difficult to control many of the variables about people that result in comparison groups of humans who are different in many ways. Third, very large numbers of subjects are needed when a trial attempts to study prevention of problems. Fourth, precision in measuring "soft" outcomes—such as quality of mother-child attachment—is lower. Funding and recognition for researchers tend to be greater when their study outcomes are "harder" and more quantifiable. Your critical analysis of clinical trials involves judgments about whether the important variables were adequately identified and controlled.

Definitions

You will need to identify, for yourself, the important terms used in the article. These will be the key concepts the study is about. They may include *breastfeeding, supplementation, multipara, infant, pain, treatment, exer-*

cise, and so on. In this section of the article, the authors should define these terms clearly enough that you know who or what was included and excluded. If the authors have studied only multiparas, were they women with previous breastfeeding experience? Or was it assumed they had previously breastfed without specifically asking them? If they were experienced breastfeeders, does it matter—to the study's conclusions—whether the previous experience was positive or negative? Does the age of the multiparas matter? What about their experience coping with other stressful situations or child rearing problems? All multiparas are not the same. You will need to keep in mind what the results were and consider how the definition of multipara in the study might affect the results. All of the possible differences in multiparas are variables. Critically reading the definitions includes being able to state how a different or clearer definition could change the results or the interpretation of the results.

Tools (Instruments)

Scales for weighing babies, survey questions, diet diaries, and pain ratings are examples of tools. Some tools can be intimidating because you are not familiar with them. You may not be able to fully critique the tool if it is new to you. Still, you want to read through it because you may encounter similar tools in later reading. Also, you will need to have some basic idea of how a defined term was measured in order to decide its applicability to your situation.

In the better studies, the tool will have been tested. Good tools should measure the dependent variable consistently. The **reliability** of the measurement from one time to the next may be reported as part of the reason the investigators chose to use this tool. Authors may assume some familiarity with the type of tool without explaining the general type in a lot of detail. For example, they would expect health care professionals to know what a **Likert scale** is and how a pulse **oximeter** is used. Although they do not describe their Likert scale in detail, they should tell how it is different from others (whether it is a 5-point or a 7-point scale, for example). They should also tell whether the pulse oximeter was placed on a finger or toe. Any details about the tool itself or how it was used should be described clearly so that you do not have serious questions about whether the quirks of their method are more responsible for their results than the explanation for the results that they expound.

It is not necessary that the authors publish the entire tool in the article. Its length, developmental status, or potential profitability may prevent its publication. Examples or short versions of a survey's questions may help you decide whether the tone or complexity of the questions could have influenced the way subjects answered them. If you have serious concerns about the quality of the questions, you can often write to the authors through the journal and request more information. Even if you agree with the study's conclusions, you may not want to use the study in a formal presentation until you have learned more about the tool so that you can adequately answer you audience's questions.

Operationalizing

When you put together the definitions and the tools, you should understand how the researchers operationalized their concepts. Suppose they are studying the change in pain after the application of a treatment. They should tell you how they define pain. Often, it will be the subject's verbal or written report of her pain. Alternatively, the definition might involve videotaping subjects before and after the treatment, and watching for changes in facial expression. Each different definition of pain will be measured by a different tool. The tool for verbal reports might be a 10-point scale in which the **anchors** (words used at specific points on the scale to describe what that number means) are "1 = no pain" and "10 = the worst pain you can imagine." You can then understand that the researchers operationalized the concept "pain" by asking the subject herself to place a mark on the scale that best represented her pain before the treatment and again at a specified time afterward.

The critical reading of this operationalization involves both the clarity of it and your judgment about its **validity**. The validity of a pain measure is often supported by expert review, or by comparing the current pain tool with an older one and finding that the two agree. Although pain is very difficult to measure because of its subjectivity, what is important is the person's own determination of the amount of pain and whether that determination changes. A scale that reflects the changes is the operationalization of pain. The construction of measurement scales is the subject of many research articles. You may want to investigate what tools have already been tested if you decide to design a scale yourself. Below are several common methodological concerns in lactation research.

Methodological Concerns in Lactation Research

◆ Uniformity of test weighing. At present, this is usually resolved by careful instruction of the people who weigh the babies and by the use of electronic balance scales.

◆ Equating volume of expressed milk to volume produced. Such volumes can be quite different unless good quality pumps are used, pumping duration is adequate, milk ejections are achieved, and time of day is accounted for.

◆ Disturbing the breastfeeding process by observing and measuring it.

◆ Obtaining a representative milk sample. Milk composition varies by length of time postpartum, time of day, proportion of breast drained, and gestation of the infant.

◆ Changing method of feeding is a one-direction change. That is, mothers do not usually switch from formula to breastfeeding (with rare exceptions). If a mother changes feeding methods, it is a change from human to artificial. So, when studies encompass babies who have been fed for any length of time, some in the group will usually have been breastfed at some point and then bottle fed. None have been fed in the reverse order. This can make it difficult to interpret growth differences. To improve growth, mothers may try to switch to formula, but they cannot switch to breastfeeding. Most researchers believe that there are ways to overcome this built-in direction, but it should be kept in mind as possibly complicating interpretation.

◆ Studies of environmental contaminants often use human milk because it is easier to obtain than blood or other body tissue, and because the milk fats promote the accumulation of some chemicals in milk. However, the media may misunderstand the use of milk, proclaiming that finding the pollutants in milk automatically means that feeding human milk is harmful.

◆ Studies of effects of breastfeeding on women's bone mineralization have sometimes been misunderstood because the time it takes to recover bone mass that was mobilized during lactation has been longer than the length of the study.

When you have read and thought about the methods, think back to the results. Do the study design, definitions, tools, and operationalizations allow for the conclusions the scientists made? How could they have done the study differently to make you believe that the conclusions were more justified? What additional information about the methods would help you evaluate the findings even more thoroughly?

Statistics

Within the methods section of the article, there is usually a brief description of the main statistical approach that was used to evaluate the data. For lactation consultants, this section may be the most difficult to decipher because the language is so specialized. As you have learned, there is a lot of meaningful critical analysis that can be done even without judging the statistical techniques used. To some extent, you must rely on the peer review process to catch any major problems in the statistics. The more you read breastfeeding research, the more you will become familiar with some of the common approaches that are used in certain research designs. The examples presented in the following sections are provided to help you understand some of these more common statistical ideas and tests.

Statistical Theory

Statistical **theory** comes from studying how chance operates when an event happens an infinite number of times. Statisticians ask, "If we flipped this coin an infinite number of times, how likely is it that the number of heads would equal the number of tails?" They also work on applications for the real world where the amount of data is less than infinite. Statistical theory tries to explain how much less accurate a test is when it is performed on only part of the infinite data. If that part is very large, the test will be more accurate. If it is very small, we cannot say as confidently that the test accurately helps make a decision.

Study Frequency

When you study the frequency of breastfeeding by mothers and their babies at 10 days of age in your city, you are studying a **sample** of the whole **population** of 10-day-old breastfed babies and their mothers (in the world, and maybe throughout human history). If your goal, in studying the frequency in this sample, was to publish in a textbook that the "normal" or "usual" or "**average**" frequency for all human babies at 10 days was X, then you would be trying to make a statement about the population by studying a sample of it. If your sample is large (500 subjects or more) there will be far less chance of an error in your estimate of X than if your sample is only 20 subjects.

Good studies will aim for the largest sample size they can reasonably get. The statistical analysis will tell what the **power** of that sample size was. Power is determined by more than sample size. However, sample size is what researchers have the most control over, so they try to maximize it. For most purposes, researchers want a power of 0.80 (80 percent) or higher. If the power of a test is low, then the reason for failing to find a significant difference between two groups could be that the sample selected was just too small for that difference to show up, not that there is no real difference. A power of 80 percent means that the data have an 80 percent probability of correctly rejecting the null hypothesis.

Statistical Tests

Statistical tests are valid only when they are applied correctly. In order to be valid, each test assumes certain things about the data. If those assumptions are not true, the test should not be used. Sometimes in the methods section there will be a brief statement about why a certain test was used and whether or not a particular assumption was met. There are few hard and fast rules in statistical analysis. Statisticians can disagree just as lactation consultants do over which should be the first solution to try.

Discussions about assumptions are often addressed to potential readers who are researchers and statisticians who might disagree with the choice of statistical test. One such discussion sometimes centers around whether or not the assumption of a **normal distribution** of the data is true. A normal distribution describes much of the infinite data we could collect about the natural world. A normal distribution, plotted on a graph, looks like a **bell curve**. Take a look at a graph entitled "How much milk the 1-month-old infant takes at a single episode at breast."

You can see that at the left end of the graph in Figure 25.1, there are a few babies who take very tiny amounts (when nursing is very frequent and short, or a "snack"). At the extreme right end, there are a few babies who take a very large amount. Most babies take somewhere around 120 ml (let's say), so in the center of the graph is the large hill (or bell) that represents what the bulk of babies do. Between the center and each extreme is a gradual **slope**.

Now, instead, suppose that the data on milk intake actually comes from a distribution that looks like the graph in Figure 25.2. Here, the bulk (greatest number of values) of the data are at one extreme, not in the middle. The left side rises quickly with a long slope off to the right. Perhaps this is a group of preterm infants at 1 month of age whose intake tends to be less than that of full-term infants. A statistical test that was attempting to predict what happens in the bulk of this distribution by expecting it to be a normal distribution would be way off. The middle in this distribution is far to the left of where it would be if the data were distributed normally. The data in Figure 25.2 would require a statistical test designed for this particular distribution. It is very impor-

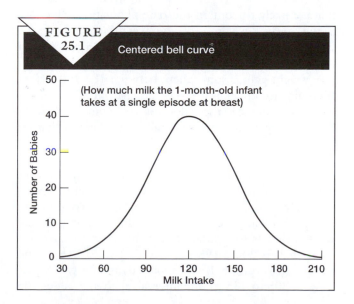

FIGURE 25.1 Centered bell curve

(How much milk the 1-month-old infant takes at a single episode at breast)

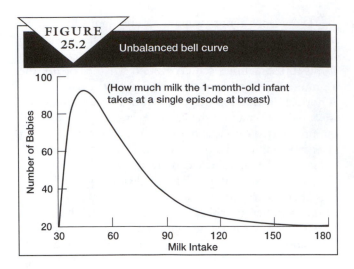

FIGURE 25.2 Unbalanced bell curve

(How much milk the 1-month-old infant takes at a single episode at breast)

tant that researchers and statisticians carefully choose which tests to use, and that they look at all the underlying assumptions, including distribution of the data.

Statistical Significance

Statistical significance, or lack of significance, is determined by applying a statistical test to a fact about the data (a result) and calculating the **probability** of obtaining that result (or a more extreme result). The probability is reported as a **p-value**. Most researchers want p-values that are 0.05 or lower. The p-value measures the risk of rejecting a true null hypothesis. Researchers only want the chance of falsely stating that there is a real difference between two groups to be 5 percent.

Confidence intervals (CIs) also provide information about the statistical significance of a result. CIs are the range within which a population's true value is expected to be found. Usually, a 95 percent CI is reported. This describes the other possible results that are close to the one that actually came from the data, and that are likely to contain the **true** population value. So, if the **mean** (average) of the weight gain from the study's sample was, say, 200 g and the 95 percent CI was 185 to 215 g, then it is likely that the population's true weight gain is somewhere between 185 and 215 g. If confidence intervals are very large (from 50 to 350 g, for this example), they do not tell you very much. Nearly every weight gain will fall somewhere in that interval, so you cannot tell the difference between a usual one and a more extreme one.

Large confidence intervals often arise when the sample size is small. Furthermore, if you are trying to compare, for example, the weight gains in two different groups and you expect them to be different, you do not want their CIs to overlap. So, if the mean for group A (breastfed) is 200 g (95 percent CI 185 to 215 g) and the mean for group B (formula-fed) is 220 g (95 percent CI 205 to 235 g), the intervals share the values 205

to 215 g. These shared values mean that the real average weight gain could be the same for both groups. These confidence intervals would not allow you to claim you had found a statistically significant difference between the two groups. (See "**odds ratio**" below, for one more example of the use of a confidence interval.)

Common Statistical Tests and Terms

This section on common statistical tests and terms is intended to help you understand some of the tests you are most likely to encounter. For greater depth, you can consult a statistics text such as one listed in Appendix B.

Chi-square. There are several slightly different versions of the Chi-square test. It is usually used to determine whether the proportions in two groups are significantly different. You may want to determine, for example, if the proportion of experienced breastfeeders who have mastitis is the same as the proportion of first-time breastfeeders who have mastitis. Large Chi-square values usually lead to low, statistically significant p-values.

Cohen's Kappa. The kappa is calculated when two observers rate the same event on a scale and the researcher wants to show that the two raters are in close agreement. Values at 0.7 or higher are considered good.

Cronbach's Alpha. A Cronbach's alpha test is often reported when the researcher is trying to give evidence of the reliability of an instrument. Values can range from 0.0 to 1.0, and the closer they are to 1.0, the better the reliability.

Odds Ratio. Odds ratio is not a statistical test. Rather, it is a way to summarize the relative proportion of illness in two different groups. For example, you may want to compare the proportion of breastfed babies who get otitis media with the proportion of artificially fed babies who do, under certain similar conditions. If you found that 2 out of 10 breastfed babies got otitis and 4 out of 10 formula-fed babies did, the ratio of those odds is 0.2/0.4 = 0.5. The odds of the breastfed baby getting an ear infection were one-half the odds of the baby who missed out on human milk's protection. The only way an odds ratio could equal 1 is if the odds for both groups are the same. CIs for odds ratios might be written like this: "0.5 (95% CI, 0.35–0.60)." This means that the best estimate of the odds ratio could be anywhere from 0.35 to 0.60. Significant CI for the odds ratio should not contain "1" (0.90–1.05, for example) because that would mean the odds ratio could be 1. This is another way of saying that the odds for the breastfed baby could have been the same as the odds for the artificially fed baby. In studies comparing breastfed and bottle-fed infants and differing risks, we hope to find that the breastfed babies had less risk.

Regression. Regression is a technique used to try to understand the relationship between variables. Simple regression relates one **predictor variable** (or independent variable) to one **outcome variable** (or dependent variable). Multiple regression relates several variables to one outcome variable. **Logistic regression** relates one or more variables to a **dichotomous outcome** (two-possibility) variable. This addresses a question such as "Do maternal satisfaction, infant weight gain, and family support with the first breastfed child relate to the decision to breastfeed or not breastfeed (dichotomous outcome) the next child?" Usually, regression methods try to estimate how much change there is in the outcome variable for a one-unit change in the predictor variable. For example, "How much change occurs in infant crying time for each additional half-hour of being carried in a baby sling?"

T-test. The t-test is used to decide between two contradictory hypotheses about the mean of a sample. For example, you may want to know if the average weight gain of breastfed infants in Hospital A is the same as the average weight gain for breastfed babies in the United States (where the national average is often considered a "norm" or "true" population value). A slightly different t-test could be used to compare the average gain of babies in Hospital A with that of babies in Hospital B.

◢ Step 7: Read the Introduction and Literature Review

You now will read the introduction and literature review to understand some of the decisions the researchers made in light of the results they found and the methods they used. You can ask yourself whether the authors' justification for doing the study seems adequate to you. Most articles start out by stating that some expert bodies recognize the superiority of breastfeeding. They may then say that, although breastfeeding by all mothers would be preferable, there is such-and-such a problem that prevents near-universal breastfeeding. They might claim that their study is going to address that problem, shed light on it, and help move humankind toward more breastfeeding. Often, they explain and reference the **theory** underlying their approach to the problem and the **hypothesis** they want to test. Somewhere in this line of reasoning is the explicit or implicit statement of why the authors chose this particular problem to study.

The literature review is used to show how their study is different from what has been done before and how their study is an improvement. If they have done a good job of this reasoning, they will convince you that (1) the problem is significant, (2) no one has adequately addressed it before, and (3) their approach is superior.

You can use your experience and your reading of other articles and books to decide whether or not they have convinced you of this. The questions to ask yourself are discussed in the next section.

Questions to Ask Yourself About the Literature Review

1. Do you think that this is a significant problem? Have they explained why? If you were a professional who is interested, but not very experienced, in lactation, would their explanation be convincing?

2. Are their summaries of the articles that they cite to explain their study accurate? If you know the studies they cite, did they do a good job of stating the conclusions? If you know any of the studies, do you think they are appropriate ones to use? For example, if the new study you are reading is about colic-like symptoms in fully breastfed babies, but the cited studies included partially breastfed babies, what parts can legitimately be compared and what parts have to be different? Suppose the new study wants to use removal of dairy products from the mother's diet as a treatment. That could be a clear change in an exclusively breastfed baby's diet. But in a baby who is also receiving some cow's milk formula, a comparable change in diet would need to have included removal of the formula. On the other hand, the older study may have found that firstborn infants suffered more colic-like symptoms and the new study might want to examine birth order. That aspect of both studies would be more similar than exposure to cow's milk because birth order is not directly related to cow's milk or maternal diet. If you do not know any of the studies cited, you will not be as able to judge their appropriateness. You will grow in your ability to do this as you read more.

3. Did they omit any studies that you would have included? Do you know about previous research (even if you do not know the exact title or authors' names) that also addresses this problem but that the authors left out? If it is an area of research in which a lot of studies have been done, that could happen due to lack of space alone. But it may happen by design if the authors do not want to mention contrary studies, especially if those studies rejected what the authors want to do. Leaving out relevant studies may also result from an inadequate literature search. However, usually peer reviewers would demand that prospective authors read and include the most important articles. Leaving out relevant studies may not be too damaging to readers who know the background information well. For those who do not, a misleading picture of the state of knowledge can be portrayed.

4. Are the methods that were used in previous studies explained fully enough that you can judge whether the authors' use or rejection of them in the new study is appropriate? For example, in a past study of infection rates in children who attend day care versus those who do not attend day care, the literature review may describe the use of "written parental diaries" as the method. The authors may tell you that they propose to use the same method, having parents record weekly whether the child had fever, sore throat, medical visits, and so on. Suppose, in the results, they find that children in day care have no different infection rates than stay-at-home children. It could be that they failed to tell you that, in the older study, parents recorded symptoms on a daily basis and received biweekly calls and cards to remind them to do so. That may explain why the older study found differences in rates while the new study does not. You are looking for ways in which the current study is different from and similar to the older studies that are cited in the literature review. The authors should be clear about those aspects that are relevant to the current study.

▼ **Step 8: Read the Discussion**

There usually is a link between the literature review and the discussion. This link may be explained in the beginning of the discussion section. You should ask yourself whether the intentions the researchers declared based on their review of the current state of knowledge were carried through in the methods and results. Did they do something different from the earlier cited studies? If so, was it an improvement?

In the discussion, the researchers may summarize their results in a less formal way. They may offer an interpretation of the results that puts their findings into the context of other studies that were done on the same problem. You should consider whether their findings are as important as the authors claim and whether the state of knowledge about the problem is now more complete or clear.

Speculation

The authors may further stretch the interpretation of their findings into a more speculative understanding of some aspect of the problem. An example of this would be a study that found that peanut butter and jelly sandwiches **correlated** with higher milk production. Suppose the authors had found evidence in the literature review that a chemical in peanuts could cause an appetite increase in lab animals. They put these two ideas together to suggest that the reason peanut butter

and jelly sandwiches are linked to higher milk production is that the sandwiches stimulate a bigger appetite in breastfeeding mothers who eat them. Their own study did not really look at either the chemistry of peanuts nor the overall calorie intake of mothers. But they speculate that such a causal mechanism exists. It is your job, as a critical reader, to judge how plausible, realistic, and rational that link is. You do not know if the link is correct but you need to think about whether it could be real, and whether further suggestions by the authors along this line of reasoning are worth considering.

Suggestions for Further Research

Often, the next step the researchers take is to suggest further research. Some suggestions will be to test the speculations that they have made. Other suggestions will be to fill in the gaps in the understanding of the problem that still remain in spite of the knowledge that was gained from their study.

Flaws or Weaknesses

Some of the flaws or weaknesses you have detected in reading the article may be acknowledged by the authors in the discussion. You can decide whether your assessment of the flaws (and their impact on the confidence you have in the results) is the same as that of the authors. If you think that the problems are more serious than the authors acknowledge, you will want to read their justification as generously as you can. On the other hand, if the authors fail to note a flaw you have uncovered, you should try to understand why. This may be just another opportunity to reinforce your critique, but it could be that the goal or methods as explained further in the discussion are different from your original understanding of them.

▼ **Step 9: Read the Results Again**

When you first read the results section, you were trying to understand what the authors claimed to have found. This time, you will read to decide whether you think those claims were justified. You probably have formed some judgments about this already, having read the methods and discussion. The following suggestions lead you to look even more closely at the logic of the relationships between variables that the authors claim to have found. Recall the three steps that were discussed previously:

1. The data needs to be consistent with the claims.
2. There must be no other equal or better explanation.
3. There must be a plausible mechanism that links the two variables.

Data Consistent with Claims

Is the data consistent with the claims? Consider again the example of the study testing the effect of discharge packs on the duration of breastfeeding. If the study had 100 subjects, (50 in the pack group and 50 in the nonpack group), and if 15 in the pack group weaned "early" but only 5 did in the nonpack group, is that a convincing difference to you? This difference would be statistically significant at $p < 0.05$. That is, there is only a 1 in 20 chance that a difference of 15 versus 5 (or a more extreme difference) would have occurred by chance. So, statistically speaking, it is probable that the difference between the number of early weaners in the two groups is a real difference and not a chance occurrence. But you could ask whether that difference is clinically important. Do 10 more "late" weaners out of 50 achieve enough additional health and relationship benefits to warrant discontinuing discharge packs? This question is not just about statistics but also about values. Many health care providers would probably consider this valid and important evidence against discharge packs. Skeptics, however, might say, "Well, if discharge packs are so bad, then how did 35 out of 50 of the mothers go on to wean late in spite of them?" Considering answers to such questions will help you think about the study, and formulate responses you could use if you presented this study to skeptics.

Another Possible Explanation for Relationship

Is there another possible explanation for the claimed relationship between variables? To continue looking at the logical steps, think about another way of presenting the numbers. Instead of defining "early" and 'late' and comparing the proportions in each group, suppose the average number of weeks of breastfeeding was computed in the pack group versus the nonpack group. If the study found that those who received packs breastfed 18 weeks and those who did not breastfed 20 weeks, would you think this was an important difference? This could be a statistically significant difference between the groups, depending on the group sizes and how much **variation** there was around the averages. Whenever an average (mean) is reported, you may want to know the **distribution and range** of each group's length of breastfeeding. An average can be misleading if one subject (or a small number) has an extremely short or extremely long duration. Figure 25.3 demonstrates the number of different ways a group could breastfeed for an average of 18 weeks.

Group 1 had many people who actually breastfed 18 weeks and four people who breastfeed for a shorter or longer amount of time. This is the kind of distribution in which the average gives a good representation of the typical behavior in the group. The range is $25 - 11 = 14$ weeks.

FIGURE 25.3	Ten subjects who breastfed an average of 18 weeks	
Group 1	Group 2	Group 3
25 weeks	50 weeks	29 weeks
20 weeks	19 weeks	27 weeks
18 weeks	18 weeks	26 weeks
18 weeks	17 weeks	25 weeks
18 weeks	16 weeks	24 weeks
18 weeks	16 weeks	23 weeks
18 weeks	15 weeks	22 weeks
18 weeks	14 weeks	2 weeks
16 weeks	13 weeks	1 weeks
11 weeks	2 weeks	1 weeks
180 weeks	180 weeks	180 weeks

Group 2 had only one person who breastfed the "average" length of time and two people whose duration was very different from the average (**outliers**), 2 and 50. The range in this data is 48 ($50 - 2 = 48$). The range in group 1 was smaller. You might legitimately question whether the extremes in Group 2 had much in common with the "average." Specifically, you might wonder whether the 2-week person had such a difficult problem (baby with ankyloglossia and a severe cardiac defect) that she would have breastfed only 2 weeks no matter whether or not she received a discharge pack. After asking yourself that question, you should look in the results section to determine whether or not the authors describe the mothers' reasons for weaning. If that information was not given (or even collected), the authors cannot claim that discharge packs alone made a difference in the groups.

Looking closely at the numbers to determine if they are consistent with the claims made has suggested a possible alternative explanation for the study's findings. At least a few mothers may have had an extremely difficult problem that would have led to short breastfeeding regardless of whether or not they received a pack. If these mothers' durations were excluded from the calculation of duration, the study's results might change. Of course, you cannot always know the results would change. But if the authors' own data make you suspicious, you might ultimately be less willing to accept and apply their findings.

Another example of looking closely at the "average" is the other extreme in Group 2. Suppose the mother who breastfed for 50 weeks was in the discharge pack group. You might ask, "If discharge packs are so bad, how did this woman manage to continue to breastfeed for so long?" Several possible explanations exist, and you might wonder whether the authors asked what the mothers did with the packs. Did they use them? If yes, how old was the baby? Did they discard the pack? If you read some of the real studies of discharge packs, you will find that the authors rarely ask this question. Instead, there is an assumption that mere receipt of a pack probably encourages formula use. Although this may be true, the results would be stronger if data were collected on actual use of the packs as well as formula use in the non-pack group.

In Group 3, no one breastfed to 18 weeks and there is quite a clear separation into two subgroups, one who nursed for 2 weeks or less and the other who nursed for at least 22 weeks. Such a split might make you think about the possibility of a major difference within the group. Perhaps, for example, there was a big difference in the amount of support the two subgroups received. The subgroup who breastfed longer may have had three or more support people, whereas the subgroup who breastfed less had two or fewer support people. So, although this entire group breastfed for an average of 18 weeks, that average does not well represent the real story about the group. By trying to explain the duration of breastfeeding using an average, the authors may have missed an alternative explanation for their findings related to differences in support.

Many studies try to avoid potential alternative explanations for their findings by avoiding major hidden differences between groups (like the difference in support cited earlier) through random assignment of subjects to groups. The idea is that if mothers are assigned, by chance, to receive a discharge pack or not, differences other than receipt of a pack between groups will be approximately the same in both groups. Differences that could confuse the explanation of findings are also called **confounding variables**. In randomized assignment to groups, there will be approximately the same number of multiparas, of people with good support, of people with inverted nipples, and so on, in both groups. Therefore, all the reasons they could have stopped breastfeeding early would be the same in both groups except for receipt of a discharge pack. Random assignment, then, allows researchers to conclude that the reason the women stopped breastfeeding must be that single relevant difference between the groups—receipt of a discharge pack.

The best studies go even further and check whether random assignment worked. In such studies, the authors will report whether the groups were different at **baseline** in some important ways. As a colleague, it is your responsibility to consider whether they checked on the right things. For example, if you think lack of support is really important in weaning early, did the scientists check their groups to be sure that, say, the average number of support people reported by mothers in the pack and nonpack groups was not statistically different? This checking for the differences and similarities achieved by random assignment is reported in the methods or results section. It is not possible to check for all differences. However, it is important to check for a few major ones

and it is up to you to decide whether the researchers omitted anything critical. If they did, you will be less likely to use the findings of the study.

Most articles related to the practice of helping women with breastfeeding do not have randomized groups. Rather they use a **convenience (nonprobability)** sample. So, for a study about discharge packs, the sample might be the first 100 breastfeeding mothers after the starting date (in which mothers 1 to 50 do not get packs and 51 to 100 receive packs). Checking the basic similarity of groups is even more important in convenience samples than in randomized ones.

All of the above-mentioned examples are meant to encourage you to take a close look at whatever numbers the authors present. Usually, you will find that they have chosen appropriate ways to measure and summarize their data. But you may find that you have questions about their numbers that make you reluctant to agree with their conclusions.

Tables, Graphs, and Charts

There is not enough space in many journals for the authors to present their "raw" data (the actual numbers they collected or measured). Rather, they resort to a summary of the quantitative information. This is done in tables, graphs, and charts; or it may be done statistically. Tables are often the simplest way to capture a large amount of quantitative information in concise form. The most helpful tables have a title that tells the main idea, a source of the numbers (e.g., from a survey or from patient charts), and clear labels on each column and row, including the units of measurement (i.e., ml, kg, sec, and so on). Some will also provide percentages of the total that each subgroup represents and statistical test results. You will want to evaluate tables first by their clarity of presentation. Then, as you read the article, make sure that the table agrees with the text. Pay particular attention to whether the number of subjects reported on in the tables is the same as the number described in the text. The number of subjects who gave consent to participate initially is often greater than the number who participated in any particular aspect of the study.

For example, the authors may have explained their study to several childbirth preparation classes and obtained consent from 50 couples to observe the first breastfeed. What could happen to reduce that number? Perhaps the researchers were out of town when two of the couples delivered. Two mothers may have been so tired after birthing that they refused permission to be observed. Three mothers may have decided not to breastfeed. This reduces the sample size to 43 couples. So, if you read that consent was obtained from 50 mothers, then see that the total number of observations was 43, you might need to reread the part of the article that describes what happened to the other seven couples. Remember to think about the effects of dropouts, as discussed previously. As long as the tables and text agree and any apparent discrepancies are explained, you will be able to use the information in the tables to decide if your clients or patients are similar to the ones studied. You will also be able to decide whether the tables and figures support the findings and reasoning that are claimed.

Graphs should have clear titles and labels. They should also be designed to portray the data accurately and to not be misleading. You will need to look carefully at the scale of the graph. In the graph in Figure 25.4, the scale goes from 0 to 20, so the height of the curved lines looks lower and less impressive than the height of the curves in the graph in Figure 25.5, in which the scale goes from 0 to 7. Either scale could be appropriate depending on how the pain scale itself was defined. However, the graphs create different feelings in the viewer. Because the slope or angle of the lines in Figure 25.5 is steeper than that of Figure 25.4, it appears that the change in pain was different than that shown in Figure 25.5. Actually, both are the same. So, although graphs can be very helpful, they can also be misleading. It is up to the reader to look closely.

Second, suppose this study was one in which each woman was her own control. That is, each one was randomly assigned to treat one nipple and to not treat the other. Suppose further that the authors claim that the treated nipple was in pain for less total time than the untreated nipple. Although you might agree with that conclusion, you might wonder if it was a fair test because the untreated nipple was already more painful than the treated nipple on Day One. This example is probably not what the authors would publish because it represents only one subject. You can see that the details of a graph can both clarify and confuse your understanding!

There are many additional kinds of tables, graphs, and charts. Their purposes range from summarizing

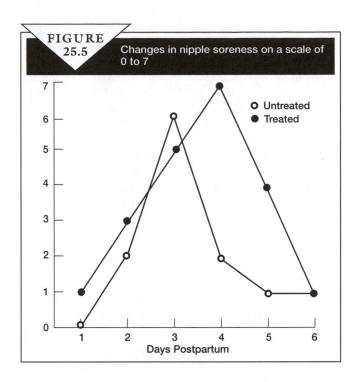

FIGURE 25.5 Changes in nipple soreness on a scale of 0 to 7

○ Untreated
● Treated

Days Postpartum

basic information to clarifying complex patterns found in the data. When you read the results to decide whether the evidence the authors present supports their claimed findings, you will want to look closely at these graphics. Critical analysis includes judging their clarity and consistency with the rest of the article.

Plausible Mechanism for Relationship

Is there a plausible mechanism for the claimed relationship between variables? This may be the most difficult of the logical steps for which to find clear evidence in the article. Sometimes authors will have addressed the reason lanolin seems to help heal sore nipples in the literature review or in the discussion section. They usually do not address this in the results section unless they have studied the possible mechanism along with the relationship between variables. For example, along with testing whether lanolin was related to faster healing, they may have taken microscopic photos of cell changes in nipple skin to see if the differences in cell changes might explain healing differences. In many studies, the mechanism itself is hypothesized and not studied directly. This is especially true when the variables are not physiologic but rather psychological or sociological.

Demonstrating a plausible mechanism for how peer support enables longer durations of breastfeeding than professional support does is not straightforward. Yet, many mechanisms for important relationships between variables related to breastfeeding are in the "not straightforward" category. Instead of dismissing research

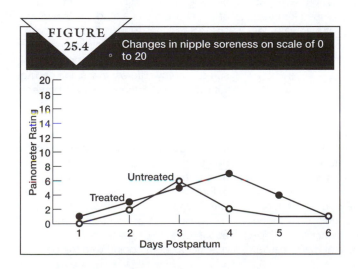

FIGURE 25.4 Changes in nipple soreness on scale of 0 to 20

Painometer Rating

Untreated

Treated

Days Postpartum

because mechanisms cannot be demonstrated convincingly, most scientists and clinicians instead require plausibility and thoughtful consideration of mechanisms. In your critical reading, you will want to consider whether a mechanism is discussed and whether you judge that mechanism to be reasonable. If there is very little consideration of how and why the variables are related as the study found them to be, you may be less likely to accept the study's findings.

Sometimes there is little discussion of mechanism because the mechanism is pretty obvious. The greatest danger in the lack of a plausible mechanism is the acceptance of a relationship that is actually **spurious**. Spurious relationships between variables are those that look statistically significant but have resulted from a correlation with no underlying meaning. Suppose that lactation consultant Lila Cecilia found that, of her last 500 clients, the ones whose babies' home nurseries were painted lavender had a statistically significantly longer duration of breastfeeding than those whose nurseries were any other color. Suppose, further, that Lila had determined that no alternative explanations adequately fit her data. She really did not know why the color of the nursery mattered but she claimed that breastfed babies should have their nurseries painted lavender. Many readers might guess that there was some explanation somewhere that Lila had just not studied hard enough. Most readers would not rush out and tell their clients to re-paint their nurseries! They would not be convinced because there is no plausible relationship between nursery color and breastfeeding duration. The numeric relationship Lila found was probably spurious.

Any time a study finds a relationship for which no plausible mechanism is discussed, it could be spurious. This most often happens when researchers just happen to notice some correlation in their data that was not the main relationship they were studying. In doing a variety of manipulations of their data, sometimes a relationship will surface that is statistically significant. Although it is considered fair to mention this "finding" in their article, it is not considered good science to claim it as a major result. Instead, mechanisms should be considered and further research should be recommended.

PRACTICING CRITICAL READING SKILLS

Now you are ready to practice using the ideas and the steps for critical reading presented earlier. Using Steps 1 through 9, read the following two mock articles in the suggested order. You will want to consider the questions presented in each section. You may find it helpful to make notes to yourself as you go through the process so that you can compare your ideas with those presented in the commentary that follows each mock article.

Sore Nipple Treatments: Gooeypaste Works Best

I.M. Wright

Journal of Supposed Things, Vol. 21, p. 5–10, 1998.

Abstract

Sore nipples are one of the obstacles many women need to overcome in order to continue breastfeeding. Thirty women began using Gooeypaste, warm water compresses, or vitamin E oil when their nipples became sore. After 3 days, Gooeypaste provided more pain relief than the other treatments as measured on the Pain Relief Self-Rating. Gooeypaste should become the standard treatment for breastfeeding-related nipple soreness.

Introduction

Breastfeeding is acknowledged by health care professionals worldwide as the best way to feed infants.[2-4] However, women who intend to breastfeed for many weeks or months are sometimes stopped by the development of nipple soreness, which makes breast-feeding intolerable.[4-5] No single measure or combination of measures has been found to reliably reduce pain and increase healing. Although prevention is surely the best policy, the need for treatment is evident. This study was designed to investigate the effectiveness of a new product against two standard treatments.

Review of the Literature

Pain with breastfeeding has been shown to be an important reason for early weaning in several studies[1,4,5] and may include pain due to engorgement or candidiasis as well as sore nipples. Positioning is important to the prevention of soreness. Sometimes, comfortable positioning is not achieved with the first few feeds and, by then, enough nipple damage is done that pain results.

Also, nipple pain may occur later in the breastfeeding relationship when the baby tries to interact with the world at the same time as he feeds, or when solid foods are introduced. Cando and associates[6] found that warm water compresses applied for 15 minutes after every feed relieved pain better than two other measures. In a study by Workhard and colleagues[7] vitamin E oil felt soothing to mothers with nipple soreness.

Relief from pain has been measured in many different ways. In keeping with Ouchless's[8] theory of pain perception, tools that measure the patient's perception of pain were reviewed for possible use. The Painometer, a self-rated 5-question scale, was believed to be the most convenient for a busy, new mother to use. The scale has been used before in postoperative patients and was found to correlate with the use of medication. In addition to the questions about degree of pain, there are three questions about coping with the pain.

Table 25.1
The Subjects of the Study

	Gooeypaste	Warm Water	Vitamin E Oil
Maternal age (mean)	22.3 yrs	25.3 yrs	24.2 yrs
Breastfed previous baby	8	5	4*
Female infants	5	7	3
Infant birthweight (mean)	3500 g	3405 g	3200 g
Number of infants who had alternative feedings prior to starting the study	1	2	3

*No statistically significant differences between groups, $p = 0.15$.

In Helpful Hospital's Mother-Baby Unit, obstetricians prescribed vitamin E oil for routine use by breastfeeding mothers. Some nurses encouraged mothers to use warm water, but mothers' actual use of these products and the relief provided by them had never been evaluated. When the new product, Gooeypaste, developed by Phunny Pharmaceuticals, became available, the staff decided it was time to conduct a study.

Subjects and Methods

Table 25.1 describes the subjects of the study. Subjects were recruited from the Mother-Baby Unit on the day of their postpartum stay when they first began to develop sore nipples. Except for mothers who had undergone cesarean births, most were discharged between 24 and 48 hours. When a nurse identified a mother with soreness who agreed to participate in the study, an envelope was pulled from the enrollment drawer. The envelopes were in random order (10 envelopes each for warm water, vitamin E oil, and Gooeypaste) and each contained instructions for the mother and nurse on which treatment was to be used. It also contained three copies of the Painometer that the mother was to complete at 24, 48, and 72 hours after she first started using her assigned treatment.

While the subjects were hospitalized, nurses reminded them to complete the scale. The nurses collected them and stored them anonymously with codes that identified the treatment used and whether this was the 24-, 48-, or 72-hour scale. For subjects who went home before all scales were completed (this included almost all subjects), nurses called mothers to remind them to complete the scales and return them in the envelopes provided. If the mother seemed especially unlikely to return her scales, nurses asked mothers the scale's questions over the phone and recorded them. Results were analyzed by **odds ratios** for the odds of experiencing less pain by Day 3 or not. Also, the mother's responses on the questions about coping were analyzed by comparing means.

Results

Thirty new mothers agreed to participate in the study. Of these, 28 went home before they completed all the scales. All mothers were called at the appropriate follow up times for reminders. As a result, all 30 had completed scales for all three measurement times.

For 15 of the mothers, pain worsened from 24 to 48 hours after the first treatment. Three of those were using Gooeypaste, 5 warm water, and 7 vitamin E oil. Pain stayed the same for 2 mothers from each group. It improved for 5 of the mothers using Gooeypaste, 3 using warm water, and 1 using vitamin E oil. By 72 hours, 8 of the mothers using Gooeypaste noted improvement, whereas 6 using warm water, and 4 using vitamin E oil reported improvement in pain.

The odds ratio for decreased pain at 72 hours comparing Gooeypaste to vitamin E was 1.3. The odds ratio comparing Gooeypaste to warm water was 2.0. Both were statistically significant at $p < 0.05$.

The average score for optimism was higher in the Gooeypaste group than in the other treatment groups. (see Table 25.2). Although that trend was nonsignificant, optimism remains an important part of pain relief.

Discussion

Although this is a small study, Gooeypaste appears to be an important measure to consider for the treatment of sore nipples. Further studies with larger groups of patients are needed to confirm these findings. Because the Gooeypaste mothers were also more optimistic, they will probably go on to breastfeed in greater numbers to meet their personal goals. The nursing staff at Helpful Hospital is currently working with the obstetric staff to include Gooeypaste as an alternative treatment for sore nipples in breastfeeding mothers.

References

1. Healthy World Alliance. Breastfeeding best for babies *HWA* 56:123–125; 1990.
2. Bet U and Wynn R. Nutrition experts endorse breastfeeding. *Nutrition Group Reports* 25:2–5; 1966.

Table 25.2
Pain Score

	Mean Pain Score at Each Time*		
	24 hours	48 hours	72 hours
Gooeypaste	7	8	5
Warm water	6	8	6
Vitamin E	7	9	7

*Mean for the 10 mothers using that method.

3. Up, G. Support for Breastfeeding grows. *Child Health Studies* 50:3–9; 1995.
4. Rocks M. A study of engorgement. *Human Nurturing* 23:21–28; 1996.
5. Complete D. Weaning from breast. *Feeding Babies Journal* 11:335–339; 1987.
6. Cando Y. Providing relief for breast-feeding problems. *HA* 58:130–140; 1992.
7. Workhard S. The many uses of vita-min E oil. *Journal of the Natural Foods Industry* 12:22–26; 1980.
8. Ouchless T. A Theory of Pain: The patient knows. *Human Nurturing* 1:70–80; 1978.

Note: The author wishes to express gratitude to Phunny Pharmaceuticals for the provision of Gooeypaste, vitamin E, and copies of the Painometer.

First Practice Article: *Sore Nipple Treatments: Gooeypaste Works Best*

Commentary

Before you read the commentary in the next section, return to the beginning of the Critical Reading section and apply the process to the article provided. Consider each part separately and in the order suggested, and make notes to yourself about the strengths and flaws you find in the article. Then compare your ideas to those that follow. You probably will have some ideas that are not mentioned here. As long as you can justify them logically, or by reference to other studies, your commentary is valuable.

Title

Your considerations of this article can begin by asking yourself what you think the article is about just from reading the title. Because this article focuses on treatment, information about the cause of the soreness will certainly be important. Will the authors have looked at causes? Will the results vary depending on the cause? Sore nipples due to continued pacifier use and resultant tongue movements would be expected to take longer to resolve than the initial tenderness of getting started. So, if the authors did not ensure that the causes were the same in the comparison groups, the results might differ for that reason alone, no matter what the treatment was.

Also consider what you already know. Because early soreness is often due to poor positioning, will they measure attempts at correct positioning? From other studies, it is known that much nipple soreness will diminish with time. But to date, no treatments have been shown to reduce that time dramatically. A group that does not use any treatment might be important to determine the baseline pain experience in order to judge whether any of the treatments is better than just the passage of time.

Does the title suggest surprises? What is Gooeypaste? It must be a new product and, so, may be available only to researchers. Does it contain lanolin? Some studies have found lanolin to relieve pain by allowing faster healing. In addition to measuring pain, will the study attempt to document wound healing as some research has done?

If you had designed a study on nipple soreness, would you have limited the ages of the babies? Would you have limited the previous experience of the mothers? Both of these factors might influence the expected duration and coping with the pain. If the groups have underlying differences in such variables, the expectation that their pain experience would be the same is not justifiable.

Authors' Names

This author is not one you have read before (since he or she is fictitious!). You would ordinarily want to keep this name in mind for future reading.

Abstract

Which of the aspects of the study that you thought about from looking at the title are clarified in the abstract? For one, the abstract does not clarify much about the mothers' experience or the babies' ages. Because the abstract recommends Gooeypaste, you would expect to find a strong relationship (documented later in the results) between its use and pain relief.

Tables and Graphs

Table 25.1 tells more about the subjects. You may have many questions after you look at this table. The average maternal age is not the same in the groups, and no statistical tests are reported to check whether or not the differences are statistically significant. The authors, and you, may decide that there is no clinically significant difference; that is, age differences like these are not likely to contribute in important ways to how the mothers respond to treatments.

You are probably more concerned about the differences between the treatment groups in the numbers who have breastfed previously. The Gooeypaste group has twice as many mothers who previously breastfed as does the vitamin E oil group. Although the statistical test showed the groups to be not statistically significantly different, that may be due to the fact that each treatment group has only 10 subjects, a fairly small sample. Before you apply the results of this study to your practice, you might want to see a study in which the experienced breastfeeders are the same (or closer to the same) in each treatment group.

A further consideration, which cannot be seen from this table and which is seldom considered in the literature, is whether or not those previous breastfeeding experiences were favorable. Many women, when asked if they breastfed a previous child, will say "Yes" even when they only breastfed one week and that week was full of problems. The level of confidence and the interpretation of pain for such women is likely to be different than for an experienced breastfeeder who met her own goals and overcame problems.

The number of female infants looks different in each group as well. But unless you know of research that links gender of the infant to pain perception or treatment effectiveness, it probably does not matter. Do you think that infant birth weight could be an important difference between treatment groups? None of these groups has an average that makes us think about preterm babies. But if you reread the abstract, there is no statement that, in fact, all babies were full term. So, it is possible that any of the groups could have a preterm baby in it. We might be especially concerned that the vitamin E oil group had more preterm babies than the other two groups. Preterm babies may take longer to learn effective suckling and, thereby, affect their mother's pain perception. We do not know for sure either (1) that there are preterm babies in the vitamin E oil group or (2) that preterm babies necessarily cause differences in healing sore nipples. But we do know that many preterm babies are more difficult to nurse in the first few days. So we wonder whether there might be a hidden difference between the treatment groups (preterm babies) that could be an alternative explanation for the reported faster pain relief in the Gooeypaste group. Such an unanswered question may be serious enough that we do not want to apply this study's findings without more information.

The authors also report the number of infants who had alternative feedings before starting the study. Were the feedings by bottle? Were they by cup? It is not clarified in the table, so we hope that it will be in the text. Because no statistical tests are reported, you have to consider the possibility that the differences are important clinically. How might having been bottle fed or cup fed affect the mothers' pain perception? Notice that the table does not tell how many times each of the babies who received an alternative feeding were fed that way. It only tells how many babies (out of ten in each group) were fed by some other method.

Now, take your critical reading one step further for this table. You may, by now, have collected doubts about the underlying similarity of the vitamin E oil group and the Gooeypaste group. That is, you may be concerned that (1) the number of mothers who previously breastfed differs; (2) there may be more small, possibly preterm, babies in the Vitamin E oil group; and (3) there are more babies who had alternative feedings in that group as well. Before reading the text of the article, you have begun to suspect that the groups may have started off different—both before they developed sore nipples and before they used treatments. These differences are potentially related to sore nipples (unlike gender of the infants, which, while different between groups, is probably not related to pain). It is possible that these differences could be an alternative explanation for the different pain perceptions between the groups rather than the different treatments. Keep these doubts in mind as you read the next table and the remainder of the text.

Table 25.2 reports average pain scores for each group. Does this seem to you to be the most meaningful way to analyze the data? Could the authors have, instead, shown a table of improvement versus no improvement? Do we know enough about the Painometer to know what a "7" means? There was no discussion of how many points that were on the scale, nor what the descriptive anchors were at each end. We would also expect a table like this to report whether the pain score averages are different for each treatment group. Looking at the numbers—without a statistical analysis—would you anticipate a clinically important difference to be demonstrated for Gooeypaste? That is, is there a really big difference between Gooeypaste and the other treatments? With experience, you will come to answer that question for yourself, even without statistics, and then can compare your impression to what the statistical tests demonstrate. In fact, there does not seem to be a very remarkable difference between the groups at any of the times. If the mothers are rating their pain on a 1–10 scale and they are reporting, on average, pain of 5, 6, or 7 at 72 hours after their pain started, they are probably still having an important amount of pain that might affect their overall breastfeeding experience.

A more difficult judgment to make is whether averaging the pain levels makes any sense. Often, when scales like this one are used in which people mark specific—defined anchor points—it is difficult to know what an intermediate point represents. It will be important to look at the instructions the author gave to the subjects about completing the scale. It could be that they were encouraged to mark a place anywhere along the line. In that event, the author would also need to explain how a quantity was assigned to a mark that fell between two points, such as between 3 and 4. Instead of averaging, some studies might try to sum the amount of time each woman spent at each pain level and compare the sums between groups.

One other aspect of the study is evident from this table. In thinking about designing a sore nipple study after reading the title, the need for a no-treatment group was identified. Yet, no such group appears to have been used for comparison. You might also wonder why the pain scores do not appear in a table because that was the focus of the study. You can reasonably expect that the author will explain this omission in the text.

Results

What do the authors claim? First, they claim that the Gooeypaste group was 2.7 times as likely to experience decreased pain at 72 hours as the vitamin E group, and 6 times as likely as the water group. This finding was statistically significant. Second, they claim that the optimism level of the Gooeypaste group was higher than that of the other groups but statistical significance was not attained.

Independent variables in this study include Gooeypaste, vitamin E, and water. Dependent variables include nipple soreness and optimism. Potential confounding variables are the cause of pain, experience of the mothers, quality of positioning, and age of the babies.

Applying the three logical steps to this article:

1. The statistical significance of the odds ratios means the data on pain is consistent with the first claim. The claim about optimism is less clear.
2. From the results section, are you reassured that the authors have ruled out other possible explanations? Probably not, because the author did not show, in the results, that the three groups were similar in their potential confounding variables. As you read the rest of the article, you will be interested to determine whether the subjects had enough in common that the only important difference between them was the treatment they were using.
3. Does the author suggest a plausible mechanism for how the treatment affects pain? Not to this point in the article, though that is often reserved for either the review of the literature or the discussion. The kinds of mechanisms you might be expecting to read later in the article are topical anesthesia, faster wound healing, anti-inflammatory effects, or others.

Subjects

We do not know whether the mothers were first-timers or experienced breastfeeders because the author did not report this. The proportion of these mothers in each treatment group could be significant if more experienced mothers persisted simply because they had been through similar pain before or had a higher level of confidence, or both. We do not know age and education level of the mothers or their intended breastfeeding duration. Both factors are related to general commitment to breastfeeding. Cesarean birth may differ from vaginal birth in several ways: (1) general rate of recovery from birth, (2) difficulty of birth, (3) more professional help with breastfeeding for mothers who have undergone cesarean birth due to longer stays, (4) and possibly later milk induction in cesarean birth mothers. We do not

know how many times each mother breastfed before pain developed. Nor do we know how often she breastfed afterward. These factors might affect pain intensity and duration, and therefore, the likelihood of relief. The effectiveness of feeding by the baby might also tell something about the quality of latch. Nothing is said about routine help with and observations of positioning.

Nurse or physician preferences for the older treatments do not seem to have prevailed, neither were they accounted for in the design. If nurses who favored warm water encouraged its use before group assignment, for example, the mothers might have continued with that as well as with their other assigned treatment.

The Painometer was not administered at a baseline time. This means that it is possible that the Gooeypaste mothers actually started the study with a lower pain level than the other groups, so their level of pain might indeed be lower at 72 hours just for that reason. Because we know little about the scale, we do not know if it tries to measure absolute levels of pain ("the worst pain I've ever felt . . . the least pain I've ever felt") or if it just measures changes in pain perception over time.

Methods

The design of this study followed the outline of a clinical trial with randomly assigned treatments. However, it is not a good example of a clinical trial because of its failure to control for several variables. Thus, the design of a study, alone, is not sufficient to guarantee the quality of the resulting evidence.

Telephoning mothers was a good way to increase compliance with the scale. However, investigators should have analyzed the scales for which the nurses asked the questions separately from the mailed ones to be sure there was no tendency to answer differently when speaking directly to a nurse. Compliance with the treatment plan was not reported as validated in any way. Often, if patients do not affirm that they have indeed followed the treatment plan 75 percent (or whatever) of the time, then it is not considered an adequate test of the treatment, so the data is discarded. Assuming that they followed the plan could lead to invalid conclusions.

What do you think of the operationalization of the variables? The independent variables were not thoroughly described. As has been addressed, the ingredients in Gooeypaste were not discussed so that we might understand its pharmacologic action. It would also have been helpful to have an explanation of the way mothers were instructed to use the warm water and vitamin E. Did they use these after every feeding or four times a day? Before the vitamin E was applied, were they instructed to air dry their nipples? Was the Gooeypaste to be removed before the next feed or allowed to soak in? (If its ingredients had been explained, we might have this answered.) In some studies, the difference between the effectiveness of treatments turns out to be related to the ease of using the treatment rather than any specific action of the treatment itself.

As already discussed, the lack of detail about the Painometer makes it difficult to judge what the measurements mean in Table 25.2. However, operationalization of "pain" and "optimism" via such a scale is an accepted way to measure these dependent variables.

The confounding variables are not defined sufficiently or even acknowledged. Even though random assignment was used, this is such a small sample that the researcher should have checked on whether some basic variables occurred in similar proportions in all the groups. In addition to the experience of the mothers and the quality of positioning already discussed, there could be several more potential influences on treatment effect that could confuse the interpretation of the data. Were any of the mothers experiencing problems establishing milk production, either because of the pain or for some other reason? If so, they might be inclined to feed more often, possibly necessitating more uses of a treatment. Conversely, they might be so discouraged that they would use the treatment less often.

Some readers of this study might ask why there is such a seemingly common problem with early sore nipples in this hospital. (It would have helped if the author had defined the percentage of all mothers that the 30 subjects represent). Could it be that the nurses have very different skills in helping breastfeeding mothers and that poor positioning is not detected early? Or, contrary to the author's intent, could it be that many of the mothers had only the initial nipple tenderness that improves without real treatment except attention to positioning? Perhaps a hospital postpartum unit was not the best place to test Gooeypaste. When critiquing a study, it is important to step back from its original premises and ask these basic questions. However, it is often difficult to answer them. Instead, we usually have to accept some of the assumptions and choices the author made and then build a critique on that. Even when the initial conditions of the study are not ideal, often the results can still have value.

Literature Review

Nipple pain is a widely acknowledged problem for breastfeeding mothers. There is no great need to establish that from the literature, although there are articles the author could have cited. Types or causes of pain may not all respond to the same treatment. It is, therefore, important that the literature review be related to the type of pain in the proposed subjects. In this study, it is not likely that Candidiasis is a common cause of pain so early postpartum, so it is unclear why the authors mentioned it. Engorgement is also not likely to be relieved by any superficial treatment, so its inclusion seems inappropriate.

The article by Cando was the only reference for warm water treatment. It is likely that the author intended to follow the protocol for its use described therein. However, details are not given for frequency of use, fabric used for application, temperature of the compresses, and air-drying afterward. These omissions make it more difficult to judge whether it was a more complex or time-consuming regimen to follow than that for Gooeypaste or vitamin E. Similarly, the protocol for vitamin E use was not described. Although the author reports that mothers found vitamin E to be soothing, there is no finding presented about its effect on healing or continuation of breastfeeding. Apparently the main reason that vitamin E was compared was that some of the obstetricians favored it. For both of these studies, it would be helpful to know whether the subjects studied were similar to those in the current study. Further, did pain relief correlate with longer term breastfeeding or more satisfaction with breastfeeding? Many studies do not report longer term outcomes such as duration or satisfaction. However, as lactation science matures, it will be important to include these as dependent variables because they are the more important goals.

The theory of pain cited (Ouchless's) may not be familiar to readers, so more description of it should be given so that its applicability to postpartum nipple soreness can be judged. Even if we agree that patient perception of pain is very important, there are other aspects of the pain that are also important—its severity, its duration, its association with an obvious wound, and its meaning to the mother. If the theory suggests that some other aspects of the mother's perception are important to the ultimate resolution of the pain, they should also have been measured as potential confounding variables.

Discussion

Readers cannot judge how adequately the author used the literature that was reviewed (see methods, earlier), so the link to the discussion is missing. Also, the author does not introduce any further literature in this section and has not delved into the problem of sore nipples to try to understand the causes. Instead, the scope of the study has been limited to treatment. This is not necessarily bad. It does mean that the implications for practice are more difficult to derive because we cannot generalize to any causes of sore nipples except those that occurred in the study. Because we are not told what those are, the best we can do is to apply the findings to patients whose soreness develops during their hospital stay. Had the author sought to define the causes of the subjects' pain, she might have used the discussion to speculate about why Gooeypaste was especially helpful to these mothers.

In light of the finding that optimism scores were not statistically significantly different between the treatment groups, is the following statement justified? "Since the Gooeypaste mothers were also more optimistic . . ." No, it is not. The lack of significance means that Gooeypaste could appear higher on the optimism scale just by chance. Watch carefully for such claims. If you had not read the results, you might be misled by the discussion. The suggestion that optimism may lead to longer nursing is reasonable. However, it would have provided even better evidence for Gooeypaste's effectiveness if the researcher had also studied the proportion of mothers in each group who breastfed until at least 3 months, for example, or who met their own goals. The author does admit the need to **replicate** these findings in a larger sample, and that is an important admission.

Results Revisited

The data do seem consistent with the claim that soreness decreases faster for those women who use Gooeypaste. But the control of confounding variables (alternative explanations) was unknown. Remember that, when they started treatment, there is no assurance that the groups were similar, and no information was provided on variables such as breastfeeding experience, adequacy of positioning, or many others. The author depended heavily on the random assignment of this small sample but did not check on its effectiveness. So there may be another explanation for the reasons Gooeypaste seemed to work so well. There is also no plausible mechanism discussed.

The data on optimism are not consistent with the claim that Gooeypaste mothers are more optimistic because of the lack of statistical significance. What are the implications for your practice? Would you want to immediately begin using Gooeypaste in your postpartum clients? It is hoped not. You might design a better randomized trial in your work setting and write up your own research report. You might investigate Gooeypaste further by contacting the manufacturer for ingredients, mechanism of action, and any studies they conducted. When you find this number of flaws in a study, and when they are so basic, you should not adopt the practice change recommended by the author.

References

Because these references are fictitious, it is difficult to determine whether important ones were included or not. Some of these references are older, but that is not necessarily bad. The most important deficiency is the lack of a reference for the Painometer. See, also, the "Note" following the reference list. It tells you that the study was partially funded by the manufacturer of Gooeypaste. Although that is not necessarily an indication of bias, you should think about that possibility. Notes about sources of funding are not always present in articles, but it is important to pay attention when they are.

Comments on the Commentary

You may have uncovered other questionable aspects of this sore nipple study that make you uncomfortable in applying its findings. That is good. Critical reading can lead to many questions. This study would probably never have been published in its present form because of the deficiencies identified. It was meant to be open to many questions so that you could take the process of critical reading in whatever direction occurred to you. You undoubtedly found still more criticism within the commentary. Peer review of this article would, no doubt, have demanded that the author provide a citation for the Painometer, additional data about the pain scores and other ways of comparing them, a change in the wording about the claim that Gooeypaste was related to higher optimism, and more information about the potential confounding variables. That is the purpose of peer review—to present to readers a good quality article without fundamental flaws so that what remains is valuable information (though not perfect), and so that the judgments required of readers are about more subtle or more arguable dimensions of the study.

> Please read the second article, using the order and questions suggested. Commentary follows this mock article as well, so that you can compare it with your own critique.

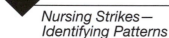
Nursing Strikes— Identifying Patterns

by Emma Halter and Makit Gogh

Journal of Intermittent Phenomena 13:44–47; 1992.

Abstract

A questionnaire was distributed to over 700 breastfeeding mothers in two suburban pediatric practices. Of this group, 200 reported having had experience with their babies refusing to nurse. There was a great deal of variation in reasons for refusing, in measures tried, in other life events, and in mothers' feelings. Stress and biting may be two types of events that precipitate refusals. Teaching mothers about possible nursing refusals in prenatal classes may help them realize that they can overcome such discouraging events.

Introduction

Breastfeeding mothers often report[1,2] that their babies display a sudden lack of interest in breastfeeding that persists long enough to cause concern about hunger and dehydration. The mothers also experience engorement. These "nursing strikes" can be the reason for the introduction of formula; and weaning may follow soon after. For mothers who

FIGURE 25.6

Appendix A: The questionnaire

Your help with this questionnaire is greatly appreciated. We are trying to understand why some babies occasionally stop breastfeeding for a few feeds. Please answer as fully as you can, and feel free to add any comments you would like.

1. Are you currently breastfeeding? ____ Yes ____ No
2. How old is your breastfed baby? ____ How old are you?____
3. Is this your first breastfed baby? ____ Yes ____ No
   A. If yes, do you have other children? ____ Yes ____ No
      If yes, how many? ____
   B. If no, how many other children have you breastfed? ____
4. With your currently breastfeeding baby, if you have had any of the following problems at *any* time, please check:
   ____ Difficulty latching on
   ____ Sore nipples
   ____ Teething
   ____ Engorgement
   ____ Breast infection
   ____ Plugged milk ducts
   ____ Baby refused to breastfeed
   ____ Baby had a cold or stuffy nose that interfered with feeding
   ____ Biting
5. Since your baby was born, have you resumed your menstrual periods? ____ Yes ____ No
   A. If yes, how old was your baby when the first period started? ____
6. Please check any of the following birth control methods you have used since this baby was born and the age of the baby when you started using it:

Method	Age of Baby when started use
____ Condoms (male or female)	____
____ Natural family planning	____
____ Lactational amenorrhea	____
____ Depo-Provera shots	____
____ Birth control pills	____
____ Intrauterine device (IUD)	____
____ Tubal ligation	____

7. Has your baby ever stopped breastfeeding for at least 24 hours? ____ Yes ____ No
   If no, you have finished this questionnaire. Thank you very much.
   If yes, how old was your baby at the time?____
   If yes, please check all of the following which you feel apply to your situation, or write a brief description of why you think the baby stopped nursing:
   Breastfeeding stopped for at least 24 hours because:
   ____ Mother needed a medicine and was advised to temporarily stop nursing.
   ____ Mother and baby were separated by a trip, a storm, or other unexpected event.
   ____ Baby had surgery.
   ____ Baby was too ill to breastfeed.
   ____ Baby was jaundiced.
   ____ Mother had sore nipples that needed rest.
   ____ Baby was teething.
   ____ Mother returned to work.
   ____ Baby had bitten mother and stopped nursing soon after.
   ____ Baby refused to nurse but would take other food.
   ____ Unknown. The reason for stopping was never clear.
   ____ Other: Please describe why you think your baby stopped nursing:
8. If your baby has stopped nursing for at least 24 hours, please check all of the following that describe your feelings during the time your baby did not breastfeed:
   ____ Concerned breastfeeding was finished for good.
   ____ Worried about hunger or dehydration.
   ____ Concerned about breasts becoming engorged.
   ____ Relieved to have a short break.
   ____ Confused about what was happening.
   ____ Confused about the cause of the refusal to nurse.
   ____ Thought baby might be sick.
   ____ Other. Please describe:

9. If your baby has stopped nursing for at least 24 hours, please check all of the following actions you tried to help resume feeding.

_____ Just kept trying to nurse in the usual ways.
_____ Just gave my baby time to feel better.
_____ Called the lactation consultant, physician's office, or breastfeeding counselor (i.e. La Leche League).
_____ Talked to a family member or friend.
_____ Nursed my baby when he/she was very sleepy.
_____ Increased the amount of skin-to-skin contact we had.
_____ Took a bath with my baby.
_____ Used a sling or pack.
_____ Tried to reduce the stress in my life.
_____ Other. Please describe:

Thank you so much for your help. If you would like to learn the results of this study, please let us know at your next appointment.

intended to continue breastfeeding longer, such unplanned weaning is emotionally difficult. Pediatric experts agree that continuing breastfeeding for 6 months to 1 year is best for infant health.[3] Some scientists have found that mothers believe that nursing strikes are related to the return of their menses[2] or to starting oral contraceptives.[4] There has been little attempt to study this phenomenon. As a first step, we collected data on breastfeeding couplets in two private pediatric practices and looked for patterns. The study was approved by the Review Board of Busy Hospital and subjects gave written, informed consent.

Subjects And Methods

Participants were mothers of currently breastfeeding infants who were recruited by lactation consultants, nurses, and nurse practitioners in two large, suburban group pediatric practices. From March 1, 1990 to May 31, 1990, all nursing mothers whose babies had appointments for any reason were invited to complete a questionnaire while they waited to see their providers. Those who needed help with child care in order to complete the survey were given that help.

The questionnaire (Appendix A—Figure 25.6) was developed by the authors after reviewing the books for mothers and professionals that suggest causes and remedies. It was designed to be concise so that mothers could finish it while they waited for their appointments (about 10 minutes to complete). Descriptive statistics were calculated for most responses. Correlations were determined for **demographic** characteristics and responses.

Results

During the 3-month period, the combined practices had 1032 breastfeeding couplet visits. Because some couplets had multiple appointments, a total of 955 different couplets were offered a questionnaire. Of those, 780 agreed to complete the survey. For various reasons, only 600 questionnaires were actually complete enough to use. Of these, 400 had never had the problem of the baby refusing to nurse for 24 hours. Of the 200 refusers, 30 had stopped nursing at a few days old because of jaundice in the infant. Medication, surgery, illness, separation, and maternal sore nipples were identified by another 50 mothers (see Table 25.3.). Teething was the cause 30 mothers indicated. These causes, although stressful and needing remedies, were not the most perplexing. The nursing strikes of interest were those which 70 mothers marked as unknown reason, other reason, or preference for another food. Of course, because these mothers were nursing at the time of the appointment, they had overcome the strike. Many of the events that occurred near a nursing strike also occurred in couplets who never experienced a strike. The two strongest correlations were an increase in family stress and biting. (see Table 25.4) However, together these included only 15 percent of couplets who experienced nursing strikes.

Discussion

Mothers need lactation professionals who are aware of the potential for a

---

Table 25.3

Reasons for Stopping Nursing as Determined by Mothers

Newborn jaundice	30
Medication	10
Surgery	12
Illness of baby	20
Maternal sore nipples	15
Separation of mother and baby	13
Teething	30
	130

Table 25.4

Correlations Between Unexplained Nursing Strikes and Recent Events in the Lives of the Breastfeeding Dyads

Event	Number of Dyads	r (Correlation)
Resuming menses within 1 week of strike ($<$3 mo old)	5	0.21
Resuming menses	3	0.15
Starting birth control within same month	2	0.09
Increase in family stress	15	0.55
Biting	16	0.59

Table 25.5

Remedies Used by Mothers to Overcome Nursing Strikes

Remedy	% of Mothers Who Used It
Time and patience	83
Calling lactation professional	80
Nursing during sleep	50
Skin-to-skin soothing	55
Bathing together	30
Sling or pack	34
Trying to reduce stress	42

emerge from this data. There is no evidence herein that resuming menses or starting the birth control pill, which have been suggested by others, is causal.

References

1. Complete D. Weaning from breast. *Feeding Babies Journal* 14:120–125; 1990.
2. Empp A. Common concerns of breastfeeding mothers in a food assistance program. *Nutrition Group Reports* 55:37–41; 1996.
3. Healthy World Alliance. Breastfeeding best for babies. *H.A.* 56:123–125; 1990.
4. Wilgot E. Postpartum menstrual cycles. *Annals of Families* 33:293–255; 1991.

nursing strike and who can encourage them to not give up. That is probably the most important message of this study. Short periods of refusal to nurse are not uncommon. Determining a cause is very difficult. Based on this survey, we suggest educating mothers in prenatal classes about possible refusals. Cautioning them against responding strongly to biting, and emphasizing the importance of stress management may be the most specific strategies that

---

▼ Second Practice Article: *Nursing Strikes—Identifying Patterns*

Commentary

Title

How will the authors define "nursing strike?" Although experienced breastfeeding mothers may speak of this phenomenon as though everyone agrees on it, a clear definition is needed in order to determine clearly associated variables. What do you think should be included and excluded? You might expect to see refusal to nurse by the baby for a certain length of time (more than one feeding) and for no obvious reason. Or would it be reasonable to allow certain probable causes and disallow others? When exploration is attempted of a previously understudied phenomenon like this, there are many possible choices for the definition, none of which is right or wrong. Rather, clarity is the most important criterion for judging the choices—so that investigators, subjects, and readers all agree on which breast refusals constitute nursing strikes and which do not.

What "patterns" does the title make you think about? Do the authors intend to see whether babies at a particular age are more likely to go on strike? Will they study whether increased bottle use or separation (common when babies start day care) often precede strikes? For mothers who have breastfed other children, is it likely that prior instances of strikes in the older child correlate with more strikes in the current nursing baby? Many patterns could be studied, so you can compare what patterns you would like to see investigated to what the researchers chose.

What study design does the title suggest? Is this a trial to determine whether certain events cause, or specific treatments cure, nursing strikes? Do you know of other studies of this phenomenon that have gained enough basic information so that such a trial could be conducted? For this exercise, the topic of nursing strikes was chosen because there is not much literature on it. So a descriptive study of some sort is more likely to be done at this point in the development of knowledge. If the authors intended to conduct a qualitative study, what kind of data might they collect? They might ask mothers to record on tape the feelings they remember having and how it affected their confidence when the baby went on strike. Alternatively, they might try to include mothers from many different cultures and compare the ways the mothers describe the experience of nursing strikes. If they do a quantitative study, they might try to find patterns by using correlation between variables as an outcome measure.

Authors' Names

Again, because this is a mock article, you will not be able to find these authors' names in any database. But for an actual article, if you wanted to know whether the authors had published on this topic previously, you could search Index Medicus or the online databases by author name. That would be a worthwhile effort if you need the most complete information available.

Abstract

The fact that 200 mothers claim experience with breast refusal might be surprising. This should start you thinking about the definition again. It could be defined in such a way that many more mothers have had strikes than your experience suggests. Alternatively, it could be that this problem is much more widespread than anyone realizes simply because no one has sought to study its **prevalence** before.

The source of subjects were two pediatric suburban practices. Will the authors provide more demographic data on maternal income, education, race, ethnic heritage, and type of insurance? If the sample population is mainly white, married, and middle class, will the results apply to mothers in other groups? The authors used a questionnaire. That requires literacy. Did they determine whether any subjects had trouble reading English? Did they provide the questions in another language? Were mothers with visual disabilities or language barriers excluded by the nature of the tool? Why did they single out biting and stress as events to mention in the abstract? Were these especially strong findings, or are they the only findings that are able to be modified by mothers? What is their reasoning for suggesting that prenatal education might help?

Table 25.3

Reasons for stopping nursing as determined by mothers: Note first that only 130 of the 900 mentioned in the abstract are tallied in this table. You will want to read why in the text. Are there reasons for nursing strikes that you had thought of that are not in this list? The investigators' reasons for these choices should be explained. Note that no descriptive statistics, such as percentages, or any tests of significance are reported for this table.

Table 25.4

Correlations: Why the focus on "unexplained" strikes and how was that defined? Why do the events listed in this table differ from the "reasons" given in Table 25.3? Although the correlation statistic r is presented, no statistical significance is reported. None of the correlations is high ($r = 0.7$ or above) in many definitions. Do moderate correlations like 0.55 and 0.59 represent the most powerful of the possible variables associated with strikes? Or has something been left out of the study inadvertently? All of the above-mentioned questions should be addressed in the text of the article. The explanations may be too complex to include as footnotes to the table.

Table 25.5

Remedies: Did all of the mothers who completed this survey successfully overcome nursing strikes? If so, they do not represent all of the mothers who have experienced strikes, because weaning occurs after strikes in some unknown proportion of cases. How would limiting the data collection to mothers who have successfully overcome strikes limit the applicability of the findings? Are there other remedies the authors should have included?

Results

First, note that the mothers who were targeted were breastfeeding at the time of the appointment. Apparently, mothers who had stopped breastfeeding after a strike were not included. Regarding the claims, the strongest correlations between variables included in the questionnaire were the correlation between strike and biting and that between strike and stress. The descriptive data appears to support the claim, but there is no report of statistical tests. In terms of ruling out alternative explanations:

1. Do the investigators offer any analysis of whether mothers who did not agree to participate were similar to or different from the mothers who participated? (This problem is similar to the "dropout" problem discussed in the Critical Reading section under "Results.") Some of these mothers may be unable to read English. Without knowing more about the nonparticipants, it is difficult to know how to apply (generalize) the results.
2. Are the preceding events of medication, surgery, jaundice, and so on listed in Table 25.3 sufficiently explanatory to exclude them from the study of nursing strikes? They are potential confounding variables if the essence of a nursing strike is that there is no "obvious" explanation. This is where definitions and the purpose of the investigation need to be very clear in order to interpret the data properly.
3. Are there plausible mechanisms suggested or investigated for the relationships that were found? The mechanism is often not discussed in the results section unless it was the focus of the study. In a descriptive study, it is important to think about how the relationships might work so that the results can be taken seriously. Even if no strong evidence can be offered for a mechanism, if it does not violate known principles of physiology or human behavior, it is plausible. Both biting and stress could be plausibly related to a nursing strike in a baby. As more of the article is read, you will be able to determine whether you believe the authors' explanations.

Methods

What is the design of this study? It is descriptive, cross-sectional, and correlational. It takes a snapshot of the couplets in one area on a limited time basis and contacts them only once, so it looks at a cross-section of the population. It is also correlational; a structured instrument was used to measure variables, and then statistically significant relationships were sought.

Was the definition of nursing strike clear and appropriate? From the questionnaire itself, rather than from the article, you can determine that the definition was "stopped nursing for at least 24 hours." Knowledgeable professionals could disagree with this definition. Some might prefer a different time period or different wording. What is crucial is that the authors and mothers mean the same thing when they use this definition. If there was a big discrepancy in understanding, the **internal validity** of the study would be in jeopardy. Because this is such a new area of research, the investigators could have done some work before this big study to be more certain about the meaning of this definition. They could have conducted a **pilot study** and talked in more depth with women about their experiences with nursing strike. They might have suggested different definitions until the mothers and researchers agreed that they were identifying the same phenomenon. They also could have asked lactation and child development experts for their opinions on the definition.

If you were to use this study to try to convince childbirth educators or pediatricians to address nursing strikes, it is very important that you discuss nursing strike as defined in this article, and that you not extend the findings to some other looser or stricter definition. The choices that are listed in the questionnaire are not defined for mothers, but most are probably reasonably clear. If you can think of multiple, significantly different interpretations for any of the phrases, you may have identified a less valuable part of the data.

Questionnaire

Take a look at the questionnaire itself. There are entire courses taught on how to design questionnaires in order to obtain the desired information. You could ask many questions about the quality of this one. Even if reasonable people would disagree, it is important to think about some aspects of it. Here are just a few ideas about specific questions:

1. Item 1 does not ask whether the mother is breastfeeding exclusively or partially. With a baby younger than 6 months of age, the nursing strike could have been the cause of a switch to partial breastfeeding. The investigators will not be able to determine such a switch from this question.
2. Questions such as Item 3 about previous breastfeeding experience often fail to ask whether the experience overall was positive or negative.
3. In Item 4, it is not clear what information or relationship the investigators were seeking with this question. It might have been useful to ask the age at which the problem was experienced in order to determine whether it was close in time to the strike. It should probably have an "other" category in case the mother wants to list problems she has had. Among ones that might bear some relationship to nursing strikes would be those in which the baby has had some frustration in getting enough milk. These may include delayed lactogenesis, delayed or overactive milk ejection, nipples that needed reshaping, or bottle feeding that led to poor breast suckling.

4. In Item 6, some of the contraceptive methods listed may not be familiar to all mothers but probably would be recognized by those who had used them.
5. Item 7 does not allow for multiple instances of nursing strikes. As a result, some mothers may list multiple causes, intending them to refer to separate events. Often, researchers ask mothers to reflect the most recent occurrence in their answer.
6. In Item 8, the age of the baby greatly influences the mother's concern about a nursing strike. With babies who are taking solid foods and other liquids, a 24-hour nursing strike may be viewed with little alarm. Therefore, it might be important to discuss the correlations separately for different age groups.

Subjects could be characterized by age, the number of children they have, the number they breastfed, return of menses, use of contraception, and problems experienced. Other variables that might influence their nursing strike experience and interpretation, such as ethnic group or planned duration of breastfeeding, are not included. This will happen often in descriptive studies. You will have to decide whether the information is useful to you even with some deficiencies.

Introduction and Literature Review

Because there is little research on this topic, the review is somewhat limited. Some authors will seek what they believe is related research from other topics that cover the hypotheses they wish to highlight. For example, if they believed that nursing strikes were related to stress in the mother, they might study other research on mother-infant stress responses. These authors chose to look for patterns in a large number of couplets without a specific hypothesis. If you knew of articles they failed to find, you might judge their effort to be less than complete.

Discussion

If this is a representative cross-section of breastfeeding mothers, the authors' statement that nursing strikes are common is probably true. However, we are not sure just what group this sample represents, and it does not represent mothers who weaned after a nursing strike. So it probably needs to be regarded as just a piece of the picture. On the other hand, if nursing strikes are very common but are handled smoothly by most nursing mothers, then it would be very important to understand how they coped in order to help those who wean as a result.

The suggestion to educate mothers about nursing strikes is difficult to argue with, although doing it in the usual childbirth class may not be the best time. Similarly, although education about biting and stress are appropriate, from this study alone, these topics cannot be expected to resolve the problems of nursing strikes greatly. Furthermore, although the authors claim to have found no evidence that resuming menses or starting birth control pills caused strikes, this cannot be regarded as the best evidence. We would believe that a prospective study that queried mothers about strikes—beginning shortly after birth—and carefully recorded other possibly relevant variables on a regular basis, would more likely detect a relationship.

Results Revisited

Depending on how convinced you are that this sample resembles your patients, you may want to initiate research yourself. At the very least, you could include questions about nursing strikes in more of your routine follow-up calls. This study, like many descriptive studies, raises more questions than it has answers. To review, the moderate correlation of stress and biting with strikes (although the statistical significance is unknown) is consistent with the claim that these are two of the more common preceding events. The biggest failure of this study is its inability to rule out alternative explanations because of study design, a not well-characterized sample, and definitions that could be better. Implications for practice have been discussed; there could be a lot of disagreement on clinical implications because of the degree of uncertainty about so many possible confounders.

References

This appears to be a relevant list. Even though the mothers in reference 2 may be a different sample than the ones in this study, the authors use that reference only to suggest what others have noted, which is appropriate.

SUMMARY

The process of critique that was presented in this chapter has been structured around the parts of a scientific article because that is the way most practicing lactation consultants will use it. However, the more general themes of the process of critical reading, as outlined in the following list, are not bounded by the article's sections. As a clinician who wants to decide whether to apply the results of a study to your work, you want to determine the following.

1. What did they choose to include and exclude in their literature review, in their subjects, in the survey questions, and in the comparisons they made in data analysis? Why did they make these choices, and did they adequately justify them? Did their choices make the sample patients or study situation so different from your practice that you cannot justifiably use the results?

2. What else could they have done? Why did they not do that? Could they have included more mothers? Could they have studied them for a longer period of time? Could the ethnic base have been diversified? Could they have included a control group?

3. For every limitation of the study identified by answering questions 1 and 2, what might have been the impact on the study's findings? For example, if you think that the authors should have included more low-income women, how might that have affected the finding that intending to breastfeed more than 12 weeks is the best predictor of continuing to breastfeed at least 6 weeks? You may be reasoning that the low-income women in your practice must return to work by 6 weeks. Therefore, very few even plan to breastfeed past 6 weeks and some other predictor variable would tell you more about what enables them to continue to 6 weeks. It is not enough, in the process of critically reading your scientific colleagues' work to say what they should have done differently. You need to justify your critique by stating how that might have changed the study's results.

Critically reading a scientific article is a skill that grows with practice. It also is a skill that strengthens your practice as a lactation consultant. Along with all the information you have learned about breastfeeding, you have now learned about learning even more! Self-direction and self-education are hallmarks of the professional lactation consultant. You are well along on the road of lifelong education.

BIBLIOGRAPHY

Candy D. Funding of research by infant formula companies. *Br Med J* 318:260; 1999.

Carr Joseph J. *A Crash Course in Statistics.* Solana Beach, CA: High Text Publishers; 1994.

Goldbeck-Wood S. Evidence on peer review—scientific quality control or smokescreen? *Br Med J* 318:44–45; 1999.

Hicks C. Bridging the gap between research and practice: An assessment of the value of a study day in developing critical research reading skills in midwives. *Midwifery* 10:18–25; 1994.

Jenken J et al. Changing nursing practice through research utilization: Consistent support for breastfeeding mothers. *Appl Nurs Res* 12:22–29; 1999.

Labbok M. Toward consistency in breastfeeding definitions. *Stud Fam Plan* 21(4):226–230; 1990.

Martens P. A mini-lesson in statistics: What causes treatment groups to be deemed "not statistically different?" *J Hum Lact* 11(2):117–121; 1995.

Massey V. *Nursing Research: A Study and Learning Tool.* Springhouse, PA: Springhouse Publishers; 1991.

Porter A. Positive messages on breast feeding would result in need for infant formula decreasing, (Letter.) *Br Med J* 318:260–261; 1999.

Rothenberg R I. *Probability and Statistics.* New York, NY: Harcourt Brace Jovanovich, Publishers; 1991.

Sackett D et al. *Evidence-Based Medicine.* New York: Churchill Livingstone; 1997.

Shaughnessy A et al. Clinical jazz: Harmonizing clinical experience and evidence-based medicine. J Fam Pract 47:425–428; 1999.

Smith G and Egger M. Meta-analyses of observational data should be done with due care. (Letter.) *Br Med J* 318:56; 1999.

vanRooyen S et al. Effect of open peer review on quality of reviews and on reviewers' recommendations: A randomised trial. *Br Med J* 318:23–27; 1999.

Waterston T et al. Researchers must recognise damage done by overt association with formula manufacturers. Br Med J 318:260; 1999.

Websites:

http://cebm.jrs.ox.ac.uk/ for Evidence-Based Medicine.

http://www.ahcpr.gov Evidence-Based Practice Centers, Agency for Health Care Policy and Research.

http://www.lalecheleague.org for LLLI Center for Breastfeeding Information.

http://www.nlm.nih.gov for MEDLINE and PubMed.

http://www.angelfire.com/in/pedscapes/index.html for journals online (links to their homepages).

26

BREASTFEEDING PROMOTION AND CHANGE

Excellence can be attained if you
Care more than others think is wise,
Risk more than others think is safe,
Dream more than others think is practical,
And expect more than others think is possible. Anonymous

Promoting breastfeeding in a society in which bottle feeding is the norm can present unique challenges. Undertaking the challenge of breastfeeding promotion requires strong, confident leadership. In order to enlist the support of colleagues and administrators, you will need to consider the cultural and societal factors involved. You can be instrumental in developing breastfeeding protocols, challenging traditional procedures, and removing barriers that erode a mother's confidence in her ability to breastfeed.

Breastfeeding promotion is a form of social marketing and will benefit from standard marketing strategies. A society that is baby friendly will require educated and committed caregivers, as well as baby-friendly practices in all areas of society. This chapter will explore the issues involved in creating real change at the local level—in hospitals, clinics, physician offices, and the general community—to empower women to nurture their babies in the manner that nature intended.

TRAITS OF A STRONG LEADER

It won't surprise you to learn that people prefer to work with people they like. We all want to associate with those who are pleasant to be around and those who are cheerful, generous, and considerate of others. Some people are fortunate to possess these qualities and, therefore, find it easy to generate cooperation from those around them. Others may need to make a concerted effort to present themselves in a manner that will achieve the same results. Likewise, there are specific things one can do to improve their leadership abilities.

Part of being an effective leader is instilling confidence in others. People naturally respond well to a leader who is self-confident, assertive, and forthright. The key to being influential is to focus on solutions, priorities, and action. An effective problem solver will look for problem areas and then focus on solutions. After establishing goals, be aware of the priorities that will help you achieve them and be willing to take risks to put your ideas into action. Be approachable, listen well, and guard against snap judgments. All of these attributes will help you build a strong team and garner support for your initiatives.

Increasing Your Effectiveness

The approach that Stephen Covey (1990) presents in his book *The 7 Habits of Highly Effective People* provides a helpful structure for examining ways to be an effective leader in breastfeeding promotion. Covey states that an effective person is proactive, establishes goals, sets priorities, and is genuinely open to other's ideas. The effective person works toward mutual benefits for both sides of an issue, promotes unity, and actively seeks self-renewal both physically and mentally. These practices will contribute to your success in facilitating real change. In the next section we will explore each of the seven habits within the context of your role in breastfeeding promotion.

Choose to be Effective

Steven Covey writes that "our behavior is a function of our decisions, not our conditions." It is human nature to react immediately to events in our lives. However, there is a gap between a stimulus and our response to that stimulus. The key to our effectiveness is how we use that gap. A reactive person responds spontaneously on the basis of feelings that are aroused because of particular conditions. The proactive person recognizes that we have the ability to choose our responses. Eleanor Roosevelt said, "No one can hurt you without your consent." It is not what happens to us but our response to what happens to us that determines the outcome. We can take the initiative to create circumstances, to make things happen by using language that is positive and proactive. When you make mistakes, acknowledge them, learn, and go on. Be careful not to give power unintentionally to others because of your reactions or responses.

Consider how you respond to policies that undermine breastfeeding . . . to coworkers who sabotage your efforts . . . to superiors who do not listen or who listen but do not *hear* you. A reactive response might be to defend what you are trying to accomplish by arguing your position and backing up your arguments with research articles and other documentation. As a proactive person, you would first try to learn the reasons for the resistance or disinterest. You would focus on practices you can change by first identifying the problem areas and then considering which ones are within your power to influence. For instance, the issue may be feeding schedules, rooming in, free formula, formula discharge packs, spending quality time with mothers, teaching staff, or starting a breastfeeding committee. Then approach the issue with a proactive, rather than reactive, stance. This may become more clear as we continue to explore this throughout the chapter.

Start with a Blueprint

The effective planner thinks first and then acts. Imagine if an architect were to begin building a new structure without first having created a blueprint. Where would a traveler be without first mapping out his route? Knowing what you want the end result to be will dictate how you plan to arrive there. Visualize the process of getting to where you want to be. Map it out on paper by establishing goals, and then determine how you will accomplish these goals in order to arrive at your destination. Leadership and vision must always precede any action, and you may very likely be the person to provide that leadership and vision to others.

Creating a mission statement will help to guide your actions. WHO and UNICEF have provided you with the blueprint for breastfeeding promotion. Their *Ten Steps to Successful Breastfeeding* will give focus to your efforts. They serve as a guide for development of breastfeeding policies and protocols. They will help you identify areas that need improvement and practices that can stay in place. Your end goal is healthy mothers and babies. Keep this end in mind, and it will help you determine how to get there.

Focus on What is Important

People often get so caught up in what they perceive to be urgent that the really important issues get little or no attention. To spend time doing what is important usually requires that you learn to say *no* to others and *yes* to yourself. An effective person practices self-management, makes decisions, and then acts on them. Learn to distinguish between what is urgent and what is important—they are not necessarily the same! Prioritize the changes to be made, then develop a time line and stay committed to the goals. Focus on what is important, and avoid becoming distracted or sidetracked by crises or obstacles. There are a variety of ways to organize and execute goals and tasks around priorities, ranging from notes and checklists to calendars, appointment books, and daily planners. You need to delegate tasks to a particular time and to other people. Becoming comfortable with delegating tasks to others requires that you trust others to come through for you. Such trust brings out the best in people and you may need to settle for things being done not exactly as you would have done them. You cannot be alone in your efforts, and the only way to build a strong team is to bring out the best in the other team members.

Teach other members of your staff how to assist breastfeeding mothers and babies so that you can delegate this responsibility to others. You cannot expect cooperation and compliance among others until you ensure that they are equipped to carry through with the appropriate practices. Time is at a premium in health care, especially in hospitals where staffing is low. With careful attention to time management, supportive breastfeeding practices need not tax the already busy day for maternity staff. Identify the essential elements that must be taught to breastfeeding mothers and focus on those areas.

Work Toward Mutual Benefit

It is important that you help create mutual benefits for both sides of an issue. All parties need to feel good about the outcome, and success cannot be achieved at the expense of others. If two opposing sides are unable to compromise, be creative and try to find an acceptable third alternative. Help others understand that, "The end result may not be your way or my way, but a *better* way." As a team, you can determine acceptable results and identify new options to achieve those results.

All members of the team need to be on an even playing field. Therefore, establish a climate in which everyone leaves their credentials and personalities at the door. Identify the key issues and concerns, and keep everyone focused on issues rather than on personalities or job titles. In planning and decision making, you want to include those who are receptive to the change as well as those who you anticipate will resist. List the needs and concerns of people on both sides of an issue and work toward the mutual benefit of everyone. If there appear to be losers on a particular issue, look for ways that both parties can benefit so that there are only winners.

Understand Other Points of View

Attempt to see an issue from the other person's point of view. In order to communicate effectively, you must first understand what is involved. People do not generally listen with an intent to understand. Consequently, the way they see the problem often *is* the problem. Effective listening involves patience, openness, and the desire to understand. If you are genuinely open to other's ideas, they will be more open to yours. Listen until you can explain their point of view as well as they can, and remain open to being influenced by them. The more deeply you understand, the more you can appreciate the other's view, thus opening the door to creative solutions.

In order to be effective in convincing another person to change, it is important that you understand their reasons for resistance. Perhaps there is a conflict between the old ways and the new ways that you are proposing. Attempt to understand specific concerns and worries and to see the issue the way they see it. One effective method for doing this is to role play the discussion of an issue with another colleague, placing yourself in the role of the resistor. Such an exercise will help you see more clearly what the concerns are and will help you determine counter arguments. Listen attentively and with an open mind to the arguments and concerns that are raised. Remember that everyone's end goal is healthy mothers and babies. There may simply be differences of opinion on how to get there. Remain open to flexibility and compromise.

Build a Strong Team

Covey tells us that the whole is greater than the sum of its parts. Work toward achieving unity and building a strong team. An effective team builds on each person's strengths and compensates for weaknesses. Help team members learn to sidestep negative energy and to not take criticism personally. Communicate back and forth until you reach a solution that is comfortable for both sides on an issue. This fosters trust and cooperation, which leads to effective communication. When others feel a problem is their problem, they become an important part of the solution. Therefore, you need the team members to take ownership of the proposed changes. Remaining open to new alternatives and compromises will help you accomplish this. Create an atmosphere in which it is safe for everyone to air differences. Differences in point of view can provide valuable resources and perceptions. Recognize that differences add to your knowledge and understanding. Two people can disagree and both can be right—they just interpret differently. So be sure to validate everyone's perspective and consider how it may help you achieve your goals.

Take Care of Yourself

Covey says that in order to be an effective person you need to be healthy both physically and mentally. This means paying attention to exercise and nutrition, and trying to keep stress at a low level. Using your value system as your guide in what you say and do will help to keep you focused in a positive direction. Find the child inside of you and stay in touch! Learn how to draw on that child's enthusiasm and energy. Continue to learn and share information with the staff, helping them stay focused on the vision and bringing out the best in each of them. Cultivate relationships, especially with adversaries, while keeping the team on track and working cooperatively.

▼ Increasing Self-Confidence

Self-confidence is an essential factor in actively promoting change. How you perceive yourself and your abilities has a tremendous influence on your level of self-confidence. Additionally, your attitude will determine your altitude. In other words, your level of success will be dependent on whether or not you view yourself as a successful person. *If* you focus on your faults rather than your strengths, you prevent yourself from soaring to great heights. The principles outlined in the next section will help you maintain perspective and increase your ability to take action in a self-assured manner (Browder, 1994).

Much of your attitude involves the vocabulary you use in self-talk. Avoid negative phrases such as, "I hope I don't . . .", and replace them with positive self-talk. Say to yourself, "I will . . ." Tell yourself how confident you are. Rather than saying, "I wish I were . . ." or "I should be . . ." tell yourself, "I am . . ." See Table 26.1 for powerful statements to replace those that convey less positive

TABLE 26.1
Powerful Language

Don't Say	Do Say
I have to . . .	I'll be glad to . . .
I'm no good at . . .	I'm getting better . . .
I failed . . .	Here's what I learned . . .
I'm going under . . .	I'm bouncing back . . .
This drives me crazy . . .	I can find a better way . . .
I can't do anything about it . . .	It's my responsibility to change . . .
We should have it ready by . . .	We will have it ready by . . .
Generally speaking, I tend to think . . .	I believe . . .
Do you have any questions?	What questions do you have?
It's not my fault. I couldn't help it.	I'm sorry. It was my responsibility.

messages. Just as positive thinking requires some re-learning, negative thinking is a learned habit as well. Simply stated, if you expect to fail, you will fail! You can recondition your mind to think positively by replacing negative thoughts with positive ones. Approach every situation with the belief that you will succeed. Focus on the best way to do the job right and visualize yourself doing it!

If you want good things to happen, you have to ask for them, and you have to make them happen. You might make some mistakes along the way. Congratulations! It means you took a risk. Learn to view your mistakes as lessons, not failures, and regard a mistake as just another way of doing things. As one lactation consultant stated, making mistakes is proof that someone out there is trying! When (you notice we didn't say if) you make a mistake, acknowledge it and regard it as a learning experience. Trust in your ability to learn and help others trust in their ability to learn as well. This concept will be especially important in your efforts to change practices that will require others to learn new skills. Coping with failure builds strength and wisdom. Help others learn from their mistakes and refuse to give up, and you do the same! Every defeat will be another step toward success.

▼ Increasing Assertiveness

Caregivers who serve breastfeeding women are predominantly women, and as we all know, women often worry that an attempt to approach something in an assertive manner may be perceived negatively as aggressive behavior. Remember that we said that attitude determines altitude. Regard assertive behavior as a strong asset and become comfortable with your assertiveness. Practicing assertive behavior will help you gain a level of comfort in presenting your ideas to others. An important first step is to analyze assertive behavior in others. Identify what it is about others that you admire. Decide which approaches or traits you would like to emulate, and observe what is said and how it is said.

Next analyze your own behavior. How do you respond in situations that call for assertiveness? Are you able to get others to comply with your wishes? Do others listen when you have something important to say? Analyze times when you were assertive, times when you were nonassertive, and times when you came across as aggressive. What language did you use? What nonverbal messages did you convey? Go one step further and record your behavior, writing down how you behave in different situations. What worked and what could you have done differently in order to be more effective?

The next step is to rehearse assertive behavior. Practice makes perfect, so practice assertiveness in your interactions with family, friends, co-workers, neighbors, and clerks in the department store. Take as many opportunities as possible to practice your assertiveness. Visualize yourself being assertive. Role play situations with others. When you have practiced and feel confident that you can approach an issue with assertiveness, then just do it! You will want to tackle an easy issue first, one that you feel confident will succeed. If it does not go as well as you had hoped, reflect on what you can do differently. Examine why it did not go as well as planned. Keep a positive attitude, and try another approach the next time. The important thing is that you not allow one setback to deter you from trying again.

▼ Becoming a Change Agent

Health care professionals are in a perfect position to plan and implement changes that will promote and protect breastfeeding. Recognizing the need for change is the first step in the process of planned change (Ellis, 1992). This recognition of the need for change may not always be easy to achieve. It is first necessary to understand how infant feeding is perceived in our culture. Regarding breastfeeding in a cultural context involves both the mother's own culture within her family and support system, as well as the cultural expectations and beliefs within her birth environment. Because most North American infants are born in hospitals, this requires attention to the culture and traditions within the hospital as it relates to infant feeding (Mulford, 1995).

Cultural beliefs evolve from the way in which members of that culture perceive their world. Covey demonstrates that two people can look at something and perceive it totally differently. Figure 26.1 illustrates this point. Most people will readily see an aristocratic young woman with a stylish hat. Now find the old hag who is wearing a scarf. The illustration can be perceived in two different ways, and neither perception is right or wrong. They are just different. One image may be more easily perceived by most people. However, another more subtle image is also present and can be seen with greater effort.

It is important to recognize that there are two very different perceptions of infant feeding in the world. In much of the Western world, bottle feeding is the readily perceived method of feeding an infant. Bottle feeding has become the norm, the expectation, of the general population. In order to achieve a strong promotional effort toward breastfeeding, society will need to change the way it perceives infant feeding. In your efforts to promote breastfeeding, you need to help others replace their perception of infants being fed formula by a bottle. You cannot persuade another person to make this change. Change must happen from the inside out and at a pace that is comfortable for those who are undergoing

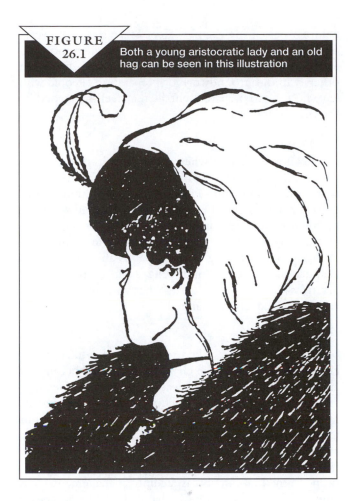

FIGURE 26.1 Both a young aristocratic lady and an old hag can be seen in this illustration

the change. What you can do is understand why others may be resistant and serve as an agent for facilitating change.

▼ Anticipating Resistance to Change

As common as change is, people do not always receive it well. A change in routine can be accompanied by tension, stress, and arguing. The changed practice may be undermined or sabotaged, and result in employee turnover, political battles, and a drain on money and time. Not everyone will share your enthusiasm for making dramatic changes in breastfeeding policies and practices. You will undoubtedly meet with some degree of resistance in your efforts to institute changes. Recognizing that this resistance is a natural part of the change process will help you capitalize on it and use it as a tool.

The Seven Stages of Resistance to Change

There is a declining scale of resistance to change. The most resistant person argues, "There is no problem." The least resistant people acknowledge the problem and enthusiastically embrace change. The seven stages of resistance to change below are adapted from educational

materials developed by SARAR International and published by *World Neighbors in Action*. They were later published in International Baby Food Action Network (IBFAN's) *Lactation Management Topic Outlines for Training Health Professionals*. Some possible arguments against breastfeeding promotion appear with each stage in the following list. With some minor adaptations from the original version, the seven stages are

1. There is no problem. I know human milk is good for babies, but artificial baby milk is perfectly safe. Babies have been raised on formula for decades. Furthermore, women have a right to choose which way they want to feed their babies.
2. I recognize there is a problem, but it's not my responsibility. I accept that breastfeeding is superior to artificial feeding. But I can't get involved. I don't have the time. Someone else will do it.
3. I accept that there is a problem, but I doubt anyone's ability to change it. We have a problem with infant feeding, but the formula companies are too strong and influential and our society doesn't see a problem. Society will never embrace a breastfeeding culture.
4. I accept that there is a problem, but I'm afraid to get involved. We have a problem, but I'm afraid to try to do anything about it. If I make too many waves, I might lose my job. I'm afraid of what others will think of me. I'm afraid of the time commitment.
5. We believe we can do something about it and I will begin to look for solutions. We have a problem with infant feeding. I want to help improve infant health and empower women. I will get involved, but I'm still unsure it will make a difference.
6. We know we can do it and obstacles will not stop us. I know I can make a difference. Working together we can change things. Let's get started!
7. We did it! Now we want to share our results with others. We finally have policies and procedures that promote breastfeeding, and our staff is following the guidelines. We have returned control to mothers and babies, and are empowering women to reach their breastfeeding goals.

It is likely that within any group of people, several stages of resistance will be represented. Expect progress with individuals in the group to take place one step at a time. Each individual must progress at his or her own rate. Notice that in Stage 5, the focus is now on a group effort and not the individual taking sole responsibility. When individuals are able to progress to this stage, they are on their way to the top! Be patient with everyone because no one can jump from Stage 1 to Stage 5 all at one time. Each individual must progress at his or her own pace and in his or her own way. It is also possible that some individuals may slide backward during the period of change depending on specific issues or information that surface. The group needs to be patient and flexible as group members proceed at a comfortable pace.

Resistance to the Ten Steps to Successful Breastfeeding

As discussed earlier, the WHO/UNICEF *Ten Steps to Successful Breastfeeding* serve as your guide to instituting changes in breastfeeding policies and practices. By anticipating the reasons that people may resist the Ten Steps, you may be able to select an approach that will help resolve those issues before they become obstacles. Table 26.2 is an example of arguments at each stage of resistance for the Ten Steps (Breastfeeding Support Consultants [BSC], 1996).

Reasons for Resistance to Change

We now can identify the stages of resistance that people experience when they are confronted with the prospect of change. Also, we have considered the types of responses they may make relative to each of the steps for breastfeeding promotion. Let us now address the various reasons they may resist the idea of change. Understanding the individual motives will help you in determining the most effective approach (Kanter, 1985). Those who resist may worry about losing control or may be uncertain about where the change will lead. Loss of face and worries about competence will also lead to resistance. The change may cause disruptions in routines, sometimes to such an extent that the job is no longer enjoyable. Unresolved past issues and grievances can also stand in the way of a person accepting change. Each of these factors are explored in the following sections.

Loss of Control

How people greet a change will depend on the degree to which they feel they are in control of it. Just as loss of control usually leads to resistance, ownership most likely will lead to commitment. It is important to keep in mind that change is exciting when it is done by us and it is threatening when it is done to us. By increasing each person's involvement and participation, and giving them legitimate choices, you can help them develop ownership of the change.

Uncertainty

People may have a sense of uncertainty about where your proposed changes will lead. You can help to allay doubts and fears by sharing openly what is happening with everyone involved. Minimize the effect by dividing a big change into small steps. In this way, people will have an opportunity to settle into one part of the change before experiencing the next step. Make sure that everyone understands what is anticipated and when more information will come. Avoid decisions that are sprung on others without groundwork or preparation. People who have no time to prepare mentally may feel threatened by the change and resist.

Difference

Acknowledge that when a change is in place, things will be different. People will be forced to question familiar routines and habits. They must begin to think about behavior that used to be taken for granted and will need to "reprogram" their daily routines. You can help others find a comfort level by minimizing the number of changes and by leaving as many habits and routines unchanged as possible. Conducting an inventory of your practices will help you identify what you are doing right and what needs to be changed.

Loss of Face

When people are asked to change, they may be inclined to believe that the change is proposed because of an assumption that the old ways were wrong. They may fear looking foolish for past actions, and may feel embarrassed and self-conscious. Help them put past actions into perspective. You all did what was perceived to be appropriate at the time. Now times are different, and the needs of mothers and babies have changed. More has been learned about breastfeeding management, and consequently, practices have changed. Praise others for their accomplishments under the old conditions and thank them for their willingness to change to meet present needs. Help them understand that you, too, have changed your practices, and help them view the change positively.

Competence

Understandably, there may be concerns about future competence. People may worry about their ability to be effective after the change. They may ask, "Can I do it?" or "How will I do it?" New ways may demand a new set of competencies, with some people finding that they are forced to "start over again." You can ensure that others will feel competent by providing sufficient training and giving positive reinforcement. Provide opportunities for them to practice new skills without judgement, through a mentorship program or other method which allows observation and practice in a nonthreatening setting.

Disruption

The proposed change may disrupt other plans or projects, intruding perhaps on people's personal time. A training program, for instance, may take place at a time

TABLE 26.2	
Responses to Arguments Against the Ten Steps to Successful Breastfeeding	
Step 1	*Have a written breastfeeding policy that is routinely communicated to all health care staff.*
STAGE OF RESISTANCE	**ARGUMENT**
There is no problem	We've had a policy for years. It's working well enough. We've been functioning well enough without one.
It's not my responsibility	I have too much to do already. I wouldn't know where to even begin writing a policy.
No one can do it	Even if we had a policy, no one would follow it. Mothers aren't motivated enough to breastfeed, so why bother.
I can't get involved	There are too many on the staff opposed to it. I wouldn't be able to get support from the supervisor or manager.
Let's begin	I can explore policies in other hospitals. I can contact ILCA to locate resources.
We can do it	Let's bring people together from all departments to work on it. Let's survey our patients to learn how satisfied they are.
We did it!	**We accomplished our goal!**
Step 2	*Train all health care staff in skills necessary to implement this policy.*
STAGE OF RESISTANCE	**ARGUMENT**
There is no problem	We have LCs, so we don't need to train the rest of the staff. Our nurses know what they need to know about breastfeeding.
It's not my responsibility	I don't have time to train everyone. I wouldn't know where to even begin with training.
No one can do it	The staff would never agree to 18 hours of training. We don't have enough money or time to train the entire staff.
I can't get involved	Staff would resent my suggesting that they need the training. I wouldn't be able to get support from the supervisor/manager.
Let's begin	I can explore how other hospitals do their training. I will take an extensive course in lactation.
We can do it	Let's survey staff to find out what they know about breastfeeding. Let's form a committee with people from several departments.
We did it!	**We accomplished our goal!**

(continued)

TABLE 26.2 (CONTINUED)

Responses to Arguments Against the Ten Steps to Successful Breastfeeding

Step 3	*Inform all pregnant women about the benefits and management of breastfeeding.*
STAGE OF RESISTANCE	**ARGUMENT**
There is no problem	We give help and advice to mothers when they are in the hospital. Teaching breastfeeding will create guilt in those who don't.
It's not my responsibility	Mothers learn what they need to know in their childbirth classes. It's the mother's responsibility to read and seek information.
No one can do it	We realize we need to, but we don't have the resources. If women want to bottle feed, it's our responsibility to help them.
I can't get involved	I don't have time to do prenatal teaching with everything else. I wouldn't be able to get support from the supervisor/manager.
Let's begin	I can explore breastfeeding initiation rates in other hospitals. I can make a questionnaire to screen mothers with difficulties.
We can do it	Let's survey our patients to find out how satisfied they are. Let's explore what we can improve in the labor and delivery department.
We did it!	**We accomplished our goal!**

Step 4	*Help mothers initiate breastfeeding within a half-hour of birth.*
STAGE OF RESISTANCE	**ARGUMENT**
There is no problem	We start breastfeeding as soon as the mother gets to her room. Most babies are too sleepy to breastfeed right away.
It's not my responsibility	If she breastfeeds after delivery, relatives will have to wait to see the baby. Babies get too cold in the delivery room.
No one can do it	The labor and delivery staff would never support such a policy. There are too many procedures that need to be done at that time.
I can't get involved	The staff is getting tired of all my suggestions about breastfeeding. I'm not very good at persuading people.
Let's begin	I can find someone in labor and delivery who will be open to change. I can teach the staff about the importance of early initiation of breastfeeding.
We can do it	Let's try it on a short-term trial basis and then evaluate it. We can find ways to keep babies warm.
We did it!	**We accomplished our goal!**

TABLE 26.2 (CONTINUED)	
Responses to Arguments Against the Ten Steps to Successful Breastfeeding	
Step 5	*Show mothers how to breastfeed and how to maintain lactation, even if they should be separated from their infants.*
STAGE OF RESISTANCE	**ARGUMENT**
There is no problem	Breastfeeding is a natural instinct; we don't need to teach it. There are plenty of support groups who will help them.
It's not my responsibility	If the baby is in the NICU, those nurses are responsible for it. I can't possibly see every breastfeeding mother.
No one can do it	We don't have enough staff to spend the time required for this. A lot of our staff don't believe in pushing breastfeeding.
I can't get involved	I wouldn't get support from my supervisor for the time it will take. Staff won't spend so much time with breastfeeding mothers.
Let's begin	I can encourage staff to accompany me on rounds. I can propose telephone follow-up for breastfeeding mothers.
We can do it	Let's survey our patients about what would have helped them. Let's explore a program to mentor staff in breastfeeding.
We did it!	**We accomplished our goal!**
Step 6	*Give newborn infants no food or drink other than breastmilk, unless* medically *indicated.*
STAGE OF RESISTANCE	**ARGUMENT**
There is no problem	We never do anything unless it is medically indicated. I am legally responsible to see that the baby is not dehydrated.
It's not my responsibility	I can't influence physician policies. Purchase of formula is an administrative decision, not mine.
No one can do it	Administration will never agree to begin purchasing formula. Formula companies will withdraw other funding if we make this change.
I can't get involved	I would not be able to get support from the supervisor/manager. What about jaundice? This could be dangerous.
Let's begin	I can explore how other hospitals have begun purchasing formula. I can teach staff the importance of exclusive breastfeeding.
We can do it	Let's review reasons we have been giving formula and water. Let's invite some mothers in to discuss how they managed.
We did it!	**We accomplished our goal!**

(continued)

TABLE 26.2 (CONTINUED)

Responses to Arguments Against the Ten Steps to Successful Breastfeeding

Step 7	*Practice rooming in—allow mothers and infants to remain together—24 hours a day.*
STAGE OF RESISTANCE	**ARGUMENT**
There is no problem	We have better security if babies are kept in the nursery.
	Babies could choke if they stay in the mother's room.
It's not my responsibility	Mothers are tired after laboring and delivering.
	That is an administrative decision.
No one can do it	If babies stay with their mothers, nursery staff will lose their jobs.
	Mothers do not want to keep their babies in the room.
I can't get involved	I will never get support from administration.
	The pediatricians will not examine babies in the mothers' rooms.
Let's begin	I can explore rooming-in policies at other hospitals.
	I can teach staff the importance of keeping babies with mothers.
We can do it	Let's invite pediatricians to meet with the breastfeeding committee.
	Let's record how much time babies spend away from their mothers.
We did it!	**We accomplished our goal!**

Step 8	*Encourage breastfeeding on demand.*
STAGE OF RESISTANCE	**ARGUMENT**
There is no problem	It is more efficient having scheduled feeding times.
	Babies need to get on a schedule as early as possible.
It's not my responsibility	I can do it with the mothers I see, but I can't see all of them.
	The babies must be fed at least two times on every shift.
No one can do it	Staff routines would be disrupted too much.
	It would be too hard to monitor babies for hypoglycemia without a schedule.
I can't get involved	Staff routines would be disrupted too much.
	This would be much too confusing.
Let's begin	I can teach staff the importance of mother and baby setting the pace.
	I can help staff learn to recognize feeding cues.
We can do it	Let's keep statistics to see if schedules make a difference.
	Let's try it for 6 months to see how it works.
We did it!	**We accomplished our goal!**

TABLE 26.2 (CONTINUED)	
Responses to Arguments Against the Ten Steps to Successful Breastfeeding	

Step 9	*Give no artificial teats or pacifiers (also called dummies or soothers) to breastfeeding infants.*
STAGE OF RESISTANCE	**ARGUMENT**
There is no problem	We have to test to see if the baby can suck and swallow. Babies have strong sucking needs and need pacifiers to keep calm.
It's not my responsibility	If parents want them it is not my position to discourage it. Everyone uses pacifiers, so what's the big deal.
No one can do it	I'm the only one in the hospital who considers this to be a problem. Pacifiers are a part of our culture just like baby bottles.
I can't get involved	The staff will think it takes too long to feed with a cup or spoon. There is nothing to document the use of cups for feeding babies.
Let's begin	I can teach staff about sucking preference and confusion. I can teach the staff how to cup feed a baby.
We can do it	Let's review why we give formula and water. Let's teach mothers to put baby to breast rather than give a pacifier.
We did it!	**We accomplished our goal!**
Step 10	*Foster the establishment of breastfeeding support groups and refer mothers to them on discharge from the hospital or clinic.*
STAGE OF RESISTANCE	**ARGUMENT**
There is no problem	We have the information at the desk if the patient requests it. They make mothers feel guilty if they wean too early.
It's not my responsibility	It is the mother's responsibility to seek help. The physician will refer her if there is a problem.
No one can do it	We don't have enough resources to start a support group here. The counselors do not always give sound advice and information.
I can't get involved	If I do this, I'll have to do it on my own time. I don't have time to keep updating the referral list.
Let's begin	I can visit community support groups and foster a strong link. I can offer to train mother-to-other support counselors.
We can do it	Let's give a name and telephone number to breastfeeding mothers. Let's explore an outpatient clinic and/or support group.
We did it!	**We accomplished our goal!**

ILCA, International Lactation Consultants Association; LC, lactation consultant; NICU, neonatal intensive care unit.
Printed by permission of Breastfeeding Support Consultants from their publication "Creating Change in the Face of Resistance," 1996.

someone had family activities planned. Be sure to introduce changes with flexibility, and be sensitive to the effect is will have on those who must implement the change and operate in a new way. People may be concerned that instituting the change will require more energy, time, and mental preoccupation. It will require that they go "above and beyond" their usual efforts. Be sure to give support and recognition for this extra effort.

Past Grievances

Although your goal is to check personalities and positions at the door, you may find that unresolved grievances from the past will surface as you approach others with your proposed changes. Perhaps one of the others had sought your support for a previous issue and was not satisfied with your response. You need to clear away past issues that could color people's response to your proposed change. After the air is cleared, everyone is better able to focus on the present issues.

Real Threat

Accept that sometimes a person's perceived threat may be real. Despite your efforts to the contrary, instituting the change may create winners and losers. People may lose status, clout, or a level of comfort. Perhaps you are proposing that 24-hour rooming in become a standard in your facility and that babies are no longer kept in a central nursery. A particular nurse has worked in the central nursery for the past 20 years and her greatest enjoyment is taking care of "her" babies. If babies spend the majority of their time in the mothers' rooms, this nurse will find that her daily routine will change dramatically. She may even consider the change to be too difficult and will choose to leave the job. It is important that you avoid any pretense or false promises. Be sensitive to the loss of routines, comforts, traditions, and relationships. People will need a chance to let go of the past and will need an understanding climate in which to do so.

▼ Conflict Resolution

Introducing change invariably will result in a certain amount of conflict. Although it may seem helpful to try to avoid conflict or pretend that it does not exist, this attitude may actually create further conflict (Calano, 1988). Accepting conflict as a natural part of the change process will enable you to manage it more rationally and productively. You need to bring conflicts out in the open in order to overcome them. This will allow you to develop honest, frank, and positive relationships with others. Conflict can actually be very constructive by getting people revved up and more receptive to creative solutions. Conflict helps us realize and validate our own values, and it is through conflict that people learn

to understand others and recognize the value of working together.

Inevitably, further conflicts will surface as the process of change continues. It is better to address these issues as they arise, no matter how minor they may be. You want to maintain a relationship in which honesty prevails and where neither side keeps an "account" against the other. Recognize that people work to satisfy their own needs, whether it be a need for money, power, or identity. People generally want to be accepted as they are, and to be liked and appreciated. In order to resolve conflict, you must meet the other person's needs as well as your own.

Be Sensitive to Others

Sensitivity to the other person's circumstances is important in any communication, and in conflict, it is critical. Never initiate a conflict in a public setting or in the presence of others who are uninvolved. Keep in mind that you are attempting to change behaviors, not people. In order to establish and maintain solid relationships, you need to keep focused on the solution rather than on individual problems. Find ways that you can all join together to work through any conflicts that stand in the way of your reaching your goals. Recognize that conflict involves both issues and feelings, and that you must get emotions out of the way before you can solve problems. When feelings are expressed, reflect them back with active listening to make sure they are resolved. You will then arrive at a point at which solutions to the problem can be addressed.

Identify Common Goals

In addressing a conflict, it may help first to determine basic goals that you share with the other person. This can set the stage for disagreeing on your respective strategies for achieving those goals. You both share a common objective of empowering mothers and babies to achieve their own goals. With that as a starting point, you can begin to discuss strategies to accomplish that goal. You know what you have in common. Now you need to figure out how you can meet on common ground on other issues. Find ways that you can both benefit. Operating in this manner sets a tone of cooperation and problem solving, and puts you on the same side instead of remaining adversaries.

Coping with Difficult People

Invariably, you will have at least one person on your team that you regard as difficult. You have tried everything in your arsenal to work with this person cooperatively. Yet, you seem to run against a brick wall continually. Consider that perhaps a change in your approach may achieve more positive results. Remember that you cannot change the person, so you may need to change the way you relate to them. Below are some suggestions for approaching a difficult person.

Approaching a Difficult Person

◆ Be positive. Give recognition and praise for accomplishments and avoid placing blame.

◆ Prepare for interactions by writing down exactly what you want to say. This will also help release any steam that has built up before any actual confrontation.

◆ Use appropriate body language. Face the person squarely, sit or stand erect, and lean forward to demonstrate a desire to communicate.

◆ Give your undivided attention and respond both verbally (I see . . . I'm with you) and nonverbally (nodding, smiling, maintaining eye contact).

◆ When you are speaking, avoid getting sidetracked. Do not focus on what you anticipate the other person will say. Focus on the goal and keep an even pace.

◆ Recycle the message to make sure the person has heard and understood what was said. After you have sent the message, wait for a response before continuing to speak.

The Aggressor

Some difficult people may be aggressive to the point of being hostile. They will have a strong sense of what others should do and how they should do it. They can be abrasive, abrupt, intimidating, and relentless. Their goal is to prove you wrong and themselves right. You need to stay as cool as possible. An angry person will not stay angry for long if you remain calm. Listen, look them in the eye, and be ready to interrupt them. On the other hand, if they interrupt you, hold your ground and say, "You interrupted me, let me finish." It is important not to allow an aggressor to take control of the discussion with negative energy.

The Saboteur

You may find yourself dealing with someone who sabotages your efforts from behind the scene. This person does not engage in direct confrontation and yet can be just as divisive as one who confronts you openly. Never ignore a sniper! Their undermining needs to be exposed, either privately or in a group setting. Otherwise they will continue to breed discontent among everyone.

The Wet Blanket

Another difficult person to deal with is the wet blanket. This person argues that "it won't work" or "it's no use," and cannot buy into what the group is trying to accomplish. Respond to this person with positive, realistic ways to solve problems. Take their complaints seriously and ask, "What's the worse possible scenario?" Put the ball back in their court and engage them in considering solutions. Be wary of these types of people because they can infect others by dampening enthusiasm and undermining positive thinking.

The Expert

Be aware of those who consider themselves to be the experts. Although they may come across as pompous and arrogant, they are usually very productive and talented. Show that you respect their opinion and ask them to explain their point further. Be prepared and accurate in your interactions with these people. Avoid trying to assert yourself as the expert too. It may be more productive to allow them to be the expert if that seems to help you accomplish your goal.

Divisiveness in a Meeting

There are some dynamics specific to meetings that can help neutralize the efforts of a difficult person. When you are dealing with such a person in a meeting, try to get involvement from others in the group. Obtain their input and support before the meeting. During the meeting, you might ask for their reactions, for example, "How would you . . . What do you think of . . . How many would agree?" Even where you sit in a meeting can help to reduce divisiveness. Whenever you expect conflict with a particular person, arrange to sit directly next to them. You want to avoid placing yourself across from the person because this heightens the possibility of conflict. It is difficult to spar with someone who is sitting immediately to your right or left!

▼ ## Using Humor as a Tool for Change

One tool that can be used for facilitating change and for diffusing resistance to change is humor. Humor makes it possible for us to survive in "the system." It leads toward a greater awareness of the strengths and weaknesses in the present system, to new ways to respond and express creativity, and to the survival and productivity of valuable human resources (Jackson, 1985). When humor is injected into a situation, the comic relief often presents a new perspective and leads to a compromising approach. A leader who maintains a good sense of humor will inspire tremendous loyalty and enthusiasm with fellow workers. Humor leads to the creation of a positive climate and fosters an energized work environment. Learn how to maintain humor in your quest for change and to infuse humor in others.

BEGINNING THE PROCESS OF CHANGE

Change takes place on a continuum, and each person involved in the change enters the process at his or her own stage. Everyone must progress at their own pace and within their own level of comfort. Many times, the greatest resister becomes one of the staunchest advocates, provided that person is permitted the time to progress through the necessary stages that will lead to understanding and embracing the change.

The Art of Persuasion

As you begin the process of change, it may be helpful to consider a lesson from Benjamin Franklin. Franklin said, "The aim of persuasion is not to confront other people, but to appreciate their points of view and try to move them generally in your direction." Franklin's success at persuasion is described by using the acronym *TALKING* (Humes, 1992). Each letter stands for one of seven keys for successful persuasion:

- Timing—It's not good enough to have the right message. You must also choose the right moment.
- Appreciation—Anyone who wants someone else to accommodate his request should learn to appreciate the other one's problems and concerns.
- Listening—Learn to listen well enough to find out what you need and how best to sell it to the other person. Feed back their own words, using their words to sell the point.
- Knowledge—Learn where the other person is coming from and how to get them where you want to go.
- Integrity—Never misrepresent your fundamental beliefs or motives.
- Need—The three most persuasive words in the English language are *I need you*. When you must ask people for something, the best way to convince them is to show them that they are uniquely qualified to give it to you.
- Giving—Learn the value of giving. If you insist on everything, you may wind up with nothing.

Do Your Homework

Your effectiveness in initiating change will depend on the amount of homework you do before you approach others with your ideas. You may have started to consider the many policies and procedures you would like changed in your facility. You next will need to collect as much supporting data as possible for each of the changes you have in mind. Appropriate and adequate preparation before beginning the process will be central to your success.

Gather Data

First, you will need to gather supporting research and lots of it! Gather any documentation you will need to support your proposed change, including collecting hospital statistics. What are your present policies and practices, and what are the consequences of the way you are operating presently? What are the success and failure rates? Find out your breastfeeding initiation rate. How many women are still breastfeeding at 2 weeks? At 3 months? At 6 months? How does that compare to the hospital across town? Survey mothers to learn how they feel about the breastfeeding support they received in your institution. What was good or bad, and what could have been improved? Record the statistics along with your goals for change. For example, if 58 percent of mothers in your hospital initiate breastfeeding, you might state that, "By October of next year, the breastfeeding initiation rate will be at 63 percent. The following year, the rate will be 68 percent, and so on." You can do the same for breastfeeding duration and any other statistics related to breastfeeding management.

Evaluate Your Facility

You next need to assess whether your present policies and protocols promote breastfeeding, and that they are research based and in line with current recommendations. Where you determine that change is needed, prepare detailed rationale for the change. Write down the anticipated arguments along with your responses to each one. Identify alternative approaches and methods in case you experience obstacles. This careful evaluation is an essential step in the process of change. It will prepare you for responding to those who present obstacles and arguments. The best defense is a strong offense! After the change has been proposed and discussed, write down any unanticipated arguments that surfaced and note changes that are needed in your approach. Then go back to the drawing board and try again!

A Model for Planned Change

An important part of your process will be developing a systematic plan for structuring the change. One such model begins by first defining the problem and the change goal, and then determining the change agent and designing a well-defined plan of action (Hales,

1981). Such a method, or one similar to it, may be helpful to you as you promote breastfeeding changes.

Define the Problem

For every change you wish to institute, define the problem or issue that makes that change necessary. Rather than stating the problem globally in terms of lack of support for breastfeeding, define each specific problem area where changes need to occur (e.g., low initiation rates, high rates of engorgement, large numbers of babies who have difficulty latching on, and so on). Next determine the change agents. In other words, which people will prove to be the most effective leaders in proposing and instituting the change? Finally, identify all the people and positions that will be affected by the change. Be sure to involve representatives from all of the affected areas in the process so that everyone has ownership to the change.

Define Goals and Strategies

Determine whether you hope to change behavior, attitudes or values, procedures, policies, or perhaps the entire structure. You will then be able to identify specific objectives and develop a time line for the planning and implementation of the change. Some objectives will be short term, some will be intermediate, and some will be long term. The goal of increasing the incidence of breastfeeding, shown earlier, may have a short-term objective of increasing the rate to 58 percent, an intermediate objective of 63 to 68 percent, and a long-term objective of 75 percent. All such objectives will be reflected in the time line. With objectives established, you will then be ready to develop an action plan and strategies. Don't forget to address the education that will be required for empowering the staff to implement the change. Also, how will the change be communicated? Which procedures and policies will need to be altered? How will changes affect people's level of authority or power? Try to think through all the issues involved in each individual objective.

Implement the Change

After you have defined the problems, goals, and strategies, you are ready to implement the change. As you do so, be sure to monitor everyone's responses to it to learn if any unanticipated problems arise. If they do, rectify them immediately so that you can maintain a high level of commitment to the change among the staff. Evaluate both the positive and negative outcomes. Too often, this step of evaluation is overlooked. Failing to evaluate the outcomes associated with the change could jeopardize long-term success. Finally, when the change has become ingrained procedurally, you can take the final step of linking it to the overall organizational structure and standardizing it.

Planning a Breastfeeding Committee

We have looked at how you can initiate change. Now we need to consider who will initiate it. Your chances of success will be greater if change is implemented through some form of concerted group effort, perhaps a breastfeeding committee or task force. If you do not already have a breastfeeding committee in your facility, you may want to consider establishing one. Even if you are not on staff in a facility, you can approach a key person (perhaps the maternity manager) to discuss how breastfeeding is going in that facility. In a low-key manner, you can ask, "Have you noticed how more and more breastfeeding mothers seem to be getting engorged?" Or, "The number of women with sore nipples seems to be much higher than mothers in the hospital across town." You might then invite that person to have lunch with you to discuss some of these issues. This is the beginning of your committee and the beginning of your initiative for change!

Members of the Team

Put a great deal of thought into the makeup of the members on a committee. You will want the committee to be large enough that if a couple of members need to be absent, the meeting can go on as planned. Each person's level of support for breastfeeding is important. You will want to include people whom you have identified as allies, those you expect will resist, and those who seem to be neutral. It is important to have this diversity in the group and to get buy-in from potential resistors. This will help avoid sabotage or a perception that the cards are stacked in favor of one group over another. Remember that many times, the greatest resistor becomes one of the most avid supporters after they understand the issues involved!

You can also find ways to use the "system" to your advantage. All hospitals that are accredited by the Joint Commission on Accreditation of Healthcare Organizations (JCAHO) are required to have a process in place for quality improvement. Therefore, hospitals are motivated to identify problem areas and make improvements. Quality improvement efforts aim to increase customer satisfaction, and the customer is the patient. And in obstetrics, the baby is the customer (Cadwell, 1997). Consequently, quality improvements in obstetrics will focus on what is best for the baby.

A quality improvement representative will be an integral member of your breastfeeding committee. You will also want the group to be representative of all the areas that will be affected by the change. In a hospital setting this may include obstetrics, labor and delivery, postpartum, neonatal intensive care, and pediatrics. Others who have contact with either breastfeeding mothers or babies should also be considered. These may include technicians, housekeeping personnel, and management; as well as community professionals such as home care personnel, a pharmacist, and a speech pathologist. Bringing all of these people together to form an interdisciplinary team will enable all those who will be affected to participate equally in the process. As Cadwell states, "Breastfeeding practices and policies in the hospital are ideally suited to Quality Improvement targeting strategies . . . lactation consultants and other breastfeeding advocates who are familiar with the Quality Improvement process are in an excellent position to facilitate positive breastfeeding outcomes for mothers and babies."

Types of personalities

You want also to consider the personalities of the specific people you have in mind for your committee. Below are descriptions of various personality types, each of which will have positive attributes to contribute to the group. There are a variety of ways to describe the differences among personalities.

Kahler (1992) has identified six basic personality types among Americans. The six types are reactors, workaholics, rebels, persisters, dreamers, and promoters. The largest group, about 30 percent of the population, are Reactors. They are emotional and react quickly to the feelings of others. Reactors will respond to assurances that you are happy to have them on your team. Workaholics comprise 25 percent of the population. They are logical and organized, and will want you to get to the point and just tell them the facts. Rebels, another 20 percent of the population, are creative, spontaneous, and playful. They enjoy stimulating contact with other people and dislike rigid schedules. Persisters are conscientious, observant, and dedicated. As 10 percent of the population, their strong beliefs make it difficult for them to accept criticism from others. It will help to let them know how much you value their character and accomplishments. Dreamers, 10 percent of the population, are imaginative and like solitude and quiet surroundings. You may need to take the initiative with them and give them personal space. The final 5 percent of the population are the Promoters. They are persuasive, charming, and action oriented, and like to bend rules. It is easy to see that each of these personalities will contribute positively to group dynamics.

Another method of comparing personality types divides them into five categories: synthesist, idealist, pragmatist, analyst, and realist. Synthesists represent 3 percent of the population. They seek conflict, are often identified as trouble makers, and provide debate and creativity. Idealists have extremely high standards, and because of this, they can suffer deep disappointments. They are good at articulating goals and providing the broad view of issues. Pragmatists look for immediate results and find it difficult to focus on long range plans. They are resourceful, adaptable, and willing to experiment. They are sensitive to what appeals to others and are willing to settle for small gains. Analysts look for one best way to do something. They rationalize, and are stubborn and strong minded. They are also methodical, accurate, thorough, and persistent. Realists provide drive and momentum, and are interested in concrete results. They are confident and practical and good at delegating. Realists focus on both facts and opinions. They can be counted on to get the job done and are rarely wrong. They are forthright, dogmatic and sometimes seem domineering. Clearly, each of these personalities have strengths to offer the group as well.

Dynamics of a Team Meeting

When the committee members are identified, you can begin to meet regularly. Recognize that, although members of an effective team may not always share a common purpose, this need not prevent them from cooperating to achieve success. Remember that the ultimate goal is to find creative solutions that are mutually beneficial. To develop a smoothly functioning team requires empathy and a willingness to encourage the best from others. Ask the members of the group to identify the problems and then to determine how and where to start making changes. Avoid the trap of entering into a discussion with your own preplanned agenda. Know when to keep quiet, sit back, and let the discussion flow. After you have stated your position or proposal, stop and let others respond. In order for group members to take ownership of the change, they each need to be a part of designing it. It is important that you learn as much as possible about the needs of each member before proposing solutions. Withholding your own agenda until the group has processed the issues will help you learn their needs. And in the process, your own agenda may take different shape, provided that you are open to hear what others say.

Take It Slow and Easy

It is important that you not try to change everything all at once. There are undoubtedly many things that are presently being done that do not need to be changed. Identify what is right with the system, and congratulate yourselves! During the process of evaluation, you will also identify what is wrong and prioritize how to make changes. You do not necessarily need to consider a total overhaul of the system. Keep those things in place that are working. Major change does not occur overnight, and you need to make sure that everyone has realistic expectations. It may take as long as 10 years for your facility to reach its full potential in protecting, supporting, and promoting breastfeeding optimally.

Starting with a change that people are likely to find most acceptable will give you a greater chance to succeed. It may be much easier in the hospital setting, for instance, to initiate regular breastfeeding rounds than to eliminate discharge packs of infant formula. In considering your priorities of proposed changes, keep in mind the anticipated level of difficulty in convincing others to support each one. Consider which proposed changes will be least disruptive to routines; these changes are likely to meet with greater acceptance. Move slowly to those issues that may be perceived as more difficult or controversial. At the same time, recognize that the change that seems easiest to you may not be the one that will garner the least resistance from others.

You need to establish a track record with several of the easier changes before going on to the big ones. Leave the toughest challenges until you have several of the less controversial and less difficult changes in place. You will find a greater level of self confidence after first having been successful in instituting the earlier changes. Also, after some of the changes are in practice, others may be better able to see the complete picture and more willing to support the tougher changes.

Give Recognition and Praise

Everyone likes to be recognized for something they do right, especially when they feel as though they have gone out of their way to provide good care. Give people positive feedback for any change you see in the right direction. Make sure others know about it, too. For example, "Did you hear how much Mrs. Robinson appreciated Pam's help in getting her baby to latch on?"

Use your creativity to provide incentives or rewards that will encourage everyone's participation and compliance. You might award a button or pen for completing a breastfeeding module or attending an inservice program, a pizza party when a breastfeeding course is completed, or a designated breastfeeding counselor of the month. You can make a breastfeeding bulletin board where you will post lactation updates, new policies that have been instituted, and minutes from the breastfeeding committee meetings. Summarize professional articles of interest and post them. Cut out articles from newspapers, magazines, and professional journals. Develop a newsletter to send to physician offices. All of these efforts can create cooperation and goodwill.

Ultimately, people have some very basic needs that must be met at work. They want work that is interesting. They want to be shown appreciation and to be involved in the overall scheme. They want job security, money, and a chance for growth. Help them meet these needs, and you will receive the support and cooperation necessary for meeting your own needs.

THE INFANT FORMULA INDUSTRY

The infant formula industry is eager to promote breastfeeding. Yes, you read that right! Breastfeeding mothers are statistically very health conscious. It stands to reason then, that when they wean their babies from the breast, they are more likely to wean to an infant formula rather than immediately to cow's milk. Their babies will probably receive formula until an older age than will babies who were fed formula from birth. Formula-feeding mothers are more likely to wean their babies to cow's milk at an earlier age. As with any industry, individual formula manufacturers are in fierce competition with one another for customers. The one that looks the best will win more breastfeeding mothers. They know breast is best, and they promote their product under the guise of promoting breastfeeding. They tell the public what they know they want to hear. That's simply good advertising.

Advertising Practices

Today, manufacturers worldwide advertise their infant foods both in medical journals and to the lay public. Free samples are given to mothers when they are discharged from the hospital. The practice of supplying infant formula to nurseries at no charge originated in the 1930s, and the practice has been criticized periodically ever since. You will be hard pressed to find any other product that is supplied to hospitals at no charge. Hospitals should be required to pay for infant formula just as they do all other supplies. If gifts are given to hospitals, they should be legitimate, documentable research, or teaching grants. Gifts should not go through the hospital's purchasing agent (Barness, 1987).

Manufacturers do not stop at giving free formula to hospitals. Families receive discount coupons and even cases of free formula at their homes (Howard, 1994). Aggressive marketing campaigns target physicians and hospital maternity units as well. Hospitals and health care providers are showered with free equipment, architectural planning, calendars, office supplies, and other giveaways. Funding is provided for airline tickets to conferences, medical fellowships, scholarships, educational grants, and other perks that are common to industry (i.e., tickets to sporting events, dinners, and fishing trips). Company representatives present themselves as experts in infant nutrition and educate both

TABLE 26.3	
The International Code of Marketing of Human Milk Substitutes	
Code Provision	**Implications to Consider**
Under the scope of the Code, items marketed or otherwise represented to be suitable as human milk substitutes can include foods and beverages such as ◆ Infant formula ◆ Other milk products ◆ Cereals ◆ Vegetable, fruit, and other puréed preparations ◆ Juices and baby teas ◆ Follow-on milks ◆ Bottled water	Whether or not a product is considered to be within this definition will depend on how it is promoted for infants. Any products that are marketed or represented as suitable substitutes to human milk will fall into this category. Since babies should receive *only* human milk for about the first six months, any other food or drink promoted for use during this time will be a human milk substitute.
Regarding advertising and information, the Code recommends that ◆ Advertising of human milk substitutes, bottles, and teats to the public not be permitted ◆ Educational materials explain the benefits of breastfeeding, the health hazards associated with bottle feeding, the costs of using infant formula, and the difficulty of reversing the decision not to breastfeed ◆ Product labels clearly state the superiority of breastfeeding, the need for the advice of a health care worker, and a warning about health hazards; and they show no pictures of babies, or other pictures or text idealizing the use of infant formula	Health workers such as lactation consultants and breastfeeding counselors need to press their legislators for measures that will implement the Code in full. This would protect mothers from advertising in parent magazines and on television. It would also prevent direct company contact with mothers through hot lines, Internet sites, mailings, home-delivered supplies of formula, and baby clubs.
Regarding samples and supplies, the Code recommends that ◆ No free samples be given to pregnant women, mothers, or their families ◆ No free or low-cost supplies of human milk substitutes be given to maternity wards, hospitals, or any other part of the health care system	Under the Code, free or low-cost supplies can be distributed only outside of the health care system and must be continued for as long as the infant needs them. In the United States, this is usually for 1 year. Elsewhere, it is for at least 6 months. The health care system encompasses health care workers, including lactation consultants *and* breastfeeding counselors.
Regarding health care facilities and health care workers, the Code recommends that ◆ There be no product displays, posters, or distribution of promotional materials ◆ No gifts or samples be given to health care workers ◆ Product information for health professionals be limited to what is factual and scientific	This provision also covers bottles that are provided and shown in advertisements by breast pump companies that are clearly feeding bottles, even when no teats are shown. Pens and pads of paper with the name of a formula company are examples of gifts.

physicians and parents through videos and literature (Young, 1990).

Accepting a "gift" implies an obligation on the receiver's part to look favorably at the giver, causing the receiver to feel a moral obligation to treat that person nicer and, ultimately, to promote his product. Michael Jenike of Harvard Medical School (1990) suggests that individual physicians should refuse to attend or speak at meetings sponsored by pharmaceutical companies. The International Lactation Consultant Association (ILCA) urges lactation consultants to refuse funding from formula companies. There is no such thing as a free lunch, and someone eventually pays. For the parents, it is in higher costs on the retail market. For the infant, it is a higher incidence of illness. For the general public, it is in higher taxes and overall health care costs.

A Global Response to Formula Advertising

Worldwide, the practice of substituting artificial baby milk whether partially or fully, has resulted in greater incidences of malnutrition, infections, diarrheal diseases, impaired growth, and even infant deaths. By the mid-1970s, health experts realized that a global effort was needed in order to stem the tide of these negative outcomes for children. This led to the adoption of the International Code of Marketing of Breastmilk Substitutes by the World Health Assembly in 1981. The Code was intended to regulate the advertising and promotional techniques used to sell infant formula, other human milk substitutes including all foods marketed or otherwise represented to replace human milk, feeding bottles, and artificial nipples. However, because of delays in national implementation of the Code, as well as continued disregard of its provisions by the manufacturers and distributors, the 1980s saw artificial feeding continue to increase and breastfeeding continue to decline.

Table 26.3 reflects the main points of the Code, which was developed by the World Health Assembly and has now been affirmed by all Member States of the World Health Organization. It still awaits enactment into legislation or enforceable regulations at the national level in many countries. The Code regulates the marketing and distribution of products that are represented to be suitable as a partial or total replacement for human milk. Breastfeeding advocates recognize that any product that is promoted for use during the exclusive breastfeeding period below the age of about 6 months will have the effect of replacing human milk in the child's intake.

Health workers can protect breastfeeding by implementing the practices outlined in this text and by urging their facilities to adhere to the International Code of Marketing of Breastmilk Substitutes. Help others in your facility develop an awareness of instances in which the facility violates the Code. Remove posters, videos, and leaflets that advertise products marketed or otherwise represented to be suitable as substitutes for human milk. Make sure that instruction on the use of infant formula is targeted only to those mothers who have chosen not to breastfeed. Videos on artificial feeding can be removed from the hospital's television channel, for instance, and loaned individually to mothers who need the instruction.

When you encounter violations of the Code, you can take action to make others aware. Ask administrators to reject anything that does not comply with the Code. Discuss the violations with colleagues, and take steps to change the practices that do not comply. Refuse any gifts or samples of formula, and prevent them from being given to mothers. Be aware that many times, sponsorship of a conference by formula companies may not be evident and you will need to ask before agreeing to participate in the program. The Code is in place to promote, protect, and support breastfeeding. You are in a good position to make sure that mothers' interests are protected.

PROMOTING BABY-FRIENDLY PRACTICES

Lactation consultants can be instrumental in developing breastfeeding protocols, challenging traditional procedures, and removing barriers that erode the mother's confidence in her ability to breastfeed. You have enormous potential to facilitate consistent nursing care by instituting care plans for managing breastfeeding problems and conducting staff inservice education. UNICEF and the World Health Organization have provided health care professionals and administrators with succinct guidelines for the establishment of policies and procedures that will promote, protect, and support breastfeeding. ILCA and other breastfeeding advocacy organizations support the UNICEF/WHO *Ten Steps to Successful Breastfeeding*. Hospitals, clinics, and physician offices throughout the world are incorporating these guidelines into their policies and practices.

Breastfeeding promotion is a form of social marketing, and marketing is a tactic used by businesses to convert people's needs into profitable company opportunities (Kotler, 1984). Hospitals, physician practices, and employers are in the business of satisfying customer needs. In this regard, breastfeeding promotion is no different from the marketing of any other health practice that improves the well-being of the consumer. An institution can add value to its services by adopting a marketing strategy that is consumer focused (Sonstegard, 1988). The use of effective marketing strategies will further the promotion of breastfeeding. Parents and infants are the consumers whose needs must be met. Baby-friendly practices will provide a framework within which they can achieve their goals.

Achieving a baby-friendly environment may seem to be a daunting task. Yet the benefits are immense. If you give more than is asked of you, you will reap great rewards. What an exhilarating feeling to be part of such a positive experience. To get where you want to go, you must have a definite vision of your overall goal. UNICEF and WHO have provided the vision through the *Ten Steps to Successful Breastfeeding* and the Baby-Friendly Hospital Initiative. The aim of the initiative is to "make health care providers the prime movers in recreating a world environment that supports, protects, and promotes the practice of breastfeeding—a world environment that is friendly to babies and their mothers (Kyenkya-Isabirye, 1992). The success of the initiative will depend on countless small changes enacted person by person, hospital by hospital, and country by country.

▼ **A Baby-Friendly Health Profession**

Changes are occurring in health care around the globe. In the United States, in response to new trends in health insurance, the length of stay following birth has changed dramatically in the past decade. Everyone working in the health care field is affected by the changes in one way or another. Promotion of breastfeeding must fit into the context of the health care system. Many mothers receive marginal in-hospital breastfeeding care. Lactation success is threatened by conflicting advice, misconceptions, inconsistencies between theory and practice, and disagreement about correct nursing care for breastfeeding mothers. Maternity nurses may acknowledge, for instance, that suckling promotes milk production, and yet advise formula supplements if a mother appears not to have enough milk. Mothers need consistent technical assistance with feeding from caregivers who will empower them to reach their goals.

The health worker is central to the encouragement and support of breastfeeding. In order to become a reality, the baby-friendly initiative will require the commitment of all health professionals. Yet, despite a universal recognition of the health benefits of breastfeeding, many physicians fail to support breastfeeding mothers (Donnelly, 1994). One study showed that 48 percent of practicing pediatricians did not recommend breastfeeding to their patients. They also reported few interventions to assist breastfeeding women. These same physicians over-whelmingly reported favorable attitudes toward breastfeeding promotion (Michelman, 1990).

Much of this lack of tangible support results from the absence of formal training in breastfeeding management. Pediatricians, obstetricians, and family practice physicians need formal instruction in breastfeeding management during their residency programs, with a focus on three main areas. First, the program must provide information regarding medical rationale, techniques, and problem solving. Second, it needs to address expectations, beliefs, and an acceptance of data that demonstrates the health benefits of breastfeeding. Finally, the program needs to focus on the physicians' confidence that they can provide effective counseling and support to breastfeeding women (Freed, 1993).

Beyond formal training, breastfeeding support also requires a genuine commitment on the part of the caregiver. Physicians need to recognize that when they distribute infant formula or vouchers to parents, they place themselves in the position of advertising and promoting a specific product. Also, this promotion contributes to the failure of women in their practice to breastfeed their infants (Howard, 1993). Those physicians who support breastfeeding can be encouraged to "convert" the doubters (Helsing, 1990). UNICEF developed a pledge for physicians to sign attesting to their commitment to protect, promote, and support breastfeeding, as presented in Figure 26.2 (Grant, 1994). Signing such a

FIGURE 26.2 Physician's pledge to protect, promote, and support breastfeeding

Recognizing that breastfeeding plays a uniquely important role in the healthy development of infants and young children;

that no substitute can provide the complex balance of nutrients, antibodies and growth factors that make human milk the perfect food for infants;

that women have the right to make infant feeding decisions based on complete and accurate information;

that my role as a physician is one of influence, authority and trust;

that current marketing practices—including the free and low-cost distribution of human milk substitute supplies to hospitals and other parts of the health care system—compete against and discourage breastfeeding;

that my Government, at the 1994 World Health Assembly, affirmed that the marketing and promotion of human milk substitutes should not be conducted anywhere in the health care system; and

that the promotion of health and the prevention of disease are my duties and the mandates of responsible health care providers everywhere;

I hereby pledge to do my part to protect, promote and support breastfeeding and to work to end the free and low-cost distribution of human milk substitutes to our health care systems.

Signature _____

pledge demonstrates the physician's desire to support breastfeeding women in his or her practice.

This support can be further formalized by the development of baby-friendly breastfeeding policies. Examples of baby-friendly policies in a hospital, pediatric practice, obstetric practice, and home health are presented in Figure 26.3, Baby-Friendly Hospital Breastfeeding Policy,

Figure 26.4, Ten Steps to a Baby-Friendly Pediatric Practice; and Figure 26.5, Ten Steps to a Baby-Friendly Obstetric Practice; Figure 26.6, Ten Steps to a Baby-Friendly Home Health Practice; and Figure 26.7, Eleven Steps to Optimal Breastfeeding in the Pediatric Unit. These policies are derived from the *Ten Steps to Successful Breastfeeding* that form the basis of the baby-friendly initiative.

FIGURE 26.3   Baby-Friendly Hospital Breastfeeding Policy

1. All pregnant women and new mothers will be informed of the nutritional and health benefits, and basic management of breastfeeding.
2. Staff will presume the mother is breastfeeding unless the mother informs the staff otherwise.
3. Mothers will be helped to initiate breastfeeding within an hour of birth unless maternal or neonatal complications intervene.
4. All nursing mothers will be given instructions on hand expression of milk. If they should be separated from their infants, nursing mothers will be given specific instructions on breastfeeding and how to maintain lactation (pumping). Mothers who have not begun breastfeeding within 8 to 12 hours of birth will begin milk expression.
5. Breastfeeding newborns will be given no food or drink other than human milk unless medically indicated and a specific order is written by the physician. A list of medical indications for using human milk substitutes is provided.
6. Breastfeeding babies will be given pacifiers only at the direction of the mother. The risks and benefits of using artificial nipples (pacifiers, bottles) will be explained to the mother.
7. Infants who need supplementation will be tube fed at the breast or cup fed unless medically contraindicted.
8. Rooming in will be encouraged; babies are to be kept with their mothers 24 hours a day. Mothers will be taught how to co-sleep with their infants safely.
9. Mothers will be taught to watch for infant feeding cues, and will breastfeed their babies on demand rather than on a predetermined schedule. Mothers will be encouraged to breastfeed their babies a minimum of eight times in 24 hours.
10. Mothers will be given information about breastfeeding support groups and lactation consultants prior to discharge from the hospital.
11. Each health care professional who cares for mothers and infants at this facility is expected to maintain the skills and knowledge necessary for implementation of this policy.

FIGURE 26.4   Ten Steps to a Baby-Friendly Pediatric Practice

1. Develop or implement a current breastfeeding protocol for use in your practice that is communicated to all staff. Provide copies to those who cover for you.
2. Arrange for all staff to attend inservices that teach the skills necessary to implement the protocol.
3. Inform all pregnant women about the benefits and management of breastfeeding. Give written, noncommercial prenatal information on breastfeeding, refer parents to breastfeeding classes, and encourage fathers to attend.
4. Help mothers initiate and maintain breastfeeding during hospital rounds. Perform newborn exam in the mother's room, showing her how well-designed her baby is for breastfeeding.
5. If mother and baby are separated due to illness, prematurity, and so on, confirm that an electric breast pump is available for expressing milk, and that milk is expressed at least eight times in 24 hours. A prescription may be written for human milk, if necessary, to cover the cost of renting an electric breast pump.
6. Avoid the use of sterile water, glucose water, or formula for breastfeeding newborn infants, unless medically indicated. Adequate amounts of milk are present at delivery in the form of colostrum.
7. Encourage mothers to room in 24 hours a day in the hospital. This protects the baby from disease in the nursery, provides opportunities for unrestricted contact and feeding, and encourages mothers to become aware of their baby's needs and rhythms.
8. Advise mothers to feed their infants on cue, 8 to 12 time each 24 hours. Teach behavioral feeding cues to avoid underfeeding or over-hunger, with resulting infant behavioral disorganization.
9. Avoid the use of artificial nipples and pacifiers in newborn breastfeeding infants. This approach decreases the incidence of nipple preference and its sequelae.
10. Have available on staff a nurse practitioner or lactation consultant whose responsibility can include prenatal teaching, hospital rounds, call-in times, and visits for breastfeeding questions or problems. Or refer such situations to a lactation consultant in the community. Refer mothers to breastfeeding support groups for mother-to-mother support.

Printed by permission of Marsha Walker.

> ▽ **FIGURE 26.5**   Ten Steps to a Baby-Friendly Obstetric Practice
>
> 1. Create and implement a breastfeeding promotion and support policy for use in your practice that is communicated to all staff. Provide copies to those who cover for you.
> 2. Arrange for all staff to attend inservices that teach the skills necessary to implement the protocol.
> 3. Inform all pregnant women about the benefits and management of breastfeeding. Give written, noncommercial information on breastfeeding. Recommend that parents attend prenatal breastfeeding classes that include fathers. Refer parents to childbirth education classes.
> 4. Help mothers initiate breastfeeding within ½ hour of birth. Place and leave the infant on the mother's chest to promote the prefeeding sequences of behavior that leads to proper latch, suck, and organization of breastfeedings.
> 5. If mother and baby are separated due to illness, prematurity, and so on, confirm that an electric breast pump is available for expressing milk; that milk is expressed at least eight times in 24 hours; that no nipple soreness, engorgement, or breast problems arise from the use of the pump.
> 6. Avoid the use of sterile water, glucose water, or formula for breastfeeding newborn infants, unless medically indicated. Adequate amounts of milk are present at delivery in the form of colostrum.
> 7. Encourage mothers to room in 24 hours a day in the hospital. This protects the baby from disease in the nursery, provides opportunities for unrestricted contact and feeding, and encourages mothers to become aware of their baby's needs and rhythms.
> 8. Advise mothers to feed their infants on cue, 8 to 12 times each 24 hours. Teach behavioral feeding cues to avoid underfeeding or overhunger, with resulting infant behavioral disorganization.
> 9. Avoid the use of artificial nipples and pacifiers in newborn breastfeeding infants. This approach decreases the incidence of nipple preference and its sequelae.
> 10. Have available on staff a nurse practitioner or lactation consultant whose responsibility can include prenatal teaching, hospital rounds, call-in times, and visits for breastfeeding questions or problems. Or refer such situations to a lactation consultant in the community. Refer mothers to breastfeeding support groups for mother-to-mother support.

Printed by permission of Marsha Walker.

> ▽ **FIGURE 26.6**   Ten Steps to a Baby-Friendly Home Health Agency
>
> 1. Create a written breastfeeding policy that is research based, and provide copies of the policy to all home health staff. Include the WHO/UNICEF Code for Marketing Breastmilk Substitutes in the policy.
> 2. Train all health care staff in the Maternal-Child Services using the WHO/UNICEF 18 Hour Course. Update staff as new or revised research-based information becomes available. New staff will be given the 18-hour course beginning during orientation and completed within 1 year.
> 3. Inform all pregnant women about the benefits and management of breastfeeding; weave breastfeeding information into every visit. Provide written information that complies with the WHO Code. Refer all pregnant women to the prenatal breastfeeding classes within the community.
> 4. Inform all pregnant women of the importance of initiating breastfeeding within the first hour of life.
> 5. If postpartum mothers are separated from their babies, be sure they have proper equipment for milk expression and provide instruction as needed. Teach hand expression to all breastfeeding mothers. Assess breastfeeding during each home visit.
> 6. Give the child (ages newborn to about 6 months) no food or drink other than human milk unless *medically* indicated. Instruct mothers (prenatal and postpartum) about the risks of artificial baby milks. A list of acceptable medical reasons for human milk substitutes is included in the breastfeeding policy.
> 7. Encourage a "rooming in" home environment. Explain the importance of close mother-infant contact 24 hours a day by the use of a sling, bathing together, sleeping together and so on.
> 8. Teach mothers the importance of their babies' cues. Explain the importance of baby-led feedings, rather than placing limitations and times on feeds. Advise mothers that 8 to 12 or more feeds in 24 hours is normal and expected.
> 9. Give no artificial teats or pacifiers to breastfeeding infants. Discourage their use, and instead direct the mother to breastfeed for suckling satisfaction. Explain the negative consequences of such devices.
> 10. Foster the establishment of breastfeeding support groups within the community, and refer mothers to them at any time.

Printed by permission of Debbie Shinskie.

FIGURE 26.7 Eleven steps to optimal breastfeeding in the pediatric unit

1. Have a written breastfeeding policy, and train health care staff caring for breastfeeding infants in skills necessary to implement the policy.
2. When the sick infant is admitted, ascertain the mother's wishes about infant feeding, and assist mothers to establish and manage lactation as necessary.
3. Provide parents with written and verbal information about the benefits of breastfeeding and human milk.
4. Facilitate unrestricted breastfeeding and frequent human milk expression by mothers who wish to provide milk for their children, regardless of age.
5. Give breastfed children other food or drink only when age appropriate or medically indicated.
6. When medically indicated, use only those alternative feeding methods most conducive to successful breastfeeding, and restrict the use of any oral device associated with breastfeeding problems.
7. Provide facilities that allow parents and infants to remain together 24 hours a day, that encourage skin-to-skin contact as appropriate, and that avoid modeling the use of artificial feeding.
8. Administer medications and schedule all procedures, so as to cause the least possible disturbance of the breastfeeding relationship.
9. Maintain a human milk bank that meets appropriate standards.
10. Provide information about community breastfeeding support groups to parents at the time of the infant's discharge from the hospital or clinic.
11. Maintain appropriate monitoring and data collection procedures to permit quality assurance and ongoing research.

Printed by permission of Maureen Minchin from *Breastfeeding Matters;* 1999.

Official Baby-Friendly Designation

Health facilities worldwide are being designated as baby friendly, with the initiative being adopted more slowly in some countries than it is in others. As of September 1998 there were 13,800 facilities globally that were officially designated as baby friendly. In the United States, action is much slower. In September 1998, there were 14 facilities with the official baby-friendly designation. Another 75 facilities had signed letters of intent and had begun the process of working toward baby-friendly designation.

A baby-friendly designation means that a facility meets high global standards and has at least 75 percent of mothers exclusively breastfeeding at discharge. The global process for receiving baby-friendly recognition involves an internal assessment, an external assessment by outside evaluators, and a presentation of the findings by UNICEF. The process may vary from one country to another as government officials make adaptations that will complement their own country's standards.

A Baby-Friendly World

The baby friendly initiative goes far beyond the health community. Breastfeeding is regarded by many as an important women's, human rights, and feminist issue. It may appear that feminism and breastfeeding are incompatible, because breastfeeding might be regarded as tying women to traditional roles. However, Van Esterick (1994) regards breastfeeding as a holistic act that is intimately connected to all domains of life—sexuality, eating, emotion, appearance, sleeping, and parental relationships. Breastfeeding confirms a woman's power to control her own body and challenges views of the breast as primarily a sexual object. Women's groups should be encouraged to commit resources and time to breastfeeding promotion. Artists can be encouraged to portray the beauty and power of breastfeeding through paintings, photographs, poems, and plays. Magazines, television, and movies can present breastfeeding as a natural part of our culture.

Promotion of breastfeeding at the governmental level has been shown to increase both the incidence and duration of breastfeeding (Parlato, 1992), with successful campaigns sharing several characteristics. They have a long-term plan for sustaining the program, sound administrative and financial management, and staff and funds devoted exclusively to the promotion program. Key obstacles are identified, along with strategies for overcoming them, and a mass media program conveys appropriate messages and materials to the target audience.

Richard Reid (1993), the then Director of Public Affairs for UNICEF, cautioned that "every culture that abandons breastfeeding is inviting upon itself sicklier children, weaker mothers, poorer families, strained national economies, and more polluted environments." He urges a global return to breastfeeding as an urgent moral, health, social, and economic imperative. Long-term strategies for achieving a baby-friendly world, developed by UNICEF, appear in the list in the next section. These efforts to return breastfeeding to its rightful place as the cultural norm will empower women to nurture their babies in the manner that nature intended.

Long-Term Strategies for Achieving a Baby-Friendly World

◆ Ensure that all maternity centers practice all of the *Tens Steps to Successful Breastfeeding*.

◆ Take action to implement fully all articles of the *International Code of Marketing of Breastmilk Substitutes*.

◆ Enact and enforce legislation to protect the breastfeeding rights of working women.

◆ Educate communities to value women's contributions to the health of their children and thus the health of the community and the world.

◆ Encourage institutions to ease the tasks of motherhood with convenient antenatal care, respect from caregivers, good obstetric services, and patient-focused delivery procedures.

◆ Provide women with counseling and clinical services for breastfeeding and birth spacing.

◆ Enlist community, health, religious, and political leaders to promote the primary health care principles of preventive health education and empowerment of mothers.

▼

SUMMARY

We wish you great success in your helping role with mothers and in your promotion of breastfeeding. We encourage you to work as an active agent for change, working toward making your community baby friendly in all areas—hospitals, clinics, health workers, and the general public. Remember that the elements of baby friendly extend beyond the baby. The practices create an environment that is mother friendly and family friendly. As stated by UNICEF, "Breastfeeding is an endangered practice. It needs an entire culture to support and nurture it back to its full, potent strength. It is time to take the baby-friendly initiative!"

▼

REFERENCES

Barness LA. Nothing is free. *Contemp Pediatri;* May, 1987.

Breastfeeding Support Consultants (BSC). *Creating Change in the Face of Resistance.* Chalfont, PA; 1996.

Browder S. Super-confidence and how to get it. *New Woman Magazine;* July, 1994.

Cadwell K. Using the quality improvement process to affect breastfeeding protocols in United States hospitals. *J Hum Lact* 13:5–9; 1997.

Calano J and J Salzman. How to turn heat into light. *Working Woman;* March, 1988.

Covey S. *The 7 Habits of Highly Effective People.* New York: Simon and Schuster; 1990.

Donnelly BW. Are we really doing all we can to promote breastfeeding? *Contemp Pediat* July 1994.

Ellis DJ. Supporting breastfeeding: How to implement agency change. Clinical Issues in Perinatal and Women's Health Nursing. *NAACOG* 3(4):560–564; 1992.

Freed GL. Breast-feeding: Time to teach what we preach. *JAMA* 269:243–245; January, 1993.

Grant JP. Physician's pledge to protect, promote and support breastfeeding. New York: UNICEF; 1994.

Hales DJ. Promoting breastfeeding: Strategies for changing hospital policy, *Stud Fam Plan* 12(4):167–172; 1981.

Helsing E. Supporting breastfeeding: What governments and health workers can do—European experiences. *Int J Gynecol Obstet* 31(Suppl. 1):69–71; 1990.

Howard C. et al. Antenatal formula advertising: Another potential threat to breast-feeding. *Pediatrics* 94:102–104; 1994.

Howard F et al. The physician as advertiser: The unintentional discouragement of breastfeeding, *Obstet Gynecol* 81:1048–1051; 1993.

Humes JC. Life lessons from Ben Franklin. Bottom Line/Personal; June 15, 1992.

Jackson M. The comedy of management. In Simms L, et al. *The Professional Practice of Nursing Administration.* New York; Wiley; pp 339–351; 1985.

Jenike MA. Relations between physicians and pharmaceutical companies: Where to draw the line. [Letter.] *N Engl J Med* 322:557; 1990.

Kahler T. Six basic personality types. Bottom Line/Personal; September 15, 1992.

Kotler P. Marketing management: Analysis, planning and control, 5th ed. Englewood Cliffs; NJ: Prentice-Hall; 1984.

Kyenkya-Isabirye M. UNICEF launches the Baby-Friendly Hospital Initiative. *MCN* 17(4):177–179; 1992.

Michelman DF et al. Pediatricians and breastfeeding promotion: Attitudes, beliefs and practices. *American Journal of Health Promotion* 4:181–186; 1990.

Mulford C. Swimming upstream: Breastfeeding care in a non-breastfeeding culture. *JOGNN* 24(5):464–474; 1995.

Parlato MB. Promotion of breast-feeding in the media, [Letter.], *World Health Forum* 15:197; 1992.

Reid R. The baby-friendly hospital initiative: A global movement for humankind, International *Child Health* 4(1):41–47; January 1993.

Sonstegard L. A better way to market maternal-child care. *MCN* 13:395–402; 1988.

UNICEF. Take the baby-friendly initiative! UNICEF House, 3 UN Plaza, New York NY 10017, page 16.

Van Esterik P. *Beyond the Breast-Bottle Controversy.* New Brunswick, NJ: Rutgers University Press; 1989.

Young D. Breastfeeding: Can it compete in the marketplace? *Birth* 17:119–120; 1990.

▼

BIBLIOGRAPHY

Apple R. The medicalization of infant feeding in the United States and New Zealand: Two countries, one experience. *J Hum Lact* 10:31–37; 1994.

Armstrong HC. Breastfeeding promotion: Training of mid-level and outreach health workers. *Int J Gynecol and Obstet* 31(Suppl 1):91–103; 1991.

Auerbach K. Breastfeeding promotion: Why it doesn't work. *J Hum Lact* 6:45–46; 1990.

Auerbach KG. The many ways of marketing artificial baby milk *J Hum Lact* 8:61–62; 1992.

Bell ML. A portrait of progress: A business history of Pet Milk Company from 1885 to 1960 St. Louis, MO: Pet Milk Company; pp 102–104; 1962.

Chezem J et al. Lactation duration: Influences of human milk replacements and formula samples on women planning postpartum employment. *JOGNN* 27:646–651; 1998.

Cypert SA. *Believe and Achieve,* New York: Avon Books; 1987.

Gunnlaugsson G and Einarsdottir J. Colostrum and ideas about bad milk: A case study from Guinea-Bissau. *Soc Sci Med* 36:283–288; 1993.

Hardin B. Project Bestfeeding receives the first ICEA Special Projects Grant. *Int J Childbirth Education* 8:15; 1993.

Harter C et al. Networking to implement effective health care. *MCN* 14:387–392; 1989.

Heinig J. Breastfeeding and the bottom line: Why are the cost savings of breastfeeding such a hard sell? *J Hum Lact* 14:87–88; 1998.

Howard C et al. Infant formula distribution and advertising in pregnancy: A hospital survey. *Birth* 21(1):14–19; March 1994.

Jacobson S. et al. Incidence and correlates of breast-feeding in socioeconomically disadvantage women. *Pediatrics* 88:728–736; 1991.

Julion B. Letter. *J Nurse Midwife* 38:179–180; 1993.

Kanter RM. Managing the human side of change. *Manage Rev;* 52–56; 1985.

Kaufman K and Hall L. Influences of the social network on choice and duration of breastfeeding in mothers of preterm infants. *Res Nurs Health* 12:149–159; 1989.

Lawrence R. Breast-feeding trends: A cause for action. *Pediatrics* 88:867–868; 1991.

Minchin M et al. Expanding the WHO/UNICEF Baby Friendly Hospital Initiative (BFHI): 11 steps to optimal breastfeeding in the pediatric unit. *Breastfeeding Rev* 4:87–91; 1996.

Minchin M. *Breastfeeding Matters: What We Need To Know About Infant Feeding.* Alma Publications; Victoria, Australia 1998.

National Association of Pediatric Nurse Associates and Practitioners. Position Statement. *J Pediatr Health Care* 7:289; 1993.

Newton E. Breastfeeding/lactation and the medical school curriculum. *J Hum Lact* 8:122–124; 1992.

Palmer G. The politics of infant feeding. *Mothering* 73–85; 1991.

Palmer G. *The Politics of Breastfeeding.* London: Pandora Press; 1993.

Radford A et al. Breast feeding: The baby friendly initiative. *Br Med J* 317:1385; 1998.

UNICEF/WHO. Breastfeeding management and promotion in a baby-friendly hospital, An 18-hour course for maternity staff; 1993.

Valaitis R and Shea E. An evaluation of breastfeeding promotion literature: Does it really promote breastfeeding? *Can J Public Health* 84:24–27; 1993.

Van Esterick P. Breastfeeding and feminism. Int J Gynecol Obstet (Supp 1): S41–S54; 1994.

Walker M. Why aren't more mothers breastfeeding? *Childbirth Instructor* W: 18–24; 1992.

Walther GR. *Power Talking* New York: Berkley Publishing Group.

Williams E and Pan E. Breastfeeding initiation among a low income multiethnic population in Northern California: An exploratory study. *J Hum Lact* 10:245–251; 1994.

Wolf H et al. First "baby friendly" hospitals in Europe. *Lancet* 341:440; 1993.

Young D. The baby friendly hospital initiative in the U.S.: Why so slow? *Birth* 20(4):179–181; 1993.

GLOSSARY

 A

abruptio placenta   Premature separation of the placenta from the wall of the uterus.

abscess   Localized collection of pus that forms from an infection because it has no opening for drainage.

acculturated   Integrated in a new culture.

acinus   Any small saclike structure, as one found in a gland. Also called alveolus.

acrocyanosis   Bluish tinge of the hands and feet.

acrodermatitis enteropathica   A rare long-term disease of infants. Symptoms are blisters on the skin and mucous membranes, hair loss, diarrhea, and failure to thrive.

active listening   A counseling skill that involves paraphrasing a message and reflecting it back to the sender.

adhesion   Tissue layers that adhere to one another.

adipose tissue   Tissue made of fat cells arranged in lobes.

afterpains   Menstrual-like pains that occur in the first few days after birth as the uterus contracts to return to normal size.

allergen   A foreign substance that can cause an allergic response in the body.

alternate massage   Technique in which the mother compresses the breast each time the baby pauses during a feed. Used to encourage suckling and increase milk production. Also called breast compression.

alveolar ridge   The bony ridge of the jaw that contains the tooth sockets.

alveoli   Tiny glands in the breast that produce milk.

amenorrhea   The absence of the monthly flow of blood and discharge of mucous tissues from the uterus through the vagina (menstruation).

amino acids   The basic building blocks of which proteins are constructed in the body. They are the end products of protein digestion.

amylase   An enzyme that aids the breakdown of starch in digestion.

analgesia   Absences of the normal sensation of pain.

anchor   A word or phrase used at the numerical endpoints of a written scale to describe the extremes of feeling or thought measured by the scale.

anesthesia   Partial or complete loss of sensation with or without memory loss as a result of disease, injury or administration of an anesthetic agent, usually by injection or inhalation.

ankyloglossia   Tight frenulum; defect of the mouth in which the membrane under the tongue is too short and limits movement of the tongue.

anomaly   Change from that which is regarded as normal; inherited problem with growth of a structure.

anovulatory   Failure of the ovaries to produce, mature, or release eggs.

anoxia   Lack of oxygen.

antibody   A protein substance that is developed in response to and interacts specifically with an antigen to form the basis of immunity.

anticipatory guidance   A form of counseling that provides encouragement, help, and guidance in order to prevent or minimize problems.

anticipatory stage   The first of four stages in role acquisition. The time in which one collects information and begins learning about the new role, as in the role of parent or lactation consultant.

antigen   A substance foreign to the body, often a protein.

antimicrobial   Preventing or destroying the development of microorganisms.

apnea   Failure to breathe.

areola   The dark, circular area surrounding the nipple.

artificial baby milk   Any food being marketed or otherwise represented as a partial or total replacement for human milk. Also called a human milk substitute.

artificial feeding   Feeding an infant anything other than human milk.

assimilate   The process of incorporating nutrition into living tissue or becoming incorporated into a culture other than one's own.

assumption   In statistics, a condition that must be true of the data in order for the statistical test to be used accurately.

asymmetry   Unequal in size or shape.

atresia   Absence of a normal body opening.

attending   A counseling skill that involves listening and observing in a noninterfering manner.

attentive listening   A counseling skill in which the listener actively focuses on the words that are heard.

autocrine control   Local control within the gland. In the case of the breast, the control agent is a secretory product from one type of cell that influences the activity of this same type of cell. This suggests that milk that is left in the breast acts to inhibit the production of more milk.

autonomic nerves   Nerves that have the ability to function independently without outside influence.

average   The sum of the values (in the group being averaged) divided by the number of members of the group. If Sally is 15, John is 20 and Bill is 35, their average age is $70/3 = 23.3$.

axilla   Pyramid-shaped space forming the underside of the shoulder between the upper part of the arm and the side of the chest. Also called the armpit.

 B

baby blues   The mild depression some women feel for several weeks following birth. This brief depression frequently appears around the third day postpartum. The mother may have bouts of tearfulness and sadness mingled with happiness and excitement. It is more common in women having their first baby.

baby friendly   Maternity care that protects, promotes, and supports breastfeeding, and is based on the Baby Friendly Hospital Initiative *Ten Steps to Successful Breastfeeding*.

baby-led weaning   Weaning initiated by the baby according to the baby's own timetable.

bactericidal   Substance that destroys bacteria.

basal   Referring to the fundamental or basic, as in the lowest body temperature or lowest prolactin level.

baseline   The starting value or values before a treatment or test is applied.

Bauer's response   Reflex in which pressure on the soles of the feet will elicit spontaneous crawling efforts and extension of the baby's head.

bell curve   The shape of the normal distribution on a graph. It looks like a bell.

bias   In statistics, unbiased estimators of the true value are usually desired because biased ones tend to consistently over estimate or underestimate the true value. In sampling, bias refers to the tendency of a sample to misrepresent the whole population because some of the sample did not answer the questions.

bifidus factor   A carbohydrate present in human milk that has anti-infective properties.

bili light   Fluorescent light used to treat jaundice.

bilirubin   A byproduct of the breakdown of the hemoglobin portion of red blood cells.

bioavailability   The amount of a nutrient, drug, or other substance that is active in the tissues.

blind   A characteristic of a study in which the treatment is kept secret from the person receiving it and, often, from those giving the treatment, as well.

blood incompatibility jaundice   A condition resulting from blood incompatibility between the mother and her baby that appears within the first 24 hours of life.

body language   Nonverbal messages sent by body position and gesture.

body mass index (BMI)   A measure of the body that takes into account a person's weight and height to gauge total body fat in adults.

bolus   A round lump of food ready to be swallowed.

bonding   Interaction between parents and infant to form a unique lasting relationship.

bradycardia   An abnormal condition in which the heart contracts steadily but at a rate below normal.

breast augmentation   Surgical procedure performed to increase the size of the breast. It can interfere with milk production.

breast compression   See *alternate massage*.

breastfeeding counselor   A lay counselor who assists breastfeeding mothers at a peer level.

breastfeeding diary   Daily log of the baby's feeds, wet diapers, and stools.

breastfeeding jaundice   Neonatal jaundice caused by mismanagement of breastfeeding. Also called lack-of-breastfeeding jaundice.

breast infection   See *mastitis*.

breast massage   Manual massage of the breast used to facilitate letdown and expression of milk.

breastmilk jaundice   See *late onset jaundice*.

breastmilk substitute   See *human milk substitute*.

breast reduction   Surgical procedure performed to decrease the size of the breast. It can interfere with milk production.

breast shell   A plastic cup worn over the nipple during pregnancy, and during and between feedings, to increase nipple protractility.

buccal pad   A fat pad in the cheek over the main muscle of the cheek. It is very evident in infants and is often called a sucking pad. It is not fully developed in preterm infants.

building hope   A counseling skill used to encourage the mother by offering hope for improvement.

burnout   A condition of becoming bored, discouraged, or frustrated.

 C

C-hold   Technique in which the mother cups her free hand to form the letter "C," with her thumb on top and her fingers curved below the breast, well behind the areola. This is used to help support the breast with positioning and attachment.

Candida albicans   A tiny, common yeastlike fungus normally found in the mouth, digestive tract, vagina, and on the skin of healthy persons.

candidiasis   A yeastlike fungal infection, commonly afflicting the vagina; producing a thick vaginal discharge; can be transmitted to the baby at birth and result in candidiasis in his mouth and digestive tract, which appears as white patches or ulcers. May also occur on the mother's nipples.

capillaries   Tiny blood vessels in the system that link the arteries and the veins.

caput succedaneum   A collection of fluid between the scalp and skull of a newborn. It is usually formed during labor as a result of the pressure of the cervix on the infant's head. The swelling begins to recede soon after birth.

case   A person who has the problem under study.

case-control study   Research in which cases (people who have the disease or problem of interest) are identified first, and then controls (people who are similar to cases but do not have the problem) are identified. The goal of the study is to find some characteristic or experience that is different between cases and controls that might explain why only the cases developed the diagnosis.

casein   Component of the proteins in milk.

case study   An article in a journal describing one (or a few) instances of a diagnosis, problem, or situation that arose in practice. The author was not designing a study; rather he or she came on the diagnosed person in practice and chose to share what was learned.

categorical data   Data that can be classified but not quantified, such as survey responses "Very satisfied," "satisfied," "unsatisfied," "very unsatisfied." Categorical data can be counted but is not measured with numbers in the same way as temperature and weight.

catheter (catheterize)   A tube inserted in the bladder to keep it empty.

Centers for Disease Control (CDC)   An agency of the U.S. Public Health Service established in 1973 to protect the public health of the nation by providing leadership and direction in the prevention and control of diseases and other preventable health conditions, and to respond to public health emergencies.

cephalhematoma   Swelling caused by the pooling of blood under the scalp. It may begin to form in the scalp of a baby during labor and may slowly become larger in the first few days after birth. It is usually a result of trauma, often from forceps or vacuum extraction.

Chi-square   A statistical term that can describe a distribution of data and can be the name for a test of categorical data. Chi-square tests can be used to tell whether observed data are what would or would not be expected by chance.

cholecystokinin (CCK)   A gastrointestinal hormone that enhances digestion, sedation, and a feeling of satiation and well-being. It is released in both the infant and mother during suckling.

clarifying   A counseling skill used to make a point clear.

clavicle   The collarbone. It is a long, curved horizontal bone just above the first rib, forming the front portion of the shoulder.

cleft lip   A birth defect consisting of one or more clefts (splits) of the upper lip. This results from the failure of the upper jaw and nasal areas to close in the embryo.

cleft palate   A birth defect in which there is a hole in the middle of the roof of the mouth (palate). The crack may be complete, going through both the hard and soft palates into the nasal area, or it may go only partly through. It is often linked to a cleft in the upper lip.

clinical practice   The day-to-day work of health care professionals rather than the kind of care that might be given in an experimental setting.

clustered feedings   Period of almost constant wakefulness and suckling at some time of the day, generally the early evening. Also referred to as bunched feedings.

clutch hold   A breastfeeding position in which the mother places the baby along her side with his feet toward her back; also known as the football hold.

Cohen's kappa   A statistical test, designed by J. Cohen, to tell whether people observing or rating the same event agree with each other more often than chance. Experts differ, but kappa = 0.7 or 0.8 or higher are considered evidence of good agreement.

cohort   A group studied together because of some characteristic or experience they have in common.

cohort study   A type of research that examines the effect or effects of belonging to a particular group on some result or outcome of interest.

colic   Extreme fussiness in the baby that is characterized by a piercing cry, severe abdominal discomfort, and inability to be comforted.

colostrum   Breast fluid secreted during pregnancy, after childbirth, and before the onset of secretion of mature milk.

community outreach   Reaching the community through programs and services.

complementary feed   New foods added to the growing breastfed infant's diet to meet the energy and nutrient needs that are not met by human milk alone. Introduction of solid foods. In some cases, this term is interpreted as "topping off" the breastfed infant with liquids other than human milk. The liquid may be water or infant formula.

complex carbohydrates   Carbohydrates that contain important vitamins and minerals. Complex carbohydrates take longer to digest and do not stimulate a craving for more foods. Foods in this category include vegetables, fruits, whole grain cereals, rice, breads, and crackers.

confidence intervals (CIs)   A statistical term that states the range within which a population's true value is expected to be found. The researcher can determine whether to use 95%, 99%, or some other level of confidence that the true value will be within that range.

confounding variable   A characteristic or attribute of the people in the study or their experiences that could confuse the interpretation of the study's results.

congenital   Present at birth, such as a congenital defect.

conjugation   The process by which the liver converts bilirubin into a form that can pass into the intestine.

contraception   A technique for preventing pregnancy.

contraindicate   To give indication against the advisability of, as in "In very few instances is breastfeeding contraindicated."

control   (1) The group in the study to whom the treatment was not given (in an experiment) or who do not have the problem of interest (in a case-control study). (2) Refers to the amount or type of regulation of study conditions the researchers can exercise.

convenience   Refers to a type of sample selected by the researcher that is not random or carefully defined but rather readily accessible.

Cooper's ligaments   Ligaments that run vertically through the breast and attach the deep layer of subcutaneous tissue to the dermis of the skin.

cord blood   Blood that remains in the umbilical cord at birth.

correlated   When two variables are correlated, they have been shown, by a specific statistical test, to be associated.

co-sleeping   Practice in which the infant sleeps with the parents. Co-sleeping infants arouse more often and in synchrony with their mothers than do separate sleepers.

cradle hold   The traditional sitting position whereby the mother sits with her baby's body across her abdomen. She places his head in the crook of her arm and supports his body with her hand.

Cronbach's alpha   A special test applied to determine whether the items on a scale or tool are internally consistent, or that they measure the same concept in a similar way. Alphas closer to 1.00 are better.

cross-cradle hold   The same holding technique as the dominant hand hold but used for the less dominant hand as well.

cross-sectional study   Research that examines a question at one point in time (such as surveys of a neighborhood all collected within the same week).

culture   The environment that surrounds us in our beliefs and attitudes.

cup feeding   Alternative feeding method in which the baby is fed with a cup.

cyanosis   Bluish coloring of the skin or mucous membranes due to low oxygen levels.

 D

Dancer hand position   Position that begins in the C-hold position. The mother then brings her hand forward so that her breast is supported with only three fingers. She bends the index finger slightly so that it gently holds the baby's cheek on one side, with the thumb holding the other cheek. This helps the baby's tongue form correctly for suckling. Originated by Sarah Danner and Ed Cerutti.

demographics   Variables that describe basic characteristics of the subjects such as age, gender, place of residence, income, education, and ethnicity.

dependent variable   The aspect or characteristic of the subjects, or of their experience, that the researcher is trying to understand or explain. In a study of the effect of calories on weight gain, weight gain is the dependent variable.

dermis   The layer of skin just below the outer layer (epidermis). It contains blood and lymph vessels, nerves and nerve endings, glands, and hair follicles.

descriptive study   Usually, a study that begins to explore a phenomenon by describing it in detail rather than trying to control any aspects of it.

detoxify   Speed up the removal of poison from the body.

diabetes   A disorder resulting from inadequate production or utilization of insulin.

dichotomous outcome   A result or answer that has only two possibilities such as "Yes, No" or "True, False".

distribution   A description of the way the values of a variable (independent or dependent) range; how many values are small, medium, and large. Often, this is shown graphically. Statisticians have names for many different types of distributions that have been studied and can summarize them with mathematical formulas.

dominant hand hold   Position in which the mother holds her baby with her dominant hand to nurse. She holds the baby's head in her hand and supports his body with her forearm. She can nurse on the nearest breast and then move her arm with the baby across her body to the opposite breast.

donor milk   Human milk that is expressed and donated to a human milk bank to be given to another baby.

dopamine   A catecholamine made in the adrenal gland that acts as a prolactin inhibitor.

doula   An experienced woman who helps other women.

Down syndrome   A form of congenital mental retardation.

drip milk   Milk that leaks from a breast that is not being directly stimulated.

duct system (ductwork)   A system of ducts and ductules through which milk flows from the point of production out to the nipple pores.

ductule   Small duct in the mammary gland that drains milk from the alveoli into larger ducts that terminate in the nipple.

dyad   Two individuals who form one unit, each dependent on the other, such as a mother and baby.

 E

eclampsia   Coma and convulsive seizures occurring in the woman between her 20th week of pregnancy and the end of the first week postpartum.

eczema   Swelling of the outer layer of skin that may be itchy, red, have small blisters, and be swollen and weeping.

edema   A local or generalized condition in which body tissues contain excessive amounts of fluid.

emergency weaning   Weaning abruptly with no preparation or forethought.

empathetic listening   A counseling technique in which the counselor listens with the intent to understand emotionally and intellectually.

endocrine   Pertaining to a gland that secretes directly into the bloodstream.

engorgement   Swelling or congestion of body tissues, overfullness of the breast.

enteral   Within or by way of the intestines.

environmental contaminant   Impurities in human milk that result from contamination of the environment by such chemicals as DDT, PBB, and PCB that then enter the food chain and are consumed by the mother.

enzyme   A protein that speeds up or causes chemical reactions in living matter.

epidermis   The outer layers of the skin. It is made up of an outer, dead portion and a deeper, living portion. Epidermal cells gradually move outward to the skin surface, changing as they go, until they become flakes.

epidural anesthesia   Anesthesia produced by injection of an anesthetic into the epidural space of the spinal cord.

epiglottis   The cartilage-like structure that overhangs the trachea like a lid. It prevents food from entering the trachea by closing during swallowing.

episiotomy   A surgical incision made to enlarge the vaginal opening during childbirth.

epithelium   The covering of the organs of the body.

erythema toxicum   Pink to red macular (raised) area with a center that is yellow or white. It has no apparent significance and requires no treatment.

estrogen   The hormone that stimulates growth of the reproductive organs, including ductwork in the breasts.

evaluating   A counseling technique used to examine the quality of the counseling contact.

evert   Protrude outward.

exclusive breastfeeding   Breastfeeding in which the baby receives no drinks or foods other than human milk, not even water; is given no pacifiers or artificial teats; has no limits placed on frequency or length of a breastfeed; and receives at least 8 to 12 breastfeeds in 24 hours, including night feeds.

excoriated   Surface of the skin that is scraped or chafed.

exocrine   Pertaining to a gland whose secretion reaches an epithelial surface either directly or through a duct.

experiment   A type of research in which the scientist plans to select a sample carefully and then apply some treatment or perform some action on part of the sample in order to measure the differences between treated and untreated parts.

extrauterine   Occurring or located outside the uterus.

 F

facilitating   A counseling technique used to direct a conversation in such a way that encourages the other speaker to provide information and define the situation.

failure to thrive   Condition in which an infant's weight is seriously compromised. Signs are failure to regain birth weight by 3 weeks of age, weight loss of greater than 10 percent of birth weight by 2 weeks of age, deceleration of growth from a previously established pattern of weight gain, and evidence of malnutrition on examination, such as minimal subcutaneous fat or wasted buttocks.

fat-soluble vitamins   Vitamins A, D, E, and K.

fat stores   Layers of fat laid down during pregnancy that provide a reserve to help nourish the breastfeeding baby.

feedback inhibitor of lactation (FIL)   A human whey protein that enables the mammary gland to regulate its milk production; it acts to inhibit milk synthesis when milk is left in the breast.

feeding cues   A progression of signs that indicate a desire to feed. The baby will begin to wriggle his body and his closed eyes will exhibit rapid eye movement (REM). He will then make mouthing movements. He will pass one or both of his hands over his head and will bring his hand to his mouth. If his cheek or mouth is touched at this stage, he will begin to root.

fibrocystic breast   A common type of benign breast condition that causes lumpiness in the breast.

finger feeding   An alternate feeding method in which the baby sucks on the mother's or examiner's finger. A 5, 6, or 8 French oral gastric tube that leads to the liquid is placed along the fat pad of the finger, extending about 1/4 inch beyond the tip of the finger. The fat pad of the finger with the tube on it is placed into the baby's mouth against the soft palate.

fistula   An abnormal passage from an internal organ to the body surface or between two internal organs.

flange (breast pump)   A portion of a breast pump that is placed against the breast to form suction.

flanged   To extend outward, to flare, as in the baby's lips being flanged when attached at the breast.

flatulence   Excessive gas in the stomach and abdomen causing pain in the abdomen, shoulder area, or intestines.

flexion   A state of being bent or curved.

flora   Normal bacteria and other microbes.

focusing   A counseling skill that is used to concentrate on a point that should be explored.

follow-up method   A counseling method used to analyze the need for further contact and/or research.

fontanel   A space between the bones of an infant's skull covered by tough membranes. Intense pressure may cause a fontanel to become tense or bulge. A fontanel may be soft and sunken if the infant is dehydrated.

football hold   See *clutch hold.*

forceps   Instruments used to help a difficult childbirth, to quickly deliver a baby with breathing problems, or to shorten normal labor. The blades of the forceps are put into the vagina one at a time and applied to opposite sides of the baby's head, with the baby's head held firmly between the blades.

foremilk   The lower fat milk that is present at the beginning of a breastfeed.

formal stage   The second of four stages in role acquisition. A time in which the role is viewed more personally. With more formalized expectations, one strives for perfection, as in the role of parent or lactation consultant.

frenulum   A fold of skin or mucous membrane that is attached to a part of the body and checks or controls its motion, as in the fold under the tongue.

▼ G

galactocele   A cyst that is caused by the closing or blockage of a milk duct. It contains a thick, creamy milklike substance and may be discharged from the nipple when the cyst is compressed. It can be aspirated, and some are removed surgically to prevent them from refilling.

galactogogues   Foods or drinks that are believed to increase milk production.

galactopoiesis   Stage III lactogenesis, which marks the establishment and maintenance of mature milk.

galactorrhea   Secretion and release of milk unrelated to childbirth or breastfeeding, excessive or inappropriate milk production; also called spontaneous lactation.

galactose   A simple sugar produced by the breakdown of lactose (milk sugar).

galactosemia   An inherited disease of galactose processing caused by lack of an enzyme.

gastroenteritis   Inflammation of the stomach and intestines.

gastroesophageal reflux (GER)   A backflow of contents of the stomach into the esophagus. It is often the result of failure of the lower esophageal sphincter. Gastric juices are acidic and produce burning pain in the esophagus.

gastrostomy   Gavage feeding in which a tube is placed through the skin directly into the stomach.

gavage feeding   A method for feeding an infant in which a tube is passed through the nose, mouth, or skin into the stomach.

generalize   A desired ability to extend the results of a study not just to the people studied but also to a larger group who are more or less similar to them.

gestation   The length of time from conception to birth.

gestational age   The age of a fetus or a newborn, usually stated in weeks dating from the first day of the mother's last menstrual period.

glucuronic acid   An agent that conjugates bilirubin in the liver.

graspability   The ability of the nipples to be grasped in the baby's mouth.

grooming   Gently stroking an infant's body during a feed. This increases a mother's prolactin level.

growth spurt   A period of sudden growth when the baby nurses more frequently than usual.

guiding method   A counseling method that provides emotional support and encourages the sharing of feelings and concerns.

▼ H

half-life   The time needed for a drug's level in the bloodstream to go down to one half its beginning level.

hand expression   Removal of milk from the breast by manual manipulation.

health consumer   An informed person who is a responsible decision maker concerning health care.

hematocrit   A measure of the number of red cells found in the blood, stated as a percentage of the total blood volume.

hemoglobin   The portion of the red blood cell that transports oxygen to all parts of the body.

Hirshsprung's disease   A condition in which a part of the infant's intestines lacks proper nerve innervation and the stool is not passed easily beyond that point. These infants frequently have large bloated abdomens from the collection of stool and gas.

high-risk infant   An infant born at risk due to a particular medical condition or social situation.

hindmilk   The high-fat milk resulting from the letdown reflex forcing milk from the alveoli and washing the fat from the walls of the ducts.

human immunodeficiency virus (HIV)   Virus that slowly weakens the body's immune system, thus allowing viruses, bacteria, parasites, and fungi that usually don't cause any problems to cause illness and death. These are called "opportunistic infections."

Hoffman technique   A technique used to train the nipple to become graspable by manually stretching the tissue surrounding the nipple.

Holder pasteurization   Heat treating at either 56°C or 62.5°C.

home visit   A form of counseling in which the counselor visits the mother in her home in order to personalize the contact and make visual observations.

homogeneity   Sameness. In studies that hope that two groups are different in important ways, finding sameness between them invalidates the results.

human milk   Milk secreted in the human breast.

human milk fortifier   Nutrient added to expressed human milk to enhance the growth and nutrient balances of very low-birth-weight infants.

human milk substitute   Any food being marketed or otherwise represented as a partial or total replacement for human milk. Also called artificial baby milk.

Human Subjects review group   Groups of people in research institutions and health care agencies who study a research proposal to be sure it does not violate people's rights nor jeopardize their safety.

humoral   Immunity against invaders, as with bacteria and foreign tissue. Humoral immunity is the result of the development and continuing presence of circulating antibodies that are produced by the body's defense system.

hydration   The water balance within the body.

hyperbilirubinemia   A yellow coloring of the tissues, membranes, and secretions due to the presence of bile pigments in the blood; a symptom in the body. Also referred to as jaundice.

hypercapnia   High carbon dioxide levels.

hyperemesis   Long-term vomiting, weight loss, and fluid and electrolyte imbalance.

hyperprolactinemia   Elevated prolactin levels.

hypertension   A common disorder, often without symptoms, marked by high blood pressure persistently exceeding 140/90.

hypertonia   Abnormally high tension or tone, especially of the muscles.

hypocalcemia   Too little calcium in the blood.

hypogalactic   The inability to produce sufficient milk.

hypothalamus   The portion of the brain forming the floor and part of the side wall of the third ventricle. It triggers the release of hormones.

hypothesis   An expected relationship between two variables expressed before a study and around which the study is designed.

hypothyroidism   A condition caused by a deficiency of thyroid secretions causing sluggishness of all functions.

hypotonia   Abnormally low tension or tone, especially of the muscles.

 I

iatrogenic   Induced by medical interference with the natural process.

ICD9   International Classification of Diseases.

identifying strengths   A counseling skill that helps the mother focus on positive qualities.

ignoring   The lowest level of listening.

immunity   The quality of being protected from disease organisms and other foreign bodies.

immunization   Any injection of weakened bacteria given to protect against or to reduce the effects of related infectious diseases; vaccination.

immunoglobulin   Group of five distinct antibodies in the serum and external secretions of the body that provide immunity. Kinds of immunoglobulins are IgA, IgD, IgE, IgG, and IgM.

immunologic   Providing immunity to disease by stimulating antigens.

independent variable   The aspect of the subjects or their experience that the researcher suspects may explain or predict the result or outcome. In a study of the effect of calories on weight gain, calories are the independent variable.

induced lactation   Initiate breastfeeding in a woman who has not given birth, as with an adoptive mother. Milk production is begun by frequent nursing and other measures rather than by the delivery of the placenta.

inert   A chemically inactive substance.

influencing   A counseling technique used to produce positive action in the mother through the use of special skills.

informal stage   The third of four stages in role acquisition. A time of modifying, blending, and individualizing ones role, as in the role of parent or lactation consultant.

informed consent   Consent to medical care based on sufficient education and information.

informing   A counseling technique used to educate the mother by offering her explanations to increase her understanding of situations and suggestions.

innervation   The distribution or supply of nerve fibers or nerve impulses to a part of the body.

insensible   Small amount, not perceptible.

instruments   Also called tools, can be a whole variety of things used to measure such as questionnaires, photographs, tape measures, stopwatches, and so on.

intercostal   Of or pertaining to the space between two ribs.

intern   In the field of lactation, one who has completed didactic education and is acquiring clinical practice hours toward becoming a lactation consultant.

internal validity   The assurance that extraneous variables are not responsible for the observed results.

International Board of Lactation Consultant Examiners (IBLCE)   A nonprofit corporation established in 1985 to develop and administer certification for lactation consultants.

International Code of Marketing of Breastmilk Substitutes   A set of resolutions that regulate the marketing and distribution of any fluid intended to replace human milk, devices used to feed such fluids, and the role of health care workers who advise on infant feeding. They were developed in 1979 by members of a joint commission convened by WHO and UNICEF. Also referred to as the *WHO Code*.

International Lactation Consultant Association (ILCA)   A global association founded in 1985 for health professionals who specialize in promoting, protecting, and supporting breastfeeding. The professional association for lactation consultants.

interpreting   A counseling skill making use of an analysis of what the mother is saying.

intraductal papilloma   Benign tumor within a duct. It is usually associated with a spontaneous bloody discharge from one breast.

intramuscular (IM)   Referring to the inside of a muscle, as of an injection into a muscle to give medicine.

intrauterine   Referring to the inside of the uterus.

intravenous (IV)   Referring to the inside of a vein, as of a tube inserted into a vein to provide nutrients or medication directly into the bloodstream.

intubation   Passing a tube into a body opening, as putting a breathing tube through the mouth or nose or into the trachea to provide an airway for anesthetic gas or oxygen.

inverted syringe   Device for everting the mother's nipple. The tapered end of a syringe is cut off and the plunger direction is reversed so as to provide a smooth surface next to the breast. The mother places the smooth end of the syringe over her nipple and pulls gently on the plunger.

involution   A normal process marked by decreasing size of an organ, as in involution of the uterus after birth.

isolette   Specialized, clear-covered infant crib that allows the infant to maintain appropriate body temperature and receive appropriate treatment; allows for continuous observation of the infant by health care providers; stablelet.

IUGR   Intrauterine growth retardation.

 J

jaundice   See hyperbilirubinemia.

Joint Commission on Accreditation of Healthcare Organizations (JCAHO)   An independent, not-for-profit organization that evaluates and accredits more than 18,000 health care organizations in the United States, including hospitals, health care networks, managed care organizations, and health care organizations that provide home care, long-term care, behavioral health care, laboratory, and ambulatory care services in order to improve the quality of health care for the public by providing accreditation and related services that support performance improvement in health care organizations.

 K

kangaroo care   Technique in which the baby is held skin to skin upright and prone between his mother's breasts, wearing only a diaper. He and his mother are then wrapped together to maintain his temperature appropriately.

kappa   See *Cohen's kappa*

Kegel exercises   An exercise to tighten muscles surrounding the vagina, urethra, and rectum.

keratin   The tough surface layer of dead skin developed in response to pressure.

kernicterus   Brain damage caused by excessive bilirubin.

Kcal   The amount of heat needed to raise the temperature of 1kg of water 1°C.

 L

lactase   An enzyme that increases the rate of the conversion of milk sugar (lactose) to glucose and galactose, carbohydrates needed by the body for energy.

lactation   Breastfeeding; secretion of human milk.

lactational amenorrhea method (LAM)   Method of contraception that must meet three conditions: the mother's menses has not yet returned, the baby is breastfed around the clock without other foods in the diet, and the baby is younger than 6 months.

lactation consultant   A health professional who is certified (IBCLC) in lactation.

lactiferous   Mammary, as in lactiferous sinus or lactiferous duct.

lactiferous sinus   Dilation in the lactiferous ducts beneath the areola that act as small holding areas of milk.

lactoferrin   An iron-binding protein that increases absorption of iron.

lactogenesis   The phase during which milk production and secretion are established. Lactogenesis occurs in three stages. Stage I is the initiation of milk synthesis and Stage II marks copious milk production. Stage III, also called galactopoiesis, refers to the establishment of a mature milk supply.

lactose   Milk sugar, the type of sugar present in human milk.

lactose intolerance   A disorder resulting in the inability to digest milk sugar (lactose) because of an enzyme (lactase) deficiency.

laparoscopy   The examination of the abdominal cavity with a laparoscope through a small incision in the abdominal wall. The procedure used for examining the ovaries and fallopian tubes.

late onset jaundice   An extremely rare type of neonatal jaundice caused by an unknown factor in the mother's milk; this condition appears between the fourth and seventh day of life. Also called breastmilk jaundice.

lay counselor   Counselor who helps others on a peer level.

leading method   A counseling method that entails directing a conversation to help identify options and resources, as well as to aid in developing a plan of action.

leaking   The involuntary releasing of human milk that usually occurs in the un-nursed breast while the baby is feeding from the other breast, the seepage of milk from the very full breast, or the expulsion of milk from the breast due to the milk letting down.

leaky gut syndrome   A condition in which the intestinal lining becomes inflamed and then thin and porous. Proteins that are incompletely digested may then cross from the intestines into the bloodstream.

lesion   A wound, injury, or other destructive change in body tissue.

letdown   Milk ejection from the breast triggered by nipple stimulation or as a conditioned reflex.

leukocytes   Cells present in human milk that fight infection.

LGA   Large for gestational age.

Likert scale   A type of commonly used attitude measure that asks respondents to "Strongly Agree" or "Strongly Disagree."

lingual   Pertaining to the tongue, as in lingual frenulum.

lipase   A digestive system enzyme that increases the breakdown of fats (lipids).

lobule   A small lobe, a cluster of 10 to 100 alveoli.

lochia   Discharge that is composed of blood, mucus, and tissue caused by the gradual renewal of reproductive structures following childbirth. Its color transforms from red to pink and then to white in about three weeks.

logistic regression   A statistical technique for studying relationships between variables that can be used when the dependent (outcome) variable is dichotomous (only two possibilities).

low birth weight (LBW)   Baby born weighing less than 2500g.

lymph nodes   Small, rounded masses that function as filters in the lymph vessels to trap bacteria and cast-off cell parts. Each is a potential dam to arrest the spread of infection. They may swell and be painful when functioning in this way.

lymph   A thin, clear, slightly yellow fluid present in the lymphatic system. It is about 95% water with a few red blood cells and variable numbers of white blood cells.

lymphatic system   Complex network of capillaries, thin vessels, valves, ducts, nodes, and organs. The lymphatic system absorbs the excess blood fluids from the tissue spaces and eventually returns them to the heart.

lymphocyte   A lymph cell or white blood cell.

lysozyme   An enzyme with antiseptic actions that destroys some foreign organisms.

 M

macular   Raised.

macrophage   Any large cell that can surround and digest foreign substances in the body.

malnutrition   Inadequate nutrition due to improper diet, regardless of the number of calories consumed.

mammary gland   Exocrine gland that functions and develops independently to extract materials from the blood and convert them into milk.

mammogenesis   Stage during which the breast develops to a functioning state.

manual expression   See *hand expression*.

masseter muscle   The muscle that closes the mouth and is the principal muscle in chewing.

mastitis   An inflammation of the breast, usually resulting from a plugged duct left untreated or a cracked nipple. Also referred to as a breast infection.

mature milk   Human milk that is approximately one-third foremilk and two-thirds hindmilk.

mean   Average.

meconium   The first stool of a newborn, greenish black to light brown with a tarry consistency.

meta-analysis   A method of putting together the results of many studies and reanalyzing them as if they had all been parts of one big study. Because some problems have only been studied with small samples that may not have enough statistical power to detect true differences, meta-analysis may be able to answer unclear questions.

metabolic   Referring to metabolism, the sum of all chemical processes that take place in the body as they relate to the movement of nutrients in the blood after digestion.

mg/dl   Milligrams per deciliter.

milk bank   A facility that collects human milk and stores or processes it, making it available to babies who have demonstrated a need for human milk.

milk ejection reflex   A normal reflex in a nursing mother, caused by stimulation of the nipple and resulting in the release of milk from the breast.

milk line   The line extending from the armpit to the inner thigh of the fetus, sometimes the site of an extra nipple.

milk/plasma ratio   The quantity of a given drug or its metabolite in human milk in relation to its quantity in the maternal plasma or blood.

milk supply   The quantity of milk that a woman is currently producing, usually compared with the baby's requirements for milk.

milk synthesis   The process of making a compound (human milk) by joining together several elements.

mini-laparotomy   A surgical incision into a cavity of the lower abdomen, usually performed using general or regional anesthesia.

minimal breastfeeding   Breastfeeding between one and three times a day, with complementary feeds providing the remaining nourishment. Typical scenario for gradual weaning.

molding   Asymmetric appearance of the baby's head after birth due to the overriding of skull bones.

monilial infection   See *candidiasis*.

Montgomery glands   Small raised areas around the nipple that enlarge during pregnancy and lactation and secrete a fluid that lubricates the nipple.

morbidity   An illness or an abnormal condition or quality.

Moro reflex   A normal reflex in a young infant caused by a sudden loud noise. It results in drawing up the legs, an embracing position of the arms, and usually a short cry.

mortality   The condition of being subject to death.

mother-led weaning   Weaning initiated by the mother without cues from the baby.

motility   Power of motion, spontaneous motion.

mucin   A glycoprotein found in mucus; it is present in human milk, saliva, bile, salivary glands, in the skin, connective tissues, tendon, and cartilage.

myelin   A fatty substance found in the coverings of various nerve fibers. The fat gives the normally gray fibers a white, creamy color.

myoepithelial cells   Smooth muscle layers that enclose the alveoli and ducts of the breast.

 N

nasogastric feeding   Gavage feeding with a tube passing through the nose into the stomach.

necrotizing enterocolitis (NEC)   Inflammation of the intestines or colon.

need feeding   Feeding the baby whenever he indicates a need, in response to feeding cues. Sometimes referred to as demand feeding.

neonate   The newborn infant up to 6 weeks of age.

networking   Communicating among people with common interests or needs.

NICU   Neonatal intensive care unit.

nipple   The protruding part of the breast that extends and becomes firmer on stimulation.

nipple, common   A nipple that protrudes slightly when at rest and becomes erect when stimulated.

nipple, cracked   A nipple that has a crack or fissure lengthwise or crosswise along it.

nipple, flat   A nipple with a very short shank that does not become erect in response to stimulation.

nipple, inverted   A nipple that remains retracted, both when at rest and on stimulation.

nipple, inverted appearing   A nipple that appears inverted but becomes erect when stimulated.

nipple pores   The 15 to 25 openings on the end of the nipple through which milk flows.

nipple preference   A preference by the baby for either an artificial nipple or the breast, resulting from sucking alternately on the breast and an artificial nipple, which require two completely different mechanisms.

nipple, retracted   A nipple that appears graspable but retracts on stimulation.

nipple shield   An artificial nipple used over the mother's own nipple during nursing.

non-nutritive sucking   Alternate bursts of sucking and resting.

nonprobability   Refers to a type of sampling other than random. Convenience sampling is nonprobability.

normal distribution   The dispersal of data that comes from measuring many natural phenomena. It is a common assumption in statistical tests.

normal fullness   Increased amounts of blood and lymph necessary for milk production that cause the breasts to become fuller, heavier, and slightly tender; not to be confused with engorgement.

nosocomial   Hospital-acquired, as in a nosocomial infection.

nursing strike   Nursing abstinence; the baby's refusal to breastfeed.

nutritive sucking   An organized continuous sequence of long drawing sucks that produce a regular flow of milk.

 O

obturator   A feeding plate placed over a cleft palate to aid in feeding the baby.

odds ratio   A descriptive measure of the association between two variables. Because it is composed of the odds of one group in the numerator and the odds of another group in the denominator, if the odds are greater in the numerator, the odds ratio will be greater than one.

oligosaccharide   A carbohydrate that is present in human milk that discourages the growth of pathogens in the intestinal tract.

open-ended question   A form of question used in counseling which cannot be answered by "yes" or "no"; questions beginning with who, what, when, where, why, how, how much and how often.

operationalize   The process of defining the concepts to be studied in terms of measurable variables and relationships, including choosing instruments or tools.

orbicularis oris muscles   Circular muscle surrounding the mouth that closes the lips.

orogastric   Gavage feeding with a tube passing through the mouth to the stomach.

osteoporosis   A loss of normal bone density, marked by thinning of bone tissue and the growth of small holes in the bone.

outcome   In the context of research, outcome is usually the same as the dependent variable. More broadly, outcomes are the results of any treatment or action, whether or not that treatment is part of a research study.

outliers   Unusually small or large values for one of the variables being measured. Outliers can distort an average. Researchers often try to offer explanations for why a few values are so different from most others.

output variable   Like an outcome variable, this data element is a result or effect. In some studies, the sample is selected based on an "effect" of interest such as jaundice. Babies would be studied only if they are jaundiced, or jaundice would be the output variable that divides babies into two comparison groups.

outreach counseling   To reach out to mothers, contacting them on a regular basis to offer support and anticipatory guidance to circumvent problems.

oximeter   A small clip-on instrument that noninvasively estimates the oxygen saturation of a person's blood.

oxytocin   The hormone that stimulates the smooth muscles to contract, specifically those surrounding the alveoli in the breast (causing the release of milk) and those in the uterus (causing uterine contractions); a synthetic form is Pitocin.

 P

p-value   This is the observed significance level of a statistical test; it measures how strong the evidence is against the hypothesis that there is no relationship. Most of the time, results are declared statistically significant when $p < 0.05$. The use of a particular p-value is usually explained in the article.

palate, hard   The hard portion of the roof of the mouth.

palate, soft   The soft portion of the roof of the mouth.

palliative care   Care that will lessen or relieve pain or other uncomfortable symptoms but not cause a cure.

paradigm shift   A change in the way in which society views.

paraprofessional   A worker trained to perform certain functions, as in medicine, but not licensed to practice as a professional.

parenteral   Nongastrointestinal, intravenous.

passive listening   A type of listening such as attending.

pathogen   Any microorganism able to cause a disease.

pathologic   That which is caused by disease.

pathologic jaundice   Jaundice that results from such conditions as infections in the blood or liver, diseases of the liver, obstructions in the gastrointestinal system, and interference with the binding of the bilirubin in the bloodstream.

peer review   A process conducted by scientific journals in which an article submitted for publication must be read and approved by several scientists with relevant knowledge. They are peers of the authors, and they can suggest improvements or reject the article.

perineum   The region between the vagina and the rectum; the floor of the pelvic region.

periosteum   A fiber-like covering of the bones. It has the nerves and blood vessels that supply the bones.

peripheral   Referring to the outside surface or surrounding area of an organ or other structure.

peristalsis   The wavelike, rhythmic contraction of smooth muscle.

personal stage   The final of four stages in role acquisition. The time in which one's style evolves to be consistent with one's personality, as in the role of parent or lactation consultant.

phthalates   Estrogen-mimicking compounds found in various plastics that infants can be exposed to by artificial feeding.

pharynx   The throat, a tubelike structure that extends from the base of the skull to the esophagus.

phenylalanine   An amino acid present in food protein which can accumulate to dangerous levels in the baby with phenyketonuria.

phenylketonuria (PKU)   A hereditary disease that, if not treated early, can cause brain damage or severe mental retardation in the baby.

phototherapy   Use of a bili light to treat infantile jaundice.

physiologic jaundice   A common type of neonatal jaundice resulting from the normal breakdown of red blood cells and the delay in removing their byproducts from the bloodstream; it appears by the third day of life.

phytoestrogen   Estrogen present in a plant, as in the phytoestrogen in cabbage (used to treat engorgement).

Pierre Robin syndrome   A condition of the newborn that consists of an unusual smallness of the jaw combined with a cleft palate, downward displacement of the tongue, and absence of a gag reflex.

PIF   See *prolactin inhibitory factor*.

pilot study   A small, trial run of a study conducted before the main study in order to test processes or instruments planned for use in the main study so that problems can be worked out.

pinch test   A test for inverted nipples, performed by gently compressing the nipple between the thumb and forefinger and observing the amount of protrusion that results.

Pitocin   A synthetic form of oxytocin.

pituitary   A small, rounded body at the base of the brain that secretes hormones. The anterior pituitary secretes prolactin; the posterior pituitary secretes oxytocin.

placenta   The spongy structure that grows on the wall of the uterus during pregnancy and through which the baby is nourished.

plugged duct   Blockage in a milk duct caused by accumulated milk or cast-off cells.

pneumothorax   Collection of air or gas in the chest causing the lung to collapse.

population   The whole group of people who have some characteristic(s) under study of which the sample actually studied is just a part.

postmature   Born after 42 weeks' gestation.

postpartum   The 6-week period following childbirth.

postpartum depression   A mild to moderate depression that lasts from 1 to 6 weeks postpartum. It is characterized by mood changes, sleep disturbances, and fatigue. The mother feels unable to cope with life and may have unexplained physical symptoms such as abdominal pains or headache. She feels no attachment to the baby and worries that something is not "right." The mother may even entertain occasional thoughts of suicide.

postpartum psychosis   Postpartum depression that can lead to a loss of control, rational thought, and social functioning. The mother may experience overwhelming confusion and hallucinations. She may even attempt to harm herself or her child.

posture feeding   Feeding position in which the baby is positioned above the breast and has better control over milk flow. The mother lies flat on her back with her baby lying tummy-to-tummy on top of her.

power   A mathematical term that represents how great is the likelihood that a given sample size and test will find a difference between comparison groups when there really is a difference.

ppm   Parts per million.

predictor variable   Independent variable; the characteristic that is believed to influence the result.

premature   Born before 37 weeks' gestation.

prepared childbirth   Conscious cooperative birth in which the woman is aware of and able to cooperate with her body.

pretending   A type of listening in which the listener gives a noncommittal response, trying to be polite and really not giving any attention to the speaker.

prevalence   Frequency of disease in the population.

primipara   A woman who has completed one pregnancy.

probability   A probability sample is one selected by random sampling.

problem solving   A counseling technique that entails following a step-by-step process to arrive at a solution to a problem.

progesterone   The hormone responsible for the development of the placenta and mammary glands.

projectile vomiting   Violent expulsion of milk, traveling 5 to 10 feet.

prolactin   The hormone that stimulates breast development and formation of milk during pregnancy and lactation.

prolactin inhibitory factor (PIF)   A factor produced in and released from the hypothalamus which prohibits the release of prolactin.

prolactinoma   A pituitary tumor that secretes prolactin.

prone   Referring to the position of the body when lying face downward.

prophylaxis   Observance of rules necessary to prevent disease.

prospective study   In this kind of study, events to be studied have not yet happened, so data can be collected as the events happen rather than from old records or memory.

prostaglandin   One of several strong hormone-like fatty acids that act in small amounts on certain organs.

protein, complete   A protein that contains all the essential amino acids.

protein, incomplete   A protein that does not contain all the essential amino acids and must be combined with a complimentary protein to become complete.

protractility   The ability of the nipple to be drawn out.

pustule   A small blister that usually is filled with pus.

pyloric stenosis   A condition in which the outflow valve of the stomach will not open satisfactorily to permit the contents of the stomach to pass through. For some reason, it is most common in firstborn white male infants. This condition is characterized by projectile vomiting.

 Q

qualitative study   A study in which the measurement of variables is less important than a description of phenomena or experiences. Statistical analysis is not usually used and changes in practice are not often recommended, except at a conceptual level. Often, such studies lead to more studies.

 R

random assignment   The process of fairly designating participants in a study to be in a treatment or control group. The fairness is achieved by a process that cannot be influenced by the scientists or participants such as a coin flip or use of a special random number chart.

randomized clinical trial   An experiment or experiment-like type of research in which the scientist controls many aspects of the study. Subjects are randomly assigned to their groups. Potential confounders are measured and analysis is planned before data collection.

range   The number that results from subtracting the lowest from the highest value in the data.

Raynaud's phenomenon   Sporadic attacks of interruptions in blood flow to the extremities (fingers, toes, ears and nose), resulting in tingling, numbness, burning, and pain.

RDI   Reference Daily Intake

reassuring   A counseling skill used to restore confidence through pointing out the normalcy of a situation.

rebirthing   Stimulating the birth experience where the baby is placed on the mother's abdomen in a bath of warm water, and allowed to find the breast on his own; remedial co-bathing.

reflective listening   See *active listening*.

relactation   Resumption of lactation beyond the immediate postpartum period.

reliability   The property possessed by good quality measurement tools that ensures that they measure a concept or characteristic the same way each time.

remedial co-bathing   See *rebirthing*.

renal solute load   Amount of solutes (ie., glucose, amino acids, potassium, sodium, and chloride) handled by the kidneys.

replicate   To repeat a study that has already been done. Often the study is conducted on a different sample of people or in a different setting.

resection   Removal of tissue by surgery.

respiratory distress syndrome   A condition present, usually at birth, that is characterized by delayed onset of respiration and low Apgar score caused by the lungs not being fully developed.

retrospective study   A study in which the result of interest is identified in a group of subjects and then the past experiences of those subjects are examined to see what might have lead to the result.

reverse cycle nursing   A nursing pattern in which the mother who has regular separations from her baby provides most or all of her baby's feedings at the breast at times when she and the baby are together.

review   In research, a type of study published in a journal that usually does not present any new results but rather summarizes several previous studies.

rooming in   Mother and baby sharing the same hospital room, beginning as soon as possible after birth.

rooting reflex   The natural instinct of the newborn to turn his head toward the stimulation when touched on the cheek.

 S

sample   The group of people or subjects that are selected to participate in a study. The sample is only part of the whole population of subjects who could be studied.

sarcoidosis   A long-term disease of unknown origin marked by small, round bumps in the tissue around the organs of the body.

sebaceous   Fatty, oily, or greasy, usually referring to the oil-secreting glands of the skin or to their secretions.

secretory   Having the function of secretion.

secretory IgA   One of the most common antibodies, found in all secretions of the body. IgA combines with protein in the mucosa and defends body surfaces against invading microorganisms.

selective listening   Form of listening in which the listener hears only certain parts of what is said.

sepsis   Infection.

seroconversion   The process by which serum shows the presence of a factor that previously had been absent, or vice versa.

seronegative   Serum that does not demonstrate the presence of a factor for which tests were conducted; tested negative.

seropositive   Serum that demonstrates the presence of a factor for which tests were conducted; tested positive.

serum   Any thin, watery fluid, especially one that keeps serous membranes wet.

SGA   Small for gestational age.

Sheehan's syndrome   A condition occurring after giving birth in which the pituitary gland is damaged. It is caused by a lessening of blood circulation after bleeding of the womb.

sibling   A brother or sister.

simple carbohydrate   The simplest sugars that cause a sudden rise in blood sugar level after ingestion. The level then drops again rapidly and can create a craving for more food. When consumed in the absence of nutritional foods, simple carbohydrate foods may cause fatigue, dizziness, nervousness, or headache.

sling   An apparatus worn by an adult to carry and comfort a baby.

slope   The slope of a line on a graph as defined by its angle relative to the horizontal axis or by making a ratio of the units of rise over the units of run.

small for date   Infants whose growth was retarded and who were delivered before 37 weeks (premature) or after 42 weeks (postmature).

smooth muscle   The type of muscle that provides the erectile tissue in the nipple and areola.

snack nursing   Shortened nursing session between regular feeding periods.

social toxicant   Mood-changing toxicant such as tobacco, coffee, tea, alcohol, marijuana, and other social drugs.

soporific   Sleep-inducing agent, e.g., warm milk.

sphincters   A circular band of muscle fibers that narrows a passage or closes a natural opening in the body.

spina bifida   A nerve tube defect present at birth that results in a gap in the bone that surrounds the spinal cord.

spitting up   Baby expelling a small amount of milk from the mouth during or after feedings; common in most babies.

spontaneous lactation   See *galactorrhea*.

spurious   Describes the relationship between two variables when statistical significance is found, but it is actually caused by some third variable that is hidden or unclear.

stablelet   See *isolette*.

standards of practice   Stated measures or levels of quality that serve as models for the conduct and evaluation of practice.

stasis   A circular band of muscle fibers that narrows a passage or closes a natural opening in the body.

statistical theory   The mathematical ideas about probability and infinite cases that underlie the applied tests commonly used by researchers.

statistically significant   Describes an outcome that did not happen by chance; but there is some underlying relationship that caused the events.

subcutaneous   Beneath the skin.

sublingual   Beneath the tongue.

suck   To draw into the mouth by forming a partial vacuum with the lips and tongue.

suck reorganization   Technique in which the examiner places the index finger in the baby's mouth pad side up and places slight pressure on the midline of the tongue, pulling the finger out slowly to encourage the baby to suck it back in.

suck training   Technique in which the therapist places the index finger in the baby's mouth and stimulates certain portions of the baby's oral anatomy to train him to suck. A baby who needs suck training must be referred to a professional who is trained and skilled in this field. It is beyond the scope of most nurses or lactation consultants.

suckle   To suck and at the same time to rhythmically compress the gums together around the areola to strip milk from the breast.

sucking pad   See *buccal pad*.

summarizing   A counseling skill that entails making a summary of the important points in a conversation.

supernumerary nipple   Extra nipple, other than the two normally found on the breasts, which may be present along the milk lines.

supine   Lying flat on the back.

supplementary feed   Foods other than human milk fed to the infant in place of or following a breastfeed. Some refer to this as "topping off" the breastfed infant with liquids other than human milk.

supply and demand   The process by which the baby increases the mother's milk production to meet his needs.

suppressor peptides   Inhibiting peptides in human milk that bring about the cessation of milk secretion during milk stasis and engorgement.

swaddle   Wrapping the baby, confining his arms and legs to inhibit the startle reflex and provide a feeling of warmth and security.

switch nursing   Frequently altering between breasts during one feeding.

syringe feeding   An alternative feeding method in which a syringe is placed into the corner of the baby's mouth. Depressing the syringe forces milk into the baby's mouth. This method is dangerous to the baby, who may be injured by the sharp tip of the syringe.

systemic Of or relating to the whole body rather than to a single area or part of the body.

 T

t-test A statistical test used on data that can be averaged, like height. It determines whether two means are significantly different from one another or not.

tail of Spence Breast tissue that extends into the axilla.

tandem nursing Describes a mother who nurses more than one sibling of different ages.

teachable moment A time of optimal attention and capacity for learning.

temporary weaning A brief interruption of breastfeeding.

tertiary Third in order of use; belonging to the third level of sophistication of development, as in a specialized, highly technical level health care facility.

thrush See *candidiasis.*

tool In research, used interchangeably with "instrument."

trachea A nearly cylindrical tube in the neck; windpipe.

transient nipple soreness Nipple soreness in the first week postpartum that is temporary.

transitional milk Milk that comes in at Stage II lactogenesis—around the second or third day postpartum. Blood flow within the breast increases, and copious milk secretion begins. The milk that is between colostrum and mature milk.

transplacental Across or through the placenta.

transplantation Removal and reattachment.

trimester A period of 3 months, particularly used when referring to pregnancy.

trough (for mother's milk) Center of the infant's tongue during suckling which forms a channel through which the milk travels.

trough levels Trough is the lowest blood or milk level achieved by the drug during its dosing period.

true In statistics, "true" value is used to refer to a population value. For example, if we knew the weight of every human baby born in the last 100 years, we could say "The true value of the mean of the population is 3020.57 grams," but since we do not know the true value of the mean, we try to estimate it using research and statistics.

tubal ligation One of several sterilization processes in which the fallopian tubes are blocked to prevent conception from occurring.

tube feeding device An alternative feeding method in which tubing that leads to liquid is placed against the mother's breast with about one-fourth of an inch extending beyond the end of the nipple. The baby suckles at the breast and the tip of the tube simultaneously. The flow of supplement from the container encourages him to continue suckling.

turgor Normal strength and tension of the skin caused by outward pressure of the cells and the fluid that surrounds them.

 U

United Nations Children's Fund (UNICEF) An agency of the United Nations, established in 1946, charged with protecting the lives of children and enabling children to lead fuller lives.

U.S. Department of Agriculture (USDA) The government agency that oversees the Special Supplemental Food Program for Women, Infants, and Children, referred to as WIC.

universal precautions Guidelines observed in health care that help control the transmission of infection.

urethra The canal for discharge of urine, located between the vagina and the clitoris.

 V

vacuum extraction Vaginal delivery of the child assisted by the use of a machine that applies suction to the child's head.

validity A property of research methods that conveys how well they capture or measure the phenomenon or concept under study.

variable A characteristic or effect of either the hypothesized "causes" or "outcomes" under study. If feeding is a partial cause of jaundice, the number and amount of feedings are variables and the possible bilirubin levels are also variables.

variation In statistics, it is expected that most phenomena will not be exactly the same when measured over time or when measured in different individuals. The variation in the number of times each day that a breastfed baby wants to nurse and the variation in the number of feedings between different babies on the same day are both examples.

vasospasms Spasms of the blood vessels within the nipple.

ventral On the abdomen, draped on the hand.

vernix The creamy protective coating on the newborn.

vertical transmission The transfer of a disease, condition, or trait from a mother to her child, either in the genes or at the time of birth, as in the spread of an infection through human milk or through the placenta, or as in mother-to-child transmission of HIV.

very low birth weight (VLBW) Infant born weighing less than 1500 g.

virus A tiny organism that can grow only in the cells of another animal.

vomiting Expelling the contents of the stomach with force.

vomiting, projectile Violent expulsion of the contents of the stomach with force enough to send it 5 feet or more.

 W

water-soluble vitamins Vitamin C and the B vitamins.

weaning Discontinuation of breastfeeding by substituting other nourishment.

wet nurse Woman who breastfeeds an infant who is not her own.

whey Clear fluid when milk stands, when curds are removed.

witch's milk Milk sometimes secreted by the newborn infant's breast which disappears shortly after birth.

WIC Special Supplemental Food Program for Women, Infants, and Children that helps pregnant women choose nutritious foods to have healthier babies and provides services to breastfeeding mothers, infants, and children up to 5 years of age.

World Health Organization (WHO) An agency of the United Nations charged with planning and coordinating global health care and assisting member nations to combat disease and train health care workers.

warm line A telephone line that is answered by a machine or voice mail, asking the mother to leave a message for a return call.

▼ **Y**

yeast infection See *candidiasis.*

A

PROFESSIONAL RESOURCES

ORGANIZATIONS

Academy of Breastfeeding Medicine
University of Rochester School of Medicine
601 Elmwood Avenue, Box 777
Rochester, NY 14642
Phone: 716-275-4354
Fax: 716-461-3614
E-mail: areglash@facstaff.wisc.edu

American Academy of Pediatrics (AAP)
141 Northwest Point Boulevard
Elk Grove Village, IL 60007-1098
Phone: 800-433-9016, 847-228-5005
Fax: 847-228-5097
E-mail: kidsdocs@aap.org
www.aap.org

American College of Nurse-Midwives
(ACNM)
818 Connecticut Avenue, NW
Suite 900
Washington, DC 20006
Phone: 202-728-9872
Fax: 202-728-9897
E-mail: info@acnm.org
www.midwife.org

American College of Obstetricians and
Gynecologists (ACOG)
P.O. Box 96920
Washington, DC 20090-6920
Phone: 202-638-5577
Fax: 202-484-5107
E-mail: resources@acog.org
www.acog.org

American Dietetic Association (ADA)
216 W Jackson Boulevard
Suite 800
Chicago, IL 60606-6995
Phone: 800-877-1600, 312-899-0040
Fax: 312-899-1979
E-mail: cdr@eatright.org
www.eatright.org

American Medical Association (AMA)
515 North State Street
Chicago IL 60610
Phone: 312-464-5000
Fax: 312-464-4184
www.ama-assn.org

American Public Health Association
(APHA)
Clearinghouse on Infant Feeding and
Maternal Nutrition
1015 15th Street NW
Washington, DC 20005
Phone: 202-789-5600
Fax: 202-789-5661

ASPO-Lamaze
1200 19th Street NW
Suite 300
Washington, DC 20036-2401
Phone: 202-857-1128, 800-368-4404
Fax: 202-223-4579
E-mail: aspo@fba.com

Association of Women's Health, Obstetric
and Neonatal Nurses (AWHONN)
2000 L Street, NW, Suite 740
Washington, DC 20036
Phone: 202-261-2414
Fax: 202-728-0575
www.awhonn.org

Baby Friendly USA
8 Jan Sebastian Way
Sandwich, MA 02563
Phone: 508-888-8044
Fax: 508-888-8050
E-mail: bfusa@altavista.net
www.aboutus.com/ba100/bbfusa

Department of Health and Human Services
Administration for Children and Families
200 Independence Avenue SW
Washington, DC 20201
Phone 202-619-0257
www.dhhs.gov

Healthy Mothers, Healthy Babies
121 North Washington Street
Suite 300
Alexandria, VA 22314
Fax: 703-836-3470
Phone: 703-836-6110
www.hmhb.org

Human Milk Banking Association of North
America, Inc. (HMBANA)
% Mothers' Milk Bank
P-S-L Medical Centre
1719 East 19th
Denver CO 80218
Phone 919-250-8599 or 303-869-1888

Infant Feeding Action Coalition
INFACT Canada
6 Trinity Square
Toronto, Ontario
Canada M5G 1B1
Phone: 416-595-9819
E-mail: infact@ftn.net
www.infactcanada.ca

Institute for Reproductive Health
Georgetown University Medical Center
3PHC Room 3004
3900 Reservoir Road NW
Washington, DC 20007
Phone: 202-687-1392
Fax: 202-687-6846
E-mail: irhinfo@gunet.georgetown.edu

International Baby Food Action Network
(IBFAN)
212 Third Avenue North
Suite 300
Minneapolis, MN 55401
E-mail: babymilkacti@gn.apc.org
www.gn.apc.org

International Board of Lactation Consultant
Examiners (IBLCE)
7309 Arlington Boulevard, Suite 300
Falls Church, VA 22042-3215
Phone: 703-560-7330
Fax: 703-560-7332
E-mail: iblce@erols.com
www.iblce.org

International Childbirth Education
Association (ICEA)
P.O. Box 20048
Minneapolis, MN 55420
Phone: 612-854-8660
Fax: 612-854-8772
E-mail: info@icea.org
www.icea.org

International Lactation Consultant
Association (ILCA)
4104 Lakeboone Trail, Suite 201
Raleigh, NC 27607
Phone: 919-787-5181
Fax: 919-787-4916
E-mail: ilca@erols.com
www.ilca.org

La Leche League International, Inc.
P.O. Box 4079
1400 N. Meacham Road
Schaumburg, IL 60173-4048
Phone: 1-800-525-3243, 847-519-7730
Fax: 847-519-0035
E-mail: lllhq@llli.org
www.lalecheleague.org

March of Dimes
1275 Mamaroneck Avenue
White Plains, NY 10605
Phone: 914-428-7100
Fax: 914-428-8203
www.modimes.org

National Alliance for Breastfeeding
Advocacy (NABA)
254 Conant Road
Weston, MA 02493-1756
Phone: 781-893-3553
Fax: 781-893-8608
E-mail: marshalact@aol.com
http://members.aol.com/marshalact/naba

National Association of WIC Directors
(NAWD)
2001 S. Street, NW
Suite 580
Washington, DC 20009
Phone: 202-232-5492
Fax: 202-387-5281
E-mail: nawdnutri@aol.com
www.wicdirectors.org

National Perinatal Association
3500 E. Fletcher Avenue, Suite 209
Tampa, FL 33613
Phone: 813-971-1008
Fax: 813-971-9306
E-mail: napaonline@aol.com
www.nationalperinatal.org

Nursing Mothers Association of Australia
P.O. Box 4000
Glen Iris, Vic 3146
Australia
Phone: 03 9885 0855
Fax: 03 9885 0866
E-mail: nursingm@nmaa.asn.au
www.vicnet.au

UNICEF
Nutrition Cluster H-8F
3 United Nations Plaza
New York, NY 10017
Phone: 212-888-7465
Fax: 212-303-7911
E-mail: addresses@unicef.org

UNICEF Canada
443 Mountain Pleasant
Toronto, Ontario
M4S 2L8 Canada
Phone: 416-482-4444
Fax: 416-482-8035
E-mail: secretary@unicef.ca

U.S. Committee for UNICEF
333 East 38th Streeet, 6th Floor
New York NY 10017
Phone: 212-686-5522
Fax: 212-779-1679
E-mail:
christyne_stuckey_at_usc@unicefusa.org

World Alliance for Breastfeeding Action
(WABA)
P.O. Box 1200, 10850
Penang, Malaysia
Phone: 604-6584-816
Fax: 604-6572-655
E-mail: secr@waba.po.my
www.elogica.com.br/waba

World Health Organization (WHO)
Avenue Appia 20
1211 Geneva 27, Switzerland
Phone: 22-791-2111
Fax: 22-791-0746
E-mail: info@who.ch
www.who.int

SOURCES FOR LACTATION RESOURCES

Resources are available from many of the organizations listed above. In addition, the
following businesses and organizations offer
a variety of resources.

BEST START
3500 E. Fletcher Avenue, Suite 519
Tampa, FL 33613
Phone: 800-277-4975, 813-971-2119
Fax: 813-971-2280
E-mail: beststart@mindspring.com

Birth and Life Bookstore
a division of Cascade Health Care Products
141 Commercial Street NE
Salem, OR 97301
Phone: 800-443-9942, 503-371-4445
Fax: 503-371-5395
E-mail: onecascade@worldnet.att.net
www.1cascade.com

Breastfeeding Support Consultants,
Incorporated
Center for Lactation Education
228 Park Lane
Chalfont, PA 18914-3135 USA
Phone: 215-822-1281
Fax: 215-997-7879
E-mail: info@bsccenter.org
www.bsccenter.org

Childbirth Graphics
Division of WRS Group, Inc.
PO Box 21207
Waco, TX 76702-1207
Phone: 800-299-3366, ext. 287
Fax: 254-751-0221
E-mail: sales@wrsgroup.com

Geddes Productions
10546 McVine Avenue
Sunland, CA 91040
Phone: 818-951-2809
Fax: 818-951-9960
E-mail:
www.geddespro.com

Hollister Incorporated (Ameda-Egnell)
2000 Hollister Drive
Libertyville, IL 60048-3781
Phone: 847-680-1000, 800-323-4060
Fax: 847-680-1017
www.hollister.com

Lactnet
e-mail to: *Listserv@library.ummed.edu*
In the body of the letter (file) put:
   Subscribe Lactnet Your Name
Put the above all on one line.

Lactnews
www.jump.net/bwc/lactnews.html
bwc@jump.net

Maginnis and Associates
(For liability insurance as an Allied Health
Therapist)
332 S. Michigan Avenue
Chicago, IL 60604
Phone: 1-800-621-3008
Fax: 312-427-7938

Medela, Incorporated
P.O. Box 660
McHenry, IL 60051-0660
Phone: 800-435-8316, 815-363-1166
Fax: 800-995-7867, 815-363-1246
E-mail: custserv@mc.net
www.medela.com

Pharmasoft Medical Publishing
4606 Oregon
Amarillo, TX 79109
Phone: 806-358-8138, 800-738-1317
E-mail: tom@cortex.ama.ttuhsc.edu

UCLA Lactation Alumni Association
Carol Follingstad
(To purchase superbill)
2021 Grismer #17
Burbank, CA 91504
Phone: 818-841-4182
Fax: 818-848-2882
E-mail: cfolling@fmsn.com

WHO Publications
49 Sheridan Avenue
Albany, NY 12210
Phone: 518-436-9686
Fax: 518-436-7433
E-mail: qcorp@compuserve.com

DRUG HOT LINES

Brigham and Women's Hospital
Boston, MA
Phone: 617-732-5500

The Lactation Center at the University of
Rochester
Rochester, NY
Phone: 716-275-0088

Rocky Mountain Poison and Drug Center
Phone: 303-893-3784 Fax: 303-739-1119

University, of California drug hot line
San Diego, CA
Phone: 900-288-8273

RECOMMENDED READING

▼ **PROFESSIONAL PUBLICATIONS**

Akre J (ed). *Infant Feeding: The Physiological Basis.* Geneva, Switzerland: WHO; 1990.

Apple RD. *Mothers and Medicine, a Social History of Infant Feeding 1890–1950.* Madison, WI: University of Wisconsin Press; 1987.

Auerbach K (ed). *Lactation Consultant Series.* Garden City Park, NY: Avery Publishing Group; 1985–1995.

Barger J and Kutner L. *Clinical Experience in Lactation: A Blueprint for Internship.* Chalfont PA: Breastfeeding Support Consultants; 1997.

Black R et al. *The Management of Breastfeeding.* Lactation Specialist Self-Study Series. Boston: Jones and Bartlett Publishers; 1998.

Black R et al. *The Process of Breastfeeding.* Lactation Specialist Self-Study Series. Boston: Jones and Bartlett Publishers; 1998.

Black R et al. *The Science of Breastfeeding.* Lactation Specialist Self-Study Series. Boston: Jones and Bartlett Publishers; 1998.

Black R et al. *The Support of Breastfeeding.* Lactation Specialist Self-Study Series. Boston: Jones and Bartlett Publishers; 1998.

Briggs G Freeman R and Yaffe S. *Drugs in Pregnancy and Lactation,* 4th ed. Baltimore, MD: Williams & Wilkins; 1994.

Chamberlain D. *Babies Remember Birth.* New York: Ballantine Books; 1988.

Fildes V. *Breasts, Bottles and Babies: A History of Infant Feeding.* Edinburgh, Scotland: Edinburgh University Press; 1986.

Fildes V. *Wet Nursing.* Oxford, England: Basil Blackwell Ltd; 1988.

Frantz K. *Breastfeeding Products Guide 1994.* Sunland, CA: Geddes Productions; 1994.

Friedman K and Gradstein B. *Surviving Pregnancy Loss.* Boston, MA: Little, Brown and Company; 1982.

Garratt S. *Going It Alone.* Hampshire, England: Gower; 1991.

Greenlagh T. *How to Read a Paper: The basics of evidence-based medicine.* London: British Medical Journal Publishing; 1997.

Hale T. *Medications and Mothers' Milk,* 7th ed. Amarillo TX: Pharmasoft Medical Publishing; 1999.

Arnold L. *Guidelines for the Establishment and Operation of a Donor Human Milk Bank.* Human Milk Banking Association of North America. Jan Sebastian CT; 1994.

Arnold L. *Recommendations for Collection, Storage, and Handling of a Mother's Milk for Her own Infant in the Hospital Setting.* Human Milk Banking Association of North America. Jan Sebastian CT; 1994.

King FS. *Helping Mothers to Breastfeed.* Nairobi, Kenya: Nairobi African Medical and Research Foundation, 2nd ed; 1992.

Klaus M et al. *Mothering the Mother.* Reading, MA: Addison-Wesley Publishing Company; 1993.

Knowles MS. *The Modern Practice of Adult Education: From Pedagogy to Andragogy.* New York, Association Press; 1980.

Knowles MS. *Self-Directed Learning: A guide for learners and teachers,* New York, Association Press, 1975.

La Leche League International. *The Breastfeeding Answer Book:* Schaumburg IL; 1997.

La Leche League International. *Topical Review and Bibliography of the Literature on Breastfeeding:* Schaumburg IL; 1990.

Lang S. *Breastfeeding Special Care Babies.* London, England: Bailliere Tindall; 1997.

Lawrence R. *Breastfeeding: A Guide for the Medical Profession,* 4th ed. St Louis, MO: CV Mosby; 1999.

Magliaro A (ed). Lactation Consultant Series Two. La Leche League, Schaumburg IL; 1999.

McKenzie JF, McKenzie JC, and Smelter J. *Planning, Implementing and Evaluating Health Promotion Programmes.* New York: Macmillan; 1993.

Minchin M. *Breastfeeding Matters.* Victoria, Australia: Alma Publications; 1998.

Montagu A. *Touching: The Human Significance of the Skin.* New York, HarperCollins, 1972.

Nutrition During Lactation, Institute of Medicine. National Academy Press, Washington DC: National Academy of Science; 1991. (Also Nutrition During Pregnancy, overview and implementation guide.)

Palmer G. *The Politics of Breastfeeding.* London: Pandora Press; 1993.

Forbes G, editor. *Pediatric Nutrition Handbook,* 3rd ed. Elk Grove Village, IL: American Academy of Pediatrics; 1993.

Riordan R and Auerbach K. *Breastfeeding and Human Lactation.* Boston: Jones and Bartlett; 1999.

Royal College of Midwives. *Successful Breastfeeding.* London, England: Churchill Livingstone; 1991.

Thevenin T. *The Family Bed: An Age Old Concept in Childrearing.* Garden City Park NY, Avery Publishing Group; 1977.

UNICEF and WHO. *Breastfeeding Management and Promotion in a Baby-Friendly Hospital: An 18-hour course for maternity staff.* New York, UNICEF; 1993.

Van Esterik P. *Beyond the Breast-Bottle Controversy.* Piscatawny, NJ: Rutgers University Press; 1989. (Published in the United Kingdom under the title, *Mother Power and Infant Feeding.*)

Van Esterik P. *Women, Work, and Breastfeeding.* Ithica, NY. Cornell Division of Nutritional Sciences; 1992.

Walker M. *Summary of the Hazards of Infant Formula.* Raleigh, NC: International Lactation Consultants Association; 1992.

Walker M. *Summary of the Hazards of Infant Formula: Part 2,* Raleigh NC: International Lactation Consultants Association; 1998.

WHO. *Breastfeeding and Child Spacing: What Health Workers Need To Know.* Geneva, Switzerland: WHO; 1988.

WHO. *Evidence for the Ten Steps to Successful Breastfeeding.* Family and Reproductive Health, Division of Child Health and Development. Geneva, Switzerland: World Health Organization; 1998.

WHO. *Innocenti Declaration on the Protection, Promotion and Support of Breastfeeding.* Geneva, Switzerland: WHO; 1990.

WHO. *International Code of Marketing of Breastmilk Substitutes.* Geneva, Switzerland: WHO; 1981.

WHO. *Protecting, Promoting and Supporting Breastfeeding: The Special Role of Maternity Services.* A Joint WHO/UNICEF Statement. Geneva, Switzerland: WHO; 1989.

Worthington-Roberts B. *Nutrition in Pregnancy and Lactation,* St Louis MO: C.V. Mosby; 1989.

▼ JOURNALS AND NEWSLETTERS

The journals and newsletters below are sources for articles about lactation and breast-feeding management.

Acta Paediatrica, Editorial Office, Building Z6:04, Karolinska Hospital, SE-171 76, Stockholm, Sweden.

American Journal of Obstetrics and Gynecology, C.V. Mosby Co., 11830 Westline Industrial Dr., St. Louis, MO 63141.

Birth: Issues in Perinatal Care and Education, 1 10 El Camino Real, Berkeley, CA 94705.

Breastfeeding Abstracts, La Leche League, P.O. Box 4079, Schaumburg, IL 60173–4048.

Breastfeeding Review, Nursing Mothers Association of Australia, P.O. Box 4000, Glen Iris 3146, Victoria, Australia.

British Medical Journal, BMJ Publishing Group, PO Box 299, London WC1H 9TD, United Kingdom.

Clinical Issues in Lactation, Breastfeeding Support Consultants, 228 Park Lane, Chalfont PA 18914-3135.

Journal of Human Lactation, quarterly professional journal published by International Lactation Consultant Association. 4104 Lakeboone Trail, Suite 201, Raleigh NC 27607.

Journal of Obstetric, Gynecologic, and Neonatal Nursing, Suite 200, 600 Maryland Ave., S.W. Washington, DC 20024.

Journal of the American Dietetic Association, 430 N. Michigan Ave., Chicago, IL 60611.

Journal of the American Medical Association, 535 N. Dearborn St., Chicago, IL 60610.

New England Journal of Medicine, 10 Shattuck St., Boston, MA 02115.

Obstetrical and Gynecological Survey, Williams and Wilkins, 428 East Preston St., Baltimore, MD 21202.

Pediatrics, P.O. Box 1034, Evanston, IL 60204.

Science, American Association for the Advancement of Science, 1515 Massachusetts Ave., N.W., Washington, DC 20005.

The Harvard Medical School Health Letter, Department of Continuing Education of Harvard Medical School, 79 Garden St., Cambridge, MA 02138.

The Journal of Pediatrics, The C.V. Mosby Co., II 830 Westline Industrial Dr., St. Louis, MO 63141.

The Lancet, North American Editor: Little, Brown and Co., 34 Beacon St., Boston, MA 02106.

Women and Health, Haworth Press, 149 Fifth Ave., New York, NY 10010.

INDEX